FOREWORD

THE BEGINNING of the twentieth century brought the birth of our
first professional journal of nursing. The mid-point in the century
brings the book, *American Nursing: History and Interpretation,* by
Mary M. Roberts. At the end of the century these two dates will
stand out in the sweep of its history. He who writes that history
will mark these signals of progress and, equally important, will find
the book and the *Journal* paramount sources for analysis and understanding of our century.

When a celebration of the golden anniversary of the *American
Journal of Nursing* in 1950 was under consideration, Miss Roberts
had completed more than a quarter of a century of service as editor
and was soon to be designated editor emeritus. In the early planning for a celebration honoring the *Journal,* the board of the
American Journal of Nursing Company listened to the story of the
Journal's founding. It was a drama of women who dared an enterprise armed only with faith and common sense, who matched sound
business judgment with sure knowledge that the time had come for
the young profession to establish a journal. We who listened knew
that the story of the founders must be written and that Miss
Roberts must write it. Accordingly, it was voted that the editor
emeritus be authorized to proceed and that she be given a free
hand in designing the scope of the work.

The board was proud of its decision and prouder still when the
scope of the project changed from a brief story of the founders to
a history and interpretation of the period. The beginnings of nursing in the United States before the date of 1900 serve as background. Miss Roberts chose 1952 as the close of the period because

in that year the momentous action for unification taken by the several nursing associations was culminated. We knew that no one held a more favorable vantage point from which to see nursing grow than did Miss Roberts, and that no one could more effectively distill the meaning of what she had seen. She had been participator, observer, and interpreter.

And now we have her book, *American Nursing: History and Interpretation.* In it are more information, deeper analyses, and a broader view of the society which nursing served and the challenges which nursing met than anyone, including the author, had envisioned as she began to write. The book is full of excitement both for the general reader whose interest is in social progress of the period, and for the nurse who will find her understanding of the familiar deepened by Miss Roberts' keen analysis and synthesis of the elements of professional progress. Miss Roberts' own aim—that the book help readers to see nursing clearly and see it whole—has been fulfilled.

The presentation for the most part is chronological. The book carries along together the development of the forces which operate to make nursing what it is today—the force of medical advance, of public health, of hospital administration, of general education. But nursing does not emerge as the creature of these forces, rather it is a force in itself, impelled to growth in accordance with its ever-expanding concept of its function in society realistically interacting with other forces. The book throws light on the complex interrelationships among the health professions and among the various components of the nursing profession. Conflicts are illuminated: from most came resolution and constructive action; from some came greater conflict and delay. History can become our wise teacher.

The stage setting of nursing history in our country is the ever-changing social scene in the United States including our implication in international affairs in times of war and of peace. Meeting human needs is shown to be the steady aim of nursing. The nature of the needs changes, and accordingly nursing practice and organization change. Nursing is seen as a major facet of the point of contact between people and health service. Nursing then grows in two directions—toward more intimate understanding of people, and toward greater mastery of their ever-expanding health services. Economic and other social conditions of the times affect the two-directional growth of nursing. It responded to changes in status of women in the half century and at the same time made striking contribution to those changes.

Miss Roberts shows this growth of nursing service and of nursing education through several periods in the 50-year time span—the early period of uncontrolled expansion, the depression years, the Atomic Age. She tells how nursing in two major wars reached incomparable heights and accomplished what seemed to be impossible. She describes health as a unifying world force and nursing as a vital component of that force. Itself a human resource, nursing is turned to account in the conservation of total human resources the world over.

Leaders in the various movements in nursing history come alive in the book, but personalities are revealed only in the account of actions. Individual action, group action, and social forces are combined in a progression which mounts to what is both an exciting climax and a prologue to the future. And throughout is the authenticity which comes from wide research and rich documentation.

Miss Roberts says she was greatly helped by a course in historical methods at Columbia University; those who know her will believe that this smoothly flowing account of a profession's development in the last half century is primarily a product of her own deep wisdom and her lifetime experience of sound analysis. She writes with a hand that is both loving and objective.

The directors of the Journal Company since 1950 can take great pride in stimulating the production of a momentous contribution to the literature of professional progress. Every nurse who reads *American Nursing: History and Interpretation* will draw from the experience of seeing nursing clearly and whole a warranted pride in her profession and her part in it, and a renewed devotion to its ideal of humane and scientific service.

LUCILE PETRY LEONE

March 12, 1954

PREFACE

THE OPPORTUNITY, made possible by the American Journal of Nursing Company, to put together the materials in this book has been the greatest privilege of an unusually long professional life. I hope the result may be useful to nurses and others who have sometimes been bewildered or frustrated, as I have been, by incomplete understanding of some of the many facets of nursing. I am deeply indebted to an impressive number of people who, through correspondence, conference, or in other ways, have assisted me in this effort to present nursing as a unity which has persistently striven to achieve the social usefulness of a profession. I regret that a comprehensive list of these friends is not possible.

I am especially grateful to Lucile Petry Leone, Kathleen M. Leahy, and Margene O. Faddis, who, as successive presidents of the Journal board, have given intellectual and moral support through the many months the book has been in preparation. Their steadfast faith in the project and their practical assistance have been a stimulant to maximum effort.

The principles laid down by Professor E. M. Hunt of Columbia University in an inspiring course in historical methods which he permitted me to audit during a very hot summer became as the inner voice of conscience! The members of an informal advisory committee were especially helpful in the planning stage of the work. They are Mary Ella Chayer, Virginia M. Dunbar, and Anna M. Fillmore. Among the many others who suggested source materials or who helped by critical reading of particular sections of the manuscript are Lavinia L. Dock, Katharine De Witt, Mrs. Bethel McGrath, Pearl McIver, Anna Heisler, Colonel Florence M. Blanchfield, Mrs. Mary W. Standlee, Louise M. Baker, Mrs. Estelle M. Osborne, Hilda M. Torrop, LeRoy M. Craig, and Charles A. Schneider. Mary Elizabeth Tennant and Mildred L. Tuttle of the Rockefeller and Kellogg foundations, respectively, have provided source materials from the files of those organizations. The director of each of the federal government nursing services and of the Red Cross Nursing Service has been generously helpful in providing factual and illustrative materials. Practically all members of the staffs at national headquarters have given assistance at one stage or another. Among those who have read portions of the manuscript are Ella Best, Leila M. Given, and Helen M. Roser of the ANA; Anna M. Fillmore, Helen Nahm, Marion Sheahan, Margaret Giffin, and Julia Miller of the NLN staff.

The cheerfulness with which the staffs of the Sophia Palmer Library and the filing departments of the national nursing organizations have responded to requests for material is beyond all praise. Thanks are due also to many other librarians, especially those of the National Health Council and the Metropolitan Life Insurance Company. Special thanks are due the McGraw-Hill Book Company for permission to make free use of material from the reprint *Nursing of the Sick—1893*, and to the American Red Cross for material from *The Red Cross Nurse in Action, 1882–1948*. The official magazines —the *American Journal of Nursing* and *Public Health Nursing*, the annual reports of the National League of Nursing Education, the transactions of the American Nurses' Association, and other official reports provided a wealth of basic source materials. Readers are reminded, however, that I alone am responsible for the interpretation of concepts and materials gleaned from so many sources.

I am grateful to the representatives of The Macmillan Company who, although embarrassed by the unexpectedly long period required for the preparation of the manuscript, have been generously helpful throughout.

MARY M. ROBERTS

New York City

TABLE OF CONTENTS

ILLUSTRATIONS

xiii

AMERICAN NURSING
HISTORY AND INTERPRETATION

SECTION I. IN THE BEGINNING

Chapter 1

THE AMERICAN SCENE AT THE
TURN OF THE CENTURY

. . . the achievements of the past provide the only means at command for understanding the present . . . . The sound principle that the objectives of learning are in the future and its immediate materials are in present experience can be carried into effect only in the degree that present experience is stretched, as it were, backward. It can expand into the future only as it is also enlarged to take in the past.

JOHN DEWEY[1]

DISSIMILAR as are the nineteenth and twentieth centuries, there is no sharp dividing line between them. Historians quite generally use the phrase "the turn of the century" rather than the year 1900 to indicate the beginning of the era in American social history in which rugged individualism gave way to cooperative and coordinated efforts. The independent pioneer nursing schools, which had made spectacular improvements in the care of the sick in the hospitals with which they were associated, had celebrated their silver anniversaries before 1900. Their success had led a considerable number of hospitals to organize schools for the primary purpose of securing student nursing service for the care of their patients. Nursing, at the turn of the century, had earnestly begun to follow the general trend toward cooperative effort through organization; and two of the professional organizations which were to have a powerful influence on the development of nursing and its adaptation to social needs had already been organized. Their official organ, the *American Journal of Nursing* (AJN), was launched in 1900 by nurses, for nurses. The

[1] Dewey, John: *Experience and Education.* The Macmillan Company, New York, 1948, Chap. 8, p. 93.

1

more than fifty volumes of that magazine provide much of the background for this book.

The United States in 1900 was a land of plenty and opportunity. The trend from predominantly rural to urban life was gaining momentum as the nation became more and more industrialized. But the US in 1900 was also a land of extremes. The stream of immigration was to continue until checked in Europe by World War I. New arrivals tended to join their countrymen in overcrowded tenements which became veritable seedbeds of communicable disease. The contrast between great fortunes and appalling poverty provided abundant stimuli for the development of humanitarianism, a social conscience, and professional services. Mounting interest in district or visiting nursing foreshadowed the development of social nursing as it was sometimes called before the inclusive term "public health nursing" was generally adopted.

A survey of the New York *Times* for October, 1900, the month in which the AJN made its first appearance, shows which events were of general interest. Much space was devoted to the November election which was to start Theodore Roosevelt on his way to the White House. An editorial commended the US Marine Hospital Service (progenitor of the US Public Health Service, 1912) on its success in having kept yellow fever out of the country for four successive years. Striking coal miners accepted a 10 per cent increase in wages and returned to work. The Boxer insurrection was causing grave anxiety about American missionaries in China. The really electrifying news of the month was a Washington report that Dr. Walter Reed and his co-workers in Cuba had confirmed by experiment the theory that the Stegomyia mosquito is the vector of yellow fever. News about women in the *Times* of 1900 was meager. The amendment to the Constitution which would give suffrage to women, it will be re-called, was still 20 years in the future. There were then only a few thousand automobiles in the whole country, and only the well-to-do had telephones in their homes. In industry, the working week in 1900 was about 56 hours. Only the most skilled workers received a wage of $3.00 per day. The census of 1900 showed that approximately 2,000,000 children were employed in wage-earning occupations, a revelation leading to a 20-year crusade for protective legislation by the National Child Labor Committee.

The majority of graduate nurses were in private duty practice. Their weekly salary was moving up from the firmly established $15.00 rate to $25.00. They were on duty around the clock, with "a little time off" for sleep and recreation at the convenience of the family. Special duty nursing in hospitals was comparatively rare. Although some professionally sponsored registries had been organized and many nursing schools conducted their own registries, considerable numbers of private duty nurses arranged to receive their calls through convenient drugstores. Private duty nurses had abundant opportunity to know their patients and their families because severe illnesses, such as typhoid and penumonia, were followed by long periods of convalescence. Skill in caring for these conditions was an important criterion of good nursing. As there were no miraculous sulfa drugs or antibiotics, the prevention of undue strain on the heart in pneumonia and of relapses in typhoid and the ultimate recovery of the patients were largely dependent on the skill of the nurse working under medical direction. Nurses who made obstetrical practice a specialty accepted engagements for from one to three months. The more successful the nurses were in adapting themselves to conditions in the homes the more they were recalled, not only for successive births but they were also remembered by appreciative families and called when needed by the next generation. Intelligent and well-informed private duty nurses exerted a very considerable influence among the families and friends of their patients. But public opinion about nursing was also influenced by the ineptitudes of the increasing number of poorly prepared nurses.

An early *Journal* carries an interesting description of the outfit of a private duty nurse in 1900. In addition to four voluminous ankle-length mutton-leg-sleeved uniforms and accessories were included two or three reference books and a variety of nursing appliances. All were packed in one or two capacious awkward-to-carry "telescope" bags. At this time the nurses of the Henry Street Settlement in New York, "after much experimentation," were carrying heavy bags containing more than a dozen bottles and porcelain jars up and down the dark stairs of East Side tenements. As nurses lugged their heavy bags on and off street cars and cindery trains, little did they dream of taxi service, of a high percentage of maternity patients being hospitalized and encouraged to return to their homes in eight days or less, that typhoid would become a rare disease in the US, or that Ford's "Model T" would facilitate the development of rural public health nursing. Their training had been highly technical with far more emphasis on the "how" than the "why" of such treatments as the various types of cold baths which were prescribed for typhoid patients or of the poultices and jackets ordered when the diagnosis was pneumonia. Some of the contrasts between nursing in 1900 and 1950 are vividly portrayed in the Golden Anniversary number of the AJN.[2]

Both private duty and visiting nurses were troubled because they knew too little about foods and had not been taught how to meet the social, psychological, and physical conditions they found in patients' homes. They did not feel secure in their knowledge of nursing. Neither they nor their leaders would have believed that, by 1950, more than 17 years would have been added to the average span of American life.[3] The brilliant work of bacteriologists which made possible the control of one communicable disease after another, the public health movement, a rising standard of living, all were to be factors in that extraordinary achievement. While it is impossible to appraise with any precision the contribution of nurses to this extension of human life, we know that it could not have been accomplished without skilled nursing for the sick; the participation of nurses in immunization and case-finding programs; persuasive teaching of health principles by nurses in homes, schools, hospitals, industries, clinics, and health centers; and public information for groups of community leaders.

Surgery was the dominant interest in most of the new hospitals which were being established across the country, although nurses

[2] Sleeper, Ruth: "Nursing Care Throughout Fifty Years," *Am. J. Nursing,* 50:586, 1950.

[3] In 1900–1902 the average length of life of the American people was 49 1/4 years . . . is now 67 1/2 years. *Statistical Bulletin,* Metropolitan Life Insurance Co., New York, Oct., 1950, pp. 2–3.

were still carefully taught how to prepare for surgery in the home. X-rays were beginning to make an important contribution to diagnosis. But it was the safety factor provided by modern nursing that made possible the extensive use of the newer scientific discoveries. Many hospitals established schools of nursing to secure care for their patients; this was done without giving consideration to the needs of students for a balanced experience which would prepare them for general practice as graduate nurses. Whereas there were only 35 schools and 471 graduate nurses in 1890, there were 432 schools and almost 3500 graduates in 1900.

The social conditions created by ignorance, poverty, and overcrowding gave rise to the voluntary organization of the humanitarian impulses of more fortunate folk. Visiting nurses were already working closely with the social settlements in the congested areas of a number of cities. By the end of the first decade of the new century, possessors of great fortunes had established some of the philanthropic foundations which were to have an important influence on the social structure of American life. Foundations were to become one of the major forces which exerted a constructive influence on the development of nursing in the new century. The evolution of nursing in the twentieth century, however, was conditioned by its past.

Early American nursing is only briefly discussed in the following chapters, because the beginnings of nursing in this and other countries and its nineteenth-century development in the US have been thoroughly presented by other writers, most comprehensively by M. Adelaide Nutting and Lavinia L. Dock.

BIBLIOGRAPHY

Barck, Oscar Theodore, Jr., and Blake, Nelson Manfred: *Since 1900. A History of the United States in Our Times*, rev. ed. The Macmillan Company, New York, 1952.

Corwin, E. H. L.: *The American Hospital*. The Commonwealth Fund, New York, 1946, pp. 122–23.

Dock, Lavinia L., and Stewart, Isabel M.: *A Short History of Nursing*, 4th ed. G. P. Putnam's Sons, New York, 1939.

Faulkner, Harold Underwood: *The Quest for Social Justice, 1898–1914.* The Macmillan Company, New York, 1931.

Hollis, Ernest V., and Taylor, Alice L.: *Social Work Education in the U.S.* Columbia University Press, New York, 1951.

Nutting, M. Adelaide, and Dock, Lavinia: *A History of Nursing,* 2 vols. G. P. Putnam's Sons, New York, 1907.

"Report of Conference of the American Association for the Study and Prevention of Infant Mortality," *Am. J. Nursing,* 11:925, 1911.

Schlesinger, Arthur M.: "The Rise of the City, 1878–1898," *A History of American Life.* The Macmillan Company, New York, 1933, Vol. X.

Slichter, Sumner H.: "How Big in 1980?" *Atlantic Monthly,* 184:39, 1949.

Sullivan Mark: "The Turn of the Century," *Our Times—The United States, 1900–1925.* Charles Scribner's Sons, New York, 1927, Vol. I.

Chapter 2

BEFORE THE TURN OF THE CENTURY

The life and work of Florence Nightingale will remain forever a beacon of the profession of nursing. Miss Nightingale did not, as is sometimes said, create the nursing profession; that was done in large measure by the Christian Church. But she reformed it and remade it, giving it a new direction and a more lively inspiration. Her service, indeed, was personal, in that she brought her vivid and alert personality into wards and dressing stations where disorder and even despair prevailed, and by her personality—compounded of courage, discipline, and a valiant faith in and love of her fellows—exorcised the evil and established a new order of goodness and mercy. Her new order has endured because it was built on the sure foundations of knowledge and experience.[1]

AMERICAN NURSES are the inheritors of great traditions which have come to us from military orders, Catholic and Anglican sisterhoods, and from the Deaconess movement which was set in motion by the Fliedners at Kaiserwerth. Most of the basic precepts of Miss Nightingale were incorporated in the plans of the pioneer schools which laid the foundation of what is now known internationally as the American system of nursing education. But sisters and deaconesses of many orders were caring for the sick in a considerable number of institutions in this country before Miss Nightingale began the reform of nursing by establishing the school at St. Thomas's Hospital in London in 1860. Some of them had given heroic service in epidemics of cholera and yellow fever. The Sisters of Charity (Daughters of Charity of St. Vincent de Paul), the first indigenous American sisterhood, in 1823 accepted responsibility for the nursing service of what is now the University of Maryland Hospital, Baltimore. In

[1] *Times* (London), July 6, 1934, quoted by the Florence Nightingale International Foundation.

7

1849 Pastor Fliedner of Kaiserwerth (where Miss Nightingale went to study a little later) at the request of the Reverend William A. Passavant brought four Lutheran deaconesses to Pittsburgh. Before the end of the century a number of Catholic and Protestant orders had established schools of nursing; a few of them for sisters only. Among the earliest were the schools inaugurated in 1889 at the hospital of the Sisters of Charity in Buffalo; Mercy Hospital, Chicago; and St. Mary's Hospital, Brooklyn. An Anglican order, the Sisters of St. Margaret, had opened schools at the Children's Hospital in Boston and at two centers in New Jersey before 1895. The first school to be established by a Lutheran order appears to have been that at Lankenau Hospital, Philadelphia, in 1899.

The need for nursing schools was recognized before Miss Nightingale's *Notes on Nursing* had begun to stir the imagination of American women. The famous Shattuck Report of 1850 to the legislature of Massachusetts recommended that:

. . . institutions be formed to educate and qualify females to be nurses of the sick . . . bad nursing often defeats the intention of the best medical advice, and good nursing often supplants the defects of bad advice. Nursing often does more to cure disease than the physician himself, and, in the prevention of disease and in the promotion of health, it is of equal and even of greater importance.[2]

In 1858 Dr. Samuel D. Gross, then president of the American Medical Association, presented a resolution to that body which read in part:

It seems to me to be just as necessary to have well-trained, well-instructed nurses as to have intelligent and skillful physicians. I have long been of the opinion that there ought to be, in all the principal towns and cities of the Union, institutions for the education of men and women whose duty it is to take care of the sick, and to carry out the injunctions of the medical attendant.[3]

The dual function of the nurse so clearly stated by Dr. Gross merited thoughtful consideration. But neither of these two forceful

[2] Shattuck, Lemuel, and others: *Report of the Sanitary Commission of 1850* (reprint). Harvard University Press, Cambridge, 1948, p. 224.

[3] Fishbein, Morris: *A History of the American Medical Association, 1847–1947.* W. B. Saunders Company, Philadelphia, 1947, p. 78.

pronouncements produced any concerted action. Prior to the introduction of Miss Nightingale's concept of nursing schools in the
United States, Dr. Valentine Seaman and other physicians had made
sporadic efforts to teach nurses. Women physicians in Philadelphia
and Boston had established elementary courses for nurses. In 1872,
the struggling school of the Women's Hospital of Philadelphia was
paying for lectures out of the "Nurse School Permanent Endowment Fund," which appears to have been the first such fund in the
United States.[4] The following year, Linda Richards, later known as
"America's first trained nurse," received the first American diploma
in nursing from the New England Hospital for Women and Children
in Boston. However, the primary interest of its founder, Dr. Marie
Zakrzewska, was in the medical education of women. Shortly thereafter, Miss Richards supplemented that experience with firsthand
study in England of Miss Nightingale's methods.

The early schools of nursing owe their inception to the initiative of groups of informed, compassionate, courageous, and influential women who had learned many important lessons from participation in nursing and other programs for the care of soldiers
during the Civil War. Many of them were familiar with Miss Nightingale's *Notes on Nursing*. So, too, apparently were some editorial
writers. *Godey's Lady's Book,* for example, advocated the preparation of the "graduate nurse" as early as 1871.

War inevitably creates need for nursing service, but the quality
and availability of the service are conditioned by many factors.
Meager records indicate that a few women were employed as nurses
to care for soldiers under Washington in the War of Independence.
A Congressional resolution dated July 17, 1775, includes "one nurse
to every ten sick" in the personnel for military hospitals. They were
to be paid "one fifteenth of a dollar per day or two dollars per
month."[5] The service could only have been that which one neighbor
might give another. Little more could have been required. As there
were no anesthetics little surgery was performed, the major opera-

[4] Hahn, Ruth E.: "A History of Nursing Scrapbook," *Am. J. Nursing,* **27**:
279, 1927.
[5] Stimson, Julia C.: "Earliest Known Connection of Nurses with Army Hospitals in the United States," *Am. J. Nursing,* **25**:18, 1925.

tions being amputations and, surprisingly, trephining. Canadian nuns cared for American soldiers wounded during the invasion of Quebec.

There was no provision for nurses in the military establishment when war broke out between the states in 1861. There were no trained nurses; but women, with and without experience in caring for the sick, volunteered by the hundreds. Many members of the sisterhoods volunteered, and some of the religious orders opened their hospitals for the care of soldiers. Clara Barton, the only woman employed by the federal government before the war (she had been dismissed by the patent office for her outspoken opinions on slavery) and who later became the founder of the Red Cross, was already in Washington giving relief to soldiers when Dorothea Lynde Dix arrived. Miss Dix had a background of 20 years of experience as crusader for better care for mental patients. She proceeded at once to the War Department to volunteer her services and those of a group of nurses. Experience with state legislatures had taught her how to put pressure on official agencies, and she received an appointment as Superintendent of Women Nurses from the Secretary of War. She was authorized to select and assign women nurses to general or permanent military hospitals; nurses were not to be appointed without her sanction except in case of urgent need. Miss Dix thus became the first woman appointed to an administrative position in the federal government. Such unprecedented action created antagonisms in the military organization. Conditions were chaotic, and Miss Dix seems not to have possessed the administrative ability required to deal with the management of supplies, with strong-willed "nurses" like "Mother Bickerdyke," and constant adaptations of personnel. Whatever the reason, orders issued in the third year of the war deprived her of much of her authority. The Secretary of War, however, wishing to honor her on her retirement, presented her with a "stand of colors." Miss Dix worked closely with both the US Sanitary Commission and the Western Sanitary Commission. In New York, Dr. Elizabeth Blackwell, working with both Miss Dix and the US Sanitary Commission, conducted one-month courses for "nurses" at Bellevue.

The US Sanitary Commission, founded by Reverend Henry W. Bellows and approved by President Lincoln in 1861, has been called the forerunner of the American Red Cross. According to Louisa Lee Schuyler, the commission aimed to secure the most healthful possible conditions in military camps, hospitals, and on transports. Its great achievement lay in the development of a comprehensive system of aid for the sick and wounded by means of the "soldiers' aid societies" which sprang up throughout all the states in the Union. Miss Schuyler, Dr. Blackwell, and other influential New York women had already organized "The Women's Central Association for Relief," which became the New York branch of the commission. Through this commission and the Western Sanitary Commission, which operated on the same principles but maintained its independence, men and women learned the value of organized effort and used the knowledge to advantage in various reform movements when the war was over.

We are here concerned only with events which had a direct bearing on the evolution of nursing. Many splendid women served as nurses during the Civil War, but no single heroic nurse figure emerged to gain popular acclaim as had Miss Nightingale after the Crimean War. The fame of Miss Dix rests on her work for the mentally sick, not on the fact that she was the first superintendent of nurses in the military establishment. Clara Barton's great work, as founder of the American Red Cross (ARC), still lay in the future. Louisa Lee Schuyler, a great-granddaughter of Alexander Hamilton, had been the organizing genius behind much of the work of the US Sanitary Commission. When the war was over, she turned her attention to conditions in her own state and founded the New York Charities Aid Association. She promptly appointed a subcommittee to make a study of conditions at Bellevue Hospital in New York.

The first publication of the State Charities Aid Association bore the title "Steps Toward the Organization of a School for Nurses to be Attached to Bellevue Hospital." The story of human degradation uncovered by the committee is effectively told by Nutting and Dock and other historians. Nor were squalor and lack of nursing peculiar to Bellevue. They existed in many institutions which purported to care for the sick. Members of the subcommittee formed the nucleus of the Board of Women Managers of the Bellevue Training School for Nurses which became famous for its stalwart support of good standards of nursing education. This school, the proud possessor of a letter of instruction from Miss Nightingale, was the first to introduce the Nightingale principles of nursing education in this country. Two other schools, which became famous, were also established in 1873 on the same general principles and added strength to the forward march in nursing. With them came the dawn of modern nursing in the United States.

In the light of later developments, when many hospitals opened schools without due consideration of the function of graduate nurses, the stated aims of these three schools have special significance, although they were often obscured by medical and other demands for service. The second of the articles of incorporation of the Bellevue school reads:

The object of this Society is the training of nurses for the sick in order that women shall find a school for their education and the public shall reap the advantage of skillful and educated labor.[6]

The Connecticut Training School, in its annual report for 1881, asserted that:

It is perhaps well to state once for all, the school is thankful they are able to relieve suffering in the hospital, but the school does not exist primarily for this purpose but for the training of nurses for the public.[7]

Vocationally, the record of the Massachusetts General Hospital Training School for Nurses is even more explicit. There the initial impetus came from the committee on industrial education of the Women's Education Association, which was "searching for new occupations for self-supporting women."[8] It should, perhaps, be noted that Smith and Wellesley colleges were founded at about the same

[6] *1873–1923, Fiftieth Anniversary*, The Bellevue Training School for Nurses, New York, 1923.

[7] Stack, Margaret K.: "Résumé of the History of the Connecticut Training School for Nurses," *Am. J. Nursing*, 23:825, 1923.

[8] Parsons, Sara E.: *History of the Massachusetts General Hospital Training School for Nurses*. Whitcomb and Barrows, Boston, 1922, p. 19.

time as the three Nightingale schools of nursing, and that there were many other evidences in the US of feminine initiative and growing independence. The Western Sanitary Commission was directly responsible for the organization of one of the earliest nursing schools west of the Mississippi at the City Hospital in St. Louis (1884) and contributed liberally to its financial support for over twenty years.

The new movement was both hampered and aided by the five-year depression following 1873. It added to the difficulty of securing funds for new ventures but it also made it necessary for many women of the comfortable classes to seek employment. It is fortunate indeed that modern nursing, in its formative years, appealed to considerable numbers of such women. By the end of the nineteenth century, when more than five million women were breadwinners in the US, ambitious young people had a wider range of occupational choices.

Recognition of need for reforms in the care of hospitalized patients was but the first step in an evolutionary process. It was no easy task to prove to unwilling minds that trained nurses were superior to the untrained. The earliest schools, and some of the later ones, met vigorous opposition from many physicians, politicians, and other influential citizens. But the pioneer schools quickly demonstrated their usefulness. They survived because the nurses who labored to establish them received the sustained and courageous support of the women who had initiated the movement for the training of nurses and who succeeded in securing the interest and support of physicians and other citizens. All honor to the women, and to the men who cooperated with them, in establishing the schools which were in the vanguard of a movement that, despite its educational weaknesses, revolutionized the care of the sick. The debt of the nation to the women who cared for the soldiers of the North and the South in the War Between the States has been memorialized in the handsome marble home of the American National Red Cross in Washington, D.C. The nation's debt to those who saw the need and initiated and supported the movement for the education of nurses has never been appropriately acknowledged. Modern nursing in the United States is the result of the dynamic compassion which gave them the insight and the determination to work for improvement of the nursing care of the sick.

By the end of 1880, a chain of fifteen schools, including the Illinois Training School in Chicago and that of the Children's Hospital in San Francisco, the latter organized in that year, had been established across the country. Many of them were directed by Bellevue graduates. The following year, the training of nurses was started at Spelman College in Atlanta as part of the missionary course "to open to Negro women a wide field of honorable, lucrative and helpful employment."[9] Experience was limited to the school's infirmary until the MacVicar Hospital (42 beds) was opened. The course was then increased to three years, and graduates received diplomas instead of certificates and ranked with the high school graduates as alumnae of the seminary. When the school was discontinued (1928) the 117 nurses who had been graduated were employed in practically all types of nursing. The Provident Hospital Training School for Nurses, established in Chicago in 1891, claims the distinction of being the first school in the world established for the sole purpose of educating Negroes as nurses. By 1900 graduate nurses and training schools for nurses had so successfully demonstrated their usefulness that the number of schools had risen to 432. With a few notable exceptions, they were completely under the control of hospitals.

The advent of the graduate nurse was quickly followed by the development of district or visiting nursing. In 1877 the New York City Mission employed a Bellevue graduate to give care to the sick poor in their own homes. The inspiration for this movement was also derived from England,[10] but was developed somewhat differently. Progress, at first, was slow, but in the middle eighties, important visiting nurse associations were established in quick succession in Buffalo, Boston, and Philadelphia. They were soon followed by those of New Bedford, Chicago, and Kansas City. By 1900 about 20 associations, including the world-famous Henry Street Visiting Nurse Service which Lillian D. Wald started in 1893, had been established.

[9] *Spelman Messenger,* March, 1908.

[10] For the origins of organized visiting nursing in England, see Seymer, Lucy Ridgely: *A General History of Nursing,* 2nd ed. The Macmillan Company, New York, 1949, p. 196.

The Instructive Visiting Nurse Association of Boston was the first to indicate the educational function of the visiting nurse by including the word "instructive" in its title. Visiting nurses were expected to make a fine art of adapting technics learned in hospitals to home situations, but they did much more than that for their patients and the public. As they became aware of the educational potential in visiting nursing, leaders in the public health movement were quick to enlist the interest of these agencies in the health crusades that were a characteristic of the budding health movement in the early part of the new century. And, as visiting nurses broadened the scope of their work, they began to press for a sounder foundation for the practice of nursing than most of the schools were providing.

Well before the end of the nineteenth century, anesthesia and scientific advances in the fields of bacteriology and pathology, together with the marked improvement in nursing, were giving tremendous impetus to the development of surgery. The Spanish-American War, with its appalling incidence of typhoid, malaria, and yellow fever, turned the searchlight of science on these and other communicable diseases. According to the American Medical Association, the number of hospitals in the United States increased from 178 in 1873 to over 4000 in 1909. This spectacular rise in the number of hospitals, many of them caring for a preponderance of surgical patients, created an extremely serious problem for nurse educators and the young national nursing organizations as they endeavored to develop an educational program designed to prepare nurses to meet the total range of needs for nursing service.

The financing of the schools was always precarious. The earliest schools, established independently, contracted to provide nursing service for a certain number of wards in affiliating hospitals, but some of them received compensation based only on the cost of the service which was being provided at the time the school was established. All of them had difficulty in augmenting such funds. As hospitals took over the administration of the schools, their identities were merged with those of the hospitals. The practice of sending student nurses to care for patients in their homes was quite generally justified on the assumption that the fees would augment the income of the schools and that the experience was valuable preparation for private duty nursing. Both arguments were fallacious. No teaching or supervision was provided in connection with such experiences, except at Dr. Alfred Worcester's Waltham school, and there was a marked tendency to prolong the experience in order to secure income which was often applied to hospital needs rather than to the education of the "pupil nurses."

Well before the turn of the century nurses were concerned with the problem of providing care in homes for patients of moderate means. Records of the efforts of groups of nurses to meet the need indicate that it was frequently assumed that private duty nurses would give a certain amount of uncompensated service each year. But charitable service, whether staffed by full-time private duty nurses or part-time visiting nurses, was not acceptable to people who wanted to pay their way in the world. An important experiment was conducted by the Illinois Training School in Chicago. The income from $50,000 provided for the purpose by the philanthropist, John Crerar, was used to supplement the sums patients could afford to pay graduate nurses. But the 24-hour schedule then in vogue for private duty nurses was ill adapted to modest homes which lacked accommodations for an extra person. When the experiment was discontinued, the fund reverted to the school.

The literature of the nineties contains many references to registries, or directories, as they were commonly called, for private duty nurses. The farseeing Miss Dock discussed the subject in two forceful articles. An ardent advocate of self-government, she indicated that self-government, as of registries by private duty nurses, would call for a higher type of self-discipline than they could be expected to accept under other auspices. The standards and dignified methods employed by the better training school directories, she pointed out, could be adapted by larger directories serving more nurses and a larger clientele.

All minor methods and heterogenous systems . . . the directory run by unprofessionals, the directory at the drug store, the directory under the control of the medical society, are to be condemned. They break down professional pride and tend to disintegration and what we need is to *unite* and, in uniting, to avoid all appearance of similarity to an intelligence office. Would it not be practicable to establish one central directory in which all the different schools would unite, and which might stand to them all in the relation of the Central Postoffice to the sub-stations? It might be so managed that convenience to the public would reach a high state of perfection. . . . [11]

Although private duty nurses were not ready for the vigorous type of self-discipline advocated by Miss Dock, nursing was fully ripe for other types of group action through organization.

BIBLIOGRAPHY

Alston, Beatrice T.: *A History of the Providence Hospital School of Nursing.* Mimeographed, 1950.

Baker, Nina Brown: *Cyclone in Calico,* The Story of Mary Ann Bickerdyke. Little, Brown and Co., Boston, 1952.

Barton, William E.: *The Life of Clara Barton—Founder of the American Red Cross,* 2 vols. Houghton Mifflin Co., Boston, 1922.

Blackwell, Elizabeth: *Pioneer Work for Women.* E. P. Dutton & Co., Inc., New York, 1914.

Brainard, Annie M.: *The Evolution of Public Health Nursing.* W. B. Saunders Co., Philadelphia, 1922.

Brockett, L. P., and Vaughan, Mary C.: *Woman's Work in the Civil War: A Record of Heroism, Patriotism and Patience.* R. H. Curran, Rochester, N.Y., 1867.

A Century of Nursing. Reprints of four historic documents including Miss Nightingale's letter of Sept. 18, 1872, to the Bellevue School; Foreword by Isabel M. Stewart and Agnes Gelinas, for the National League of Nursing Education. G. P. Putnam's Sons, New York, 1950, p. 175.

Corwin, E. H. L.: *The American Hospital.* The Commonwealth Fund, New York, 1946.

Dock, Lavinia L.: "A National Association for Nurses and Its Legal Organization," *Third Annual Report of the American Society of Superintendents of Training Schools for Nurses,* 1896, p. 42.

———: "The Question of Nurses' Directories," *The Trained Nurse,* Oct., 1894, p. 177.

Doyle, Ann: "Nursing by Religious Orders in the United States," *Am. J.*

[11] Dock, Lavinia L.: "Directories for Nurses," *First and Second Annual Report of the American Society of Superintendents of Training Schools for Nurses,* 1895, p. 59.

Nursing, **29:**775, 1929 (Part I, 1809–1840); **29:**959, 1929 (Part II, 1841–1870); **29:**1085, 1929 (Part III, 1871–1928); **29:**1197, 1929 (Part IV, Lutheran Deaconesses, 1849–1928); **29:**1331, 1929 (Part V, Deaconesses, 1855–1928); **29:**1466, 1929 (Part VI, Episcopal Sister-hoods, 1845–1928).

Duncan, Louis C.: *Medical Men in the American Revolution, 1775–1783.* Medical Field Service School, Carlisle Barracks, Pa., 1931.

Gardner, Mary S.: *Public Health Nursing,* 3rd ed. The Macmillan Company, New York, 1936, p. 28.

Gerberding, G. H.: *Life and Letters of W. A. Passavant, D.D.* Young Lutheran Co., Greenville, Pa., 1906.

Giles, Dorothy: *A Candle in Her Hand, A Story of the Nursing Schools of Bellevue Hospital.* G. P. Putnam's Sons, New York, 1949.

Goodrich, Annie W.: "Louisa Lee Schuyler, An Appreciation," *Am. J. Nursing,* **15:**1079, 1915.

Goostray, Stella: *Fifty Years, A History of the School of Nursing, The Children's Hospital, Boston.* Alumnae Association of the Children's Hospital School of Nursing, Boston, 1940.

Greenbie, Marjorie Barstow: *Lincoln's Daughters of Mercy.* G. P. Putnam's Sons, New York, 1944.

"Lady Nurses," *Godey's Lady's Book and Magazine,* **32:**188, 1871.

Livermore, Mary A.: *My Story of the War,* A Woman's Narrative of Four Years Personal Experience in the Civil War. A. D. Worthington and Co., Hartford, Conn., 1889.

Marshall, Helen E.: *Dorothea Dix—Forgotten Samaritan.* University of North Carolina Press, Chapel Hill, 1937.

Nutting, M. Adelaide, and Dock, Lavinia L.: "The Development of Nursing in America," *A History of Nursing.* G. P. Putnam's Sons, New York, 1907, Vol. II, pp. 326–69.

Oates, Louise: "Civil War Nurses," *Am. J. Nursing,* **28:**207, 1928.

Schryver, Grace Fay: *A History of the Illinois Training School for Nurses, 1880–1929.* Published by the Board of Directors, Illinois Training School, Chicago, 1930, pp. 64–66, 82, 85.

Schuyler, Louisa Lee: Letter to the New York *Times,* July 3, 1923.

Sellew, Gladys, and Nuesse, C. J.: *A History of Nursing,* 2nd ed. C. V. Mosby Co., St. Louis, 1951.

Stimson, Julia C.: "Earliest Known Connection of Nurses with Army Hospitals in the United States," *Am. J. Nursing,* **25:**18, 1925.

Stimson, Julia C., and others: "The Forerunners of the American Army Nurse," *Mil. Surgeon,* Feb. 1926.

Stimson, Julia C., and Thompson, Ethel C. S.: "Women Nurses with the Union Forces in the Civil War," *Mil. Surgeon,* Jan., Feb., 1928.

Tiffany, Francis: *Life of Dorothea Lynde Dix*. Houghton Mifflin Co., Boston, 1890.

Trenholme, Louise Irby: *History of Nursing in Missouri*. Missouri State Nurses' Association, Columbia, Mo., 1926, pp. 33–34.

Vietor, Agnes C.: *A Woman's Quest: The Life of Marie E. Zakrzewska*. Appleton & Co., New York, 1924.

Wald, Lillian D.: *The House on Henry Street*. Henry Holt & Co., New York, 1915.

————: *Windows on Henry Street*. Little, Brown & Co., Boston, 1933.

Williams, Blanche Colton: *Clara Barton, Daughter of Destiny*. J. B. Lippincott Co., Philadelphia, 1941.

Woodham-Smith, Cecil: *Florence Nightingale*. McGraw-Hill Book Co., Inc., New York, 1951.

Woolsey, Abby Howland: *A Century of Nursing with Hints toward the Organization of a Training School*. Reprinted in cooperation with the National League Nursing Education. G. P. Putnam's Sons, New York, 1950.

Worcester, Alfred: "The Waltham Training School for Nurses," *Nurses and Nursing*. Harvard University Press, Cambridge, 1927, Chap. X.

Chapter 3

THE GENESIS OF ORGANIZED NURSING

A profession can only be said to exist when there are bonds between the practitioners, and these bonds can take but one shape—that of formal association.

A. M. CARR-SAUNDERS AND P. A. WILSON[1]

By 1890 nurses in key positions were keenly aware that the success of the early schools in improving the care of the sick and in cleaning up hospitals had stimulated an unwholesome mushroom growth of training schools, as they were rightly called, and of short courses for nurses. Graduates of the better schools were available to fill only a fraction of the new positions for which nurses endowed with leadership characteristics were needed. Many of the new schools were started without any conception of Miss Nightingale's principles or of what a school should be and without qualified graduates to direct them. The excellent history of nursing in Kansas gives a vivid picture of conditions which were disturbing nurse leaders in many parts of the country.

Lacking a model, the majority of the hospital founders conceived of the trained hospital nurse as a substitute for the competent mother or neighbor who cares for the sick in the home. Primarily she should be a "good housekeeper" of the neighborly type. Since the average housewife of Kansas was still scrubbing her own floors and doing the family washing, it was assumed that these and similar chores were part of the work of a nurse. Even after it became apparent that there was much waste in using educated women for such labors, hospitals continued to spend every available cent to add to their number of student nurses . . . the stu-

[1] Carr-Saunders, A. M., and Wilson, P. A.: *The Professions.* Oxford University Press, New York, 1933.

20

dents, promised an education, would work for little or for nothing except room and board . . . . Humanitarians, quite as much as the physicians who founded hospitals as money-making ventures, shared in the exploitation. . . . It simply did not occur to them that they were perpetuating one wrong in correcting another.[2]

The 1893 World's Fair in Chicago provided an admirable forum for considering the development of national standards of organization and administration of nursing schools. The scope and ebullient spirit of the Fair attracted people from all over the world, and many organizations seized the opportunity to hold meetings in Chicago. Dr. Henry M. Hurd, superintendent of Johns Hopkins Hospital, was secretary of the Section of the International Congress of Charities, Correction, and Philanthropy which was to meet there in June, 1893. He was also responsible for a program on hospitals, nursing, dispensaries, and first aid. Mrs. Bedford Fenwick, brilliant leader of nursing in Great Britain, and editor of a publication which was soon to be renamed the *British Journal of Nursing*, came to this country in 1892 to arrange for a nursing exhibit at the Fair. Isabel Adams Hampton (Robb),[3] superintendent of nurses at Johns Hopkins, was Mrs. Fenwick's hostess. The meeting of two such minds must have been an exciting experience for both. As kindred spirits, they collaborated on plans for the inclusion of nursing in the Congress program. Miss Hampton was appointed chairman of the committee on arrangements for a subsection on nursing. The program set out in 1893 was international in scope but specific in content.

The period was one of tremendous vitality and nascent social change. The climate of the times was favorable for the development of the seeds of national and international nursing organizations which were sown there. Miss Hampton, a Bellevue graduate, who had been a teacher before she entered the school at Bellevue, had developed the first graded course for nurses in the United States at the Illinois Training School for Nurses in Chicago, leaving there to

[2] *Lamps on the Prairie—A History of Nursing in Kansas*, compiled by the Writers' Program of the Work Projects Administration in the State of Kansas, sponsored and copyrighted by the Kansas State Nurses' Association. Emporia Gazette Press, Kansas, 1942, p. 93.

[3] Miss Hampton married Dr. Hunter Robb in 1894.

organize the school at Johns Hopkins Hospital in Baltimore. Speaking in Chicago on "Educational Standards for Nurses" she said:

The object of schools for nurses is primarily to secure to the hospital a fairly reliable corps of nurses; and it is in order to insure a continuous source of supply that such schools are established and certain inducements are offered to women to become pupils in them. These inducements are set forth in the circulars of general information published by each school. But when one compares these circulars, the teaching methods of no two schools will be found to be alike, all varying according to the demands of the various institutions and their several authorities. Each school is a law unto itself.

As a result of the lack of any standard, she pointed out that ". . . 'trained nurse' may mean then anything, everything, or next to nothing . . . and public criticism is frequently justly severe upon our shortcomings. . . ." According to Miss Hampton, private duty and district nursing were "the two great fields in which the nurse will be principally occupied." Apparently she did not perceive that a program, no matter how good, designed solely to provide care for hospitalized patients could not adequately prepare nurses for either of those fields. Had she done so, such was her extraordinary capacity for leadership, the evolution of American nursing might have more nearly paralleled that of other professions. Miss Hampton advocated a three-year course; arrangements between smaller schools and large institutions to "supplement their teaching"; an eight-hour day; definite admission dates; a school year divided into terms comparable with those of high schools and colleges; a high school education or its equivalent for admission; and careful selection of students with special reference to intelligence, character, and upbringing.[4] But many years went by before all schools had established definite admission dates and had given up the practice of accepting probationers as need arose or as vacancies occurred.

The paper, "Sick Nursing and Health Nursing,"[5] prepared by Miss Nightingale and read at the nursing section by Miss Hampton, left no doubts as to the principles in which she believed, or that we

[4] Hampton, Isabel A., and others: *Nursing of the Sick, 1893.* McGraw-Hill Book Co., New York, 1949, p. 4.
[5] *Ibid.*, pp. 24–43.

were then "only on the threshold of nursing." In summary the criteria are:

1. A well organized hospital associated with a medical school, with a matron (superintendent of nurses) herself a trained nurse;
2. A special organization for the purpose of giving systematic technical training;
3. Provision for supervision and for records;
4. A well supervised student residence where the students are steadily "mothered";
5. Ward sisters (head nurses) "not constantly changing—for they are the key to the whole situation."

The emerging American system, it was pointed out at that Chicago meeting by Louise Darche (who gave her life to the struggle to establish the City Hospital School of Nursing on Blackwell's Island, New York City), was not in agreement at several points with the criteria laid down by Miss Nightingale. In the Nightingale plan, teaching was a primary function of head nurses. Those who would be expected to perform that function were carefully chosen in advance, whereas the democratic principle of equality of opportunity was a prime characteristic of the American plan. Advancement depended upon demonstrable ability. In the early days of the schools, undergraduates of necessity acted as head nurses since there were no graduates. "But," said Miss Darche, "by degrees what was at first regarded as a misfortune came to be regarded as a part of the system, and it was found that by extending the course of training from one year to two, the services of the nurses after they had obtained the practical training of the first year could be retained and utilized as head nurses."[6]

In the Nightingale school, nurses who had completed the course (originally one year) remained under the jurisdiction of the school for three years with the understanding that employment might then be found for them in other institutions. This provided a substantial background of graduate staff nurses. Not for almost a half century after the Chicago meeting did American nurse educators recognize the fundamental importance of the graduate staff nurse in relation to nursing education and the stabilization of nursing service.

[6] *Ibid.*, p. 96.

In the British hospital system, the matron had more authority and carried far more responsibilities than the superintendents of nurses in American hospitals. In the Nightingale school, the educational functions of the matron and the ward sisters were well defined. They received salaries, provided by the school's endowment fund, which were additional to the salaries paid them by the hospital for service to the institution. Isabel M. Stewart has carefully analyzed the American version of the Nightingale system in her admirable history of nursing education. Further discussion here is therefore unnecessary.

The report of the Chicago Congress, in a volume entitled *Hospitals, Dispensaries, and Nursing,* is one of seven historic publications by which the nursing profession now measures its progress. Fortunately, the material on nursing in this out-of-print volume has been reprinted. (All references in this book are to the reprint).[7]

The Congress was so successful that, seven years later, the AJN closed its first volume with the statement that it "produced a complete revolution in the relations of training schools and nurses. Movements for the higher education of the nurse in training date from that time. . . . "[8] Although it produced something less than

[7] Hampton, Isabel A., and others: *Nursing of the Sick, 1893.* Papers and discussions from the International Congress of Charities, Correction, and Philanthropy, Chicago, 1893. Reprinted under the sponsorship of the National League of Nursing Education, McGraw-Hill Book Co., New York, 1949.

The other documents are:

Nutting, M. Adelaide: *Educational Status of Nursing,* Bulletin #7, Whole #475. US Bureau of Education, US Government Printing Office, Washington, D.C., 1912.

Nursing and Nursing Education in the United States, Report of the Committee for the Study of Nursing Education, and Report of a Survey by Josephine Goldmark. The Macmillan Company, New York, 1923.

Nursing Schools—Today and Tomorrow. Final Report of the Committee on the Grading of Nursing Schools, New York, 1934.

Brown, Esther Lucile: *Nursing for the Future,* a report prepared for the National Nursing Council. Russell Sage Foundation, New York, 1948.

A Program for the Nursing Profession, by the Committee on the Function of Nursing (Teachers College, Columbia University, New York). The Macmillan Company, New York, 1948.

Nursing Schools at the Mid-Century. National Committee for the Improvement of Nursing Services, New York, 1950.

[8] *Am. J. Nursing,* 1:941, 1901.

a revolution, the Congress of 1893 is a milestone in American nursing history second only to 1873. The Congress program clearly foreshadowed coming events. Before the nursing section adjourned, Miss Hampton suggested that superintendents of nurses might like to meet before leaving Chicago to consider the organization of a national society. Some twenty persons enthusiastically did so. A preliminary organization was set up which adopted resolutions calling for a convention of training school superintendents in New York in January, 1894. At that meeting, the American Society of Superintendents of Training Schools for Nurses of the United States and Canada, renamed the National League of Nursing Education in 1912, was organized. The primary purposes of the new society were to advance the best interests of the nursing profession by establishing and maintaining a universal standard of training, and by promoting fellowship among its members by meetings, papers, and discussions on nursing subjects and by interchange of opinions. A curriculum committee was promptly appointed, and a report was published in the proceedings two years later.

Contrary to the usual practice of young organizations, action on matters of immediate concern was deferred, and major consideration was given to the development of a second organization which should have an inclusive nurse membership. Miss Dock, endowed with one of the keenest and most versatile minds in the profession, made a careful study of the laws under which professional organizations could operate, also of the organization and purposes of the American Medical Association and other national associations having local units. The most striking characteristic of all such organizations, she told the convention of 1896, was "provision for a systematic division and subdivision of work and responsibility." National bodies, Miss Dock found, were policy making; their principal asset was moral force. Their real work was done locally. Medical schools, she noted, did not lead the march of progress but were urged to go forward by the purposes of the professional organization. "We labor," said Miss Dock, "under the very serious practical disadvantage of having no recognized standard of work or requirements."[9] At that time, there were believed to be 225 training schools but only some 40 alumnae associations.

As a result of the action of the Society of Superintendents, delegates from ten alumnae associations met at Manhattan Beach, New York, in the autumn of 1896 for the purpose of organizing a national association of professional nurses. The following year the constitution and bylaws were completed and the Nurses' Associated Alumnae of the United States and Canada was organized. When the association was renamed the American Nurses' Association in 1911 and chartered by the state of New York, Canadian membership had been discontinued. Then began concerted efforts, which were to absorb most of the energy and resources of the new association for many years, to create a smoothly functioning organization and to secure legal recognition of nursing in all states. Mrs. Robb was elected president of the new society. Her contemporaries invariably used superlatives in describing Mrs. Robb; they spoke of her majestic beauty, the charm of her personality, of her vision, and her contagious enthusiasm. "She held us in her hands; tense with excitement. I sat on the edge of my chair and drank in every word." Thus a younger nurse described her reaction to Mrs. Robb as she presided at an early meeting of the Associated Alumnae. She was the radiant center of the magnetic force which brought the two national organizations into existence before 1900.

M. Adelaide Nutting, a member of the first class graduated from the Johns Hopkins School, who was to be designated "one of the most useful women in the world,"[10] brought to nursing a cultural heritage, a scholarly mind, and a dynamic personality. Already a collector of rare editions and historical materials, she was keenly aware of the potential value of a publication which could be devoted to the development of the profession. She lost no time in reminding the new association of earlier discussions in which they had decided that a medium of communication was needed between

[9] Dock, Lavinia L., "A National Association for Nurses and Its Legal Organization," *Third Annual Report of the American Society of Superintendents of Training Schools for Nurses*, 1896, p. 42.
[10] From William Lyon Phelps' citation when Yale awarded Miss Nutting an honorary master of arts degree in 1922. *Am. J. Nursing*, **22**:875, 1922.

nurses. How this was accomplished is recounted in the next chapter.

Having launched the Associated Alumnae, the Society of Superintendents began at once to work toward the improvement of educational standards and methods. Following the presentation of a paper in 1898 in which she advocated the development of a course in pedagogy for nurses who expected to teach, Mrs. Robb was appointed chairman of an education committee. This was the forerunner of the hospital economics committee which persuaded Dean James E. Russell of Teachers College, Columbia University, to open the doors of that young and pioneering institution to graduate nurses. Years later, Miss Dock described Mrs. Robb at the time the idea of a collegiate program for graduate nurses first came to her: "I saw it dawning in her eyes at breakfast; at dinner time it was nearing completion and at supper time it was finished in all its details.[11] Unable to secure a meeting of her committee, Mrs. Robb discussed her idea at length with the one available member, Miss Nutting, who had succeeded her at Johns Hopkins. Together they approached Dean Russell, who, believing that progress is dependent on successful experimentation in new lines, agreed wholeheartedly that nurses destined to teach nursing courses should be taught how to teach.

Mrs. Robb's contagious enthusiasm and Miss Nutting's burning zeal were supported by a strong committee. The desired course, they were told, could be given only if an endowment of $50,000 could be secured or an enrollment of 12 students could be ensured the college. These were impossible goals. The agreement to go forward in 1899 was based on a pledge by the Society of $1000 per annum, although its annual income was less than half that amount. Gifts were sought, and received, from alumnae associations, nurses, and friends of nurses. As funds trickled in, the ardent supporters of the plan not only held fast to the shining dream of a chair of nursing endowed in the amount of $50,000, but they began collecting the nucleus of a fund for that purpose. Thus modestly was begun a work which was destined to have an influence on the development of nursing throughout the world, second only to that of

[11] *Am. J. Nursing,* **9:**955, 1909.

the school which Miss Nightingale had established 40 years before. The AJN had pride in publishing in its first volume the complete outline of the course in Hospital Economics offered in 1900. Only two students were enrolled that first year. One of them, Anna L. Alline, later the first inspector of nursing schools for a board of nurse examiners (New York), became so interested that she consented to serve as secretary of the education committee and director of the course for an extremely modest stipend. Nurse lecturers, some of them from Boston and Philadelphia, received reimbursement for travel expenditures only. As in many later developments, the voluntary unpaid service of a few farseeing, energetic, and determined nurses was an extremely important factor in the development of a foundation for the profession.

The Spanish-American War, brief though it was, gave prestige to the work of graduate nurses and set in motion forces that were to have an important influence on the further development of the profession.[12] When war was declared there was no Army or Navy Nurse Corps and no enrollment of Red Cross nurses. This was still the era of Queen Victoria. Medical officers were opposed to the development of any feminine services, some of them because they sincerely believed that adequate provision for women could not be made in the military establishment. They were to find that good nurses are both determined and adaptable. There were few battle casualties, but tropical fevers in Cuba and the epidemic of typhoid which swept through the camps in the United States could not be dealt with effectively by hospital corpsmen, many of whom were raw recruits. Many women's organizations offered assistance, among them the Nurses' Associated Alumnae. To the chagrin of the association, the Daughters of the American Revolution (DAR) had already been authorized to procure nurses. In perspective, although bitterly resented at the time, this seems to have been fortunate for the Army and an incentive to the nursing organization.

The DAR was a young, energetic, well-financed organization with

[12] Spain declared war April 24, 1898, the US the following day. August 12 was Armistice Day, and the Peace Treaty was signed at Paris, December 10, 1898.

an efficiently active office in Washington, D.C. The Associated Alumnae had no such resources. Dr. Anita Newcomb McGee, a vice-president of the organization and a friend of the Surgeon General, had made the original suggestion to him. She was made chairman of a committee to pass upon applications. This was no small task as more than 8000 women, nurses and non-nurses, applied during that summer of 1898. Dr. McGee was an alert-minded person of high personal and professional standards coupled with plenty of energy and initiative. The application forms she worked out, and the records of nurses accepted as contract nurses for service with the Army, provided the basis for permanent records when the Army Nurse Corps was organized. Only nurses who were approved by the directors of the schools from which they had been graduated were accepted. Dr. McGee worked so efficiently that by early autumn she had been appointed Acting Assistant Surgeon General and almost 1200 contract nurses were caring for patients in general and field hospitals in the US and in Cuba. This, however, does not mean that all patients had received prompt attention.

The ARC at that time was still under the direction of Clara Barton, who had founded it in 1881. It was loosely organized and interested chiefly in relief. But some of the state and local Red Cross societies became very much interested in nursing. This was especially true of New York's Auxiliary No. 3, also known as the Red Cross Society for the Maintenance of Trained Nurses. This organization recruited a high percentage of the nurses who served during the war, not all of whom were assigned by Dr. McGee. A considerable number remained under Red Cross jurisdiction and were financed by it. In some instances, they gave more prompt service than would otherwise have been possible. Anna C. Maxwell and a little band of nurses brought order out of the chaos created by the epidemic of typhoid at Chickamauga for which the Army was unprepared, and Mrs. L. W. Quintard[13] did likewise at Montauk Point, N.Y. Some of the conditions with which they had to cope were all too reminiscent of those encountered by Miss Nightingale

[13] Superintendents of nurses and principals of the training schools of the Presbyterian and St. Luke's hospitals of New York respectively.

at Scutari and by Mother Bickerdyke and others in the War Between the States. Under such divided authority, misunderstandings were inevitable. Consideration of them paved the way for the liaison between the Army Nurse Corps and the Red Cross which was established (1909) some years before the nation was again at war. Dr. McGee repeatedly expressed appreciation of the assistance received from superintendents of nurses, registrars, and sisterhoods. Many Sisters—Charity, Mercy, and the Holy Cross—were permitted to sign up as contract nurses. Nurses proved their worth and were soon to have a place in the US Army!

With the war over, Dr. McGee began work on the fundamentals of a permanent organization, and the Associated Alumnae undertook a very active program to secure Congressional action on a bill authorizing an Army Nurse Corps. The bill failed to pass, a second blow to the pride of the Associated Alumnae. But the Army was undergoing reorganization, and Dr. McGee, at the request of the Surgeon General, wrote the section of the Army Reorganization Act of 1901 which established the "Army Nurse Corps, Female," under the direction of a graduate nurse. Dr. McGee had been well aware of the determined effort of the professional organizations to have military nursing directed by a nurse. She resigned late in 1900 after having chosen Mrs. Dita H. Kinney, a member of the corps, as her successor. Mrs. Robb, then president of the Associated Alumnae, realizing that time and effort would have been saved and the soldiers better nursed had the nursing profession been better organized, promptly began taking the first steps that led to an effective liaison between the Associated Alumnae and the ARC nursing service.

BIBLIOGRAPHY

Ashburn, P. M.: *A History of the Medical Department of the United States Army.* Houghton Mifflin Co., Boston, 1929.

Best, Ella: *Brief Historical Review and Information about Current Activities of the American Nurses' Association, including Certain Facts Relative to the National League of Nursing Education.* American Nurses' Association, New York, 1940.

Blanchfield, Florence A., and Standlee, Mary W.: *Organized Nursing and the Army in Three Wars.* Unpublished manuscript on file, Historical Division, Office of the Surgeon General of the Army, Washington, D.C.

Dock, Lavinia L.: "The Growth of Nursing in the United States," *A History of Nursing.* G. P. Putnam's Sons, New York, 1912, Vol. III, Chap. 2, pp. 116–236.

First Annual Report of the American Society of Superintendents of Training Schools for Nurses, 1897.

"First Superintendent of the Army Nurse Corps Passes," *Am. J. Nursing,* **40:**1308, 1940.

Gibbon, John Murray, and Mathewson, Mary S.: *Three Centuries of Canadian Nursing.* The Macmillan Company, New York, 1947.

Kernodle, Portia B.: *The Red Cross Nurse in Action, 1882–1948.* Harper & Brothers, New York, 1949.

Kinney, Dita H.: "Dr. Anita Newcomb McGee and What She Has Done for the Nursing Profession," *The Trained Nurse and Hospital Review,* March, 1901.

Maxwell, Anna C.: "The Field Hospital at Chickamauga Park," *Sixth Annual Report of the American Society of Superintendents of Training Schools for Nurses,* 1900, pp. 76–80.

Munson, Helen W.: *The Story of the National League of Nursing Education.* W. B. Saunders Co., Philadelphia, 1934.

Nutting, M. Adelaide: "The Course in Hospital Economics at Teachers College," *Am. J. Nursing,* **8:**125, 1908.

Palmer, Sophia F.: "Women in War" (including DAR report, Sept. 25, 1898). *Sixth Annual Report of the American Society of Superintendents of Training Schools for Nurses,* 1900, pp. 68–75.

Quintard, L. W.: "The Field Hospital at Camp Wikoff," *Sixth Annual Report of the American Society of Superintendents of Training Schools for Nurses,* 1900, pp. 81–89.

Seymer, Lucy Ridgely: *A General History of Nursing,* 2nd ed. The Macmillan Company, New York, 1949, pp. 124–25 (The American System).

Stewart, Isabel M.: *The Education of Nurses.* The Macmillan Company, New York, 1943, pp. 90–134.

Stimson, Julia C., and associates: *History and Manual of the Army Nurse Corps.* Medical Field Service School, Carlisle Barracks, Pa., Oct. 1, 1937.

West, Roberta Mayhew: *History of Nursing in Pennsylvania.* Pennsylvania State Nurses' Association, Harrisburg, 1939.

Williamson, Anne A.: *Fifty Years in Starch.* Murray & Gee, Inc., Culver City, Calif., 1948.

Chapter 4

AMERICAN NURSES IN OTHER LANDS

Western ideals in nursing are the guiding star in the East.

ALICE FITZGERALD [1]

THE SCOPE of this book does not permit consideration of the evolution of nursing in other countries. But nursing, which has been molded by the opposing forces of Christian ideals and war, is a response to a universal need. The book would be incomplete without recognition of the missionary spirit in which American nurses began, at an early date, to care for the people of other countries and to participate in efforts to develop modern nursing as a service to societies which had previously been without it. Early nurses had in abundance that pioneer spirit which was a marked national characteristic in the nineteenth century. Coupled with the driving forces of compassion and spiritual motivation, that spirit carried considerable numbers of nurses to mission stations in non-Christian countries. When assigned to remote stations infrequently visited by doctors they seem to have combined an elementary type of medical care with nursing and evangelistic work. Where medical missionaries were well established, the ground was usually ready for some type of nursing education program. Among the doctors were women who had defied convention to secure a medical education. In the Orient, especially in India and other countries where veiled women (purdah) could under no circumstances be treated by men, they found abundant opportunity for opening up channels of sympathetic understanding for the practice of their profession and for the teach-

[1] Fitzgerald, Alice: *Western Influence on Nursing Education in the Orient,* Annie W. Goodrich Lecture. Teachers College, Columbia University, New York, 1931, p. 128.

32

ing of Christianity. The early development of medical missions was a Protestant movement, sponsored by the Mission Boards of many denominations in this and other countries. Although Catholic sisterhoods traditionally gave devoted care to the sick in mission lands, it was not until the 1920's that medical missions, as such, were developed under Catholic auspices.

According to Dr. Edward H. Hume, secretary of the Christian Medical Council for Overseas Work, modern professional nursing began in China in 1884 with the arrival at Shanghai of Elizabeth McKechnie who promptly undertook the organization of a school of nursing. Missionary nurses from this and other countries had already made tentative efforts to develop a national organization in China when Nina D. Gage, who was to be president of the International Council of Nurses twenty years later, arrived (1909) to establish the Yale-in-China Nursing School at Changsha. By 1912 the National Association of China had adopted a curriculum and a plan for the registration of nurses, adapted to China's needs, which closely resembled the American "system."

The year after Miss McKechnie arrived in China, Linda Richards established the first school in Japan in connection with the Doshisha University Hospital at Kyoto. This she accomplished in addition to her missionary work for, she has told us, ". . . strictly missionary work was expected of me outside of as well as in connection with my training school work."[2] Miss Richards, as became her custom, remained only long enough to establish the school. When a wave of antiforeign feeling swept Japan, the school and hospital were placed under native auspices. It was the modest school established in 1903 at St. Luke's Hospital, Tokyo, by Araki San, graduate of a mission school that, with American aid, was to become an important center of nursing education in the Orient prior to World War II.

The work of missionaries in the cholera epidemics of the eighties helped to break down the resistance of Koreans to Western medicine. The first Korean schools of nursing were started early in the new century by American nurses—Margaret J. Edmunds at the

[2] Richards, Linda: *Reminiscences of America's First Trained Nurse.* Whitcomb and Barrows, Boston, 1911, p. 81.

Methodist Hospital and by Esther L. Shields at the Severance Hospital, both in Seoul. Missionaries of many faiths and nationalities were working in the Near East when Jane E. Van Zandt established the school of nursing at Beirut in 1905 which was to become an influential international center of nursing education. American nurses have a long record of usefulness in India, but British nurses, quite naturally, were the pioneers in that field. Miss Nightingale, it will be remembered, had begun writing on the need for sanitary reforms in India before she had established the school at St. Thomas's Hospital. The translation of nursing texts and the preparation of other instruction materials has been no small part of the complicated task of nurses who endeavor to teach nursing to men and women of different cultures and traditions. The work of nurses in mission fields, begun in the nineteenth century, continued to be of such interest throughout the profession that for some years the *Journal* devoted a department to it in the early part of the new century. The histories of early schools have recorded with pride the work of their graduates in the mission field. The first school of nursing established under Seventh-day Adventist auspices (1884) was organized solely for the preparation of missionary nurses.

The Spanish-American War, brief though it was, began the transformation of the United States from an isolationist country to one aware of world-wide responsibilities, and provided new opportunities for nurses which extended into the twentieth century. Victory brought not only Cuba and Puerto Rico, but also Guam and the Philippines into the orbit of American responsibility and interest. Communicable diseases were rife, but the age of preventive medicine was dawning. The heroic story of the conquest of yellow fever by Dr. Walter Reed and his associates in Cuba is too well known to require repetition. So, too, is that of the sanitary engineering of General Gorgas which made possible the construction of the Panama Canal. The story of Clara L. Maass, the ex-Army nurse who sacrificed her life that others might be spared the scourge of yellow fever, might have remained forever buried in official records had it not been for the painstaking researches of a nurse and the publication of her findings by the AJN.

At mid-century, a bronze plaque was unveiled in the Gorgas Hospital in Ancon which honors Mary Eugènie Hibbard—"nurse, patriot, gentlewoman, humanitarian, friend, who rendered outstanding service to the development of better health in the tropics." Canadian-born Miss Hibbard was the director of the Grace Hospital School of Nursing (Detroit) when she volunteered for service in the Spanish-American War. Following the war, she was superintendent of nurses on the hospital ship *Maine* which sailed under the flags of the United States, Great Britain, and the Red Cross to aid the South Africans in the Boer War. When an American military government was established in Cuba, the members of the sisterhoods who had been in charge of the hospitals returned to Spain. Miss Hibbard and other American nurses were invited to participate in the development of a national health program. She became a leader in the development of Cuban nursing in which Mrs. L. W. Quintard, who had served at Montauk Point, also participated. Mary O'Donnell, who had been the first director of the nursing school at Charity Hospital, New Orleans, remained in Cuba, as director of a school, for many years. In swift succession, seven schools of nursing were established under the Department of Charities. The stated aim of those concerned with the organization of schools was to "establish a standard that would at once command the respect of the people and the self-respect of the accepted student, defining emphatically a position for the nurse in a country until recently ignorant of her existence."[3] The schools were organized as state institutions attached to hospitals for mutual benefit but with their own budgets. The regulations, based on those principles, which were established early in the period of military government remained unchanged after Cuba had gained her independence. Provision for state licensure was secured in 1902, thereby antedating the first nurse practice acts in the United States. To complete the story, it may be noted that, after a four-year period in the Panama Canal Zone, Miss Hibbard returned to Cuba as Inspector General of Nurses. With Miss O'Donnell, she was instrumental in establishing the first tuberculosis dispensary in 1909.

[3] Hibbard, M. Eugènie: "The Establishment of Schools for Nurses in Cuba," *Am. J. Nursing*, 2:985, 1902.

The work in Panama, although it was developed after the turn of the century, is so much a part of the post-Spanish-American War story that it is also included here. Under the Isthmian Canal Commission, Panama, in which General (then Colonel) William C. Gorgas was Chief Surgeon, Miss Hibbard developed nursing services in the hospitals required by the commission. The Ancon (now Gorgas) Hospital, which had been started by French Sisters, was taken over by the commission. The question of starting a school in order to secure inexpensive service was considered. The decision to employ graduate nurses under civil-service regulations has never been rescinded. Miss Hibbard's modern-mindedness was again revealed in the time schedules she established, eight-hour days and ten-hour nights, and in her plans for recreation for nurses working under pioneer conditions in tropical heat and humidity. A nursing school was established, however, by presidential decree in the Republic of Panama in 1908. Santo Tomas, one of the oldest hospitals on the continent, was chosen for the location of this school and was reorganized by agreement between the United States and the Republic of Panama. Louise Brakemeier, a graduate of the Philadelphia General Hospital School of Nursing, organized and for many years directed the school which was destined to become an educational center to which students could be sent from the Central American countries.

Conditions in Puerto Rico were quite unlike those in Cuba where the military government had expedited the development of nursing. Nurses were already at work there under Presbyterian mission auspices when Amy E. Pope, coauthor with Anna C. Maxwell of *Practical Nursing*, was appointed to organize the Government Insular Training School for Nurses in 1909. As in Cuba before the American occupation, untrained members of Catholic sisterhoods were responsible for hospital nursing services in Central and South America. There were no schools of nursing at the turn of the century when the United Fruit Company began the health service which was to call on North American nurses to establish nursing services in its hospitals and health centers. By the time that the United States entered World War II, it had so expanded that 15 of them were stretched in a 2,000-mile chain through the Caribbean area. When other North American industries, such as the Standard Oil Company, began working in the Southern Hemisphere and found it necessary to establish health services for their workers and their families, they too continued to depend chiefly on North American nurses after the slow development of nursing schools in Latin America had begun.

In the Philippines, plans for caring for the sick, after the period of military occupation, called for the building of hospitals and the training of native doctors and nurses under the direction of the Bureau of Health. To inaugurate nursing under government auspices on a socially acceptable level, the first school was established in connection with the normal school. Charlotte Layton was responsible for the theoretical work, and several hospitals were used as practice fields for the first two years. But careful plans were not enough. Not until a drama interpreting nursing was performed before an audience of the socially elite was sufficient interest aroused to attract the desired type of young woman. The story is amusingly told by Dr. Victor Heiser in *An American Doctor's Odyssey*.

Scholarships in the Philippines were made available by the government and private sources. At the end of two years (1910), the school was transferred to the then new Philippine General Hospital under the direction of Mabel E. McCalmont, who was also the supervising nurse for the Bureau of Health. This 500-bed hospital, which had a very active outpatient department and a communicable disease hospital, provided a wealth of experience for the students. The curriculum was well planned, with the university providing the science courses. Many of the graduates of the first two classes of Filipino nurses were added to the staff of forty American nurses, and plans were made for the time when the American nurses could turn the school and the nursing services over to its own graduates. The number of eligible candidates steadily increased as the school progressed.

When the second class had been graduated, the Bureau of Health considered that the time had arrived to provide public health nurses for the provinces. The enthusiasm with which the young graduates interested mothers in infant welfare programs and the skill with which they cared for obstetrical patients on the mud floors of the huts, in which many of their patients lived, were a matter of pride to their instructors. They were making some headway with the maternity and infant welfare program when an epidemic of amebic dysentery occurred. The nurses rose so splendidly to that challenge that the "last vestige of prejudice disappeared."[4]

Other nursing schools were developed in Manila during this early period. A mission school under Presbyterian auspices had already made a struggling beginning when the government school got under way. The French sisters who operated the 200-bed St. Paul's Hospital employed American graduate nurses to organize a school for Filipino nurses. At the same time the school of the Mary Johnston Memorial Hospital was well under way. Nursing in the Philippines was later influenced by the political ups and downs of the Islands, but the general pattern of American nursing had been well established. The government school became in time, as its promoters had hoped, a center to which other oriental countries might send young women for an education in nursing.

BIBLIOGRAPHY

Adams, Sara E.: "Santo Tomas Hospital School for Nurses," *Am. J. Nursing,* **26:**109, 1926.

Dengel, Anna: *Mission for Samaritans,* The Bruce Publishing Co., Milwaukee, Wisc., 1945.

Dock, Lavinia L.: "Nursing Sisters of the Orient," Chap. 5, pp. 229–87; and "Some Island Hospitals and Nurses," Chap. 6, pp. 288–322; *A History of Nursing.* G. P. Putnam's Sons, New York, 1912, Vol. IV.

Dock, Lavinia L., and Stewart, Isabel M.: *A Short History of Nursing,* 4th ed. G. P. Putnam's Sons, New York, 1938.

Guevara, Martina: *Proceedings of the American Nurses' Association,* 1928, p. 37.

———: "Tuberculosis Nursing in Cuba," *Am. J. Nursing,* **40:**1219, 1940.

Guinther, Leopoldine: "A Nurse among the Heroes of the Yellow-Fever Conquest," *Am. J. Nursing,* **32:**173, 1932.

---

[4] Wheeler, Margaret M.: "Provincial Nurse Corps of the Philippines," *Am. J. Nursing,* **14:**513, 1914.

Heiser, Victor: *An American Doctor's Odyssey.* W. W. Norton & Co., Inc., New York, 1936, pp. 151–56.

Hibbard, M. Eugènie: "With the 'Maine' to South Africa," *Am. J. Nursing,* 1:319, 395, 615, 1901.

Hume, Edward H.: *Doctors Courageous.* Harper & Brothers, New York, 1950, p. 245.

Keeler, Floyd: *Catholic Medical Missions.* The Macmillan Company, New York, 1925.

Korea: "A Few Notes on the History of Nursing in Korea, . . ." *The I.C.N.,* Official Organ of the International Council of Nurses, 2:237–38, 1927.

McCalmont, Mabel E.: "Hospitals and Nursing in the Philippines," *Am. J. Nursing,* 10:89–94, 1909.

Norelius, Jessie P., and Schwarte, Johanna J.: "Panama's Nursing School," *Am. J. Nursing,* 40:515, 1940.

"Nurses for Panama," *Am. J. Nursing,* 5:11, 1904.

Seymer, Lucy Ridgely: *A General History of Nursing,* 2nd ed. The Macmillan Company, New York, 1949.

Shields, Esther L.: "Work in Korea," *Am. J. Nursing,* 8:368, 1908.

Simpson, Cora E.: *A Joy Ride through China.* Kwang Hsueh Publishing House, Shanghai (no date), p. 12.

Socorro, Salamanca: "Public Health Nursing in the Philippine Islands," *The I.C.N.,* Official Organ of the International Council of Nurses, 2:107–15, 1927.

Standard Oil Company (N.J.) and affiliates: *Medical Bulletin, Standard Oil Co., U.S.* Thirtieth Anniversary Issue 1918–1948, Vol. 8, 1948.

Van Zandt, Jane E.: "A Training School for Nurses in the Turkish Empire," *Am. J. Nursing,* 9:274, 1909.

Walton, Harold, and Nelson, Kathryn Jensen: *Historical Sketches of the Medical Work of Seventh Day Adventists.* The Review & Herald Publishing Co., Washington, D.C., 1948, p. 145.

Chapter 5

THE AMERICAN JOURNAL OF NURSING   1900

When the first number of our nursing journal appeared, those who had wrestled with the problem of getting it started, those who had given what they could to help establish it, those who had written for it, those who had skirmished for subscribers for it, could look upon it with joy and pride and say: "I am glad I was in that battle."

KATHARINE DE WITT[1]

THE *American Journal of Nursing* is now taken for granted by those for whom it was created. It was, however, produced by the determined and sometimes painfully misunderstood efforts of a few far-seeing nurses. The budding profession had attracted able women whose educational backgrounds, personal characteristics, and life experiences were widely varied. In addition to those whose primary interest was in improving the care of the sick, there were those who also welcomed the opportunity to become economically and socially independent. American nursing owes the foundation of its flexible but durable structure to the collective courage, intellectual force, breadth of vision, and the varied talents of the founders of the American Nurses' Association and the National League of Nursing Education.

Two independent magazines (not sponsored by professional organizations) had made their appearance in 1888. This was also the year in which Mrs. Bedford Fenwick (who subsequently became the founder of the International Council of Nurses) launched the publication which became the *British Journal of Nursing.* A short-lived monthly, *The Nightingale,* was the property of its editor, Dr. Sarah

[1] De Witt, Katharine: "The Opportunity and Responsibility of the Graduate Nurse of Today," *Am. J. Nursing,* 2:77, 1902.

Post, a Bellevue nurse who had also graduated in medicine. Quite unaware of the *Nightingale's* existence, Margaret Francis (Mrs. Sirch), then superintendent of nurses and head of the training school of the Buffalo General Hospital, in the same year secured financial support and began publishing *The Trained Nurse* which, at mid-century, was renamed *The Nursing World*. There may have been other early independent publications but an "official organ," from the earliest discussions of organized effort, was considered essential to the development of the profession and the organizations which were designed to promote it.

Edith A. Draper, superintendent of the Illinois Training School, Chicago, had pointed out the need of the profession for such a publication in a paper, "The Necessity of an American Nurses' Association,"[2] presented at the meeting in 1893. Louise Darche discussed the subject at an early meeting of the American Society of Superintendents. That farseeing group deferred action, believing that such a project would require the backing of the whole profession as represented in the proposed organization of associated alumnae associations. By the end of its second year, the Nurses' Associated Alumnae of the United States and Canada had a membership of 26 associations representing about 2500 graduate nurses. When the need for a professionally sponsored publication was raised at the annual meeting of the association, the idea was received with enthusiasm by Mrs. Robb, the presiding officer. It was supported with fervor by influential members. However, for almost three years after the Associated Alumnae was organized, the proposal hung fire. Only women of great courage and tenacity of purpose could have accepted responsibility for what must have seemed a Gargantuan task for so small an organization. It is probable that not many of the members really understood the functions of an official publication. The timorous feared financial responsibility; wishful thinkers longed for philanthropic assistance.

When the Committee (of the Associated Alumnae) on Ways and Means of Producing a Magazine was reorganized in 1899, with Mary

[2] Hampton, Isabel A., and others: *Nursing of the Sick, 1893*, McGraw-Hill Co., New York, 1949, p. 152.

E. P. Davis as chairman, things began to happen. After ten years of successful administration of the University of Pennsylvania Hospital, Miss Davis had resigned. She generously contributed her time to the work of the committee. Supported by a group of stalwarts, which included Mrs. Robb and Miss Nutting, Miss Davis went to work. Like Miss Palmer, who was to edit the magazine for twenty years and who had taken an especially lively interest in the project from the beginning, Miss Davis had been graduated in the Massachusetts General's class of 1878. Experienced in hospital administration, these two were good businesswomen and were keenly aware of both the fiscal and professional responsibilities the organization was undertaking. The other members of the committee were concerned principally with the professional aspects of the proposal. In retrospect, it is clear that nursing was extremely fortunate in having attracted women of such diverse capacities and backgrounds as the members of that committee. They did not always find it easy to agree, but they were women of vision, integrity, and purposeful devotion to their profession. They shared a keen sense of destiny.

The report Miss Davis presented at the annual meeting of the Associated Alumnae in 1900 is a remarkable document. It must have amazed those who listened to it. Four methods of producing a magazine had been explored. Having decided on a stock company, the committee did not merely recommend that a company be organized; it had already sold shares of stock! Stock was sold only to nurses or to alumnae associations, thus ensuring professional control of the magazine. Linda Richards, America's first trained nurse, purchased share No. 1. Five hundred and fifty subscriptions to the still unauthorized and unborn magazine, with encouraging promises of more, had been secured. Those who subscribed because they believed in the enterprise provided the only working capital available to the committee. They had been informed that if the magazine failed to materialize there would be no refunds. Admitting frankly that it had "exceeded the bounds of its duty," the committee now requested power to act! There were two reasons for urgency. Miss Davis could not be expected to give her time indefinitely without compensation to the project. More important, the development and promotion of standards for the rapidly mounting number of nursing schools and provision for the legal control of the practice of nursing, neither of which could be effected without a general sharing of information through the medium of a publication, could no longer be deferred by the two organizations.

Authorized to proceed, Miss Davis secured the interest of the J. B. Lippincott Company of Philadelphia, and arranged for the production of the magazine and the administration of all business pertaining to it. This fortunate relationship was maintained for about 20 years. (Responsibility for the business administration of the magazine—contracts for printing and paper, maintenance and promotion of circulation, and the like—was then delegated by the board of directors to the editor.) Work proceeded apace. The first issue of 2500 copies of the magazine was ready for mailing in October, 1900. But the Philadelphia post office refused to accept it as the masthead carried no statement of responsible ownership. Quite undaunted, Miss Davis, "having no skirt to hang on," went to the postal authorities and made herself and Miss Palmer (without Miss Palmer's knowledge) responsible for the magazine in accordance with postal regulations. Years later, the National League of Nursing Education made Miss Davis a life member, in appreciation of her progressive work and sacrifices for the ideals of nursing education.

Sophia F. Palmer began the work of editor-in-chief, to which she was to devote the last twenty years of her life, while still superintendent of the Rochester City, now General, Hospital (New York). The *Journal's* first "office" was a trunk in which she kept manuscripts and other materials related to the magazine. She wielded a trenchant pen and was assisted by an able corps of departmental editors, which included Lavina L. Dock, Mrs. Robb, Miss Davis, Mary M. Riddle, Louise C. Brent, Isabel McIsaac, Linda Richards, Lucy L. Brown, and Mary E. Thornton. Even a cursory review of the earlier volumes of the *Journal* reveals the depth and scope of Miss Dock's contribution to the profession through the magazine. In addition to providing material on nursing in other countries for the Foreign Department, she contributed some of the most important articles the magazine has ever published on the structure and purpose of the professional organizations and on a variety of social problems. For almost a year, there was no financial outlay for salaries or other expenses for the editorial department. For almost a dozen years, space for the editorial office was set apart in Miss Palmer's home without cost to the magazine. Human nature being what it is, the judgment and motives of the prime movers in the enterprise were sometimes challenged by equally honorable nurses holding different points of view. The fact remains that without a penny of subsidy from either of its parent organizations, the magazine was safely launched. In discussing preliminary plans for the *Journal* with Mrs. Robb, Miss Davis wrote: "I have always contended that if the foundation was laid securely along proper lines there was not much danger but what the superstructure would be a success." At the end of a half century, it could be recorded that the foundation was, indeed, securely laid.

The *Journal's* appointment of a highly qualified private duty editor in 1906 was made in frank recognition of the professional and numerical importance of private duty nurses. Katharine DeWitt, a graduate of Mt. Holyoke and the Illinois Training School, who was to remain on the editorial staff and to serve the profession faithfully and with sympathetic understanding for twenty-five years, had already contributed a number of valuable articles based on her long and successful experience in private duty and on her participation in the work of alumnae and other professional organizations. Her dominant characteristics of faith in a divine providence, compassion, loyalty, unswerving integrity, and devotion to the best in individuals and in nursing helped to enrich many a page of the magazine.

Then and later, however, the editors had difficulty in persuading nurses to write on the actual practice of nursing. However, news and articles on the policies and programs of the organizations were fairly well balanced by articles on nursing practice. The development of initiative was definitely inhibited by the repressive discipline and adherence to routines imposed by the schools. The extremely long hours on duty (72 hours a week on night duty and approximately 60 on day duty) provided a frequently used alibi.

Despite all this, the first ten or twelve volumes of the *Journal* contain a fair percentage of well-written material on the care of patients, "Five Hundred Cases of Pneumonia"[3] is the arresting title of an article published in 1902. Forty-seven of these patients (of the Henry Street Nurse Service) were sent to hospitals. The care given the others in their homes, with excellent results, was graphically described. Adaptation to the variations in orders of many physicians was emphasized; so was the importance of teaching some member of the family the essential elements of the care to be given between calls. Thus there was early recognition of some of the basic principles of public health nursing. "New Ways of Nursing in Typhoid Fever"[4] described the very different methods in use in three institutions. Although the author did not so designate it, it is a fine example of material on comparative methods. The didactic teaching of the period with its emphasis on "our way" did not, however, encourage emulation.

Preparation for surgery in a home was an important and recurring subject in those days, as was preparation for travel with patients. Among the illustrated articles many were on the types of cold baths used for the reduction of temperature in typhoid. Poor souls! How the patients hated those baths, and how ravenously hungry most of them became on diets planned, with relatively little consideration of nutritional needs, to avoid strain on inflamed Peyer's patches. The term calorie did not appear until a later date. Typhoid patients were "pulled through" their six-weeks' trial by nurses who gave the icy baths and other treatments conscientiously and helped to maintain the morale of the patient and his family during the long siege. By the end of the first decade the effectiveness of typhoid vaccine had been demonstrated in the Army, and sanitary and milk commissions were helping to reduce the incidence of the disease by improving water and milk supplies.

The author of "Hospital Sketches," written diary-fashion, provides a delightful and unself-conscious pen picture of a student nurse who

[3] Hitchcock, Jane Elizabeth: "Five Hundred Cases of Pneumonia," *Am. J. Nursing*, 3:169, 1902.
[4] Lawler, E. M.: "New Ways of Nursing in Typhoid Fever," *Am. J. Nursing*, 4:438, 1904.

enjoyed working with patients as people who needed her care.[5] Then as now the powers of observation of the nurse and skill in giving ordered medications and treatments were of the utmost importance to physicians. Patients, however, judged nursing care by the skills that brought them comfort. Nevertheless, in the case of abdominal surgery patients, whose backs ached intolerably because of long periods of lying on poorly padded operating tables, who also suffered from nausea and gas pains, immobilization for the first few days was virtually the law. Neither they nor the nurses could possibly have foreseen dangling or early ambulation. Such postoperative procedures would have been considered nothing short of malpractice.

Although private duty nurses constituted by far the largest group within the profession, relatively few were personally interested in the work of the organizations. One of the devoted few has described how she contrived a light in a closet off her patient's room by which she wrote alumnae and other reports while the patient slept. In retrospect, it is amazing that the professional organizations did not perceive that demonstrations of nursing procedures at national and state meetings could have been an effective means of attracting larger numbers of the practitioners of the art of nursing.

By 1912 the initial purpose of the founders of the magazine, who were equally interested in the National League of Nursing Education and the American Nurses' Associations, had been fulfilled. The ANA became the sole owner of *Journal* stock. Some of it had been contributed to the association; Miss Dock, for example, presented a share in 1904. Most of it had been purchased. The board of directors of the ANA, therefore, when functioning as the representative of the sole stockholder, became responsible for electing the board of directors of the *Journal* company. The success of the magazine has been due to the extraordinary perspicacity with which the foundation was laid. The board is directly responsible for the financial policies of the company. It delegates broad powers to carefully chosen nurse edi-

[5] De Witt, Katharine: "Hospital Sketches," *Am. J. Nursing*, 6:455, 591, 610, 1906.

tors who can be depended upon to deal with the rapidly changing conditions in nursing within the frame of reference of accepted editorial policies. The NLNE, as an organization, took no part in the financing or planning of the magazine. It had definitely referred that responsibility to the younger organization. So closely interwoven were the interests of the two organizations and so thoroughly was it understood that the magazine existed to serve the profession and the organizations that some years went by before either of the organizations made provision in its bylaws for recognition of the *Journal* as its official organ. Through its continuous promotion and integration of the programs of the two organizations, the AJN became a powerful coordinating force within the profession.

BIBLIOGRAPHY

Ashburn, P. M.: *A History of the Medical Department of the United States Army.* Houghton Mifflin Co., Boston, 1929, p. 274.

Dock, Lavinia L.: *A History of Nursing.* G. P. Putnam's Sons, New York, 1912, Vol. III, p. 119.

Palmer, Sophia F.: "A Resume of the Early History of the American Journal of Nursing," *Tenth Annual Report of the American Society of Superintendents of Training Schools for Nurses,* 1904, pp. 82–84.

Pennock, Meta Rutter: "Margaret Francis Sirch," *Makers of Nursing History,* 2nd ed. The Lakeside Publishing Co., New York, 1940, p. 106.

Report of Committee on Ways and Means of Publishing a Magazine: "Proceedings of the Third Annual Convention of the Associated Alumnae of Trained Nurses of the United States," *Am. J. Nursing,* 1:80, 1900.

Story of the American Journal of Nursing (pamphlet), 4th ed. The American Journal of Nursing Co., New York, (March) 1950.

Records in the *American Journal of Nursing* files.

SECTION II. A PERIOD OF
UNCONTROLLED EXPANSION   1900 – 1912

Chapter 6

THE STATUS OF NURSING AND RELATED
PROFESSIONS IN 1900

Principal among the triumphs of nursing I hold to be this: that you have created a demand for your services even before you knew them all, and then met the demand in a fashion to create still more calls upon you.

ALAN GREGG[1]

NURSING is now an essential element in any comprehensive health and medical care program. But, in 1900, the services of "trained nurses" were usually available only to patients in general and a very few mental hospitals, to the well-to-do, and, in the larger cities, to the poor in their homes. Nurses had a tendency to congregate in the cities where they had received their training. Some of them had endeavored, without success, to find an effective method of providing care for patients of moderate means. Rural folk were almost wholly dependent on friendly neighbors or persons described as "experienced" or "practical" nurses. Hospitals were being established at an increasingly rapid rate but without any planned relationship to each other or to total community needs and resources. Many of them were privately owned. The potential function of hospitals in relation to the education of doctors and nurses was not generally recognized; other types of professional and technical workers who would also be dependent upon them for some type of student experience were still to be born.

For years after the earliest nursing schools opened their doors,

[1] Gregg, Alan: "An Independent Estimate of Nursing in Our Times," *Am. J. Nursing,* **40**:743, 1940.

the term "professional" was applied and accepted without question
by nursing schools and their graduates, quite without regard to
the extraordinary range of their educational offerings. Miss Nutting
analyzed its use early in the century, as follows:

The criticisms of us as members of a profession are constant, severe, and
searching. We claim, and I think justly, the status of a profession; we
have schools and teachers, tuition fees and scholarships, systems of instruction from preparatory to post-graduate; we are allied with technical schools on the one hand, and here and there a university on the other;
we have libraries, a literature, and fast-growing numbers of periodicals
owned, edited, and published by nurses; we have societies and laws. If,
therefore, we claim to receive the appurtenances, privileges, and standing of a profession, we must recognize professional responsibilities and
obligation which we are in honor bound to respect and uphold.[2]

Miss Nutting spoke for the vanguard. The state boards of nurse
examiners, then just coming into existence, were to discover that
many nursing schools fell appallingly far short of the professional
standard she described.

When Dr. Gross reminded the American Medical Association
(AMA) in 1868 of the nation's need of schools for nurses, he made
a clear distinction, it will be recalled, between the nurse's obligation
to the physician—"to carry out the injunctions of the medical attendant," and to the patient—"to take care of the sick." Organized
medicine took no step to promote the development of schools of
nursing. Nursing was then, and indisputably continues to be, ancillary to medicine in the area of therapy. But the skillful and intelligent execution of the doctor's orders is only one segment of the
function of the professional nurse.

The rise of nursing toward the stature of a profession has sometimes been stimulated, sometimes retarded, by the rate of progress
of the other health professions. The relation of nursing to them is
therefore of some interest. In 1900, the National League of Nursing
Education was six years old and the American Nurse's Association
barely four. Nursing literature of the period indicates keen interest

[2] *Eleventh Annual Report of the American Society of Superintendents of
Training Schools for Nurses, Including Report of the First Meeting of the
American Federation of Nurses,* 1905, p. 137.

not only in surgery and the widely prevalent communicable diseases but also in psychiatric nursing and the care of patients suffering from tuberculosis. The American Psychiatric Association (APA) had been in existence more than half a century, and the development of psychiatric nursing was to be much more strongly influenced by that organization than has nursing, in general, been influenced by the AMA. This appears to have been due to the administrative function of the physicians who were leaders in the care of psychiatric patients. A mental hospital was usually a self-contained cosmos. The example of Dr. Edward Cowles, who established the first school of nursing in the world in a mental hospital (McLean Hospital, Waverly, Mass.) was followed by the state hospitals of New York and a few other eastern institutions before the turn of the century. The American Medical Association had already passed the half-century mark and had been publishing an official magazine for twenty years. It had promoted the control of medical practice by licensure through state legislation. Its form of organization and its example in relation to licensure were to be closely followed by the nursing organizations. Medicine, with divinity and the law, was considered a learned profession. The fact that medical schools then ranged from excellent educational institutions to worthless commercial enterprises or "diploma mills" was not to be revealed until 1910 when the "Flexner Report,"[3] plus massive sums of money from foundations and other sources, began to revolutionize medical education. Miss Nutting and other nurse educators yearned for a comparable study of nursing.

The unevenness of medical standards inevitably created problems in relation to the evolution of nursing and nursing education. "Loyalty to the physician" was a cardinal principle in the ethical code of nursing. The better nursing schools stressed intelligent obedience. Well-prepared nurses, when called upon to work with relatively less well-prepared physicians, needed the wisdom of a Solomon. This fact was recognized by the visiting nurse associations and provided

[3] Flexner, Abraham: *Medical Education in the United States and Canada,* a report to the Carnegie Foundation for the Advancement of Teaching, Bulletin #4, Merrymount Press, Boston, 1910.

the basis for some of their fundamental policies. A medical advisory committee was found to be essential to effective administration of such services, with a city or county medical society usually making the nominations for membership. These committees assist with the formulation of standing orders and help to solve such problems as arise through misunderstandings, changing situations, and the like.

The American Medical Association established its Council on Medical Education and Hospitals in 1901. It was influential in securing the passage of the Pure Food and Drug Act of 1906. Upton Sinclair's novel, *The Jungle,* although it had been written to arouse interest in the social problems of stockyard workers, aroused an indignant nation to action about the quality of the foods they produced. At the turn of the century, the American Public Health Association (APHA), established in 1872, was more concerned with sanitary science than with conditions which would require the service of nurses. But the age of preventive medicine, which was to broaden and deepen the scope of nursing, lay just over the threshold of the new century, with that of health preservation only a little further in the future. The National Tuberculosis Association (NTA), organized under a slightly different name in 1904, was the first of many voluntary health associations whose programs influenced, and were influenced by, the evolution of public health nursing. The National Committee for Mental Hygiene, an outcome of Clifford W. Beer's book, *A Mind That Found Itself,* was established in 1909 as was the American Association for the Study of Infant Mortality.

The New York School of Philanthropy, which became the New York School of Social Work, had been giving short courses since 1898. It began offering a full year's course in 1904. This was the first school of its kind in the country. Hospital social service was inaugurated by Dr. Richard C. Cabot in the Out-Patient Department of the Massachusetts General Hospital, Boston, early in the century. Bellevue Hospital, New York, was a close second. Ida M. Cannon in Boston and Mary E. Wadley in New York, both nurses, were pioneers who helped to lay foundations for the profession of medical social service. The growing pains of social work as a profession were sometimes painful for both nurses and social workers.

The Chicago conference of 1893, which had provided a point of departure for the organization of nurses, started a similar movement among hospital superintendents. The forerunner of an association, renamed the American Hospital Association (AHA) in 1906, was organized four years later than the Society of Superintendents of Training Schools for Nurses. The two national nursing organizations had already launched well-considered programs for developing standards of nursing education and for securing legal control of nursing practice. A committee composed of three eminent medical superintendents of hospitals was appointed by the AHA in 1908 to study the whole question of training schools for nurses, to prepare a model curriculum, and to consider to what extent hospitals should prepare a class of nurse helpers or assistants. The report of that committee is discussed in the next chapter.

Hospitals were then highly individualistic institutions. Nursing schools, with a few notable exceptions, were embedded in them, but there was neither an established hospital system nor a generally accepted code of administrative and fiscal policies on which to build either a system of nursing education or one of nursing service. Therein lay a fundamental weakness which was to plague both groups. For many years, lack of generally accepted fiscal policies for hospitals and the complete identification of schools with hospital nursing services had a seriously inhibiting influence on the development of nursing schools and therefore on the evolution of nursing practice in relation to the changing needs of individuals, institutions, and communities.

BIBLIOGRAPHY

Aikens, Charlotte A.: "Report of Special Training School Committee (1909)," *Hospital Management*. W. B. Saunders Co., Philadelphia, 1911, Appendix I.

Beers, Clifford W.: *A Mind That Found Itself*, twenty-fifth anniversary edition commemorating the foundation of the National Committee for Mental Hygiene. Doubleday, Doran and Co., Garden City, N.Y., 1935.

Fishbein, Morris: "Recommendation for Establishment of Training Schools for Nurses," *A History of the American Medical Association*. W. B. Saunders Co., Philadelphia, 1947, p. 78.

Flexner, Abraham: *Medical Education in the United States and Canada,* a report to the Carnegie Foundation for the Advancement of Teaching, Bulletin #4. Merrymount Press, Boston, 1910.

A Half Century of Public Health, Jubilee Historical Volume, edited by Mazyck Ravenel. American Public Health Association, New York, 1921.

Hamilton, Samuel W.: "The History of American Mental Hospitals," *One Hundred Years of American Psychiatry*. Columbia University Press, New York, 1944.

Hollis, Ernest V., and Taylor, Alice L.: *Social Work Education in the United States*. Columbia University Press, New York, 1951.

Washburn, Frederic A.: *The Massachusetts General Hospital—Its Development, 1900–1935*. Houghton Mifflin Co., Boston, 1939.

Worcester, Alfred: *Nurses for Our Neighbors*. Houghton Mifflin Co., Boston, 1914.

Chapter 7

TRAINING—OR EDUCATION?

Whether the freedom of the training school is brought about by means of endowments or by state or municipal aid does not matter. The thing to be secured is a separate government for the training school. . . .

M. ADELAIDE NUTTING[1]

THOUSANDS of Americans in 1900 had never seen a trained nurse. The splendid response of nurses to military needs during the Spanish-American War had briefly thrown an aura of flattering publicity about the profession. But the public was poorly informed about nursing and tended to sentimentalize it. Parents might admire self-sacrifice, but not for their own daughters. Nursing schools did not possess the characteristics of schools as parents understood them, and the long hours and tales of scrubbing and other menial services required in some schools were a further deterent to the recruitment of sufficient numbers of qualified students. Men were admitted to three schools of nursing in the late eighties,[2] and a few institutions have followed that example, but American nursing has been essentially a vocation and a profession for women. The popular concept of nursing as a calling of particular interest to young women whose romances had been blighted was played up in the original *Life* magazine by one of the best-known artists of the day, Charles Dana Gibson. More helpful was the comment of Finley Peter Dunne's

---

[1] Nutting, M. Adelaide: *Educational Status of Nursing*, US Bureau of Education, Bulletin #7, Whole #475. US Government Printing Office, Washington, D.C., 1912, p. 52.
[2] See "Men Nurses," Chap. 31.

socially alert humorist, "Mr. Dooley," to his friend "Hinnessy": "I think," said Mr. Dooley, "that if th' Christyan Scientists had some science an' th' doctors more Christyanity, it wuddn't make anny diff'rence which ye called in—if ye had a good nurse."[3]

The American Medical Association reported that, in 1909, there were more than 400,000 hospital beds for the care of acute and sub-acute conditions. The total number of beds in all institutions for persons requiring some type of nursing service was double that number. Only a few of the hospitals were tax-supported. Many were privately owned. A considerable number of the voluntary hospitals were established under religious auspices. There is no evidence of any systematic coordinated effort to provide hospital service for the American people. The institutions were wholly unrelated and highly individualistic. Under such circumstances, there was no consensus of medical, hospital, and nursing opinion as to how so many patients might be nursed. The success of the earlier schools of nursing had been due, in part, to the fact that they were developed in connection with established hospitals caring for a sufficient number of patients and varieties of conditions to provide good experience for the student nurses. This fact was often overlooked or ignored as the number of nursing schools shot up from 432 to 1129 in the first decade of the new century,[4] regardless of clinical and other limitations.

The prescient Mrs. Robb had pointed out that there were five methods for providing nursing services and threw the weight of her influence toward the development of "cooperative nursing." "Exclusive of training schools," she said, "the nursing could be undertaken: (1) by the graduates of smaller schools willing to give their services in return for a postgraduate course under competent instructors; (2) by paid competent graduate nurses; (3) by attendants under the supervision of trained nurses; (4) by adopting the system of cooperative nursing; (5) by members of religious orders, previously

[3] Dunne, Finley Peter: *Mr. Dooley's Opinions: Christian Science.* R. N. Russell, New York, 1901, pp. 3–9.

[4] Burgess, May Ayres: *Nurses, Patients, and Pocketbooks,* Report of a Study of the Economics of Nursing. Committee on the Grading of Schools of Nursing, New York, 1928, p. 36.

trained for these duties."[5] This analysis antedated the organization of the American Hospital Association. There were no established channels for the sharing of the group thinking of nurses with that of hospital administrators.

The "system of cooperative nursing" that Mrs. Robb advocated was based on the principle that a central school could utilize the clinical resources of more than one institution for teaching students while concurrently providing the participating institutions with nursing service. She cited a half-dozen examples of such arrangements then in operation in New York, Milwaukee, Syracuse, and San Francisco. Emphasis, however, seems to have been on the provision for nursing service.

Many new institutions started schools of nursing for economic reasons only. Few had any demonstrable interest in the future of the nurses they graduated. The service of students, as schools were then operated, was much less costly than any other type of service. It was also more stable. Students did not drop out of "training" as frequently as employed personnel changed their jobs. Those who completed the training accepted, often with mental reservations that later bore fruit outside the field of institutional nursing, the repressive discipline of the times as a necessary attribute of "training." The contribution of the better schools to the hospitals was two-fold. They provided an economical type of nursing service and they created a wholesome atmosphere throughout the institutions. This was commonly attributed to the presence of young people. We now know that it was a combination of youthful resiliency and the subtle influence of learning situations in which both teachers and students are stimulated. Institutions in which there is no teaching quickly become static. At the turn of the century, when there was little medical teaching in most hospitals, the presence of a nursing school created a more dynamic situation than would otherwise have been possible in many institutions.

The rapid increase in the number of schools sharpened the aware-

[5] Robb, Isabel Hampton: "Nursing in the Smaller Hospitals and In Those Devoted to the Care of Special Forms of Disease," *Fourth Annual Report of the American Society of Superintendents of Training Schools for Nurses*, 1897, pp. 59–68.

ness of the two nursing organizations to the need for state control of nursing education. The early reports from state boards of nurse examiners confirmed the conviction that "trained nurse can mean anything or nothing." They worked on the premise that the basic functions of professional organizations are to set progressive standards of education and of practice for the professions they represent, and to promote the welfare of the members. During this period, the leaders of both associations, although they did not state it so simply, were necessarily concerned with the development of an educational system which would provide the basic preparation of nurses for service where needed—in hospitals, homes, or communities. They were so much occupied with that fundamentally important task that they ignored the necessity for setting standards for nursing services in institutions without schools and promoting alternative types of service such as Mrs. Robb had suggested. As time went on, this concentration on the basic education of nurses, because it was believed to be fundamental to any sound development of nursing services, caused critics to state that leaders in nursing were more interested in the education and advancement of nurses than in the development of nursing services.

Hospitals and nursing have indissoluble mutual interests. The institutions are dependent on nursing for a very large portion of their total service to patients. Schools of nursing are dependent on hospitals for the major practice field for their students. But there was no concept of an American hospital system with which a system of nursing education could be coordinated. The schools, with the few exceptions previously noted, had been established by the hospitals to ensure a low cost supply of nursing service. They had neither endowments nor budgets. The profit motive dominated many privately owned or commercially controlled institutions. The fiscal policies of voluntary institutions were still beclouded by old concepts of hospitals as charitable institutions. Their deficits were usually made up by benevolent members of the boards of trustees. Hospitals that operated schools viewed nursing only in terms of the immediate needs of their own patients. The nursing organizations, accepting responsibility for guiding the development of nursing education as well as of nursing service, were necessarily concerned with the needs of patients in their homes as well as in hospitals. As the public health movement began to gain momentum, the organizations, especially the Society of Superintendents, became concerned with the education of nurses for participation in community and industrial health programs.

The Society of Superintendents of Training Schools had begun working in 1895 for a three-year curriculum and an eight-hour day for pupil nurses. There were many unemployed private duty nurses. The time seemed auspicious for increasing the basic training in order to prepare pupils adequately for the work they would be expected to do as graduates. Few schools had succeeded in securing the eight-hour day, although Mrs. Lystra E. Gretter had established that schedule at Harper Hospital in Detroit the year before the Superintendent's Society came into existence. The development of pre-clinical (then called preliminary) courses was advocated as part of a three-year program. As the number of schools increased, it became difficult to obtain students in some areas. The shortage of applicants, which created serious friction between hospital administrators and nurse educators, was attributed to the three-year course and the high (!) entrance requirements, rather than to the opening of more and more hospitals and schools of nursing, and to the growing variety of vocational opportunities for women. One year of high school work, or its equivalent, was then the minimum requirement of the board of examiners of New York, a state in which the lack of sufficient numbers of candidates was causing concern to some well-established hospitals. The concept of the pupil nurse as a worker rather than as a student is well illustrated by the following excerpt from a book, presumed to be one of the first of its kind, which was intended to promote the enrollment of students. "In some schools it is the custom for the superintendent to give the probationer certain instructions before going to the ward, and to draw her attention to the Hospital and Home rules. She is then taken to the ward at a rapid gait and introduced to the head nurse who will be too busy to waste any time in desultory conversation, but will at once call attention to the schedule of the ward routine posted for the guidance of all the ward workers and allow her to study what her duties will be."[6]

The American Hospital Association took cognizance of the unwholesome situation. A committee composed of some of its best-known members was appointed to study "the training school" with special reference to the curriculum and to the advisability of undertaking the preparation of nurse helpers or assistants. The widely distributed report of that committee is remarkable for its clarity and awareness of a need for some method of grading schools of nursing. The preparation of a secondary type of worker is not mentioned. The dichotomy that continued to plague both hospitals, which are service agencies, and nursing schools, which are responsible for the education rather than limited in-service training of nurses, was frankly faced:

. . . the Committee has been careful not to lose sight of the interests of the training school as a school . . . has tried to consider the interests of the school apart from the hospital whenever possible. At the same time the Committee recognizes that the training school is an integral part of and subordinate to the hospital.[7]

The report was highly commended by the AJN which, however, failed to point out that it did not touch the core of the problem, namely, the distinction between a nursing school and a nursing service and the need of both for budgets. The committee's condemnation of the establishment of schools by very small hospitals was encouraging to nurse educators. The report pointed out that very small general hospitals could not be considered from the same standpoint as large city institutions "whose functions of late years have broadened and diversified along special and sociological lines." The committee approved preliminary courses as advocated by the Society of Superintendents of Training Schools. It approved a three-year curriculum for schools in large general hospitals only and recommended a 27-month minimum course for smaller institutions. Hospitals of

[6] Hodson, Jane (ed.): *How to Become a Trained Nurse*, 3rd ed. William Abbott, New York, 1911, p. 18.

[7] Aikens, Charlotte A.: "Report of Special Training School Committee to the American Hospital Association," *Hospital Management*. W. B. Saunders Company, Philadelphia, 1911, Appendix I, p. 427.

25 beds or less were considered unsuitable for nursing schools unless affiliations could be obtained. This committee was of the opinion that pupil nurses should not be called upon to give more than 63 hours per week to their work, including class hours. Shocking as it now seems, that recommendation, by including class hours in on-duty time, represented a far more liberal point of view than that of many institutions. Night duty was then usually a full 12 hours and often seven nights a week. Many classes were held at the end of a long day on duty.

The report included a suggested form letter which might be sent by the schools in response to inquiries. Significantly, it contained no reference whatever to opportunities that might be anticipated by those who would receive diplomas and be allowed to wear the badge of the school. At that time, nursing education was so subordinated to institutional need for nursing service that it was not uncommon for schools to graduate students who, it had already been decided, should never be employed by the parent institution or recommended to an employing agency. An appendix to the report includes a list of 21 "Instructions for Special and Graduate Nurses" which throws a revealing light on the long hours and other administrative practices of the period. Among the more significant was one that required special nurses to have cots in the patient's rooms on which to secure such sleep as their patient's condition (and their own) permitted; the cots had to be removed from the patient's room by 8:00 A.M. Patients were charged for the board of their special nurses and for the use of the cots, without reference to the fact that the institution had given them far less than the normal amount of nursing care. Excellent though it was considered at the time, the report dealt only with symptoms. It failed to make and act upon a diagnosis. There is no reference whatever to the financing of nursing schools, most of which could accurately be described as indigent since they had no visible means of support. At least one influential hospital administrator had endorsed the principle that nursing schools should be endowed;[8] however, there was a strong but subtle

[8] Hurd, Henry M.: "Shall Training Schools for Nurses be Endowed?" *Am. J. Nursing,* 6:843, 1906.

and pervasive resistance to efforts to secure any measure of independence for the schools.

"It seems tolerably clear," wrote Miss Nutting in her comprehensive analysis of nursing in this period, "that the principle of dependence upon the student body for all of the actual nursing work and for a very considerable amount of other work, some purely domestic in nature, some supervisory and executive, is so universally accepted and so deeply rooted as to render hospitals generally unwilling to tolerate any conditions which affect this principle and which require a modification or frank abandonment of the plan and system upon which it is based. . . . While hospital and training school are fundamentally 'interdependent,' there is no more reason why the hospital should own and control the training school than the medical school. The basis of relationships should be one of close and efficient cooperation."[9]

No other profession has been developed on the assumption that an education can be secured in exchange for service. Some of the diplomas granted by schools organized for the sole purpose of providing service for a few hospital patients were as worthless as those of the "diploma mills" which were castigated in the Flexner report on medical schools. But condemnation by nurses of such schools had no comparable support and was often misinterpreted and resented as condemnation of all hospitals which operated training schools. Regardless of the extraordinary nature of its educational origins, American nursing began at an early date to demonstrate two characteristics of a profession: (1) Continuous effort toward the improvement of nursing education, as a basis for nursing service, has consistently been based on what were believed to be the needs of those to be served, namely, patients, actual or potential, as individuals in relation to their families and communities. These efforts have not been restricted to the area of technical care in which nursing is ancillary to medicine nor to the immediate needs of hospitals and other institutions. (2) Acceptance of responsibility for handing on an ever-increasing body of knowledge.

[9] Nutting, M. Adelaide: *Educational Status of Nursing*, US Bureau of Education, Bulletin #7, Whole #475. US Government Printing Office, Washington, D.C., 1912, p. 51.

Through the years the profession's struggles for educational improvement have been based upon the social vision of its leaders and the dissatisfaction of practicing nurses with their basic preparation. Before the end of the first decade of the new century, the successes of visiting nurses had created a variety of opportunities for nurses in connection with the growing public health movement. Leaders in the movement for the education of nurses, rather than apprentice training on the job, believed that institutions called schools should be expected to have definite educational standards and objectives. They could look back upon substantial evidence of progress toward acceptance of that principle. The addition of the title "principal of the school of nursing" to that of "superintendent of nurses," which Mrs. Robb had insisted upon when she was invited to organize the school at Johns Hopkins Hospital, by an increasing number of institutions indicates that the dual function of these administrators and educators was gaining recognition. The better schools were responding to the influence of the work at Teachers College which the Society of Superintendents had brought into existence. The day when a busy superintendent of nurses was expected to do all the classroom teaching, exclusive of doctors' lectures, was passing.

Which school first appointed a full-time instructor? We do not know. A search for "firsts" is a fascinating but often also an exasperating experience. Due in part to incomplete records, the available histories of schools vary considerably in scope. They conform to no one pattern. This adds to their interest but detracts from their value as sources of comparative information. The history of the school of the University of Pennsylvania Hospital notes that Jane A. Delano was "elected to the position of instructor to the nurses and assistant superintendent" (to Mary E. P. Davis) in 1890. Her duties seem to have included those of principal of the school as well as those of assistant superintendent of the hospital. Isabel McIsaac, principal of the Illinois Training School for Nurses and a superlative teacher, is believed to have been first to institute "instruction in nursing procedures by clinical demonstrations" in 1895.[10] Annabella

[10] Schryver, Grace Fay: *History of the Illinois Training School for Nurses, 1880–1929.* Published by board of directors of Illinois Training School, Chicago, 1930, p. 73.

McCrae, one of the earliest to achieve distinction as a teacher of nursing, was an assistant and part-time instructor in the Massachusetts General Hospital School of Nursing from 1902 until 1912, when she was relieved of administrative responsibilities to devote full time to the organization and teaching of the basic course in nursing procedures.

The Johns Hopkins Hospital School of Nursing is unique in that the founder of the hospital, Johns Hopkins, instructed his trustees to establish, in connection with the hospital, a training school for female nurses. There is nothing in Isabel Hampton's inaugural address at the opening of the school (1889) to indicate that she then perceived that a school should have a broader objective than the provision of a continuous supply of nursing service for the hospital. However, under her direction and that of her successor, Miss Nutting, the nursing school, like the medical school, established standards that were to have world-wide influence. A preliminary (preclinical) course was established by Miss Nutting in 1901. In 1903, the school had two instructors in nursing arts and was in the vanguard of the movement to remove the preparation of nurses from the field of mere apprenticeship. Carrie J. Brink, who was to become famous for her teaching of bedside nursing at Bellevue, was appointed instructor of probationers in 1903. Amy E. Pope, who also gained recognition as a teacher, was appointed by the Presbyterian Hospital School, New York, the following year. Affiliations with educational institutions were developed in several cities at about this time. Among those still in existence at mid-century are the Children's Hospital of Boston with Simmons College (1904) and Evanston (Illinois) Hospital with Northwestern University (1911). Slowly but surely the stronger schools were acquiring some of the characteristics of educational institutions.

Appended to the first curriculum committee report to the Society of Superintendents (1896) was a brief list of reference books and a list of about 50 textbooks which was headed by Miss Nightingale's *Notes on Nursing.* Less than a dozen of the authors were nurses, but it represented the beginnings of the professional literature of nursing. Several manuals were included but, surprisingly, the two

of most lasting influence were not. These were the Bellevue handbook published by Putnam & Sons and that of the Connecticut
Training School which Lippincott published in 1878. The latter
book paid royalties to the school until 1913. The first textbook
by an American nurse was Clara S. Weeks' (Shaw) *A Textbook of Nursing for the Use of Training Schools, Families, and
Private Students,* published in 1885, last revised in 1916. Royalties
from this book were paid into a special fund for the New York Hospital School of Nursing well into the new century. Harriet Camp
Lounsberry's *Ethics of Nursing* (1889) had a place on that list, as
had Miss Dock's *Materia Medica.* The latter was the standard text
in its field for many years. It was written in 1890 while the author
was on night duty at Bellevue. Mrs. Robb's *Nursing, Its Principles
and Practice,* published in 1893 and twice revised before her tragic
accidental death (1910), is of special historical significance. Written
before there were any courses for administrators she included chapters on the organization and management of nursing schools and on
ward administration. The current (1948) edition of Kimber's *Anatomy*[11] bears little resemblance to the book Miss Kimber wrote while
assisting Louise Darche with the extremely difficult task of developing the City Hospital School of Nursing on Blackwell's (Welfare) Island in New York City.

A growing sense of responsibility for the development of a professional literature is an important characteristic of this period.
Isabel McIsaac retired from the Illinois Training School to write a
series of elementary texts. Some of the early instructors of nursing
procedures, considered martinets by their students because of their
insistent emphasis on precision of technic, became the authors of
widely used textbooks. The publication of two volumes (1907) of
the now classic four-volume *History of Nursing* was an epochal
event. It contributed an extremely important element to the foundations of the emerging profession. Miss Nutting had already begun
collecting historical materials for her classes when she and Miss

[11] Kimber, Diana Clifford, and Gray, Carolyn E., revised by Stackpole,
Caroline E., and Leavell, Lutie C.: *Textbook of Anatomy and Physiology,*
12th ed. The Macmillan Company, New York, 1948.

Dock became collaborators. The publisher to whom they took the completed manuscripts declined them on the ground that such a work would not pay its way. The intrepid pair secured a bank loan to cover the cost of publication. Their belief that nurses would be interested in the history of their profession was fully justified and the loan was repaid within a year. The two later volumes (1912) were edited and in part written by Miss Dock. Their title pages indicate that the International Council of Nurses receives all proceeds from the sale of these volumes. Rights to the first two volumes have been willed by Miss Dock to the American Nurses' Association.

There are two educational landmarks in this period—one in undergraduate, the other in graduate education. They are the establishment of the University of Minnesota School of Nursing in 1909, which proudly claims the distinction of being "the first university school of nursing in the world," and the expansion of the work at Teachers College. Dr. Richard Olding Beard, who had fathered the movement for a school on a collegiate level, not without vigorous opposition from some members of his own profession, announced the opening of the new school at a meeting of the American Federation of Nurses in Minneapolis in 1909. In a historic paper, "The University Education of the Nurse," he made prophetic reference to the function of a state university. "It is, and it should be, peculiarly interested in providing for the highest and most selective training of those who are to engage in the pursuits by which human life, human development, and human health are conserved. In a word, it should bring the full emphasis of its nurture upon the value of human life itself." The announcement was hailed with joy. For the first time, a basic program in nursing education was to be conducted and controlled by a university in accordance with sound principles of education. Student nurses paid tuition for the preliminary course and found living accommodations for themselves as did other students on the campus. Probably few who listened to that announcement realized what vision and fortitude would be required of the directors of the new school. Facilities for teaching nursing practice were extremely limited. "Makeshift" seems to be the only term which describes the place in which patients were cared for until the university hospital was completed in 1911. Standards of admission were those of the university, and there were few applicants. But Louise M. Powell, the gentle Virginian who had studied at Teachers College and succeeded frail Bertha Erdman as director of the school in 1910, possessed lionhearted courage. Dr. Beard, thoroughly convinced of the rightness of placing nursing education under university auspices, gave unfailing support. Ten years of pioneering effort went into the upbuilding of the school before it offered a degree-granting basic program (1919). In the meantime, the University of Cincinnati had assumed control (1916) of the School of Nursing and Health which had been organized by Laura R. Logan to succeed the earlier school of the city's general hospital.

The statement that the Minnesota school was the first undergraduate school for nurses in a university has sometimes been challenged. The catalog of the School of Medicine of the University of Texas, 1896–1897, announced that the Board of Ladies which had sponsored the John Sealy Hospital School for Nurses could no longer support it. Therefore, "to save it from going out of existence . . . the Regents of the University recently adopted this branch as one of the regular schools of the Medical Department." Class work was the responsibility of the college, but admissions "at any time from May to October" and all other administrative details were delegated to the hospital. It is of some interest that the catalog quoted indicates that "Mental and Nervous Diseases and Medical Jurisprudence" were included in the program. The school was saved; however, it would seem that it was a hospital school sponsored by the university and of superior quality for its times but not a collegiate school in the mid-century meaning of the term. Happily it secured that status at a later date.

The one-year course in hospital economics which had been established in 1899 at Teachers College, Columbia University, was extended and enriched to cover two years in 1905. The following year, Miss Nutting was called from Johns Hopkins to establish a new department of household administration in which was included the division of hospital economics. Miss Nutting took office in the fall of 1907 after a year of European travel, and was the first nurse in the world to become a professor in a university. The influence of her keen intelligence and forceful personality was felt throughout the college, and some of the most eminent members of the faculty became interested in contributing to the program of the department. Miss Dock and Miss Wald were added to the roster of nurse lecturers, which had previously included institutional nurses only, to teach the history and the social aspects of nursing. Isabel M. Stewart who had left teaching, or so she thought, to study nursing at the Winnipeg General Hospital, was appointed assistant to Miss Nutting in 1909. Loyal, generous, imaginative, and indefatigable, she began at once to develop special courses for nurse-teachers, although there was only a dawning demand for nurses with such preparation. Thus began a career that was to exert an extraordinary influence on the development of nursing education in this and other countries.

By 1910 there was obvious need for nurses with special preparation in administration and teaching in visiting nursing and other types of public health nursing. An endowment of $150,000, subsequently increased to $200,000, by Mrs. Helen Hartley Jenkins, a trustee of Teachers College, made it possible for the college to transfer all nursing programs to a new Department of Nursing and Health. Dynamic and socially minded Ella Phillips Crandall, a graduate of "Old Blockley" (Philadelphia General), was appointed to the faculty to develop the courses in district nursing and health protection. In 1912 summer courses were first offered. By this time the department was growing rapidly in scope and enrollment. The term "public health nursing," created by Miss Wald when she prefaced Miss Nightingale's "health nursing" with the word "public," was adopted in that year. A clear distinction was made between the courses for administrators and teachers in nursing schools and those for public health nurses. The NLNE, which had been responsible for the inauguration of the department and (assisted by the ANA) for its financial support, could now with pride relinquish that obligation. The work, begun in hope and faith in 1899, was now firmly and independently established in an institution of higher education. For years, however, in acknowledgment of its origins and the continuation of mutual interests, reports of the work of the department were presented at the annual conventions of the NLNE.

Efforts to supplement inadequate or outdated preparation for nursing were not wanting. In the mid-nineties, the Illinois Training School under Isabel McIsaac's leadership had begun offering postgraduate courses chiefly to graduates of the school. Early in the new century, they were more formally developed and made generally available. When Annie W. Goodrich became superintendent of nurses at Bellevue and Allied Hospitals, she promptly grasped the opportunity to assist graduates of small schools by offering postgraduate courses based on the abundant clinical resources available for teaching. Maternity, children's, and other special hospitals offered "postgraduate" courses in order to secure nursing service. In fairness to them it must be noted that the professional organizations did not attempt to set standards for such courses.

In the first decade of the new century, the larger visiting nurse associations were overwhelmed with requests for nurses to establish new services. To help meet this need, the Instructive District Nursing Association of Boston[12] was the first (1906) of several such organizations to offer postgraduate courses. This was definitely a response to need, not a means for supplementing the existing staffs of these agencies. As service agencies, the visiting nurse associations (VNA's) realized that they were not well equipped to take on the teaching of graduate nurses or to provide affiliations for student nurses, as a few of them were attempting to do. It was in recognition of a need which could not be met adequately by such efforts that the work at Teachers College was expanded in 1910.

As previously stated, the fundamental problem of the schools was rooted in the fact that there was no hospital system and no generally accepted standards of administrative practice and fiscal policies for the hospitals which operated them. It must not be forgotten, however, that the voluntary hospitals, which were the standard bearers in their field, were burdened with the tradition of gratuitous service to the sick poor. Both hospitals and nurses had to cope with the

[12] "A School for the Training of District Nurses," *Am. J. Nursing*, 6:836, 1906.

deep-seated psychological reluctance of human beings to pay for their illnesses and with the hard economic fact that many could not do so. Nurses were thus attempting to establish a system of education and of service on a structurally and financially unstable foundation. Despite its financial, educational and social weaknesses, the system established by farseeing nurse leaders, working through the media of the national nursing organizations, has withstood the pressures of two wars and a catastrophic depression.

BIBLIOGRAPHY

Beard, Richard Olding: "The University Education of the Nurse," *Fifteenth Annual Report of the American Society of Superintendents of Training Schools for Nurses, Including Report of the Second Meeting of the American Federation of Nurses*, 1909, pp, 111–25.

Corwin, E. H. L.: *The American Hospital.* The Commonwealth Fund, New York, 1946.

Dock, Lavinia L.: "The Growth of Nursing in the United States," *A History of Nursing.* G. P. Putnam's Sons, New York, 1912, Vol. III, Chap. II.

Fillmore, Anna: "Scene—U.S.A. 1900," *Am. J. Nursing*, **41**:913, 1941.

Goostray, Stella: *Fifty Years, A History of the School of Nursing, The Children's Hospital, Boston.* The Alumnae Association, Boston, 1940.

Gray, James: *The University of Minnesota, 1851–1951.* University of Minnesota Press, Minneapolis, 1951.

A Handbook of Nursing for General and Family Use, published under the direction of the Connecticut Training School for Nurses, State Hospital, New Haven, Conn. J. B. Lippincott, Co., Philadelphia, 1878.

Handbook on Nursing, compiled by a committee of the Bellevue School of Nursing. G. P. Putnam's Sons, New York, 1878.

Lee, Eleanor: *History of the School of Nursing of the Presbyterian Hospital, New York, 1892–1942.* G. P. Putnam's Sons, New York, 1942.

Ludlum, George P.: "The Reaction in Training School Methods." Address at the Convention of the American Hospital Association, Chicago, Sept. 17–20, 1907.

Keith, Mary L.: "The Introduction of District Nursing into the Training-School Curriculum" (Eleventh Annual Report of the National League of Nursing Education), *Am. J. Nursing*, **5**:104, 1905.

"Mrs. Clara S. Weeks Shaw," *Am. J. Nursing*, **40**:356, 1940.

Robb, Isabel Hampton: "The Three Years' Course of Training in Connection with the Eight Hour System," *First and Second Annual Reports of the American Society of Superintendents of Training Schools for Nurses*, 1897, p. 33.

Schryver, Grace Fay: "Post-Graduate Training," *A History of the Illinois Training School for Nurses, 1880–1929*. Published by the board of directors of the Illinois Training School for Nurses, Chicago, 1930, p. 74.

Smith, Clare Louise: "The Establishment of the Affiliation with Northwestern University, 1909–1914," *The Evanston Hospital School of Nursing, 1898–1948*. The Lakeside Press, Chicago, 1948, p. 30.

Stack, Margaret K.: "Résumé of the History of the Connecticut Training School for Nurses," *Am. J. Nursing*, **23**:825, 1923.

Third Annual Report of the American Society of Superintendents of Training Schools for Nurses, 1896, pp. 10–17.

Twenty-five Years of Nursing Education in Teachers College, 1899–1925, Teachers College Bulletin, 17th Series, 3, Feb., 1926, Columbia University, New York.

Washburn, Frederic A.: *The Massachusetts General Hospital—Its Development, 1900–1935*. Houghton Mifflin Co., Boston, 1939.

Chapter 8

THE NURSING ORGANIZATIONS BUILD
FOR THE FUTURE

These societies are splendid schools in which to learn to disagree without quarreling.

SOPHIA F. PALMER[1]

A CONSIDERATION of the evolution of nursing cannot readily be fitted into decades or other conventional time units. One of the most fertile periods of American nursing reached its climax at the epochal convention of 1912 at which the National Organization for Public Health Nursing (NOPHN) was brought into existence. Like the two older associations, it was created by leaders of nursing thought who had what has been called the power to realize the future.

All three groups were excitingly aware of the expanding fields of social usefulness which were opening up for qualified nurses. They were deeply conscious of the danger to society, and to the profession, of inadequate preparation for nursing. The influence of the hundreds of young women who had dropped out, or had been dismissed, from nursing schools was having a deleterious effect on nursing as a whole. Those who entered the then wholly unstandardized field of practical nursing might, or might not, become dependable workers. The frustrations of graduate nurses who, for lack of information, had entered substandard schools were having an inhibiting influence on the enrollment of desirable students.

The primary purpose of the Society of Superintendents (renamed the National League of Nursing Education in 1912) was to further the best interests of the nursing profession by establishing and

[1] *The Trained Nurse,* Sept., 1895, p. 151.

71

maintaining a "universal" standard of training.[2] The purpose of the
Associated Alumnae, as stated in its constitution, was to "strengthen
the union of nursing organizations, to elevate nursing education,
and to promote ethical standards in all the relations of the nursing
profession."[3] The third organization (NOPHN) was given a broader
base: its object was "to stimulate the general public and the visiting
nurse associations to the extension and support of public health
nursing service, to facilitate harmonious cooperation among the
workers and supporters, to develop a standard of ethics and technic,
and also to act as a clearing house for information for those interested in such work."[4] The NOPHN is discussed in the following
chapter.

The only method through which the standardization of nursing
schools, so earnestly desired by the professional organizations,
might be secured was through the medium of legislation. Although
a national standard was discussed, it was realized that the power to
regulate the practice of professional and other workers is a function
of state governments. When, therefore, the Associated Alumnae
undertook the task of securing legislation to control the practice of
nursing as a protection to the public and as a means of standardizing or upgrading the preparation of nurses, it had first to promote
the organization of nursing in the states. By 1912, 38 state nurses'
associations had been organized and 33 of them had secured nurse
practice acts. The Associated Alumnae had been renamed the
American Nurses' Association in 1911.

For several years, a highly competent (and unsalaried) interstate
secretary had assisted the alumnae and other groups of nurses with
their organizational problems, chiefly through correspondence. Even
the cheerful and inexhaustible patience of Sarah E. Sly must often
have been taxed by repetitive reviewing of constitutions and bylaws, insistence on the study of parliamentary procedure, and as-

[2] *First Annual Report of the American Society of Superintendents of Training Schools for Nurses,* 1897, p. 10.
[3] "Report—Fifth Annual Convention of Nurses' Associated Alumnae of U.S.," *Am. J. Nursing,* 2:766, 1902.
[4] Wald, Lillian D. (chairman): "Report of the Joint Committee Appointed for Consideration of the Standardization of Visiting Nursing," *Am. J. Nursing,* 12:897, 1912.

sistance with other pioneer work in relation to state legislation. Isabel McIsaac came out of retirement in 1910 to serve her profession as a traveling interstate secretary. The basic unity of purpose of the organizations is shown in this connection. Responsibility for the salary was shared by the Associated Alumnae, the Society of Superintendents, the *Journal,* and the American Red Cross nursing service, which had been established the previous year. Travel expenses were borne by those state and local associations which requested visits. Miss McIsaac has recorded a charming story of a nurse, working in complete isolation from her own kind, who cheerfully paid out of her own pocket the not inconsiderable cost of a visit from the interstate secretary. That nurse was rewarded by an overflowing measure of stimulating information from the astonished and always generous Miss McIsaac. The "Progress of State Legislation" was a major head in the *Journal* for almost a quarter of a century.

Attendance at the convention of the two associations in 1912 far exceeded expectations, due largely to preliminary work by Mary S. Gardner and other representative public health nurses. The ANA then represented some 20,000 nurses. The exceedingly long hours of the private duty nurses, who made up the largest group within the profession, were a deterrent to attendance at meetings. Also, the discussions of educational standards and of legislative and organizational procedures were of little interest to many nurses who might have flocked to demonstrations of nursing procedure and discussions of the care of patients. Miss McIsaac's report of two years of field work, in which she had traveled up and down and across the country, is an illuminating document.[5] For the first time a substantial cross section of the nursing schools had been visited. "The common good for which we strive," said Miss McIsaac, "can be stated in six words—better schools, better nurses, better service." A highly competent judge of nursing schools, she was also frank. In almost every city she had found the source of many nursing problems to be substandard schools. She considered it significant that a start had

[5] McIsaac, Isabel: "Report of Work of Interstate Secretary of the American Society of Superintendents of Training Schools for Nurses and the American Nurses' Association," *Am. J. Nursing,* 12:875–84, 1912.

been made toward creating an informed public opinion on major nursing issues within the profession.

At an earlier date, Miss McIsaac had pointed out that securing and improving nurse practice acts was by no means the sole function of the state associations. Observing their tendency to sit back, when that objective had been achieved, she spoke feelingly on the subject. Although sympathetically aware that the welfare of nurses required attention, she recommended that newer methods in nursing should be given a major place on the programs of the professional organizations. "Study courses" had been outlined and recommended at an early date. There were, however, no national or state staffs to promote such programs by providing stimulating suggestions and follow-up materials. There is, unfortunately, little evidence that Miss McIsaac's advice on that point was followed to any appreciable extent. For many years, the profession was to be subjected to the criticism that the two older organizations were more concerned about nurses and nursing education than about the care of patients. This opinion tended to create a climate unfavorable to the development of wholesome relationships with other groups. By 1912, however, American nurses had laid sound foundations for the professional cohesiveness which was a necessary first step in the development of the embryonic profession.

In a still cogent article, "What We May Expect From the Law," Miss Dock stated a profound truth when she wrote: "Restrictive legislation affecting the professions . . . is not to be gained once and forever; . . . It does not mean just one effort, but continuous efforts for the rest of time."[6] Nurses were novices in legislative matters. Some of them, according to Miss McIsaac, had acted in zealous haste rather than on the basis of sound judgment and careful planning. Consequently, many of the early nurse practice acts were ineffective. A session of the 1912 convention was devoted to consideration of state registration. Annie W. Goodrich, (New York Hospital Training School), who had directed four important schools of nursing, including Bellevue, had recently suc-

[6] Dock, Lavinia L., "What We May Expect From the Law," *Am. J. Nursing,* 1:8, 1901. (Reprinted, *Am. J. Nursing,* **50:**599, 1950.)

ceeded Anna L. Alline as inspector of nurse training schools in New York. She led off with an analysis of 33 laws, at least one of which had already been amended. Only one other state, Illinois, had appointed an inspector. A considerable number of the acts made no provision for any type of helpful supervision of the schools. Lack of specificity about the qualifications and methods of selection and appointment of members of boards of nurse examiners was another serious weakness. Laws are not self-operative! Time was to reveal that, granted power to act, the success of the movement for state registration depended chiefly on the scope of the professional knowledge and the administrative ability of the persons selected to execute the nurse practice acts. The tone of that conference in 1912 was extremely optimistic. Sufficient information had been accumulated about the schools to provide a substantial basis for constructive work in some of the states. One, at least, of the seven so-called mandatory laws was having a wholesome influence on the schools, but it also had the negative effect of driving unqualified nurses out of the state to practice where legal barriers to their practice as graduate nurses had not yet been set up.

Opposition to standard-setting legislation was not wanting. Proprietary hospitals and those which added to income by sending student nurses out, ostensibly for practice as private duty nurses in the homes of patients, were often influential opponents. Much time and effort were wasted on endeavors to secure legal protection for use of the word "nurse" by graduate registered nurses only. The word, in its many connotations, is so deeply embedded in the English language that the nurse practice acts can protect only such titles as "registered nurse," "registered graduate nurse," and the like. A quarter of a century was to pass before the legislative committee of any state nurses' association worked toward the inclusion of a definition of nursing in a nurse practice act. Truly, Miss Dock had spoken with the voice of a prophet.

It was in this nascent period that the affiliation was effected (1909) between the American Red Cross nursing service and the American Nurses' Association which was to be a constructive force in American nursing for over twenty years. The success of Red

Cross Auxiliaries in enrolling nurses for the Spanish-American War led the reorganized ARC (1905) to consider nurse enrollment a proper function of the national organization, and the now widely known nurses' pin was devised. But when no effective plan for maintaining an enrollment of reserve nurses had been developed by either the ARC or the Army Nurse Corps, Mrs. Robb and other leading spirits in nursing became concerned. As chairman of a committee appointed by the American Federation of Nurses, Mrs. Robb presented an elaborate plan to the ARC for maintaining an enrollment through affiliation with the American Federation of Nurses.[7] The plan was rejected, but the principle of affiliation was accepted and developed with the Associated Alumnae.[8]

A national committee on Red Cross nursing service was appointed (1909) by the ARC, with Jane A. Delano chairman. Membership was representative of the nursing organizations, the Army, the Navy, and the Red Cross. Miss Delano had worked with the Red Cross in a yellow fever epidemic. She had been the principal of her alma mater, the Bellevue School. She was then superintendent of the Army Nurse Corps and also president of the Associated Alumnae. She resigned from the Army in 1912 to give full time, as a volunteer, to the work which was to make her one of the commanding figures in American nursing. In cooperation with the ANA she developed a system of state and local committees which were responsible for securing and evaluating the credentials of nurses in preparation for their enrollment in the nursing service of the ARC. The professional standards for enrollment and other policies worked out by Miss Delano and supported by the national committee were to have a powerful influence on the development of nursing in the period when the nursing organizations were still weak and legal requirements for practice as registered nurses were lamentably low in many states. In this connection, Miss Palmer, editor of the AJN, seems to have possessed that most desirable of editorial qualities, namely, an awareness of what is about to become important. The magazine had

[7] *Fifteenth Annual Report of the American Society of Superintendents of Training Schools for Nurses, Including Report of the Second Meeting of the American Federation of Nurses*, 1909, pp. 204–14.
[8] "The Red Cross," *Am. J. Nursing*, 10:77, 1910.

established a department, "Notes on Red Cross Nursing," two years
before the affiliation was effected. It was to be continued for some
thirty years as the "Department of Red Cross Nursing."

In 1912 the American Society of Superintendents of Training
Schools for Nurses was renamed, after some years of discussion, the
National League of Nursing Education. "League," Miss Nutting
averred, "is a good strong word!" And so it proved to be since its
use is continued by the National League for Nursing which was
formed by the fusion of the NLNE with two other organizations in
1952. In its formative years, the League membership included a
high percentage of women who were convinced that education must
be the foundation on which any professional superstructure could
safely be built and who accepted their responsibility as educators
with an almost religious zeal. Having no office or staff, the organization's work was carried on by officers and committees. Early records
indicate that questionnaires were freely used to secure information
by busy women who had no secretarial assistance. They established
an extraordinary pattern of industry and of devotion to their profession.

The League had two solid achievements to its credit by 1912,
notably the organization of the ANA and of the Department of
Nursing at Teachers College. Its annual reports became one of the
major assets of the profession. The convention program of the historic year reveals both sustained effort and prophetic insight. The
rallying cry of the keynoter, Miss Goodrich, was: "Our place . . .
has been found in the institutions of the sick, but we shall never
render our full service to the community until our place is also
found in the university."[9] It was at that meeting that Miss Nutting,
chairman of the Education Committee, sorrowfully reported that the
Carnegie Foundation recognized the importance of the society's request for a study of nursing education comparable to that of medical education but could not then undertake it. Its interests were
centered in other fields. (Several years were to pass before the
Rockefeller Foundation met the profession's need for a study of

[9] *Eighteenth Annual Report of the American Society of Superintendents of
Training Schools for Nurses,* 1912, p. 43.

nursing education.) Methods of cooperating with educational institutions were a major topic at that convention. So was the question of introducing some basic concepts of visiting nursing in the curriculum. The preparation, status, and functions of a newcomer to the educational scene, the *instructor,* received considerable attention. Two papers on scientific management were presented. The suggestion of Frank B. Gilbreth, a brilliant pioneer in that field, that nurses might lead the way to scientific management in hospitals fell on unprepared soil.

Problems of organizational structure, a subject of primary importance at the half century, were not unknown in the early part of the century. The American Federation of Nurses (1901–1912), of which Miss Nutting was president, was an association of the two national organizations to provide for representative membership in the National Council of Women. But that affiliation was discontinued in 1905 in favor of membership in the International Council of Nurses (ICN). The only meetings of the federation were held conjointly with the two older organizations in 1905 and 1909. The programs differed little from those of the two components. The federation was discontinued after the American Nurses' Association made provision for membership on its board of directors of the presidents of the League and of the newly organized NOPHN (1912). The ANA became the American representative of nurses in the International Council of Nurses. An interesting report of a Committee on Closer Union of the Nursing Societies had been presented at the meeting of the Society of Superintendents in 1910. The members present favored closer union but feared loss of identity in any merger.[10] It was agreed, however, that it would be desirable to hold the meetings at the same time and place as the Associated Alumnae. This principle was agreed upon by the three organizations at the harmonious and forward-looking 1912 convention.

The story of the National Association of Colored Graduate Nurses (NACGN) is in many ways similar to that of the older organizations. It owes its inception to the vision, wisdom, and initiative of

[10] *Fifteenth Annual Report of the American Society of Superintendents of Training Schools for Nurses,* 1909, p. 26.

Martha Franklin, a graduate of the school of the Woman's Hospital of Philadelphia. Miss Franklin made a two-year study of the status of Negro nurses before sending out 1500 letters to explore their interest in forming a national organization. As a result, 58 nurses who met in New York at the Lincoln Hospital in August, 1908, organized the National Association of Colored Graduate Nurses. The first volume of the *Journal* records some of the experiences of Jessie C. Sleet (Mrs. John R. Scales), a graduate of the pioneer Provident Hospital School of Nursing, Chicago, who was the first Negro nurse to enter the field of public health nursing. She was employed by the Charity Organization Society of New York. A few years later, the Henry Street Nurses' Settlement reported its good fortune in securing the services of two graduates of the Freedmen's Hospital school in Washington who were "especially alive to social movements and organized preventive work."[11] Because the organization had no headquarters office or permanent staff, work progressed slowly for the first ten years. The annual meetings, however, were a source of inspiration and growth. Graduates of the pioneer schools for Negro nurses, such as those of Provident Hospital, Chicago (1891), and Freedmen's in Washington (1894), were destined to become leaders in nursing and in the promotion of democratic interracial relationships.

Reference has been made to the International Council of Nurses. Busy though they were with the internal affairs of American nursing, some of the founders of the two older national nursing organizations were very active in the organization of the ICN. Historically, the 1899 meeting in London of the International Council of Women has much the same relationship to the ICN as that of the Chicago World's Fair to the NLNE. A number of representative American nurses attended the meeting in London at which a one-day program was devoted to nursing. Mrs. Bedford Fenwick, as editor of the *British Journal of Nursing*, was already crusading for state registration. Her agile mind quickly grasped the possibilities inherent in the development of strong professional organizations. She presented her concept of an International Council of Nurses at a

[11] "Nurses' Settlement News," *Am. J. Nursing*, **6**:832, 1906.

meeting of the Matrons' Council of Great Britain and Ireland, following the adjournment of the International Council of Women. Nurses from a number of countries attended on invitation. The group accepted the idea and appointed a provisional committee to work out a plan of organization. Mrs. Robb and Miss Dock were members of that committee which was ultimately enlarged to include representative nurses from nine countries. At a meeting of the provisional committee in London in 1900, the International Council of Nurses was brought into existence by the adoption of a constitution. The preamble to it well states the purpose of the council:

We, nurses of all nations, sincerely believing that the best good of our Profession will be advanced by greater unity of thought, sympathy, and purpose, do hereby band ourselves in a confederation of workers to further the efficient care of the sick, and to secure the honour and the interests of the Nursing Profession.[12]

Thus, with high hopes, but practically no funds, was born an international organization of nurses that antedates by many years the international hospital and medical associations and which by mid-century could claim to be the largest international organization of professional women in the world. Mrs. Fenwick, who became known as the founder of the ICN, was elected president, and Miss Dock, secretary. The early development of the ICN was largely due to Miss Dock's creative and enthusiastic devotion to its purposes, her linguistic ability, and the fact that it was possible for her to make relatively frequent journeys across the Atlantic. The provisional committee accepted an invitation to hold the first congress of the ICN in connection with the two American organizations in Buffalo (1901). The meetings concluded with a detailed resolution which stressed the importance of securing suitable legislation to control the practice of nursing in all countries or, as Mrs. Bedford Fenwick put it, to provide for a "one portal entry" to the profession.

At the Berlin congress in 1904, representatives of the national organizations of Great Britain, Germany, and the United States re-

[12] Breay, Margaret, and Fenwick, Ethel Bedford: *The History of the International Council of Nurses, 1899–1925.* Published by the ICN, Geneva, 1931, p. 12.

ported that their organizations were ready and eager to affiliate with the International Council of Nurses. Memberships of individual nurses were abolished, and the ICN became a federation of national organizations (one only in a country) of professional nurses. The official magazines of the respective organizations were designated official organs of the ICN in their own countries. Miss Dock, already the editor of the *Journal's* "Foreign News," continued to provide the magazine with a wealth of informative material on nursing in other countries. At the congress in London in 1909, Mrs. Robb was elected chairman of the Standing Committee on Education which was destined to become one of the strongest arms of the ICN. Following Mrs. Robb's sudden death the following year, Miss Nutting accepted the chairmanship.

By 1912, ten national nursing organizations were members of the ICN.[13] Public health nursing was gaining ground in many countries, and papers on "the social service of the nurse" were a feature of the program.

The basic problems of nurses then, as now, were universal. Excessively long hours were causing anxiety everywhere. One of the resolutions adopted at Cologne reads:

Resolved, that we earnestly beg hospital authorities to give the same consideration to the problem of overwork among nurses that industrial leaders are giving to the question of overwork among workers in industry, in order that the present grievous destruction of the health of nurses may cease.[14]

This was the first meeting of the ICN held after the death of Miss Nightingale in 1910. Mrs. Fenwick, having conferred with Miss Nutting and other members of the congress, proposed that the nurses of the world should cooperate to found an educational memorial in memory of Miss Nightingale, which would benefit the nurses throughout the world. Miss Nutting supported the recommendation with impressive enthusiasm. Miss Goodrich was elected president of the ICN, and the congress adjourned in an aura of

[13] The national organizations of Great Britain and Ireland, the US (ANA), Germany, Holland, Finland, Denmark, Canada, India, New Zealand, and Switzerland.

[14] *Ibid.*, p. 98.

good will and high hopes that plans for the memorial would be completed at the next congress. This, it was anticipated, would be held in San Francisco in 1915. The conflagration in Europe wrecked the plans for that congress and delayed action on a Florence Nightingale Memorial for many years. The subsequent developments of the ICN and the Florence Nightingale Foundation are discussed in Section IX. The exciting beginnings of the NOPHN, which promptly embarked on an active and forward-looking program, are discussed in Chapter 9, which follows.

BIBLIOGRAPHY

"The American Federation of Nurses," *Am. J. Nursing,* **2:**764, 1902.

Best, Ella: *Brief Historical Review and Information about Current Activities of the American Nurses' Association, including Certain Facts Relative to the National League of Nursing Education.* American Nurses' Association, New York, 1940.

Breay, Margaret, and Fenwick, Ethel Gordon: *The History of the International Council of Nurses, 1899–1925.* The International Council of Nurses, Geneva, 1931.

Dulles, Foster Rhea: "Formation of a National Committee on Red Cross Nursing Service," *The American Red Cross, A History.* Harper & Brothers, New York, 1950, p. 96.

Goodrich, Annie W.: "A General Presentation of the Statutory Requirements of the Different States," *Eighteenth Annual Report of the American Society of Superintendents of Training Schools for Nurses,* 1912, pp. 212–22.

Lesnik, Milton J., and Anderson, Bernice L.: "Enactment of Laws—By Whom and by What Authority," *Legal Aspects of Nursing.* J. B. Lippincott Co., Philadelphia, 1947, p. 18.

McIsaac, Isabel: "What Shall the State Societies Do After Registration Is Secured?" *Am. J. Nursing,* **8:**684, 1908.

Munson, Helen W.: "The American Federation of Nurses," *The Story of the National League of Nursing Education.* W. B. Saunders Co., Philadelphia, 1934, p. 37.

"A Successful Experiment," *Am. J. Nursing,* **1:**729, 1901.

Thoms, Adah B.: *Pathfinders—A History of the Progress of Colored Graduate Nurses.* Kay Printing House, New York, 1929.

Woodham-Smith, Cecil: *Florence Nightingale.* McGraw-Hill Book Co., New York, 1951.

Chapter 9

THE RISE OF PUBLIC HEALTH NURSING

Nowhere, . . . has the growth of opportunity for nurses been so great as in the field which may be broadly termed that of social welfare. Under the form and title of district and visiting nursing, a system of activities has been developed which makes of the nurse not only a skilled agency for the relief of suffering, but a teacher of sanitary and healthful living, and a power for the prevention of disease. This is looked upon as one of the most promising movements of modern times for social betterment.

M. ADELAIDE NUTTING[1]

MARY S. GARDNER found, in 1912, that approximately 3000 nurses were engaged in what we now call public health nursing, whereas less than 200 were known to have been so employed in 1900. Within that period, according to Dr. C.-E. A. Winslow, the visiting nurse had become the most important figure in the modern public health movement. How had the visiting nurse attained such stature? By making herself a welcome visitor in the homes of the sick. Her demonstrable nursing skills gave her an entree to households confused by the sudden onset of illness. Her insight into the social and economic problems that caused or were contributory to the illness and her skill in helping families to care for the illness and to solve some of the underlying problems made her a dependable family friend. Broadly speaking, the visiting nurse services at the turn of the century were giving what was later to become known as a generalized service. Many of them included the care of tuberculosis patients in their programs. But the age of specialization in public health nursing was at hand with tuberculosis nursing, school nursing, and infant welfare work taking the stage in quick succession.

[1] Nutting, M. Adelaide: *Educational Status of Nursing*, US Bureau of Education, Bulletin #7, Whole #475. US Government Printing Office, Washington, D.C., 1912, p. 11.

The employment of special tuberculosis nurses has been signalized as one of the outstanding contributions of the United States to the movement for the control and eradication of that disease. It was through the influence of the great Osler, then professor of medicine at Johns Hopkins, that the first nurse, Reba Thelin, was appointed in 1903 to devote her time exclusively to the home care and instruction of tuberculosis patients in Baltimore. This event preceded by a year the organization of the society later renamed the National Tuberculosis Association. "The trained tuberculosis nurse, in her relation to physician and patient, has a much greater sphere of activity, than in any other branch of medical work. In no other case is she as equal a partner of the medical man as in supervising the treatment of a tuberculous patient, as without her the application of a proper method of treatment is frequently impossible and the services of the physician are almost useless. . . . The effective management of the campaign against tuberculosis in New York, Boston, Philadelphia, at present in Chicago . . . and in other large cities would be impossible without the trained nurse on the firing line."[2]

Discussions of nursing care of the tuberculosis patient with emphasis on fresh air, rest, and food are a distinguishing characteristic of the AJN in its early years. The problem of including the care of tuberculosis patients in the curriculums of nursing schools was recognized as early as 1903, when the school of the Metropolitan Hospital in New York made a study of current practice. That school decided, with the majority of the institutions studied, to make it "a voluntary service of pupils in training" while employing nurses especially interested in the work to care for the patients.[3] Although there were few institutions for the care of tuberculosis in 1900, the number increased rather rapidly. The organization and administration of these institutions, like those for the care of mental patients, tended to keep them aloof from the main stream of nursing interest.

[2] Sachs, Theodore B.: "The Tuberculosis Nurse," *Am. J. Nursing*, 8:597, 1908.
[3] Annual Report and Curriculum, Metropolitan Hospital Training School, New York, 1906.

Miss Wald was familiar with school nursing as it had been developed in London before 1900. But it was the plight of a bright 12-year-old boy excluded from school because of an untreated skin condition that crystallized her thinking and caused her to discuss with health authorities the wastefulness of medical inspection of school children without a follow-up service. She offered the city of New York the services of a Henry Street nurse for a demonstration of one month in 1902. The results, especially in increased school attendance, were so convincing that within a few weeks an appropriation had been secured by the Commissioner of Health, and 12 nurses were appointed. School nursing rather quickly became an essential component in the health resources of city after city. A report to the board of health of conditions in tenement homes where children were freely exposed to scarlet fever, measles, and diphtheria resulted in the appointment of a special staff of nurses to supervise the care of the patients and to instruct the parents. New York, however, was not the first city to put nurses on the municipal payroll; that honor belongs to Los Angeles, which made its first appropriation for the salary of a visiting nurse in 1897.

It was just before the turn of the century that nursing opened the door of opportunity for industrial medicine which was to become one of the phenomena of the twentieth century. The first industrial nursing service established by a Vermont marble company in 1895 was a visiting nurse service inspired by an employer's paternalistic and humanitarian interest in the welfare of his workers and their families. It was so successful that the service was continued; also a hospital was opened within a year in a community which had lacked any such facility.

The economic value to industry of a service which helped to reduce the time lost through accidents and illness quickly became apparent. An audience of nurses was told in 1908 that nursing had become "a paying proposition . . . to the business world."[4] This was three years before the passage by the state of Wisconsin of the

---

[4] Bannister, Lucy A.: "A New Field, The Nurse's Opportunity in Factory Work," *Fourteenth Annual Report of the American Society of Superintendents of Training Schools for Nurses*, 1908, p. 104.

first Workmen's Compensation Act. With the application of the insurance principle came a new emphasis on the prevention of accidents and illness. In common with visiting nursing, the development
of the early services was very largely dependent upon the initiative,
character, and professional background of the nurses who pioneered
in the new field. But the "factory" or "industrial welfare" nurses
were employed under conditions quite unlike those which pertained
in visiting nursing. Nursing was the primary interest of the visiting
nurse agencies. It was quite incidental to the major purpose of the
employers of industrial nurses, since many employers were unaware
of or indifferent to any existing standards of nursing practice.

A few visiting nurse associations provided service for industries
at a relatively early date, but most of the new services were developed by widely divergent types of commerce and industry on an
individualistic basis. Then, as now, industrial nurses combined in
varying proportions functions characteristic of both institutional
and public health nursing. The significance of that duality was not
clearly understood for many years. Miss Waters' historic report published in 1909 groups all types of part-time nursing services, as distinguished from full-time private duty and hospital nursing, as visiting nursing. Among the 66 commercial and industrial agencies
which were employing nurses at the time of that study were a number of department stores in San Francisco and other cities which
had followed the lead of the Wanamaker store in New York. First
aid and some degree of hospitalization for customers had an important place in their programs.

When the American Society for the Study and Prevention of Infant Mortality held its first meeting, visiting nurses had done such
effective work in milk stations that a speaker declared that the
quarts of pure milk dispensed were secondary to the instruction
nurses were giving the mothers in the care of their children. The
organization in 1909 by the Metropolitan Life Insurance Company
(MLI) of a nursing service for its industrial policyholders climaxed
a decade of rapidly increasing opportunities for "social welfare"
nursing. Within three years, the company had arranged affiliations,
that is, it had made contracts for service with over 400 visiting nurse

services in the United States and Canada. When no satisfactory service was available, nurses were employed directly by the company. For the first time, nursing care in acute illness, together with special services for women during the months of pregnancy and the post-partum period, was made available for the wage-earning group as such. The MLI set high standards and contributed an element of fundamental importance to the whole public health nursing movement. The concept of utilizing existing services was born in the fertile mind of Lillian D. Wald and was developed by Dr. Lee K. Frankel, the practical idealist who inaugurated the new service. As a basis for estimations of results and of costs, the company required careful records of the services rendered. Nothing more wholesome could have happened. Public health nurses, acceding reluctantly at first, came to acquire a healthy respect for records and statistics. Some of them were to gain real competence in the collection and analysis of data. MLI studies became an authoritative source of information on nursing for the profession and for other public health workers, just as the statistical department of the company became one of the nation's major sources of data on health.

Visiting nurses discovered that they were poorly equipped for the work which they had chosen. An early *Journal* commented on the "growing need for a national society of district and settlement nurses." But despite the very considerable volume of public health nursing materials it was publishing and editorial awareness of the importance of the movement, the magazine did not provide space for a "Visiting Nurse Department" until 1908. In the meantime, visiting nurses were seizing every chance to get together for discussions of their rapidly increasing opportunities for service. Opinion began to crystallize at a meeting arranged by the Chicago Visiting Nurse Association. By 1912 the growth of new services was so rapid that national standards, as had been the case with nursing schools two decades earlier, were urgently needed. Early in that year, a joint committee of the two national organizations was appointed with Miss Wald as chairman and Mary S. Gardner as secretary. They sent a stimulating summary of the growing opportunities in public health nursing to over 1000 agencies which were then employing visiting nurses and invited them to send representatives to a meeting to be held in connection with the annual conventions of the American Nurses' Association and the National League of Nursing Education. The response astonished even the energetic enthusiasts who had planned the meeting. At that June convention in Chicago, the National Organization for Public Health Nursing came into being.

The name was selected with the utmost care to emphasize the fact that the new organization was not composed solely of nurses and that it would be concerned with the development of *nursing*. Three classes of membership were agreed upon: corporate (agency), individual (active public health nurses), and associate. The associate members would be non-public health nurses and lay persons, privileged to participate in discussions but with no voting power. That restriction was removed at an early date when fear of lay domination or interference with strictly professional matters had been found to be quite groundless. The Cleveland Visiting Nurse Association promptly and generously transferred the ownership of its excellent *Visiting Nurse Quarterly* to the new organization and provided for its maintenance for a period of years. Six years later (1918) the *Quarterly* was converted into the monthly *Public Health Nurse* magazine, which still later was renamed *Public Health Nursing*, and finally lost its identity but not its purpose as a part of *Nursing Outlook* when the NOPHN was fused with the other organizations to form the National League for Nursing (1952).

Miss Wald seems to have been foreordained to be the first president of the new organization. Endowed with charm, an encompassing love of her fellow men, and the possessor of a creative and statesmanlike mind, Miss Wald had not only created the Henry Street Settlement Visiting Nurse Service but she had provided successively the intellectual and emotional sparks that set in motion the development of school nursing, the MLI Nursing Service, the US Children's Bureau (1912), and the Town and Country Nursing Service of the American Red Cross (1912). Miss Wald also helped to secure the inclusion of preparation for public health nurses in the program at Teachers College. Having a gift for public relations, she promoted the agencies which came into being as a result of her social vision and extraordinary gift for friendship. Miss Gardner, who was to acquire renown as the author of *Public Health Nursing* and who was already on the way to becoming the wise and gently firm guide, counselor, and friend of thousands of nurses and lay people interested in the development of public health nursing, was elected secretary. Preventive medicine had begun to develop rapidly along a broad front. With the organization of the NOPHN, an important and enthusiastic segment of the profession became a potent factor in the over-all public health movement. The immediate effect on the nursing profession was tangential. For a number of years the new organization appeared to be moving away from the main body of the profession, although its leaders had foreseen this threat to unity and had endeavored to forestall it through affiliation with the American Nurses' Association. The year 1912 is now recognized as one of the most important milestones in the history of American nursing.

BIBLIOGRAPHY

Brainard, Annie M.: *The Evolution of Public Health Nursing.* W. B. Saunders Co., Philadelphia, 1922.

Chayer, Mary Ella: *School Nursing.* G. P. Putnam's Sons, New York, 1937.

Dublin, Louis I., and Lotka, Alfred J.: *Twenty-five Years of Health Progress.* Metropolitan Life Insurance Co., New York, 1937.

Duffus, R. L.: *Lillian Wald, Neighbor and Crusader.* The Macmillan Company, New York, 1938.

Fulmer, Harriet: "History of Visiting Nurse Work in America," *Am. J. Nursing*, 2:411, 1902.

Gardner, Mary S.: *Public Health Nursing*, 3rd ed. The Macmillan Company, New York, 1936.

Haupt, Alma C.: "Thirty Years of Pioneering in Public Health Nursing," *Am. J. Nursing*, 39:619, 1939.

Knox, J. H. M., Jr.: "The Opportunity of the Nurse in Reducing Infant Mortality," *Visiting Nurse Quarterly*, July, 1910, p. 7.

McGrath, Bethel J.: *Nursing in Commerce and Industry.* The Commonwealth Fund, New York, 1946.

Markolf, Ada Stewart: "Industrial Nursing Begins in Vermont," *Pub. Health Nursing*, 37:125, 1945.

"Report of the Fifteenth Annual Convention of the A.N.A.," *Am. J. Nursing*, 12:982, 1912.

Rogers, Lina L. (Struthers): "What the Public School Nurse Is Doing," *Visiting Nurse Quarterly*, April, 1910, p. 14.

Struthers, Lina Rogers: *The School Nurse*. G. P. Putnam's Sons, New York, 1917.

Wald, Lillian D.: *The House on Henry Street*. Henry Holt and Co., New York, 1915.

Waters, Ysabella: *Visiting Nursing in the United States*. Charities Publication Committee, New York, 1909, p. 42.

Winslow, C.-E. A.: "The Role of the Visiting Nurse in the Campaign for Public Health," *Am. J. Nursing*, 11:909–20, 1911.

SECTION III. NURSING IN
THE PREWAR PERIOD   1913 – 1917

Chapter 10

NURSING ORGANIZATIONS AND
RELATED INTERESTS

The United States of 1914 certainly presented as unwarlike a spectacle as the sun ever shone upon. The problems of politics were economic problems, concentrating on the "quest for social justice," not questions of foreign policy.

PRESTON WILLIAM SLOSSON[1]

WITH THE CONVENTION of 1912, the profession passed out of the period of unpremediated expansion into an era in which, through the medium of the three national organizations, it assumed more and more responsibility for its own development. The country was peaceful and prosperous. Philanthropic foundations had begun giving impressive financial and moral support to the reform of medical education and to some phases of public health work. The increasing tempo of the public health movement was exerting a powerfully stimulating influence on the development of nursing. One of the gravest problems of the profession, the very long hours on duty required of most student nurses, was brought into the open by a law passed in California in 1913, which regulated the hours of female workers and restricted the hours of student nurses to 8 per day and 48 per week. Legislators asserted that the exploitation of students had so aroused public opinion that action was required of them. Discussion pro and con rocked the state. Hospitals operated for profit, of which California had many, were bitterly opposed be-

[1] Slosson, Preston William: *The Great Crusade and After, 1914–1918.* The Macmillan Company, New York. 1930, p. 2.

91

cause the income from the special duty service of students was financially important to them. Their appeals to the American Hospital Association for support in opposing the legislation were fruitless. The graduate nurses of California were torn between the need for reasonable hours for nurses and distaste for arbitrary regulation of hours and for increasing the cost of nursing to patients. At a mass meeting in San Francisco, they approved the inclusion of students, and the exclusion of graduate nurses, in the provisions of the act. The act was considered so radical that it did little to accelerate reform in other states. Many years later (1930), California nurses worked for and secured the eight-hour day for special duty nurses in many hospitals; they also led the movement for reasonable hours for all nurses which is still going on.

The public health movement, while still concerned with preven-. tive measures, was becoming more and more concerned with the preservation of health. The National Tuberculosis Association had demonstrated the value of health education. Nurses in milk stations had discovered that the ignorance of mothers was often as lethal as impure milk. The Metropolitan Life Insurance Company had demonstrated the practical financial value of the promotion of health and was becoming a potent force in the development of good standards of visiting nurse service.

The increasing demand for nurses with varied backgrounds of preparation and experience hereafter to be included in the generic title "public health nurse" could not be met by the well-established visiting nurse services alone. One of the most significant signs of the times was provision by law, in 1913, for a Division of Public Health Nursing in the New York State Department of Health. This was not only the first state division; it antedated the Division of Nursing in the United States Public Health Service by many years.

At the first program meeting of the National Organization for Public Health Nursing in Atlantic City in 1913, Miss Wald described the characteristics of public health nursing as follows:

This body of nurses, we must remember, is primarily designed to work in the homes of the people, and the approach to them must often be taught in order that sympathy and understanding may light the way for the nurse, that the latent quality of sympathy may be brought out through understanding of social conditions and of the need of help in the most basic institution on earth, the home and the family. We cannot properly send nurses into the homes unless they comprehend the economic problems and the social needs of the people whom they serve. Contact with the immigrant and with those others, whether in cities or in remote rural regions, whom the nurse visits should be made understandingly. There is a technique in visiting nursing and all phases of public health work which we are comprehending is essential for the utmost development of the worker, and which has a wide range, from psychology to the best card cataloging.[2]

From 1912 to 1920, the three organizations held annual joint conventions, a custom which had been adopted by the two older organizations in 1910. From that time until 1952 joint meetings have been held biennially, leaving the smaller and highly specialized organizations free to concentrate on their own programs and those of other health organizations in the intervening years.

Through the affiliation of the American Nurses' Association with the American Red Cross, provincialism gave way to the concept of nursing as a national service and as a means of promoting international understanding and good will. The requirements for ARC enrollment—membership in the ANA and professional preparation well above the minimum requirements of many of the state boards of nurse examiners—tended to expedite the organization of state nurses' associations in laggard states, usually those with relatively few nurses, and to encourage improvement in state legislation.

The mission of the "Mercy Ship" in September, 1914,[3] was reminiscent of that of the *Maine* which, flying the flags of the US, Great Britain, and the Red Cross, had sailed for South Africa in 1899. The real name of the Mercy Ship was *Red Cross*, and it carried about one-half of the 250 nurses who were assigned in units of twelve nurses and three doctors to work with the Red Cross societies of England, France, Russia, Germany, Austria, and Hungary. Equipped by the ARC, they set up hospitals in such buildings as could be made available to them. There is no more dramatic story

[2] *Public Health Nurse Quarterly,* **5**:7, 1913.
[3] World War I began when Austria declared war on Serbia July 28, 1914.

in the annals of the ARC than that of the units assigned to Serbia where the ravages of an epidemic of typhus were added to military casualties. The volume of service performed in one year by these small units bore no relation to the magnitude of the needs of the warring countries. The honors bestowed on nurses by some of the governments were tangible evidence of good will. The experiences of these nurses provided the ARC nursing service with information which was very useful when the US began intensive preparation for participation in World War I.

The joint convention programs of the three organizations developed bonds of professional interest between nurses and helped to broaden the profession's concept of its function in society. Health insurance, for example, was an outstanding topic in 1917 when many state legislatures were considering the subject. A comprehensive article on the organization of central schools, presented at the same convention by Mary C. Wheeler, was based, in part, on her experiences as principal of the Illinois Training School. Hourly nursing, household nursing services, and the training of attendants were subjects of interest to all groups in this period. The problem of providing care for patients of moderate means runs like a continuous thread in the warp of the proceedings of the professional organizations; so also does the distribution of nursing service but under a wider variety of titles. Socially experienced nurses were beginning to realize that neither problem could be solved by nurses alone.

Two highly significant committee reports were presented to convention audiences in this period by Katharine Tucker, who was to become a distinguished executive director of NOPHN. The first, "Nursing Care of the Insane," was the report of a committee of the ANA. The second report, to which we shall return, was prepared by a committee of the NOPHN. The National Committee for Mental Hygiene financed the study reported by the ANA committee and assisted with the preparation of a questionnaire which was sent to all mental hospitals. Apparently this was related to the studies then being made for the young (1909) mental hygiene organization by Dr. Thomas W. Salmon. The report contains no reference to the much older American Psychiatric Association which was interested in nursing from an administrative rather than an educational point of view. It was found that 41 mental institutions were operating training schools for nurses. Standards of administration and teaching and for admission to the schools were, in general, much lower than those for schools in general hospitals. In many of the state hospitals, the superintendent of nurses had so little authority that the schools were operated, to all intents, by the non-nurse superintendents. In some of the schools some students were eligible to sit for state board examinations, some were not. In many instances, hours were even longer than the prevailing long hours in general hospitals. Living conditions were usually very poor. "Speaking generally," says the report, "neither doctors, nurses, nor the public have felt the need of nurses in this branch of medical work." The committee goes on to say that "nurses themselves should be educated to the needs of the mentally sick, for until nurses see their opportunity they can scarcely expect the doctors and the public to recognize it." Psychiatric nursing had no crusader to do for the schools what Dorothea Dix had done for the hospitals, although Linda Richards, Sara E. Parsons, and Mary E. May struggled with the problem. The public health field was ripe for the mental hygiene movement, but only a few administrators of mental hospitals were constructively interested in the education of nurses for the care of psychiatric patients. The American Psychiatric Association had inaugurated a program for the standardization of nursing schools in mental hospitals in 1906, but no evidence has been found of collaborative efforts between that association and the nursing organizations until a later date.

The new NOPHN in structure and program was quite unlike the two older nursing organizations. It was organized with nurse, lay, and agency members, whereas the other two restricted their membership to graduate nurses. It was interested in stimulating the use of public health nursing services, in standardizing the practices and personnel policies of public health nursing agencies, and in the education of nurses for their special functions in this growing field. One of its distinctive characteristics was interest in the development of cooperative relationships with other health and social agencies. In addition to income from membership dues, the organization was subsidized by interested lay members. Also, beginning at a fairly early date, it received support from the Rockefeller Foundation, on a decreasing scale, for a period of years. The NOPHN was exceedingly fortunate in being able to start its career with a well-established publication as previously noted. Ella Phillips Crandall, endowed with physical energy, crusading zeal, a winning personality, and social vision, who resigned from the faculty of Teachers College to serve as executive secretary of the new organization, set up an office in New York. The NOPHN, although the youngest, was therefore the first of the national organizations to establish a headquarters. The work expanded so rapidly that Mary E. Lent had been appointed assistant to Miss Crandall before the United States entered World War I.

The NOPHN almost inevitably took on some of the characteristics of a pressure group in relation to the older organizations. Its leaders were quick to see the many opportunities for the development of nursing services which were being opened up by the public health movement. The organization was responsive to the social pressures created by the programs of the new health agencies which required well-prepared graduate nurses with initiative and a social point of view. The basic concepts for which it pressed were not new. Miss Nutting had frequently reminded League audiences that community needs should be considered in planning curriculums. But the schools were harrassed by the increasing demands of the hospitals for service without budgetary provision for nursing education. The state boards were encountering many difficulties as they labored to implement the nurse practice acts.

Miss Tucker's second report was made, as chairman of NOPHN's Committee on Education, to the NLNE. The schools, the committee assumed, should provide the foundations for skilled and intelligent care of the sick. Such care called for nurses with knowledge of the causes and the methods of preventing disease. It suggested that five lectures on illness as a social problem, coupled with a few days spent in observation with visiting nurses, should be added to the first-year curriculum so that students should ". . . be able at the very start to visualize the homes from which the patients come, something of the forces at work that brought the patient to the hospital should, and does, where tried, vivify and humanize all that otherwise might be impersonal and detached technic." In the second year, the committee suggested, students should be given information about the work of health organizations in relation to the clinical study of the care of such conditions as tuberculosis, psychiatric conditions, and venereal disease. In the third year, it was felt that, just as the schools endeavor to give the students some idea of the openings in other fields of nursing, five lectures should be given on the various fields of public health nursing. The committee also asked for the inclusion of lectures on morale and on social problems such as immigration, labor conditions, housing, et cetera. The recommendations of the NOPHN were unanimously accepted by the NLNE. Securing the interest of any but the more advanced schools in putting them into effect was quite another matter. A determined and increasingly cooperative effort was thus modestly begun in 1916; an effort to develop basic curriculums upon which any type of specialization could be built, as might be required by changing medical and social needs.

The alumnae associations were the basic units of the American Nurses' Association as that organization was originally planned. But nurses are migratory folk. In some places organizations of like-minded nurses, who were not members of locally centered alumnae associations, had sprung up almost spontaneously. The legislative program of the national organization had quickly demonstrated the need in each state for an organization with an inclusive membership which could work for a nurse practice act, since licensure is a function of state governments. As previously noted, the name of the national association had been changed to the American Nurses' Association in 1911 to indicate the inclusive nature of its membership and program. By 1916 it had become an unwieldy aggregation of alumnae, local, and state organizations. Duplication of membership made any estimates of total membership worthless. But the alumnae associations, the original units of the organization, were resistant to change. Fortunately, at this juncture, Miss Goodrich was elected president of the association and was subsequently re-elected. Working hand in hand with a strong and conscientious revision committee, Miss Goodrich led the membership to understand the feasibility and desirability of a federation of state nurses' associations. During those years, Miss Goodrich became one of the best-known and most popular leaders in American nursing. Respect for her comprehensive knowledge and sympathetic understanding of nurses and nursing was blended with affectionate admiration for the dynamic force and luminous quality of her personality. Reorganization of the association was begun in 1918 and completed in the postwar period. The new structure provided representation for the individual nurse at all levels—alumnae, district, state, national—and, since the association was affiliated to the International Council of Nurses, at the international level. The House of Delegates became the voting body of the ANA. Provision was made for sections, the private duty and mental hygiene sections being the first to be organized. In connection with the reorganization, the National League of Nursing Education made membership in the ANA a prerequisite to League membership.

The ANA, in 1912, had made provision for ex-officio membership on its board of directors of the presidents of the other two national nursing organizations in order to facilitate the close working relationship desired by all three. When this was found to be illegal in the state of New York in which the association was incorporated, the possibility and desirability of securing a national charter was investigated and found not feasible. The ANA and the NLNE were incorporated in the District of Columbia in 1917 and 1918 respectively. In 1914, the ANA had created a central bureau of legislation and information to facilitate the legislative programs of the state nurses' associations. To implement its work, the first list of schools approved by state boards of nurse examiners was compiled in 1915. Procuring protective, standard-setting legislation was an uphill task, complicated by the resistance of selfish medical and other interests and lack of resources for nursing education in many states. The public at this time was quite generally uninformed about the several types of persons who were known as nurses, whether registered, graduate or practical, with or without training. Under such circumstances it is not surprising that it was, generally speaking, critical of nurses. But it was often extremely difficult to persuade the representatives of the public in state legislatures that the primary function of a nurse practice act was the protection of the public rather than the creation of a privileged class of workers.

A continuous interest in the technics of patient care and the practice of individual nurses is revealed in the earlier issues of the AJN. From 1912 to the beginning of American participation in World War I, the upgrading of nursing by means of improvement in nursing schools and strengthening of the nurse practice acts were dominant themes. A few schools were making notable advances, just as some of the state boards were having a degree of success in their efforts to improve the level of preparation of nurses in their states. Discussion of the individual nursing care of patients was subordinated to consideration of over-all methods for improving practice. The difficulty of interesting many competent practitioners of the art of nursing in the forward-looking work of the organizations caused some anxiety to leaders of nursing thought, but there is relatively little evidence of interest in this period in the provision of programs for nurses as practitioners in addition to those designed to secure collective action in improving the conditions in which nursing was taught and practiced.

As we have seen the NOPHN had established a headquarters office shortly after it was organized in 1912, but the two older organizations were still without national offices. The office of the AJN in Rochester (New York) had provided a base of operations for the interstate secretary who served the two older organizations on a part-time basis from 1909 to 1912. After Miss McIsaac's resignation to succeed Miss Delano as superintendent of the Army Nurse Corps (1912) there was no field work until Adda Eldredge was appointed in 1917 to serve the ANA and the *Journal* with the office of the magazine as her headquarters. In the interval, however, Katharine De Witt, assistant editor of the *Journal*, had been elected secretary of the ANA and devoted half time to that work. With the appointment of Miss Eldredge (St. Luke's, Chicago), a nurse with a fine platform presence and unusual breadth of professional experience, the ANA began to gain stature. A fluent speaker, Miss Eldredge had effectively spearheaded a program which overcame opposition to the passage of a nurse practice act in Illinois. As the nation, and the nursing profession with it, moved toward war, nurses had need for the stimulating and practical guidance she could give on professional and organizational matters. Her slogan, "The A.N.A. is where *you* are," stimulated effective organization of state associations and helped to bring many nurses into membership.

The National League of Nursing Education had learned that a membership composed of individuals cannot be effectively served by publications and an annual meeting only. Furthermore, its membership included only a fraction of the principals of nursing schools. In order to interest more of the nurses qualified for membership, there was need for affiliated state and local organizations. The earliest state leagues were organized in 1912. A little later the base of membership was broadened to include instructors and supervisors with membership remaining on an individual basis.

The publication in 1917 of the League's *Curriculum for Schools of Nursing* established this organization as the authoritative source of information on nursing education. Preparation of the *Curriculum* had been an extremely difficult task, carried out over a three-year period by the organization's committee on education of which Miss Nutting was chairman and Isabel M. Stewart secretary. The concept of nursing upon which the *Curriculum* was based is that of a national service which requires nurses to be equipped to meet conditions as they may find them in any type of community. Although Miss Nutting had publicized her dream of autonomous nursing schools which would carry on much of their work in hospitals, the *Curriculum* was based on the premise that training schools would be established in hospitals. The type of hospital which provides a suitable teaching field was carefully defined. Most of the "standards" had already been tested by a few schools which had good clinical and teaching facilities and well-qualified faculties. Such a guide as the *Curriculum* was urgently needed by schools, state boards of nurse examiners, and by trustees and others responsible for the hospitals which operated nursing schools. It frightened poorly prepared persons who were administering "schools" with very limited resources. It was welcomed by most of the state boards of nurse examiners and by the better schools. It was a godsend to the faculties of the 31 units of the Army School of Nursing which was organized the year following its publication.

Abraham Flexner's epochal paper, *Is Social Work a Profession?*, presented at the National Conference of Charities and Correction in 1915 brought a fundamental issue into sharp focus. Social work had already gained the interest of at least one of the philanthropic foundations. Nursing, it will be recalled, had tried and failed to secure such assistance although the need for a definitive study of nursing and the preparation of nurses for their special functions in society was keenly felt by Miss Nutting and other leaders in the profession. The criteria postulated by Dr. Flexner and widely publicized were:

. . . professions involve essentially intellectual operations with large individual responsibility; they derive their raw material from science and learning; this material they work up to a practical and definite end; they possess an educationally communicable technique; they tend to self-organization; they are becoming increasingly altruistic in motivation.[4,5]

His conclusion that social work, like nursing, was in a twilight zone since it could measure up to some but not all of the criteria was a stimulating challenge to the social workers to whom the paper was addressed. It was a direct challenge also to public health nurses who were working in the same broad field of human welfare. Dr. Flexner suggested that since public health nursing seemed to provide more opportunity for the development of initiative and independence of action, such nurses might more readily develop professionally than nurses working "in the sickroom under orders."

[4] Flexner, Abraham: *Is Social Work a Profession?* Proceedings of the National Conference of Charities and Correction. Reprinted by the New York School of Philanthrophy, New York, 1915.

[5] For further consideration of these criteria see Brown, Esther Lucile: *Nursing for the Future.* Russell Sage Foundation, New York, 1948, p. 76.

The question of status was less important than determination of the functions of the several groups as a basis for the development of educational programs. The nation was to go through two wars before the nursing profession was to feel the full impact of the criteria that had promptly provided potent yeast for the rise of social work.

A number of new national associations were organized in this period with which the nursing organizations were to develop cooperative relationships. Among them was the College of Surgeons (1913) which launched its hospital standardization program in 1918. Surgeons to a very large extent had been responsible for the rapid expansion of hospital facilities. The standardization program, designed to improve the quality of surgical practice in hospitals, had a pervasive and constructive effect which indirectly influenced nursing.

By 1915, when the Catholic Hospital Association was organized, many of the sisterhoods were operating schools of nursing. Relatively few of the graduate nurse sisters were contributors to nursing publications or participants in professional programs. The new association, by bringing many sisters out of their professional anonymity, helped to broaden and enrich the main stream of nursing.

It was in this period that the first school for nurse anesthetists was established at Lakeside Hospital in Cleveland, Ohio. The administration of anesthetics by nurses was by no means new. A nurse had been appointed anesthetist at the Mayo Clinic in 1889, and other institutions had also found them a dependable asset. Mrs. Robb had devoted a chapter of her textbook on nursing to the subject. But the organization of the school aroused medical opposition. In 1917 an appellate judge in Kentucky ruled that nurse anesthetists were not practicing medicine when working under the direction and receiving renumeration from a physician, a ruling which indicated growing interest in the subject although it settled the question of legality for one area only.

The profession as a whole was unaware of the growing pains of two younger groups of workers as they struggled upward toward professional status. These were the medical social workers and the dietitians who were then splitting off from the general field of home economics. Leaders in nursing were beginning to perceive that nursing and younger professions, as they grew, would all find it necessary to define functions and to develop cooperative relationships with the other members of the growing family of health professions. These two used the term "profession" in relation to their status and their work, just as nursing had done from its inception, to indicate a vocation requiring special preparation. Both projected their programs into areas which had been of at least marginal interest to nurses. Indeed, gifted nurses, as we have seen, had headed the pioneer work in hospital (medical) social service. But as hospital social service grew toward professional stature services originally staffed by nurses employed more and more social workers. As Ida M. Cannon pointed out, much of the technical training of the nurse was unused in social work and much medical information, such as the causes and progress of disease as well as the treatment of long convalescence, then frequently omitted from the basic nursing course, was essential to the practice of medical social work.

American nurses had made great progress in their efforts to meet the nation's need in the 20-year period between the Spanish-American War and President Wilson's declaration of war on Germany April 6, 1917. The ANA was well started on the reorganization which was to make it a federation of state nurses' associations. It had published the first printed list of schools accredited by the state boards of nurse examiners. Forty-five states, with the District of Columbia and Hawaii, had secured nurse practice acts. The National League of Nursing Education was becoming a definitely constructive force in the upgrading of basic nursing education. So too was the Department of Nursing and Health of Teachers College. The National Organization for Public Health Nursing had greater administrative resources than either of the other national nursing organizations, and was beginning to have a constructive influence on the adaptation of nursing to changing social and health conditions in American society. In 1917, largely through its influence, four universities in addition to Teachers College were offering courses in public health nursing to graduate nurses for which the ARC was providing scholarships. The nursing service of the Red Cross and the American Nurses' Association had perfected a relationship which was to be of tremendous assistance to the armed forces. Finally, in the AJN and the *Public Health Nurse Quarterly*, the profession possessed the media for intercommunication between nurses which were to be of the utmost importance when it became necessary to adjust and readjust policies and programs to meet the mounting needs for military and civilian nursing service.

BIBLIOGRAPHY

Best, Ella: *Brief Historical Review and Information about Current Activities of the American Nurses' Association, including Certain Facts Relative to the National League of Nursing Education.* American Nurses' Association, New York, 1940.

Cannon, Ida M.: *Social Work in Hospitals,* rev. ed. Russell Sage Foundation, New York, 1923.

Dunwiddie, Mary: *A History of the Illinois State Nurses' Association, 1901–1935.* Illinois State Nurses' Association, Chicago, 1937.

Eldredge, Adda: "How to Organize for Registration," *Am. J. Nursing,* 7:839, 1907.

Fife, Gertrude L.: "The Nurse as an Anesthetist," *Am. J. Nursing,* 47:308, 1947.

Gardner, Mary S.: *Public Health Nursing,* 3rd ed. The Macmillan Company, New York, 1936.

Gladwin, Mary E.: "Experiences of a Red Cross Nurse in Serbia," *Am. J. Nursing,* 16:902–11, 1916.

Hampton (Robb), Isabel Adams: *Nursing: Its Principles and Practice for Hospital and Private Use,* 3rd ed. E. C. Koeckert, Cleveland, 1909.

Haupt, Alma: "Thirty Years of Pioneering in Public Health Nursing," *Am. J. Nursing,* 39:619, 1939.

Hibbard, M. Eugènie: "With the Maine to South Africa," *Am. J. Nursing,* 1:1, 1900.

Kernodle, Portia B.: *The Red Cross Nurse in Action, 1882–1948.* (The Serbian Units, pp. 99–102.) Harper & Brothers, New York, 1949.

List of Schools of Nursing Accredited by the State Boards of Nurse Examiners. American Nurses' Association, New York, 1916.

Munson, Helen M.: *The Story of the National League of Nursing Education.* W. B. Saunders Co., Philadelphia, 1934.

Nutting, M. Adelaide: *A Sound Economic Basis for Schools of Nursing.*
G. P. Putnam's Sons, New York, 1926.

One Hundred Years of American Psychiatry. Published for the American
Psychiatric Association by Columbia University Press, New York, 1944.

Pacific Coast Journal of Nursing, 1909 and 1913.

Packard, Francis R.: *Some Account of the Pennsylvania Hospital from Its
First Rise to the Beginning of the Year 1938.* The Pennsylvania
Hospital, Philadelphia, 1938.

Poupore, Elizabeth S.: "Mrs. Horatio Walker Who First Introduced the
Eight-Hour Day for Special Duty Nurses," *Am. J. Nursing,* **33:**1154,
1933.

Russell, William Logie: *The New York Hospital—A History of the Psychiatric Service, 1771–1936.* Columbia University Press, New York, 1945.

Standard Curriculum for Schools of Nursing. National League of Nursing
Education, New York, 1917.

Tucker, Katherine: "Nursing Care of the Insane in the United States,"
Am. J. Nursing, **16:**198, 1915.

————: "The Training School's Responsibility in Public Health Nursing
Education," *Twenty-second Annual Report of the National League of
Nursing Education,* 1916, p. 115.

Washburn, Frederic A.: *The Massachusetts General Hospital—Its Development, 1900–1935.* Houghton Mifflin Co., Boston, 1939.

Wheeler, Mary C., and Wood, Mrs. Ira Couch: "A Central School of
Nursing and Public Health," *Am. J. Nursing,* **17:**1042, 1917.

Chapter 11

NURSING LEGISLATION AND
NURSING PRACTICE

At the present juncture, it behooves the profession of nursing to rise to its waiting occasion, to follow in the footsteps of the related profession of medicine in dictating the terms upon which schools for nurses shall be legalized and their graduates received into practice.

RICHARD OLDING BEARD[1]

IN THE FIVE-YEAR PERIOD under consideration, 1913–1917, more than 500 new schools of nursing were established! The three-year course had been generally adopted, and the schools were graduating a markedly smaller percentage of the enrolled students than had been the case at the turn of the century. Indeed, they were pouring out a stream of partially prepared "nurses." As the nation moved toward war many a graduate nurse was shocked by the discovery that she was not eligible for enrollment in the nursing service of the ARC. Thirty-nine per cent of the schools were operated by hospitals with a daily average of less than 50 patients, the basic requirement for ARC enrollment.[2] In every state nurses continued to work tirelessly to secure or to improve the nurse practice acts. The effort was bringing increasing numbers of graduate nurses into the orbit of concerted effort, through membership in the state nurses' associations, to improve first the standards of nursing education and later those of nursing practice. Ten years after the passage of the first acts in 1903, 38 states had such laws on the statute books. All were the re-

[1] Beard, Richard Olding: "The Social Development of the Nurse," *Am. J. Nursing,* **12**:785, 1912.
[2] *Nurse Training Schools, 1917–1918,* Bulletin, US Office of Education. US Government Printing Office, Washington, D.C., 1918.

sult of inexperience and compromise. In some states success had
been won only after the defeat of one or more bills. Campaigning
for legislation was arduous and often disappointing work. The outstanding personalities in the state registration movement were
Sophia F. Palmer, Adda Eldredge, and Annie W. Goodrich. Miss
Palmer, editor-in-chief of the AJN, many years president of the
New York State Board of Nurse Examiners, was credited with
having first suggested the appointment, by state boards, of training school inspectors. The general acceptance of that idea caused
the boards to place primary emphasis on the upgrading of the
schools rather than on the practice of individuals, as is the case with
other professions. This was an obvious point of attack for the improvement of nursing; also the state boards lacked the facilities for
investigating individual violations of the law. The representatives
of medicine and hospital administration were well aware of the
significance of the movement. Nursing had the philosophical and
moral support of influential members of both groups, but considerable numbers in both were hostile to it. "In getting publicity for social legislation," said an adviser, "we can count more and more on
the growing public sentiment for the advancement of human life
as opposed to the protection of property interests."[3] But most nurses
were too unskilled in public relations to make very effective use of
that assumption in their efforts to create a favorable public opinion.

For more than two decades, the *Journal* gave a dominant place in
its pages to state legislation and the administration of the nurse
practice acts. The New York State Board published the first state
curriculum (syllabus) in 1908. State-accredited schools were required to provide 236 hours of theory and demonstration. The provisions of the acts varied widely; such variations resulted from the
marked differences in political and economic conditions, as well
as differences in the hospital, medical, nursing, and educational
resources of the several states. Representatives of state associations
had encountered almost unbelievable opposition in some areas. Also,
in their inexperience, some of the others had secured the passage

[3] Baldwin, Roger: "The Preparation of Bills and Publicity Methods,"
Twentieth Annual Report, NLNE, 1914, p. 112.

of acts that were so ineffective that early amendment was necessary. Nurses were also beginning to learn that legislation which controls licenses to practice must be amended at intervals to retain its usefulness lest it become an obstacle to progress. Some of the laws, for example, specified that the entire period of preparation for practice as graduate nurses (or other specified titles) should be spent in hospitals. This was done originally to put a stop to the practice of sending unsupervised students into homes as private duty nurses in response to the demands of influential persons or as a means of augmenting hospital income. The retention of that provision, after it had served its purpose, came to be a serious obstacle to progress when schools began to realize that students, being prepared to practice as graduate nurses in a wide variety of situations, needed a broader preparation than could usually be provided by a hospital alone.

Adda Eldredge (St. Luke's, Chicago), who was later to become widely known as interstate secretary and as president of the American Nurses' Association, presented a report in 1914 which indicated that in many states marked progress was being made. But nurses were encountering serious legislative opposition in some areas, especially in states in which women could not legally hold office, or in which powerful vested interests were opposed to any type of control of nursing practice. She urged unity of effort toward a universal standard, closer intercommunication between the examining boards, a spirit of fraternal helpfulness, and a strong *esprit de corps* which would bind the groups together for efficient progress. Legal requirements for licensure are necessarily minimum standards. It is a responsibility of those who guide the development of legislation, that is, of the state nurses' associations, to be constantly aware of the relationship between the minimum standards and changing educational, medical, social, and economic conditions. They learned, but slowly, that in a changing society a law which gives power to act with provision for the setting up of board rules for the execution of the purposes of the act can be more effectively administered than one which contains many specific details.

As the number of states having nurse practice acts increased, it became more difficult for poorly prepared or pseudo nurses to evade the law by moving from state to state. Hospitals continued to increase in number. By 1912 many doctors had become concerned lest legal requirements interfere with a free-flowing supply of student nurse service. The New York state requirement of one year of high school was vigorously attacked. Between 1909 and 1916, three committees of the American Hospital Association brought in reports on nursing. The report of 1909, noted previously, was in substantial agreement with the aims of the nursing organizations at that time. The committee of 1913 reported that it had surveyed the field and found no less than nine types of workers who were calling themselves nurses. It discovered, as Mrs. Robb had pointed out many years earlier, that the word "nurse" could mean anything or nothing in the way of preparation for practice. The proposals of the committee bear a marked family resemblance to matters under consideration at mid-century. It suggested a system of grading nurses which would include all those who nursed for hire. The grading was to be based on preparation for three recommended categories, all to work under the supervision of some responsible representative local organization. The recommended grades were registered graduate nurses, certified nurses (those who had taken courses of not less than one year in special or very small general hospitals or had acquired experience under certain specified conditions), and household nurses, which included all nurses not eligible for either of the other grades. This report indicates keen awareness of the needs of patients in their homes and the desirability of developing centralized agencies for meeting such needs. A similar proposal, put forward by the New York Academy of Medicine at about the same time, was discussed from many angles; the whole question was referred back to the council of the Academy.

Miss Goodrich, then inspector of the nurse training schools for the state of New York, in one of the forceful papers for which she was to become famous, pointed out the need for clarification of the existing situation. The New York law, conceded to be one of the best in force, protected the title "registered nurse" but it did not prevent persons who had dropped out of the training schools nor

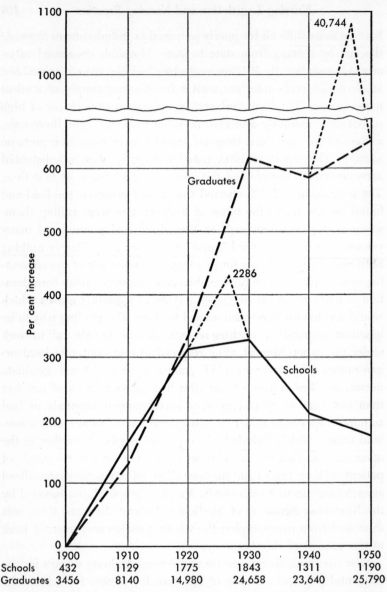

Chart 1. Per cent change each ten years since 1900 in number of nursing schools and in number of students graduated. It will be noted that the peak in number of schools and in number of graduates came in 1927 and 1947 respectively. (Prepared by Ella E. Taylor, NLNE Department of Studies, 1951.)

the possessors of correspondence school diplomas from offering themselves as nurses to an uninformed public. Miss Goodrich cited one correspondence school which reported that it had turned out 12,000 "graduates" in 10 years, whereas the number of nurses graduated in 1912 from all state-accredited schools in New York was slightly less than 1200. She took a firm stand on the principle that the scope of the work of professional nurses must be clearly defined and regulated by law before the status and work of attendents could be equitably dealt with.

The AHA plan for three grades of nurses was carefully considered at a joint meeting of the three national nursing organizations. They went on record as approving two classes of workers for the care of the sick—"the nurse with the proper training under suitable conditions and the trained attendant, the minimum educational qualifications for each being determined by law."[4] The ANA was requested to transmit a resolution, supported by the three organizations, to the AHA requesting cooperation in an effort to secure suitable preparation for both nurses and attendants. A joint meeting of representatives of the AHA and the three national nursing organizations was held in 1916, but no formal action was taken. There appears to have been general agreement that any attempt to grade nurses would obscure the issue and that the real need was for grading the hospital schools of nursing in such a way as to bring about a constant and effective influence toward the affiliation of small and special hospitals with large institutions for the purpose of providing an adequate education for both medical and nurse students. There was general agreement that satisfactory education, both practical and theoretical, could be secured in a three-year course, if the student nurse were free to pursue her education unhampered by institutional requirements for non-nursing service. The next AHA committee to study the nursing problem (1916) supported the fundamental principles of state registration as established by the nursing profession. It also advocated the licensing of registries as a safeguard to the nurse-employing public. Such agreements stimulated rapport but did not lead to action. None of these reports included

[4] *Twentieth Annual Report, NLNE,* 1914, p. 224.

consideration of the fundamental problem, "How shall nursing education be financed?" Almost 30 years elapsed before the problem of home versus hospital care (stated, as follows, in the report of 1916) led to positive action by a few socially alert institutions and public health nursing agencies. (See Chap. 46.)

Whether it is wise to ask for public funds or private capital to provide hospital accommodations for patients who could be as efficiently and safely cared for at home as in a hospital, and for the same rates or less, given reasonable provision for meeting the needs of the patient and home, is an important and unsettled question relating to hospital and home economics, which has a definite bearing on the organization of nurses, on how many kinds of nurses should be trained and how they should be trained. These questions suggest the magnitude and complexity of the problem of the development of nursing facilities in relation to the needs of each community and of the responsibilities of hospitals in connection with the problem.[5]

A general résumé of the accomplishments of the state boards of nurse examiners, based on the laws of 37 states, clearly shows that the result of the 10-year effort fell far short of the hopes of pioneers in that movement, but some gains could be counted. An increasing number of affiliations of small and special institutions with larger ones was considered especially noteworthy since in only New York and Illinois did the schools receive assistance from state board inspectors. Six states required a three-year course; twenty-six a two-year course. Other requirements are not stated. Among the controversial issues of the times were bed capacity and range of clinical services in hospitals and the limited requirements for admission to state-accredited schools. The age for registration varied from 18 to 23. Chronological age was beginning to be recognized by nurse leaders as an unreliable measure of maturity.

Reciprocity between the state boards, described as a sickly infant requiring proper food and careful handling, was still only a partially solved problem at mid-century. Six states required high school graduation or an equivalent education for admission to nursing schools, but the equivalent was more often assessed with chari-

⁵ *Transactions of the American Hospital Association,* 1916, Report of Special Committee on Grading and Classification of Nurses, p. 67.

table liberality than with academic precision. At the lower end of the scale, seven states required only grammar school graduation. The individual schools were, of course, free to adopt requirements in advance of those set by law and a substantial number did so.

The NLNE voted in 1913 to recommend that the minimum legal requirement for admission to a nurse's training school should be one year of high school, or a definite equivalent. By 1915 the entrance requirement should be two years. The NLNE could set desirable standards, but it had no power to enforce them.

The urgency and magnitude of the problem of providing nursing service for patients of moderate means in their own homes received attention in many quarters. Nurses, it was often stated, had been so conditioned by their hospital training that they were generally quite unaware of, or even indifferent to, the care which patients needed in their homes, and to the problem of keeping the household mechanism functioning. Nursing, on a visit basis, was the obvious answer to part of the need since it could be provided through insurance, or on a cost per visit basis by the visiting nurse services and hourly nurses. But the stigma of charity, which still clung to organized visiting nursing, tended to inhibit its wider use. The subject was presented from every angle at the San Francisco convention in 1915. Richard H. Bradley of the Thomas Thompson Trust of Boston, a crusader for economic and humanitarian realism in meeting this problem, based his arguments for the employment of nongraduate nurses on a study of nursing needs and services in Dutchess County, New York. Many of the thousands of such workers could be more effective, he believed, if their work could be coordinated with that of graduate nurses and supervised by them. Legally and professionally nurses were generally still too insecure to willingly accept responsibility for a subsidiary group. However, two states did take action. Mississippi in 1913 and Virginia in 1918 (as a war measure) secured legislation which provided licensure for subprofessional workers.

Between 1907 and 1917, the *Journal* published a fairly representative cross section of the questions used by state boards of nurse examiners. They provide an interesting basis for comparison with

later developments in medicine and nursing. Responsibility for
ward housekeeping, an important function in the pioneer period,
was unwisely retained long after the principle had been established
that the order and cleanliness of their surroundings are important
factors in the care of the sick. The history of nursing in a midwestern
state notes, ironically, that precedence in an early examination on
nursing practice was given to a question on how to dust a ward.
Recurrent questions on poisons, their antidotes, and burns and scalds
are a reminder that ignorance and carelessness in the home accounted for many accidents. Visiting nurses tried to teach mothers
in crowded homes to keep lye and other dangerous substances out of
the reach of little children. In this connection, it may be noted that
the National Safety Council, organized in 1913, specifically included
(as it continues to do) the prevention of accidents in the home in
its comprehensive program. Questions on rickets and chorea appeared frequently. Not until the end of the period do we find a question on how to provide diversion for a sick child. Arthritis, Bright's
disease, and cardiac conditions were of secondary interest, if judged
by the number of questions asked about them. The communicable
diseases received far more attention than all else, with questions on
intubation and tracheotomy an inevitable corollary. Questions on
quarantine and methods of terminal disinfection of the room, the
patient, and of the person of the nurse herself appeared frequently.

But this was the period in which the science of immunology was
catching up with bacteriology. Questions on the vaccines occurred
more frequently as typhoid and other vaccines and antitoxin came
into general use. The results of the soon-to-come mass wartime im-
munizations would make radical changes in nursing practice. Questions on surgical nursing were surprisingly limited in scope. How
to change the mattress under a patient the third day after an abdominal section now seems fantastic, but keeping such patients quiet,
almost immobilized, was a test of the skill of nurses in the earlier
part of the century.

The growth of nursing had been so rapid that many members of
the boards of nurse examiners were as poorly qualified for their important functions as were many of the nurses who were directing

the schools. There were, therefore, wide variations in the scope and quality of the essay-type examination questions in common use. A good question, a convention speaker pointed out in 1916, should compel reflection, should not be ambiguous, should not contain the answer, and should be within the experience of the student. The subject was timely. Boards of examiners worked slowly; the results of examinations were not received promptly. When war had been declared, the Red Cross suggested to the state boards that examinations be held at more frequent intervals and reports expedited in order that young nurses might become eligible for military service at the earliest possible moment. It was necessary to repeat that lesson in World War II.

There were, however, some significant evidences of progress in this dark period of nursing education in the United States. They were due to the initiative of individual nurses in the better established schools, to the work of Miss Goodrich and Mary C. Wheeler as training school inspectors in New York and Illinois, to preliminary courses offered by 25 colleges and universities, to the growing number of nurses who were securing preparation at Teachers College for administration and teaching in schools of nursing, and to special preparation for public health nursing at Teachers College and a few other universities. The educational highlight of the period was the conversion of a hospital school into a professional school of nursing at the University of Cincinnati in 1916 through the brilliant leadership of Laura R. Logan. The low standard of nursing education in many parts of the country explains why a proposal to prepare a supplementary type of worker became the most bitterly contested issue of the war period.

BIBLIOGRAPHY

Aikens, Charlotte A.: "Training School Regulations and Suggestions, Report of Special Training-School Committee to the American Hospital Association," *Hospital Management*. W. B. Saunders Co., Philadelphia, 1911, Appendix I.

Boyd, Louie Croft: *State Registration for Nurses*, 2nd ed. W. B. Saunders Co., Philadelphia, 1915.

Bradley, Richard M.: "Household Nursing in Relation to Other Similar Work," *Am. J. Nursing,* **15**:968, 1915.

Eldredge, Adda: "The Progress of the Past Year in Nursing Legislation and Some Lines of Future Effort," *Twentieth Annual Report of the National League of Nursing Education,* 1914, p. 93.

Goodrich, Annie W.: "The Need of Orientation," *The Social and Ethical Significance of Nursing.* The Macmillan Company, New York, 1932, p. 27.

————: "A General Presentation of the Statutory Requirements of the Different States," *The Social and Ethical Significance of Nursing.* The Macmillan Company, New York, 1932, pp. 159–69.

Lesnik, Milton J., and Anderson, Bernice E.: *Legal Aspects of Nursing.* J. B. Lippincott Co., Philadelphia, 1947.

McKee, Caroline Vincent: *Essentials of Nurse Registration.* Ohio State Nurses' Association, Columbus, 1933.

"Meeting of Committee on Grading of Nurses of the American Hospital Association and Representatives of the Three National Associations of Nurses," *Twenty-second Annual Report of the National League of Nursing Education,* 1916, p. 170.

Peebles, Allon, and McDermott, Valeria D.: *Nursing Services and Insurance for Medical Care in Brattleboro, Vermont.* Publications of the Committee on the Costs of Medical Care, 17. University of Chicago Press, Chicago, 1952.

"A Resolution," *Twentieth Annual Report of the National League of Nursing Education,* 1914, p. 224.

Chapter 12

PRIVATE DUTY NURSES AND THE DISTRIBUTION
OF THEIR SERVICES

*The medical adviser sees [that] the family needs the aid of a skilled hand,
a thoughtful mind, a will to act, with consciousness of soul. . . .*

*The afflicted people request their doctor to send or recommend such
a person, . . . the arrival of the nurse is looked for with the utmost
anxiety. The doctor telephones to Miss A.; her 'phone is out of order and
he gets no answer. He then tries Miss B. . . . Miss B. is out; . . . he
then with a sigh refers to his note-book for the address of Miss C. . . . ;
she has just gone on a case. The doctor by this time begins to whistle.
He again refers to his memorandum of nurses and calls Miss D. . . . ,
she is engaged by Doctor So-and-so. . . . In despair the doctor calls up
the superintendent of the hospital training-school, wants her to send him
one of her best pupil nurses. . . . The superintendent tells the poor
doctor that "The . . . State Association does not allow sending out pupil
nurses." He is by this time in a frenzy of impatience and wants to know
what the . . . State Association has to do with it. . . .*

*The superintendent after much delay secures a graduate nurse for the
case.*

SISTER M. IGNATIUS FEENY[1]

IN THE PREWAR PERIOD we have been discussing, there were serious
shortages of nurses qualified for the rapidly expanding field of public health nursing and for positions in institutions which operated
schools of nursing. Conversely, there was such a plethora of private
duty nurses that there was serious unemployment in that group from
1915 until after the United States had entered the war. Conditions
for graduate nurses in this field were complicated by the competition

[1] Feeny, Sister M. Ignatius: "Central Directories," *Am. J. Nursing*, 4:797,
1904.

of large numbers of partially trained nurses, graduates of short courses and of correspondence schools.

The outstanding event of the period for private duty nurses was the announcement in 1916 by Miss Goodrich, then president of the ANA, that the reorganized association would have a private duty section. Private duty nurses far outnumbered all other nurses in the ANA. They could be counted on to support the major programs of the organization but they had yearned for this recognition as a special service group. They had not, however, offered any clear statement of purpose or program. They had no plan for the upgrading or standardization of private duty nursing comparable to the programs for the improvement of nursing education and public health nursing of the NLNE and NOPHN.

Private duty nurses are independent practitioners of the art of nursing. They cherish their independence but have often paid the price of economic insecurity for it. Those who have achieved distinction in their own communities, and fortunately there have been many, have done so because they had the character, interest, and intellectual ability to develop wholesome interpersonal relationships and to acquire new skills as required by changes in medical practice. The ANA has worked continuously to secure improvement in the conditions under which nurses practice their profession, but no method has been devised for rewarding, financially or socially, the nurse who becomes an expert practitioner. Those who take academic or other postgraduate courses therefore do not commonly remain in the field of nursing practice.

The question of a sliding scale of fees for private duty nurses had been considered and rejected early in the century in connection with the problem of providing care for patients of moderate means. Would a sliding scale of fees for private duty nurses provide an answer to two needs: that of patients for care and that of private duty nurses for a tangible incentive to develop expertness in their chosen field? Why, said the exponents of a sliding scale, shouldn't Mrs. Millions pay a nurse more than Mrs. Modest Purse? The system worked well for doctors, why not for nurses, they argued? Why should recently graduated nurses receive the same compensation for a day or a week or a month on duty as would the nurses who had already demonstrated their professional competence and personal adaptability? A professional person, it was argued, continues to add to her knowledge and skills and should, therefore, be able to command a higher fee. The basic problems in the administration of such a scheme, it was pointed out, would inevitably be: How shall a nurse's competence be evaluated? How shall the patient's ability to pay be determined? Most nurses believed a sliding scale undesirable. Their decision might have been stated in Gertrude Stein fashion—a nurse is a nurse is a nurse.

Discussions of private duty nursing in the prewar years emphasized the fact that nurses in that group were making few contributions, in relation to the practice of nursing, to the literature of the profession. Two books on the subject had been published about 1912. The periodical literature of the time indicated growing concern about the conditions under which private duty was practiced but relatively little about how it was carried out. The terms, "private duty" and "registry," which appeared frequently were like two sides of a coin which represented service to society. One of the important characteristics of the prewar period we are discussing was a marked interest in the development of central registries. For that story, we shall have to go back to the days when graduate nurses were pioneers in an untried field and trace developments up through the prewar period.

The graduates of the earliest classes had no choice other than to enter the field of private duty nursing if they were not needed, or were not interested, in helping with the organization of new schools of nursing. Leadership in the development of channels for the distribution of the service of private duty nurses was of several types. It was at the graduation exercises of the New York City Hospital's first class in 1879 that the mayor of New York urged the valedictorian of the class to plan a central headquarters in the city where graduate nurses could be found by the public. Adelaide Mabie thereupon organized The New York Agency for Trained Nurses. This she turned over to the Philomena Society, the first organization of graduate nurses in the United States, which unfortunately "died of inanition" in 1887. The registry, however, was continued as a commercial venture by one of the nurse members of Philomena.[2] Registries were established by Bellevue, the Illinois Training School, and other early schools as a convenience to themselves and as a means of helping their graduates. There were those who came to think of such registries, operated from the training school offices, as a primary source of nurse power for the institution and its clientele but also as a form of paternalism which prevented the graduates from attaining real stature as independent practitioners of nursing. Some of the alumnae associations organized for the primary purpose of establishing registries. The alumnae of what is now the Rochester (New York) General Hospital School of Nursing organized for that purpose about 1896. It is believed to have been the first to undertake such a project. Because two of its members had already developed successful practices as hourly nurses, such service on a larger scale was offered by the registry. In 1912 this registry was merged with a new central registry. At about the time the Rochester registry was being developed, a group of alumnae associations in Brooklyn banded together to organize the first central directory (registry). Eminent doctors promoted the use of the new service although a medically sponsored registry was already well established.

Beginning in the eighties, a considerable number of medical societies organized registries which were a convenience to the physicians and often an important financial asset to the libraries of the societies. Some of them were continued well into the new century. The number of nurses continued to increase. As Miss Dock and other leaders in the development of the national nursing organizations pointed out, it was important that the principle of self-government should be applied in all professional undertakings, including the development of registries. The potential efficiency of a central service appealed to spacious thinkers like Mrs. Robb and Miss Dock. It was frequently discussed at meetings of both of the professional organizations. They were opposed to the control of the

[2] Correspondence in the *American Journal of Nursing* files, Adelaide Mabie and Sophia F. Palmer, 1906.

placement of private duty nurses by the medical societies because they had little or no interest in the standardization and upgrading of nursing. Some of the medically controlled registries made no distinction between graduate and nongraduate nurses. Even so, it may be assumed that, in the interest of the patients, they were more discriminating than the registries operated solely for profit, which seemed to have sprung up at an early date.

The transition from medical to nursing leadership in the field of registry development was effected in a variety of ways. Generally speaking, the idea took hold more rapidly in western than in eastern cities. In Minneapolis, for example, the existence of a medically sponsored nursing bureau which listed on an equal basis graduate, partly trained, and practical nurses stimulated nurses to organize a county nurses' association in 1901. Three years later, through the efforts of farsighted leaders, control of the registry had been transferred to the association, which subsequently became a district of the Minnesota State Nurses' Association. In St. Paul, a central registry was achieved at about the same time, but the circumstances were different. Since there was no medical directory, each school had its own placement service. Graduates of out-of-town schools registered at a cooperative drugstore. Again the first step was the organization of a county nurses' association, which in time became a district of the state nurses' association. Within a few years all but one of the schools had abandoned their registries in favor of the professionally sponsored central service. The reluctance, in some cities, of the "caste conscious" alumnae of the better known schools to participate in such cooperative planning was frequently referred to as an obstacle to progress in providing community-wide services through central registries.

Mary E. P. Davis, whose financial acumen and staunch devotion to her profession had made the *Journal* possible, applied her intellectual gifts and forceful personality to the development of a professionally sponsored central registry in Boston where the medical society had, for years, maintained its library on the proceeds of its nursing bureau. The substantial contributions of a few nurses to a sinking fund, raised to support the bureau in its experimental years, were returned to the donors within a few years after the establishment of the registry in 1912. Prominent citizens of Boston, many of them physicians, served on an advisory board. The registry flourished, and some years later the state nurses' association established its headquarters in connection with it. At about the same time, the registry of the Illinois Training School, one of the oldest and most firmly established in the country, announced that with the registry of the Presbyterian Hospital of Chicago it would join the central registry of the district nurses' association. The example of these two influential schools was followed by most of the other schools which were operating registries in the Chicago area. In accordance with a growing trend, a nurses' club was established in connection with this registry. The next 20 or 30 years saw the rise and fall of nurses' clubs. Rarely built for the purpose and sometimes established in donated mansions, they showed a marked tendency to become static. As residents stayed on year after year the clubs, instead of becoming the dynamic centers of activity the founders had anticipated, became static and more of a liability than an asset.

From the standpoint of service to the public, all arguments favor the development of central registries. But the fact that private duty nursing is a specific service rendered by one nurse to one patient was not conducive to group action in relation to community needs. Neither had nurses generally begun to think of themselves as citizens contributing to the common good nor of all nursing as a response to community needs. Deep-seated loyalties to hospital, alumnae, and other registries, and the inertia in relation to the development of the profession of those who were well served by them, were deterrents to the development of central registries. But the trend was definitely toward the centralization of these important services. An ANA committee made a study of registries in 1914 which marks the beginning of the association's effort to implement broad service aims by promoting effective organization of professionally sponsored registries. There were then more than 40 central registries.

The success of a registry is dependent upon three things: the leadership of its parent body and the scope of the policies it formulates to govern the agency, the professional and personal characteristics of the registrants, and the preparation and personal characteristics of the registrar—the administrative officer appointed to implement the policies. Many of the early registrars were poorly paid for 24-hour service "with a little time off duty during the day," in accordance with the early formula for private duty nurses. Their service was often incidental to home-making responsibilities. Many of them were faithful, if not constructive, servants of both the profession and of the public.

In the period when the word "nurse" might mean anything, employment agencies recognized an opportunity for increasing their business. Registries for nurses sprang up which were not in any way connected with the profession. The range in the quality of the service they rendered may be assumed to have been at least as great as the range in preparation of those who called themselves nurses. There were many graduates of correspondence schools and other short courses, and many practical nurses of varying abilities including those who had dropped out of the schools of nursing. When professionally sponsored registries restricted their service to graduate nurses only, they inadvertently strengthened the position of the more discriminating commercial agencies which provided a wider range of service to the public. As the number of central registries increased, *Journal* editorials waxed eloquent about their potentialities as community centers for the distribution of nursing service and as sources of comprehensive information about nursing. Some of those which had developed cordial relationships with the hospital nursing services helped to break down the traditional 20- or 24-hour schedules for private duty nurses. Many of them won high praise for their effective cooperation with the ARC when its enrollment program went into high gear in 1918. But the concept of a central registry as a bureau of nursing service for a community had not been accepted by a majority of nurses. Registries continued to be a matter of major concern to the ANA. But, at mid-century the scope of their services and methods of integrating them with other professional services was still not clearly defined.

BIBLIOGRAPHY

Bouton, Florence L.: "Registries as a Part of the Professional Counseling and Placement Service," *Am. J. Nursing*, 52:1206, 1952.

"Central Directories," (report of Annual Convention of the Nurses' Associated Alumnae of the United States), *Am. J. Nursing*, 4:791–799.

Darche, Louise: "Training School Registries," *Third Annual Report of the American Society of Superintendents of Training Schools for Nurses*, 1896, pp. 22–28.

De Witt, Katharine: *Private Duty Nursing*. J. B. Lippincott Co., Philadelphia, 1913.

Dock, Lavinia L.: "Directories for Nurses," *First and Second Annual Reports of the American Society of Superintendents of Training Schools for Nurses*, 1895, pp. 56–60.

Dunwiddie, Mary: *A History of the Illinois State Nurses' Association, 1901–1935*. Illinois State Nurses' Association, Chicago, 1937.

Foster, Reba Thelin: "The Organization of Nurses' Clubs and Directories under State Associations," *Am. J. Nursing*, 9:247, 1909.

A History of Nursing in West Virginia. West Virginia State Nurses' Association, Charleston, 1941.

Holmes, Grace: "An Ideal Central Directory," *Am. J. Nursing*, 6:606, 1906.

Lounsberry, Harriet Camp: *Making Good on Private Duty*. J. B. Lippincott Co., Philadelphia, 1912.

Merrill, Bertha Estelle: *The Trek from Yesterday—A History of Organized Nursing in Minneapolis, 1883–1936*. Minneapolis Nurses' Association, 1944.

Merritt, Isabel: "The Brooklyn Associated Alumnae Registry," *Fourth Annual Report of the American Society of Superintendents of Training Schools for Nurses*, 1897, pp. 14–17.

"Report of Special Registry Committee (A.N.A.)," *Am. J. Nursing*, 15:1121, 1915.

Robb, Isabel Hampton: *Nursing Ethics*. E. C. Koeckert, Cleveland, 1900.

Rodabaugh, James H., and Rodabaugh, Mary Jane: *Nursing in Ohio*. Ohio State Nurses' Association, Columbus, 1951.

Roth, Anna: *Thirty-five Years of the Massachusetts State Nurses' Association (1903–1938)*. Massachusetts State Nurses' Association, Boston, 1938.

Smith, Virginia Jeffrey: *A Century of Service—Rochester General Hospital, 1847–1947*. Rochester, 1947.

Trenholme, Louise Irby: *History of Nursing in Missouri*. Missouri State Nurses' Association, Columbia, 1926.

Chapter 13

EARLY PUBLIC RELATIONS PROGRAMS

The Supply and Demand principle, taken alone, is a fallacy. It leaves out altogether the most important element, viz., the state of public opinion at the time. You have to educate public opinion up to wanting a good article. Patent pills are not proved to be good articles because the public pays heavily for them.

FLORENCE NIGHTINGALE[1]

WHEN THE BELLEVUE SCHOOL was still in the planning stage, a member of the committee was asked how work would be found for the graduates of the school. The spirited reply was, "Our school will not train nurses only. We shall train the public at the same time."[2] The public was not wholly uninformed. *Godey's Lady's Book,* for example, had already discussed the potential usefulness of graduate nurses as portrayed in British publications. Bellevue was not alone in securing the interest of the press, the gateway to the public. The women who served as members of the boards of managers of other early schools were also energetic and resourceful. They, too, had social prestige and did not hesitate to use it in a good cause. Influential national magazines, such as the *Century* and *Scribner's,* gave space to articles on the new vocation for women which attracted such women as Lavinia L. Dock, who was then "at home just having a good time." The Connecticut Training School was organized and chartered before any steps were taken to interest potential students. That problem was solved by newspaper articles supplemented by circulars which were printed in large type and

[1] Cook, Sir Edward: *The Life of Florence Nightingale.* The Macmillan Company, New York, 1942, Vol. II, p. 269.
[2] Giles, Dorothy: *A Candle in Her Hand,* A Story of the Nursing Schools of Bellevue Hospital. G. P. Putnam's Sons, New York, 1949, p. 217.

bright colors, then distributed to railroad stations and post offices. More applications were received than could be accepted. Opportunistic exhibits were used at an early date by both schools and nursing organizations. The Model Ward displayed at the World's Fair in Chicago in 1893 by the new school of the Presbyterian Hospital, New York, greatly increased the number of applications. There are, however, no records of sustained efforts to keep the public informed about the schools or about the availability of nursing services. As they became known, the larger schools received applications by the hundreds. When other occupations began opening up for women, the number of desirable candidates began to decrease. But a tradition that it was undignified for schools to advertise grew up which persisted until World War I.

Early journals contain many references to favorable and unfavorable comments on nursing in newspapers and medical publications. The efforts of the professional organizations to establish good standards of preparation for the practice of nursing through legislation were resisted by very vocal representatives of selfish interests, such as correspondence schools and proprietary hospitals. Nurses had been taught to "keep out of the papers," and the profession of public relations was still unborn when the state nurses' associations began their campaigns to secure nurse practice acts. Very few had any conception of technics which might be used to create an informed public opinion, but some of them learned rapidly in the school of experience. When the Illinois State Nurses' Association, for example, had twice failed to secure the passage of a nurse practice act, it was decided that the matter must be put before the public. Adda Eldredge was appointed to undertake the task. She developed a highly successful legislative program which at a later date would have been described as a public information program. The interest of editors was secured through interviews. The Federation of Women's Clubs, of which the state association was a member, gave wide publicity to the purpose of a nurse practice act. Traveling up and down the state Miss Eldredge addressed an extraordinary variety of audiences including the medical societies. As a result, the third bill sponsored by the Illinois nurses became a law in 1907!

Some of the unfavorable publicity directed at nursing in the early part of the century was due to the steadily increasing numbers of partially trained persons and poorly prepared graduate nurses who were offering their services to the public. They were undermining the reputation of nursing as a budding profession. By 1912, when vocational guidance was beginning to emerge as a field of professional interest, there was a serious shortage of qualified candidates for the schools. The NLNE appointed no less than three committees to work on the several aspects of the problem of vocational guidance. The organization became a member of the newly formed National Vocational Guidance Association the following year. Plans for a vocational program were based on an initial study of conditions in New York State which was made in cooperation with a committee of the New York Academy of Medicine. Half of the schools lacked the desired number of candidates. The study revealed the startling fact that the great mass of women in the state who aspired to become nurses could not be considered even fairly well educated. High school students, it was found, possessed distorted ideas about nursing and the preparation for it. But the greatest opposition to nursing as an occupation for well-bred, well-educated young women came from parents who had heard of the long hours, the rigid discipline, and hard work commonly associated with the concepts "hospital" and "nursing." No method had been provided by which they could differentiate between good and poor schools, and few had any conception of nursing as a service to society.

The collegiate and vocational committees were combined to work with state leagues, state associations, or other appropriate organizations or individuals in developing programs to interest high school and college students in nursing. Talks in high schools had been given sporadically over a period of years. This was the first national effort to develop a coordinated program of prevocational information about nursing. The advice of a consultant on guidance was sought. This summed up was: Secure the interest of the editor of a women's magazine in publishing a provocative article on nursing; provide traveling exhibits that can be placed in libraries, high schools, and other suitable places; prepare inexpensive information leaflets which can be freely used in connection with both. An article in the *Delineator,* a widely read magazine for women, brought highly gratifying results. The recommended exhibits were not planned, doubtless because funds were lacking. The Barnard *Bulletin* published an article, "Nursing as a Profession," by Miss Nutting. Copies of the publication were sent to a selected list of colleges and universities.

While the League committees were getting under way, members of the alumnae of the Department of Nursing and Health of Teachers College had also become interested in vocational guidance. This group was responsible for the preparation and publication in 1913 of *Opportunities in the Field of Nursing.* For two decades this pamphlet, written by Isabel M. Stewart, and revised at intervals, was a major mailing piece in vocational programs sponsored by the profession.

The publicity committee recommended that the excellent programs of the other committees should be continued but that a more fundamental task should be undertaken. This was nothing short of "educating the people who manage and support hospitals on the duty of the hospital to the school!"

"We must also show," says the report, "that our schools are improving and that the nursing profession has opportunities worthy of the best womanhood in our country." There is no evidence that even the most prescient dreamed that the war raging in Europe would become a means for adding some of the nation's best educated young women to the ranks of nursing; or that these committees were laying a groundwork that would be extremely useful in connection with the nation's participation in World War I.

BIBLIOGRAPHY

Dunwiddie, Mary: *A History of the Illinois State Nurses' Association, 1901–1935.* Illinois State Nurses' Association, Chicago, 1937.
Jones, Mary Cadwalader: "The Training of a Nurse," *Scribner's,* November, 1890.
"Lady Nurses," *Godey's Lady's Book,* **82:**188, (Jan. to June) 1871.

Lee, Eleanor: "Chronological List of Events," *History of the School of Nursing of the Presbyterian Hospital, New York, 1892–1942.* G. P. Putnam's Sons, New York, 1942.

North, Franklin H.: "A New Profession for Women," *The Century Magazine,* November, 1882.

"Report of the Collegiate Committee," pp. 37–40; "Report of the Vocational Guidance Committee," pp. 41–59; "Report of the Publicity Committee," pp. 74–76, *Twenty-first Annual Report of the National League of Nursing Education,* 1915.

Stack, Margaret K.: "Résumé of the History of the Connecticut Training School for Nurses," *Am. J. Nursing,* 23:825, 1923.

SECTION IV. WORLD WAR I   1917 – 1918

Chapter 14

WARTIME EXPANSION AND CONSERVATION
OF NURSING RESOURCES

. . . we pledge our best service to the nation wherever called upon to render it, either in home or foreign field, in the daily routine of civil or military hospital, or in the equally great effort to conserve, protect and strengthen the health and endurance of the citizen population, the men, women and children at home in our land.[1]

PRESIDENT WILSON terminated his courageous and persistent efforts to keep us out of war by signing a declaration of war with Germany and its allies on April 6, 1917. Three weeks later representatives of the three national nursing organizations were assembled in convention in Philadelphia. Resolutions expressing the loyalty and readiness of nurses to serve their country were sent to President Wilson. They adjourned, however, without formulating a wartime action program. Within a month, Miss Nutting, the far-seeing dean of American nurses, called an informal meeting at which a committee designating itself a National Emergency Committee on Nursing was organized with Miss Nutting serving as chairman, and Ella Phillips Crandall, executive secretary of the NOPHN, as secretary. Shortly thereafter the committee became the Committee on Nursing of the General Medical Board of the Council of National Defense. Under Miss Nutting's forceful and informed leadership, it became the dynamic center of basic professional information and action throughout the war. The Council of National Defense was composed of six members of the President's Cabinet. Dr. Franklin H. Martin, a founder of the American Col-

[1] *Am. J. Nursing,* 17:762, 1917.

lege of Surgeons, was chairman of the medical board. In addition to Miss Nutting's committee, as it came to be known, subcommittees on nursing were attached to two other committees of the council. The subcommittee on public health nursing of which Mary Beard, president of the NOPHN, was chairman became extremely active. Miss Crandall was released and financed by the NOPHN to serve in Washington as secretary of the committee on nursing and as coordinator of the three nursing committees. She developed effective working relationships between the committees and the nursing service of the Red Cross. It was a complicated situation in which Miss Crandall served with distinction. Major Winford H. Smith, one of the two hospital administrators who were members of the committee on nursing, was chairman of the committee on hospitals of the council. Despite this effort to coordinate the interests of nursing and hospitals, civilian hospitals felt that they were not consulted by the committee on nursing.

The stated purposes of the committee on nursing were:

To ascertain through a census the real nursing resources of the country; to find an effective way of making them readily available for service where needed; to increase the supply of pupils in training schools for nurses; to conduct a serious educational campaign with that end in view; to secure cooperation from hospitals in enlarging their training schools and teaching forces; to consider and advise upon problems of nursing as they may, from time to time, arise during the war.[2]

Both the Red Cross and the committee on nursing were harried by persons who were eager to set up short courses in nursing. But Miss Nutting and some of the members of her committee were acutely aware of the conditions discussed in Chapter 11, "Nursing Legislation and Nursing Practice." They were unshakably convinced that standards of preparation of nurses must be maintained and improved if the nation was to be adequately served. Opposition to this point of view, some of which came from important sources, was met with lionhearted courage. An extremely influential member of the general medical board, for example,

[2] Nutting, M. Adelaide: "Statements of Purposes and Plans of the Three Committees on Nursing of the Council of National Defense," *Public Health Nurse Quarterly,* 9:325, 1917.

made no secret of his opinion—which was held also by some of his confreres—that in the committee on nursing the preservation of educational standards took precedence over the nation's need for nursing service. Such opinions did not abate the zeal of Miss Nutting and like-minded nurses who realized that a breakdown in the nation's system of nursing education, unsatisfactory though they knew it to be, would have a disastrous effect on both war and postwar medical and health programs. They were keenly aware of the council's obligation to ensure their country, insofar as the profession itself could do it, an increased supply of good nursing service, both military and civilian.

Private duty nursing, in which there had been serious unemployment, was the only field which had adequate numbers of qualified nurses to meet current civilian needs at the time the United States entered the war. Placement services reported that they had been unable to fill 90 per cent of the positions calling for special preparation for administrative positions, teaching, or for public health nursing. The problem, which recurred in World War II, was that of finding ways and means for ensuring maximum use of existing resources, of making the most effective use of the services of nurses with special preparation, and of devising ways and means for increasing nursing resources.

Miss Beard's subcommittee on public health nursing moved quickly to ensure efficient use of the limited supply of public health nurses of whom there were only 6000 in the US in 1916. The Red Cross was asked to set up a special roster of public health nurses and to call the nurses on it, unless they specifically requested otherwise, only for public health nursing. When this had been done, the NOPHN urged all its members to enroll, hoping to develop a national roster of public health nurses. There were three good reasons for this plan: the growing dependence of the civilian population on public health nurses which had caused the ARC in the middle of the war to replace its Town and Country Nursing Service with the more spacious Bureau of Public Health Nursing; the unanticipated call for public health nurses for overseas service; and the development of nursing services in the sanitary zones the United States Public

Health Service (USPHS) established around the cantonments. The NOPHN having loaned its executive secretary to the committee on nursing then loaned her assistant, Mary E. Lent, to the USPHS to establish the first public health nursing service that governmental agency ever had. No two zones were alike in needs or resources. Skilled public health nurses were needed to help coordinate the work of existing agencies and to supplement it, when possible. Emphasis was placed on educational programs for the control of communicable disease. The country was not then crisscrossed with bus lines, and automobiles were not in common use. Miss Lent reported as "unique" a need discovered in one zone where the wives of some sixty service men required maternal care. She did not live to see how that problem, multiplied by many hundreds, was met by the Emergency Maternity and Infancy Care (EMIC) program of the Children's Bureau in World War II.

Nurses who conscientiously remained in administrative, educational, and public health positions, such as were to be designated "essential" in World War II, were subjected with embarrassing frequency to the spoken or implied epithet "slacker." The ARC expanded its special enrollment to include instructors and other nurses in educational positions. A chevron bearing the words "Special Service" above the symbol of the Red Cross was provided for their use. Only nurses who were fully qualified for military duty, but who were performing important nonmilitary service, were granted this privilege. At this time, also, the ARC set up a roster of nurses who, for family or other reasons, were not eligible or available for military service. They wore with pride the Red Cross nurse's pin with a bar attached which bore the words "Home Defense."

Since knowledge of existing conditions and resources is a preliminary step to intelligent planning, the council on national defense, through the committee on nursing, planned for a survey of national nursing resources and for a survey of nursing in military hospitals. The American Nurses' Association, which was asked to make the national survey, delegated the task to the states nurses' associations. The committee sought from the Surgeon General of the Army an invitation to make the study of military nursing.

A census was a formidable undertaking for the state associations, since none of them had offices or staffs of trained workers. The results, made available in March, 1918, while not considered statistically accurate, indicated that the total number of registered nurses was probably nearer 65,000 than the 98,000 which had been estimated by a publicity committee. The data seemed to provide a reasonable basis for both wartime and postwar planning. The assumption that postwar demand for nursing service would greatly exceed the prewar employment of nurses proved to be correct. A later compilation of data from schools accredited by state boards of nurse examiners indicated that the total number of student nurses in schools was slightly more than 50,000. Enrollment of students had been increased by over 7000 despite the inability of many schools to increase the number admitted, due to lack of housing facilities for larger classes. The New York State Nurses' Association made a more comprehensive study than was possible in many states. The results published in a hospital magazine revealed many types of "nurses" and attendants. The findings stiffened the resistance of nurse leaders to complicating the situation further by extensive employment of ARC volunteer, or paid, nurses' aides.

The committee conceived one of its major functions to be the promotion of methods for recruiting and teaching student nurses. Emphasis was placed on securing greatly increased numbers of students with superior qualifications since is was assumed they could be prepared more quickly for some of the positions of responsibility which were going begging. Three major projects were developed through the leadership of the committee. These were the Vassar Camp, the Army School of Nursing, and the Student Nurse Reserve.

Shortly after the US declared war, the Provisional Alumnae Council of Vassar College began considering plans for patriotic use of the facilities on the campus during the summer of 1918. Guidance was sought from Miss Nutting's committee on nursing. To the lasting credit of Vassar and the permanent enrichment of nursing, it was decided that "the fundamental need at the present moment for women is in the department of nursing."[3] The war added the name of Mrs. John Wood Blodgett, a trustee of Vassar, to the roster of alert-minded and socially perceptive lay women to whom the nursing profession is forever indebted. The original concept of a camp at Vassar was hers, and she promoted the nursing program wholeheartedly. A 12-week preliminary course in nursing offered to graduates of approved colleges was sponsored by the Red Cross, which received a gift of $75,000 for the purpose, and the Council of National Defense. When the council asked the NLNE for assistance in planning the program an advisory committee on curriculum was appointed. The members were: Isabel M. Stewart; Elizabeth Burgess, who had succeeded Miss Goodrich as state inspector of training schools for nurses in New York; and Anne Strong, assistant professor at Simmons College, an inspired teacher of public health nursing. The principle that the three-year course in nursing could be shortened for college graduates (with proper recognition of the requirements of the nurse practice acts) had already been accepted by the nursing committee and adopted by some of the stronger civilian schools. Arrangements were made for a two-year period of theory and practice following the preliminary course in selected schools of nursing for Vassar Camp students. Not all could be admitted to the schools of their first choice.

The opportunity for patriotic service and participation in an educational experiment attracted a faculty remarkable for the distinction of its members. The Vassar alumnae put on such an effective recruitment program that over 400 graduates, of 115 colleges scattered throughout the length and breadth of the US and Canada, enrolled for the course. It was believed to be the largest group of college women gathered together anywhere for a single type of patriotic service. Many of the Vassar campers had given up teaching and other positions to take the course. They wore the probationary uniforms of the civilian schools in which they expected to complete their training. Time schedules corresponded with those of the nursing schools. The students quickly grasped the real sig-

[3] *The Training Camp for Nurses at Vassar College.* National Council of Defense and the American Red Cross, Poughkeepsie, New York, 1918, p. 12.

nificance of the camp. As one of them put it in their student publication:

. . . when our blundering awkward fingers have grown deft and skilful, we shall find our place. Overhere or Overthere? It does not matter and this is the wonderful lesson which Vassar has taught. In the lecture, in the classroom, in the very atmosphere of the camp there has come to us this message. Service is greater than war, or peace, greater even than death. It is the very soul of life. We are talking less of France these days. Most of us realize that ours may be the sacrifice of "those who stay at home," but because of these wonderful weeks we are ready to serve either over here or over there."[4]

A very high percentage of these students reported for the period of hospital affiliation, but, as in the Army school and civilian schools, many dropped out after the Armistice. It was no secret that the educational methods and authoritarian personnel policies of some of the civilian schools disaffected some of the Vassar campers. But the 42 per cent who completed the course justified the high hopes of the Vassar alumnae and the educators who had so enthusiastically participated in the program. The names of many of them could be found on mid-century rosters of distinguished nurses.

Stimulated by the example of Vassar and encouraged by the American Council on Education in cooperation with the Council of National Defense, 50 institutions of higher education were planning similar programs when the Armistice abruptly halted all wartime plans. However, five widely scattered universities gave preparatory courses somewhat similar to the Vassar program during the summer of 1918, but not on a graduate basis. The ten-week course at Western Reserve, for example, which was given in cooperation with the local league of nursing education, was offered to high school graduates enrolled in Cleveland's schools of nursing. It was financed by the city through a special wartime committee. Both the quality of the teaching and the selection of students were well above the standards of some of the participating schools. Most important, in terms of wartime patient care, the students were assigned to duty in the wards some three months in advance of the usual date.

[4] *The Thermometer,* Vassar College, July 17, 1918, Vol. 1, No. 4, p. 2.

Miss Goodrich was asked by Miss Nutting's committee to make the survey of nursing in military hospitals. No other nurse could have brought so rich a background of experience to that task. She had been director of four schools of nursing and inspector of the schools in the state of New York. She was well acquainted with many of the doctors who were serving as national advisors on matters pertaining to military and civilian health. She was granted a leave of absence from the faculty of Teachers College and from her position as director of the Henry Street Visiting Nurse Service to serve her country. All of her work had been animated by the driving conviction that the adequate development of nursing service to meet the changing needs of society depended upon careful selection of students and the utilization of educational technics and resources. She was animated by the zeal of a crusader. The survey was made in the spring of 1918 when American troops had just begun to participate on a massive scale in the titanic struggle in Europe. At Miss Goodrich's request, action on a plan, which had been authorized by the Surgeon General for the employment of ARC nurses' aides in military hospitals, was delayed until her study could be completed. Having completed the survey in record time, Miss Goodrich recommended the establishment by the Army of a school of nursing. The matter was under consideration in the War Department at the time of the annual convention in Cleveland of the three national nursing organizations. This made it possible for a large and representative segment of the profession to hear the pros and cons of Miss Goodrich's proposal and Miss Delano's discussion of the ARC program for nurses' aides. It was a discussion of epic proportions. A historian later wrote of it: "The nursing profession may well be said to have stood on this May morning at the crossroads. Miss Goodrich beckoned at one fork for them to follow her, Miss Delano at the other."[5] Because strong personal loyalties to a few leaders was a marked characteristic of nursing in that period, the situation was fraught with emotion.

[5] Dock, Lavinia L.; Pickett, Sarah Elizabeth; et al., *History of American Red Cross Nursing*. The Macmillan Company, New York, 1922, Chap. X by Miss Pickett, p. 962.

Miss Delano and Dora E. Thompson, superintendent of the Army Nurse Corps (ANC), were acutely aware that the demand for a greatly increased volume of nursing service might come at any moment (as it did!). The plan for the use of aides had been carefully developed over a period of years with the understanding and support of the National Committee on Red Cross Nursing Service of which representatives of the nursing organization were members. Miss Delano had, therefore, felt confident that she had the understanding and support of her profession. She had secured for the Red Cross nursing service a status not accorded to professional nursing by any other Red Cross Society in the world, and thought of herself as representing the profession and upholding its standards in the Red Cross. Both Miss Delano and Miss Thompson had good reason to know that time is required for organizational changes in the military setup. The plan for aides was ready for action, and they feared delay in securing the additional service which they knew would inevitably be requested at an early date. They were firmly opposed to the Army school plan as a substitute for aide service, and were supported in that stand by distinguished members of the American Hospital Association.

The plan for an Army school was presented to the convention with the approval of Miss Nutting's committee. It had not yet received official approval from the War Department, but although aware that there was both military and civilian criticism of the plan, Miss Goodrich believed that approval would be forthcoming. The plan as approved by the committee was for a central school to be established in the office of the Surgeon General with units, each with its own faculty and instructional resources, in designated military hospitals. Completion of high school or its equivalent was the entrance requirement. The *Standard Curriculum* published in 1917 was providentially available. The arguments for the school in terms of wartime service were: It would attract a high type of young women who would appreciate the opportunity to acquire a professional education while giving patriotic service; since the service of student nurses was an acceptable method of providing civilian hospitals with nursing service it could be assumed that such service could provide equally satisfactory care for military patients; because affiliations would be required for experience not available in military installations some civilian hospitals could anticipate sharing the service of the Army school students; the graduates of the school, whether they remained in the ANC or not would constitute an important addition to the nursing resources of the nation. Few subjects, according to the records of the national nursing organizations, had ever received such concentrated attention at a convention as the plan for an Army school. When all sides had been presented, approval of the plan by the nursing organizations was recorded by vote. That decision was a blow to the volunteer services of the ARC. It was characteristic of Miss Delano that she wasted no time repining about the profession's repudiation of the aide program. She proceeded at once to plan a recruitment program which enrolled additional thousands of nurses for military service.

When Miss Goodrich returned to Washington she found that her plan for an Army school had been disapproved by the Secretary of War, but she and Miss Nutting refused to accept defeat. Through a special committee, of which Mrs. Frances Payne Bolton (who was to sponsor the Cadet Nurse Corps in World War II) was a member, a conference was sought with the Secretary of War, Newton D. Baker. Mrs. Bolton, who was chairman of the War Program Committee of the NOPHN, was a neighbor in Cleveland of Mr. Baker. He granted a special hearing for a delegation headed by the Surgeon General of the Army and including Mrs. Bolton and Miss Goodrich. He gave approval to the Army school program after being assured that the Student Nurse Reserve would also provide students for civilian schools of nursing.

There were many nurse educators in the ANC but most of them were overseas. The faculty of the school, therefore, was largely made up of nursing school administrators and instructors who secured leaves of absence in order to work with Miss Goodrich, who was appointed dean in May, 1918. They had pride in serving with such a distinguished leader. In 1923, Miss Goodrich was awarded the Distinguished Service Medal for the organization and administration of the school. The school, however, had barely been started at the time of the Armistice. But over 10,000 applications had been received, so great was its popular appeal as a war service activity. When assignments were discontinued on December 21, 1918, more than 5000 applications had been accepted. There were 1578 students on duty in 32 military hospitals, the great majority of which were of a temporary nature. As the cantonment hospitals closed, units of the school were combined. The ARC allocated $40,000 to defray the costs of an affiliation in public health nursing. Many students resigned to be married or to return to some former occupation. But 512 nurses, the largest class in American nursing history, were graduated in two units in June and July, 1921, at the Walter Reed General Hospital in Washington and the Letterman General Hospital in San Francisco, respectively.

By 1923 only the unit at Walter Reed was in operation. Two classes and a list of accepted students were transferred to the Army school from the school which the USPHS had established at Fort McHenry in 1922. In 1931, partly as a result of economic conditions and the relatively high cost of affiliations, and partly because it had never been wholeheartedly accepted by the ANC, the school was closed. Miss Goodrich wrote in 1919 that the number of students had made no appreciable contribution to nursing service during the war but that the experiment was valuable because "it demonstrated without doubt the great asset a well-established school under the Medical Department would be in the rapid expansion of nursing service required by a similar emergency." To her bitter disappointment, the experiment of establishing a school in an administrative agency had not been as convincing as she had believed. When plans were in the making for an increased number of nurses to meet the anticipated shortages of the World War II period, there was little or no support from nurse leaders to reopen the Army school. From the civilian viewpoint, it seemed more practical to provide for an increased registration of nursing students to fill gaps in the graduate staffs of civilian hospitals which would otherwise be unable to secure assistance. From the viewpoint of the Army's Medical Department, an all-graduate staff was an economy. The Army School of Nursing had not provided, as it had been anticipated, a sufficiently large percentage of regular Army nurses to justify repeating the experiment. Statistics that included the final graduating class showed that of the 940 who graduated between 1921 and 1933 only 269 nurses, or 28.6 per cent, had at some time accepted the usual three-year appointment as Army nurses. Only 42 of this number were on active duty in 1940, among them Mary G. Phillips, who became chief of the ANC following World War II. A considerable number of graduates of the school achieved distinction comparable to that of Vassar campers in various fields of nursing.

The Army school was a brilliantly conceived expedient for meeting the critical situation in nursing in 1918. Obviously, it would not have been authorized had the War Department foreseen the early termination of the war. But, such was the administrative genius of Miss Goodrich, that the school, authorized on May 25, 1918, and discontinued on August 12, 1931, played a significant part in the evolution of nursing. Through the accident of war, the government had provided a demonstration school in which the accepted principles of organization, administration, and teaching were effectively applied.

Many of those who participated in the earlier phases of the development of the Army school returned to civilian schools with a clearer concept of what a nursing school could be, and with the courage to make use of their new knowledge. Stirred by the incandescent enthusiasm and inspired leadership of Dean Goodrich, they had learned that with courage, plus knowledge, seemingly insuperable obstacles can be overcome.

On request of the committee on nursing of the Council of National Defense, the Women's Committee of the council, in cooperation with the National Association of Collegiate Alumnae, undertook a campaign to recruit 25,000 students for the Army and civilian schools. The Army and Red Cross cooperated with the council in the Student Nurse Reserve program for which offices were opened in Washington. To provide space for new students and to make the earliest possible contribution to military needs, civilian schools were urged "to crowd forward the theoretical instruction of senior students . . . to hold final examinations and graduation exercises as early as possible in 1918, . . . to release their graduates, providing the government needs them and they consent to enter directly into government service."[6]

Circular letters were extensively used to secure the interest of the 1917 graduates of high schools and colleges, of the deans of colleges, and other influential persons. Isabel M. Stewart, a generous and productive writer who was then assistant to Miss Nutting at Teachers College, prepared most of the materials used in the campaign.[7] Of approximately 14,000 eligible candidates, a little less than one-third were referred to the Army school, over 5000 were directed to civilian schools, and there was a substantial waiting list when the campaign closed late in 1918. The needs of all schools in some states were met. The weaknesses of some of them were revealed as the campaign progressed, and those which, although accredited by state boards of nurse examiners, were considered definitely undesirable for the training of student-nurse-reserve candidates were dropped from the list. Regional differences in educational standards and resources created difficulties for agencies which operated on a national basis, as they did again in World War II.

BIBLIOGRAPHY

Blanchfield, Florence A., and Standlee, Mary W.: *Organized Nursing and the Army in Three Wars.* Unpublished manuscript on file, Historical Division, Office of the Surgeon General of the Army, Washington, D.C.

"Committee on Nursing of the General Medical Board of the Council of National Defense," *The Public Health Nurse Quarterly,* 9:325, 1917.

Crandall, Ella Phillips: "Report of the Secretary of the Committee on Nursing," *Am. J. Nursing,* 18:1078, 1918.

Delano, Jane A.: "Red Cross Aid Versus the Short-Term Course," *Twenty-fourth Annual Report of the National League of Nursing Education,* 1918, p. 159.

[6] Crandall, Ella Phillips: "Report of the Secretary of the Committee on Nursing," *Am. J. Nursing,* 18:1079, 1918.

[7] Among them were: *Opportunities in the Field of Nursing* (revised); *A Message to Secondary School Principals and Teachers; Preparatory Courses for Nurses in College and University; The Nation's Call for Nurses* (Notes for Speakers).

Dock, Lavinia L., and Pickett, Sarah Elizabeth: "Mobilization" (The Student Nurse Reserve Campaign), *Official History of American Red Cross Nursing*. The Macmillan Company, New York, 1922, pp. 293–96.

Goldwater, S. S.: "The Nursing Crisis: Efforts to Satisfy the Nursing Requirements of the War," *Twenty-fourth Annual Report of the National League of Nursing Education,* 1919, p. 132; also *Am. J. Nursing*, **18**:1030, 1918.

Goodrich, Annie W.: "The Plan for the Army School of Nursing," *Twenty-fifth Annual Report of the National League of Nursing Education,* 1918, p. 171.

———: "The Contribution of the Army School of Nursing," *Twenty-fifth Annual Report of the National League of Nursing Education,* 1919, p. 146.

Kernodle, Portia B.: *The Red Cross Nurse in Action, 1882–1948.* Harper & Brothers, New York, 1949.

Martin, Franklin H.: *The Joy of Living,* An Autobiography. Doubleday, Doran & Co., New York, 1936, Vol. II, p. 359.

"Report of the Vassar Nursing Conference," *Am. J. Nursing,* **21**:237, 1921.

Smith, Winford H.: "How Nurses Are Meeting Present Needs," *Am. J. Nursing,* **18**:979, 1918.

Stewart, Isabel M.: *Preparatory Course for Nurses in Colleges and Universities* (pamphlet). Committee on Nursing, General Medical Board, Council of National Defense, Washington, D.C.

Stimson, Julia C., and associates: *History and Manual of the Army Nurse Corps.* Medical Field Service School, Carlisle Barracks, Pa., Oct. 1, 1937.

Summer Preparatory Courses for Nurses at Western Reserve University, 1918.

"Vassar Nursing-Preparatory Course: A New Experiment in Nursing Education," *Am. J. Nursing,* **18**:1155, 1918.

Chapter 15

NURSES FOLLOW THE FLAG

It is a fearful thing to lead this great peaceful people into war, into the most terrible and disastrous of all wars, civilization itself seeming to be in the balance. But the right is more precious than peace, and we shall fight for the things which we have always carried nearest our hearts—for democracy, for the right of those who submit to authority to have a voice in their own governments, for the rights and liberties of small nations, for a universal dominion of right by such a concert of free peoples as shall bring peace and safety to all nations, and make the world itself at last free. . . .
WOODROW WILSON, APRIL 2, 1917

WHEN WAR was declared on April 6, 1917, the United States had only the nucleus of an army and of a navy. The swift growth of the Army within a year from 100,000 to 4,000,000 men presented a problem of previously undreamed of magnitude to the nursing profession. The Army Nurse Corps had only 400 nurses on active duty, and the Navy approximately two-fifths of that number. The corps were well established but they were almost completely isolated from the main stream of professional nursing. When the war ended, they had a total of 21,000 regular and reserve nurses. Including those who served directly under the American Red Cross, some 24,000 nurses had been in war service. This was well over one-fourth of the estimated total of graduate nurses in the country.

Nurses, in common with other Americans, had gone through the successive stages of isolationism, neutrality, and rising indignation at stories of wanton brutality and reports of the shocking destruction resulting from submarine warfare. Not all of them perceived at once that the declaration of war had personal significance for every member of the profession. By virtue of their special skills nurses may be said to have been in a privileged class. They were to learn that the obverse of privilege in a democratic society is responsibility. The response of the profession as a whole to the calls for service during "the Great War" is a legitimate source of pride.

Credit for the withdrawal of so many thousands of nurses from their regular pursuits without destroying the American system of nursing was due to two agencies. These were the well-established nursing service of the American Red Cross, inaugurated and directed by Jane A. Delano, and the war-born Committee on Nursing of the General Medical Board of the Council of National Defense of which M. Adelaide Nutting was chairman. Under Miss Delano's leadership, with the support of a strong national committee, the nursing service of the American Red Cross had become a powerful force in American nursing. The requirements for enrollment in the nursing service had made it, in effect, a standardizing agency. Many nurses thought of it as the equivalent of a fourth national nursing organization. No other Red Cross society in the world had done so much to promote the development of professional nursing. Historically, as Miss Nutting often pointed out, this was quite contrary to the usual practice of Red Cross societies which base their programs on voluntary (unpaid) service. The nursing service was featured at all conventions of the ANA. Many nurses were responsive to the patriotic and professional idealism of Miss Delano's concept of nursing as a service which could extend its usefulness by affiliation with the Red Cross and which would in turn strengthen that great organization. In her benign and majestic presence they saw a dedicated person, a living embodiment of their own aspirations. The War Department had formally accepted the Red Cross enrollment as a reserve for the Army Nurse Corps in 1913. By tacit agreement it also provided a reserve for the Navy Nurse Corps. Excellent collaborative relationships had been established with both.

When war was declared, the enrollment of 8000 nurses provided the only available roster of nurses (they were classified later) whose credentials had been evaluated. Enrolled nurses were assumed to be available for military service and for a variety of Red Cross activities. These included the provision of nurses for participation in ARC disaster relief programs, for the development and teaching of courses in elementary hygiene and home care of the sick, and for the rural public health nursing service established in 1912 as the Town and Country Nursing Service.

Foreseeing the need for a greatly expanded enrollment after the passage of the National Defense Act, Miss Delano persuaded Clara D. Noyes late in 1916 to relinquish the congenial position of superintendent of nurses at Bellevue and Allied Hospitals in New York in order to become associated with her as director of a bureau of nursing service under the Department of Nursing. Miss Noyes was then president of the NLNE and thoroughly familiar with the work of that organization and of the ANA. A somewhat austere daughter of New England, she was deeply devoted to her profession. She was an excellent administrator in the authoritarian tradition. Standing shoulder to shoulder with Miss Delano in the midst of a seeming whirlpool of activity she assumed responsibility for an ever-swelling stream of enrolled nurses. By accepting enrolled ARC nurses as a reserve, the heavily burdened offices of Dora E. Thompson, superintendent of the Army Nurse Corps, and of Lenah S. Higbee of the Navy Nurse Corps, were relieved of enormous amounts of detail. Before the declaration of war, when the Red Cross was concentrating on recruitment of reserve nurses for service with the armed forces when needed, there were no warning signs to suggest that nurses, especially public health nurses, would also be required for civilian services overseas. Increasing demands for public health nurses, at home and abroad, caused the ARC to discontinue the limited Town and Country Nursing Service in 1918, establishing in its place a Bureau of Public Health Nursing under the direction of Mary S. Gardner. However, administration of the bureau was taken over at an early date by her associate, Elizabeth G. Fox, in order to release Miss Gardner for special service in Italy. Henceforth, for more than a decade, the forceful and clear-thinking Miss Fox exerted a powerful influence on the development of public health nursing.

When the national nursing organizations met in Philadelphia in an atmosphere of tense expectancy a great audience was told that the nursing service of the ARC was ready, perhaps better prepared, for war than any other official or nonofficial agency of the United States. But it was not a time for complacency. In the course of that convention week the chief nurses of three base hospitals received instructions from the War Department to mobilize their units at once. Within six weeks of the declaration of war six base hospitals were crossing the submarine-infested Atlantic for service with the British Expeditionary Forces (BEF). (They were later transferred to the American Expeditionary Forces [AEF].) Nurses were thus in the vanguard of the nation's war effort.

In her comprehensive history of the Red Cross nursing service, Mrs. Kernodle gives the following description of the personnel of the base hospitals that were organized by medical schools or large general hospitals. Most of them were not called until the mass movement of trained troops got under way in 1918.

Before the United States entered the European War, the organization of 25 base hospitals was well under way, and several had been completed. The local chapter provided the equipment for the unit at a cost for each of between $25,000 and $75,000. The personnel included 23 doctors (later raised to 50); 50 nurses (later raised to 100); 25 nurses' aides (never called out); 15 reserve nurses (later raised to 25); 25 reserve nurses' aides (never called out); and other personnel needed to care for a 500-bed hospital (later raised to 1,000 beds). To the chief nurse was delegated the selection of nurses, the dietitian, and the nurses' aides, all of whom must be secured through the Red Cross nursing service.[1]

The total of 49 base hospitals that were sent over, according to Ashburn, constituted the backbone of the American hospitalization system. They were expanded to care for many more patients than had been planned for originally. Some of them were grouped together in great hospital centers. The base hospitals were supplemented by a variety of Army, Navy, and Red Cross installations. Nurses were concentrated in the base hospitals; but they were also assigned to camp, evacuation, and mobile hospitals as well as to hospital trains. Many more volunteered for service close to the front than were needed. Those assigned gave superb service.

[1] Kernodle, Portia B.: *The Red Cross Nurse in Action, 1882–1948.* Harper & Brothers, New York, 1949, p. 109. Quoted by permission, The American National Red Cross, Washington, D.C.

While the War Department was putting its plans for an enormously increased Army into effect, the Red Cross began to mobilize the "vast capacity for unselfishness" of the American people. As a golden stream began flowing into the treasury of the national organization in the early summer of 1917, the chairman of the ARC War Council asked General Pershing, commander-in-chief of the American Expeditionary Forces, what the Red Cross could do to help. The French people had already endured the agonies of three years of war on their own soil. Families were scattered and thousands of children were fatherless and homeless. Tuberculosis was taking a terrible toll. "Buck up the French," was the General's cabled reply. In response, an ARC commission "bent on clearing away a mountain of misery" landed in France in early June. Commissions were also established in Great Britain, Russia, Rumania, Serbia, and Italy.[2]

The miseries of the French civilian population and the tragic plight of the children, in particular, were self-evident. The commission, according to the chairman of the War Council, promptly began giving needed assistance without waiting to perfect an organization. This statement seems to explain some of the perplexities and misunderstandings which gave Miss Delano and other eminent nurses many anxious moments. Nurses were being pressed into service without clearance from the ARC headquarters in Washington, which was also receiving and doing its best to meet insistent requests for nurses. Cabled requests to Miss Goodrich, asking her to take charge of all ARC nursing in France, were not cleared with Miss Delano and became known to her many weeks later. The results of that contretemps were extremely disconcerting on both sides of the Atlantic! When Miss Delano approached Miss Goodrich she found that Miss Goodrich would go to France only under the highest governmental authority. Miss Delano felt the Red Cross could not ask that privilege and the subject was dropped. (This unfortunate incident is fully documented in Harriett Berger Koch's biography of Miss Goodrich.) Subsequent developments seem to

[2] Davison, Henry P.: *The American Red Cross in the Great War.* The Macmillan Company, New York, 1920.

indicate the soundness of Miss Goodrich's thinking. In March, 1918, Julia C. Stimson, then in France as chief nurse of a base hospital, was appointed chief nurse for the ARC in France while retaining Army status. Some months later she was appointed chief nurse of the American Expeditionary Forces.

The ARC organized its civilian program in France in three bureaus, all of them charged with responsibility for developing cooperative relationships with both governmental and other voluntary relief agencies. The programs of the three bureaus—Children's, Refugees and Relief, and the Bureau of Tuberculosis—required nurses. That of the Children's Bureau, directed by Elizabeth Ashe of the Telegraph Hill Neighborhood Association, San Francisco, was the most extensive. There was a constant demand from the bureaus for more public health nurses and more French-speaking nurses' aides than the Washington office could supply. However, a high percentage of exceptionally well-qualified American public health and other nurses were active in the civilian program. Nurses and aides of nine nationalities participated in the Children's Bureau program which left behind, as permanent installations, a number of hospitals, dispensaries, and child welfare agencies.

Along with the many administrative problems related to the assignment and equipment of nurses, two problems arose in connection with the status of enrolled Red Cross nurses. They had a sentimental attachment to the insignia of the Red Cross nursing service and had been permitted to wear the badge when, as reserve nurses, they became members of the ANC. When it was found that the custom tended to divide loyalties in the rapidly growing ANC, it was discontinued by the War Department. The decision was based on the sound administrative principle that identification with the corps and loyalty to it were of greater importance than the method by which membership in it had been attained.

The second problem had to do with eligibility for War Risk Insurance. Only nurses who had been militarized, that is, had become members of the Army or Navy Nurse Corps were eligible. Non-militarized nurses, of whom there were about 1000 who served directly under the ARC were not eligible. Nurses who might have been militarized (there were some who, in their eagerness to serve overseas, had accepted Red Cross appointments rather than risk assignment by the ANC to cantonment hospitals in the US) had reason to regret their decision. The situation was not unlike that following the Spanish-American War when only nurses who had been identified with the Army as contract nurses were eligible for pensions.

In the summer of 1917, while the civilian program in France was requiring more and more nurses, 32 cantonments or "soldier cities" sprang up like mushrooms throughout the US. Planned for an average of 48,000 soldiers each, they were indeed cities. Each one had a 1000-bed base hospital planned for expansion as needed. Hardly had young men from the cities, towns, and villages, from mountains, hills, and plains begun to pour into the camps, then those hospitals were needed. Patients were admitted almost as soon as the roofs were on the buildings, when they were only partially staffed and incompletely equipped. Nurses who arrived before quarters were ready for them later boasted that they had known "the base" at its crudest and muddiest. Prophylactic vaccines and serum protected the men from smallpox, typhoid, paratyphoid, and diptheria, but fatigue, exposure, and crowding made the draftees, especially those from rural areas, susceptible to the communicable diseases for which there were no protective measures. Meningitis, mumps, and measles filled many wards. After measles and influenza came pneumonia and, too often, empyema. It will be remembered that this was before the introduction of the sulfonamides and antibiotics. The extensive use of Carrel-Dakin solution for infected wounds was one of the medical highlights of that war. Many of the men were critically ill, but the needs of soldiers in the making made no such emotional appeal to nurses as the care of those wounded in battle. Many insisted, in the highly charged spirit of the times, that they were available for overseas service only.

As the numbers in the armed forces increased, so did the need for nurses. The Army's requirements were based on a ratio of one nurse to ten hospital beds. Beginning with an estimated need for the Army alone of 10,000, the number was increased later in 1917 to

22,000. The goal of the ARC was raised to 50,000 enrolled nurses by July, 1919.

In the spring of 1918, thanks to the Navy's antisubmarine warfare, convoy after convoy of American troops was landed in England and France without the loss of a man. The great allied offensive began in July. The Surgeon General of the Army called for 1000 nurses a week for a period of eight weeks, and nurses responded! But a response to a Surgeon General's call for nurses is one thing, securing military transportation for women is quite another. At the height of the troop movement the chief nurse at the Army Mobilization Center in New York had 1300 nurses on her waiting list. Then, as in World War II, it was difficult for civilians to understand the complexities of mass military movements. The psychological effect of long waiting periods on recruitment was not good. The dramatic figure of the Red Cross nurse in scarlet-lined cape was used so extensively in an intensive recruitment program that summer that many people came to think of "Red Cross" and "nurse" virtually as synonymous terms. This concept was manifestly unfair to the many thousands of volunteers who performed a variety of services and kept vast quantities of surgical and other supplies moving toward the front throughout the war. Negro nurses had offered their services through the ARC late in 1917. But almost a year went by before two units of nine nurses each were assigned by the Army to cantonment hospitals in Ohio and Illinois. A few others served during emergencies at training camps in Arkansas and South Carolina.

The ARC, with the approval of the ANC, lowered the age requirement from 25 to 21, temporarily discontinued membership in the ANA, and admitted graduates of state-approved schools with less than a daily average of 50 patients. The chief nurse of an Army base hospital wrote sympathetically of the 15 nurses comprising a mobile unit which arrived at an extremely active, tented base hospital in France after midnight in a pouring rain. Very young and inexperienced, they were assigned to crowded wards which needed many more than the 15 additional nurses to care for the wounded men just admitted from casualty clearing stations. "It seemed a heartbreaking thing to thrust them into this unbelievable hell," she wrote, but a day or so later she found them "adjusting wonderfully and . . . making themselves felt. . . ."[3]

The smaller, although greatly expanded, Navy Nurse Corps maintained its standards throughout the war. When the Armistice was signed, the Navy had base hospitals in both Great Britain and France, and some Navy nurses had been assigned to transport service.

Shock, hemorrhage, infection, and the care of gassed patients challenged the powers of observation as well as the technical skills of nurses who, of necessity, limited their services to bare essentials. Their very presence was encouraging to wounded men. For the first time in military situations, nurse anesthetists demonstrated their usefulness. Nurses proudly volunteered for service with surgical teams at the front. When a drive was on, nurses worked with the doctors until exhaustion demanded relief. Those on hospital trains helped to speed patients on the way to base hospitals and to the transports which brought those with long-term conditions back to hospitals in the US. Even though it had been difficult for some of them to adjust to military situations, nurses almost invariably responded magnificently to the needs of wounded men. When granted leave of absence, they were grateful for the rest homes provided by the ARC.

Just as the Allies were reaching the crescendo of their war effort in the autumn of 1918, Spanish influenza, associated with pneumonia, struck like a plague out of the Middle Ages. It was no respecter of persons. Incidence in the civilian population was highest in congested areas. For the same reason it was appallingly high among the troops in the cantonments. Transports buried many victims of "flu" at sea. One ship alone landed 2000 soldiers with "flu" and pneumonia at Southhampton at a time when casualties from Flanders were pouring into the hospitals of the AEF in Britain. One base hospital landed with its personnel so unfit for duty that it was never organized for service. The incidence in France, however, was lower than in the cantonment hospitals in the US, none

[3] Stimson, Julia C.: *Finding Themselves.* The Macmillan Company, New York, 1927, p. 217.

of which escaped. The census of one 2000-bed hospital rose to 8000 and at one time 90 of the 300 regular nurses were sick.

As the cantonment and other military hospitals began to overflow, they called for help. Home defense nurses (enrolled ARC nurses not available for military service), nurses' aides, women who had taken the home nursing courses, and others with no preparation whatsoever responded to the call of the Red Cross local committees. Many of them gave splendid service. Some became patients, as did nurses and Army school students, and in every group there was some loss of life. Ashburn states that influenza, combined with pneumonia and other respiratory diseases, caused 82 per cent of the deaths of the Army during World War I. The lessons of that pandemic were kept in mind when doctors and nurses were again called to the colors.

In the autumn of 1918, Carrie M. Hall, chief nurse of the ARC in Great Britain, and Miss Stimson in France were reporting serious shortages of nurses. The Surgeon General reversed a previous decision and called for hundreds of nurses' aides. However, nothing had been done about the preparation and transportation of aides when the Armistice abruptly stopped all warlike activity and focused attention on plans for returning patients and personnel to the US. The ARC had fallen far short of the projected enrollment of 50,000 nurses; chief nurses had often needed more nurses than were immediately available to care for their patients. But there had never been a time throughout the war when nurses were not waiting for transportation overseas.

BIBLIOGRAPHY

Ashburn, P. M.: *A History of the Medical Department of the United States Army.* Houghton Mifflin Co., Boston, 1929.

Barck, Oscar Theodore, Jr., and Blake, Nelson Manfred: "From Peace to War," Chap. 8; "War for Democracy," Chap. 9; *Since 1900. A History of the United States in Our Time,* rev. ed. The Macmillan Company, New York, 1952.

Blanchfield, Florence A., and Standlee, Mary W.: *Organized Nursing and the Army in Three Wars.* Unpublished manuscript on file, Historical Division, Office of the Surgeon General of the Army, Washington, D.C.

Dock, Lavinia L., and others: *History of American Red Cross Nursing.* The Macmillan Company, New York, 1922, p. 228.

Dulles, Foster Rhea: *The American Red Cross, A History.* Harper & Brothers, New York, 1950.

Higbee, Lenah S.: "The Work of the Navy Nurse Corps," *Twenty-fifth Annual Report of the National League of Nursing Education,* 1919, p. 126.

Kernodle, Portia B.: *The Red Cross Nurse in Action, 1882–1948.* Harper & Brothers, New York, 1949.

Koch, Harriett Berger: *Militant Angel.* The Macmillan Company, New York, 1951, pp. 84–88.

The Medical Department of the United States Army in the World War, Vol. 13, Part II, "The Army Nurse Corps," by Julia C. Stimson. US Government Printing Office, Washington, D.C., 1927.

Slosson, Preston William: *The Great Crusade and After.* The Macmillan Company, New York, 1937.

Thompson, Dora E.: "How the Army Nursing Service Met the Demands of War," *Twenty-fifth Annual Report of the National League of Nursing Education,* 1919, p. 116.

Wadsworth, Eliot: "The Work of the Red Cross in the Event of War," *Am. J. Nursing,* **17**:1153, 1917.

Washburn, Frederic A.: *The Massachusetts General Hospital—Its Development, 1900–1935.* Houghton Mifflin Co., Boston, 1939, p. 534.

Chapter 16

CONTINUING SERVICE OVERSEAS

. . . circumstances made the association of nursing service with European countries more lasting than that of other services.

PORTIA B. KERNODLE[1]

WHEN THE ORDER "Cease firing!" terminated hostilities on November 11, 1918, American nurses on the far side of the Atlantic were participating in the civilian relief and health programs of a number of agencies in which they were often associated with nurses of other countries. The American Red Cross had commissions at work all the way from western Europe to Vladivostok on the eastern border of Siberia. Many other relief agencies were also at work. Among those with which American nurses were working were the American Women's Hospitals (AWH), the American Committee for Devastated France, the Joint Committee on Distribution, the Near East Relief, Hadassah, and the Rockefeller Foundation. Work with sick, malnourished, and often homeless people, many thousands of them children, tested the courage and initiative while it challenged the skill, resourcefulness, and compassion of the participating nurses, a considerable number of whom later received governmental and other awards in recognition of their service. The preparation of workers to assist with the emergency programs and to carry on some type of health program, when foreign assistance should be withdrawn, was an important feature of most of the programs.

Following the Armistice, the ARC appointed a director of nursing

[1] Kernodle, Portia B.: *The Red Cross Nurse in Action, 1882–1948.* Harper & Brothers, New York, 1949, p. 180.

service in Europe, a position held successively by Carrie M. Hall, who had been chief nurse for the ARC in Great Britain; Alice Fitzgerald, who had been supervisor of some of the ARC activities in France; and Helen Scott Hay, who had been a member of the ARC staff in Washington and chief nurse of the "Mercy Ship" in 1914. What turned out to be a four-year postwar program went through several stages. In France, the programs of the ARC and of the Rockefeller Foundation for the control of tuberculosis, to which Elisabeth Crowell had made a brilliant contribution, were turned over to local authorities or agencies as rapidly as possible. Under Anne Morgan's Committee for Devastated France, Mary Breckinridge established (1919) in the Aisne a visiting nurse service which became a permanent agency. Some 600 nurses were still on overseas duty in several countries under the ARC. They represented a cross section of American nursing—institutional, public health, and private duty—and were serving in hospitals, dispensaries, and in various types of public health nursing. By June, 1922, when all activities, except assistance to new nursing schools, were terminated, the program had gone through the successive stages of emergency hospitalization and relief, a general health program, and, in the final stage, child welfare. Except in the new schools only public health nurses were employed in the concluding stage in which several hundred child welfare centers were established in the hope that they could be continued by national or local agencies. The time had been very short for so ambitious a project, but Miss Noyes found some evidence of its continuing usefulness when she visited Europe in 1925. In Austria, where 100 child health centers had been established, much of the effort might have been lost had not the Commonwealth Fund undertaken a child welfare program in time to build on the earlier work. This was a demonstration in which Alma C. Haupt directed the nursing program. When it was over, it was believed that American initiative had helped to clear the way for Austrian enterprise.

When ARC work in Siberia was discontinued early in 1920, eight of the fourteen hospitals originally set up to care for Czechoslovakian and Russian soldiers were still in operation. Some of this work was turned over to the Russian Red Cross. Most of the 150 nurses still on duty were at Vladivostok. Nurses of the Siberian commission had helped to check an epidemic of typhus in Siberia and one of cholera at Mukden in Manchuria. They had cared for homeless and starving orphans, and had taught their Russian aides some of the principles of elementary nursing, using translations of excerpts from Miss Delano's *Elementary Hygiene and Home Care of the Sick*.

During the war Italy had received assistance from the ARC Commission on Tuberculosis to which Mary S. Gardner and a group of public health nurses were assigned. Tuberculous men were being returned by the trainload from prison camps to a country which had a mere handful of graduate nurses and practically no public health nursing. Three schools were set up to teach the rudiments of public health nursing to demobilized "war nurses." This expedient, adopted on the basis of all the factors in the situation, was a violation of the concept generally accepted in the United States that preparation for public health nursing should follow a basic training. But, so carefully was the work planned that it created among influential Italians an interest in nursing under lay auspices which, it is believed, had a constructive influence on the subsequent development of professional nursing in Italy.

When the programs in Western Europe were being closed, the ARC turned its attention to the countries of Eastern and Southern Europe where thousands of people were homeless, and poverty and disease were depressing whole populations. Nurses served in varying capacities in practically all of those countries. In the Near East, an area in which missionary nurses of various nationalities had long been at work, the ARC turned its work over to the more permanent Near East Relief shortly after the Armistice. Nurses were assigned to that agency and supplies turned over to it. The Near East organization had cared for over a hundred thousand children and had operated "the largest children's hospital in the world," an improvised 3000-bed institution for the care of trachoma patients. There, in Armenia, American nurses supervised the work of Russian and Armenian "sisters." It was under the Near East Relief also that Alice Carr made history by teaching the people of Corinth how malaria,

the historic scourge of Greece, could be controlled through elimination of the breeding places of Anopheles mosquitoes. In one year
malaria among orphaned children under her care was reduced from
60 to 3 per cent.

Most of the work of the American Women's Hospitals, organized by women physicians denied the privilege of military
service who were eager to help alleviate wartime suffering, was concentrated in the Near East. When the Christian section of Smyrna
was burned by the Turks in 1922, a flood of refugees poured into
Greece. The ARC based a special program on the child welfare program it had previously conducted there. The AWH and the Near
East Relief also rose magnificently to the challenge of the appalling
health and medical needs of the tragically displaced persons. To
provide occupational preparation for orphaned girls, as well as to
enhance the health resources of the area, a school of nursing was
established with primitive equipment at Salonika (later transferred
to Kokkinia) by the AWH. Many of the refugee students had been
educated in American and English mission schools in Asia Minor.

The work of the ARC in Palestine was taken over at an early date
by the Near East Relief, but Hadassah, an American Zionist organization, continued with nursing and health work for which two
American nurses had begun laying the groundwork in 1913. In 1918,
in cooperation with other Hebrew organizations, Hadassah sent a
medical unit including nurses for emergency service to develop a
long-range program in Palestine. A school of nursing was established
which graduated its first class in 1921 and, under the direction of
native nurses, was an important center of nursing education until
the partition of Palestine.

As each country faced the monumental task of rehabilitation, it
quickly became apparent that economic recovery would, to a considerable extent, be dependent upon improving the health of the
people. This could not be accomplished without public health nursing. Sound planning called for schools of nursing which would provide the necessary basic training. The ARC rounded out its service
in Europe by sponsoring the organization of five schools of nursing.

It also provided short courses in some other countries, as had been done in France and Italy, to meet the urgent need for health workers. The new republic of Czechoslovakia was the first country to request such assistance, and a school was established in Prague under ARC auspices by American nurses (1919). Schools were opened in Poznan and Warsaw in Poland (1921). The Warsaw school has an especially interesting history. An Army school student, Dorothea Hughes, contributed the funds administered by the ARC which made it possible. Under the direction of Helen Bridge (Pohlman) this school, subsequently given substantial assistance by the Rockefeller Foundation, was outstandingly successful. The fourth school was opened in Sophia, Bulgaria (1922). Hazel A. Goff, who achieved distinction in a variety of international positions, joined the faculty at an early date and became the director of the school. With the aid of scholarships, graduates of these schools were prepared to take over the administration of them in a relatively short time. Such nurses became leaders of nursing in their own countries and frequently represented them in international nursing affairs. The fifth school which received ARC assistance was developed under quite different circumstances. The request for help was received from the American Hospital in Constantinople just as the ARC was terminating its program in the Near East. Nurses were available to assist in establishing it, and both the ARC and the Near East organization contributed supplies to it. Unlike the other schools it was not anticipated that it could quickly be turned over to native auspices since Turkish women were still veiled. Many of the students were Armenian.

While the ARC was promoting the development of these schools, the Joint Distribution Committee sponsored the very successful school which was organized by Amelia Greenwald at the Jewish Hospital in Warsaw. Like the ARC schools, it was autonomous. It had the great advantage of affiliation with a 1200-bed city hospital whereas the Red Cross schools had some difficulty in securing an entree to hospitals in which adequate opportunities for the nursing practice of students could be secured. Scholarship aid made it possible for graduates of this school to assume responsibility at an early date for its further development. (The section of Warsaw in which the school was located was reduced to rubble in World War II.)

Accounts of the work of American nurses in Europe and the Near East filled many pages of the professional journals in the postwar years. Only the more colorful highlights of their services under various auspices could be considered here. Any lasting values derived from their services have been woven into the fabric of nursing in other countries. The influence of the extraordinary range of foreign experience in connection with World War I on American nursing has been far reaching. When the war was over, many Americans reverted to their previous isolationist attitudes. But nurses, through the International Council of Nurses and the League of Red Cross Societies, which was organized in 1919, proceeded at once to strengthen the relationships that bind the nurses of the world together in a service which is a response to universal need. Consideration of international relationship is deferred to a later chapter.

BIBLIOGRAPHY

Barton, James L.: *Story of Near East Relief, 1915–1930.* The Macmillan Company, New York, 1930.

Breckenridge, Mary: *Wide Neighborhoods.* Harper & Brothers, New York, 1952, Chaps. IX and XI.

Dulles, Foster Rhea: *The American Red Cross, A History.* Harper & Brothers, New York, 1950.

French, William J., and Smith, Geddes: *The Commonwealth Fund Activities in Austria, 1923–1929.* The Commonwealth Fund, New York, 1929.

Gardner, Mary S.: "The Influence of International Organizations and Contacts of Nursing Education from the Standpoint of Public Health Nursing," *International Aspects of Nursing Education.* Annie W. Goodrich Lectureship Fund, Teachers College, Columbia University, New York, 1931.

Kernodle, Portia B.: *The Red Cross Nurse in Action, 1882–1949.* Harper & Brothers, New York, 1949, pp. 164–231.

Knowlton, Elizabeth: "The Largest Children's Hospital in the World," *Am. J. Nursing,* 22:829–31, 1922.

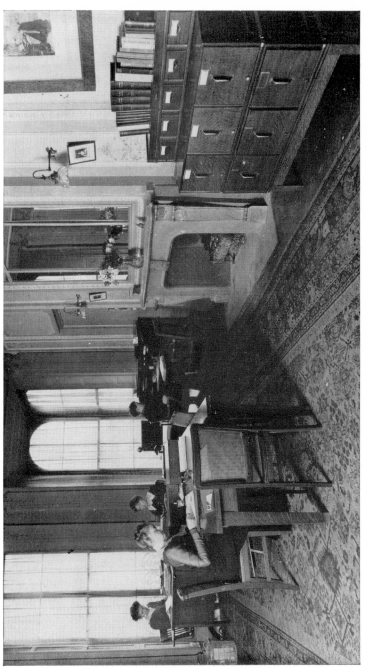

Plate I. First national nursing office. Ella P. Crandall, director, NOPHN, 1912–1920, at right. Ysabella Waters in foreground.

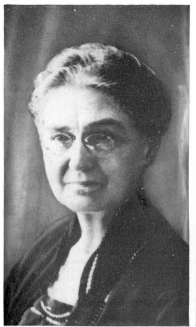
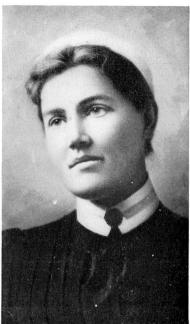
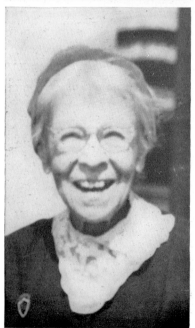

Plate II. Mary Adelaide Nutting (*upper left*), scholar, historian, and educator, was the first nurse in the world to receive an appointment on the faculty of a university. Isabel Hampton Robb (*upper right*), nurse educator and leader in the movement for an organized nursing profession, was the first president of the American Nurses' Association. Lavinia L. Dock (*lower left*), student of social forces, crusader, and historian, was secretary of the ICN, 1899–1922.

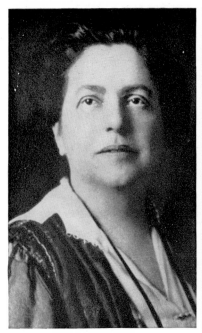

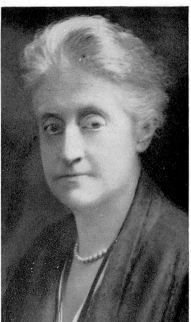

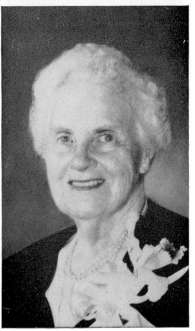

Plate III. The concern of Lillian
D. Wald (*upper left*), for humanity
led her to found the Henry Street
Visiting Nurse Service. Annie W.
Goodrich (*upper right*), Dean
Emeritus, Yale School of Nursing,
crusaded for a place for nursing in
institutions of higher education
while contributing to many phases
of the evolution of nursing. Mary
Sewall Gardner (*lower right*),
prime mover in the organization
and development of the NOPHN,
encouraged its fusion with the
NLNE and the ACSN.

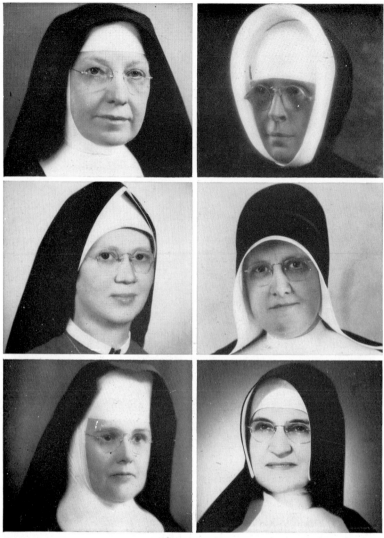

Plate IV. Among the many Catholic Sisters who have promoted the development of professional nursing are (*left, top to bottom*) Sister M. Domitilla, O.S.F., M.A. (*Kenneth M. Wright Studios, St. Paul*); Sister M. Theophane, S.C.M.M.; Sister Olivia Gowan, O.S.B., M.A., LL.D. (*Bradford Bachrach*). (*Right, top to bottom*) Sister John Gabriel, F.C.S.P., M.A., Hon. F.A.C.H.A.; Sister Cyril, S.C., Sc.D.; Sister Mary Geraldine, S.S.M., M.S. (*Vincent Price, St Louis*).

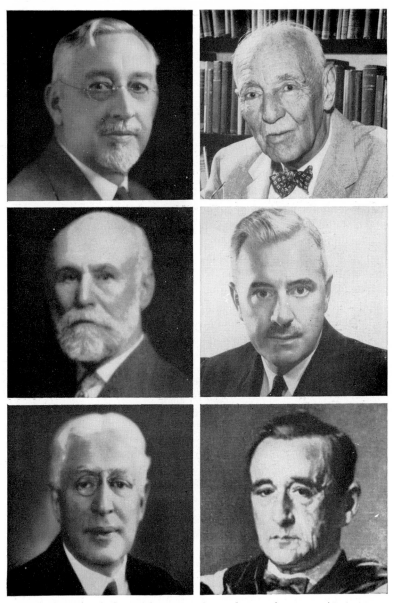

Plate V. Distinguished contributors to the evolution of nursing. (*Left, top to bottom*) William E. Russell, Ph.D. (*photo by Blank-Stoller, Inc.*); Richard Olding Beard, M.D.; Lee K. Frankel, Ph.D. (*Right, top to bottom*) C.-E. A. Winslow, D.P.H.; Thomas Parran, M.D., D.P.H.; and Milton C. Winternitz, M.D. (*Yale University News Bureau*).

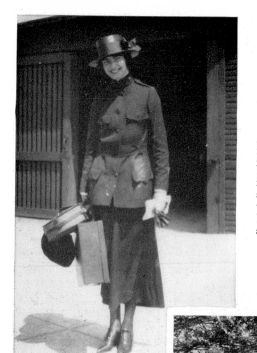

Plate VI. During World War I, Army school students wore blue chambray indoor uniforms with white "butcher" aprons. The outdoor uniform was a somber dark blue relieved only by white collar and cuffs.

Plate VI. Members of the US Cadet Nurse Corps during World War II wore the indoor uniforms of the schools of their choice, with the insigne of the corps on a sleeve. The gray outdoor uniform with its touches of scarlet was especially designed for teen-age students (*photo by US Public Health Service*).

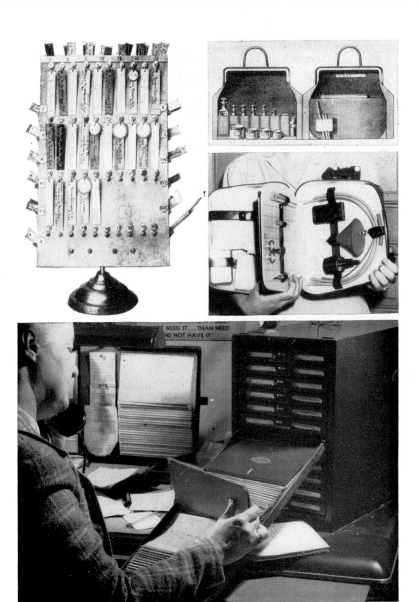

Plate VII. (*Upper left*) Registry board, 1910 (*courtesy of the Professional Nurses Registry, Minneapolis*). (*Upper right*) Visiting nurse bag, 1900, weight 15 pounds. Mid-century bag, weight 4 pounds (*courtesy of the Visiting Nurse Association of Brooklyn; photographed by* Publicity Photographers, Brooklyn). (*Below*) Vertical file system, 1950 (*Milwaukee Journal photo*).

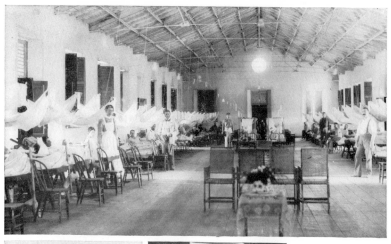

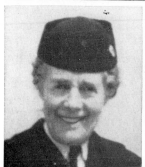
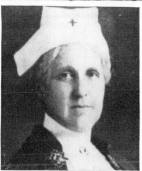

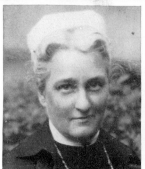
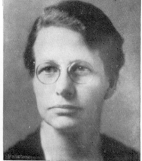

Plate VIII. (*Top*) Cantonment hospital, World War I (*Army Nurse Corps photo*). (*Center*) Florence M. Johnson, international hostess, ARC and ANA, and Jane A. Delano, director, ARC Nursing Service, 1909–1919 (*ARC photo*). (*Bottom*) Clara D. Noyes, director, ARC Nursing Service, 1919–1936, and Elizabeth Gordon Fox, director, ARC Public Health Nursing Service, 1921–1930 (*ARC photos*).

Lovejoy, Esther Pohl: *Certain Samaritans.* The Macmillan Company, New York, 1933.

Noyes, Clara D.: "The Red Cross—Withdrawal of the Siberian Commission," *Am. J. Nursing,* **20**:480, 1920.

———: " 'Health Courses' as Temporary Measures," *Am. J. Nursing,* **22**:825, 1922.

Phillip, M. C.: "The American Women's Hospital," *The International Nursing Review,* Oct., 1927, p. 305.

Seligsberg, Alice L.: "A Modern Training School for Nurses in Jerusalem," *Am. J. Nursing,* **21**:721, 1921.

Smith, Mabell S. C.: "American Public Health Methods in the Near East," *Am. J. Nursing,* **28**:463, 1928.

Willms, Emilie: "A First Graduating Class," *Am. J. Nursing,* **30**:1281, 1930.

Chapter 17

AFTER THE GREAT CRUSADE

*The present somehow does not seem to fit with the past, and the great
future of useful and remunerative work seems very distant. This attitude
is, of course, to a great extent, the reflection of the world's unrest, but
the people who stayed at home have advanced along different lines from
those who went overseas and they cannot see why the daily round cannot
easily be taken up again.*

LAURA HARTWELL[1]

THE SIGNING of the Armistice in November, 1918, shut off the tremendous unifying force of the war effort so abruptly that it created
a spiritual and emotional vacuum in which many Americans seemed
to lose their sense of direction. Along with several million ex-servicemen, most of the 24,000 nurses who had served with the armed
forces and the Red Cross returned to their homes within a year.
Some of the nurses were physically and emotionally exhausted. Wartime experiences had changed both the veterans and the people in
their home towns in unanticipated ways which were disconcerting to
both. As a veteran nurse put it: ". . . the first private duty case,
when one returned to the white uniform, brought a certain amount
of satisfaction, but soon one's thoughts turned wistfully back to the
days when slithering around in the mud, wearing rubber boots, was
the usual method of going on duty."[2] Remembrance of the dis-
orientations of this period caused farsighted leaders in all fields of
endeavor to encourage postwar planning at a relatively early stage

---

[1] Hartwell, Laura; "The Returned Nurse," *Am. J. Nursing,* **20**:295, 1920.
[2] *Ibid.*

of World War II. Such planning will have an important place in later chapters of this book.

Before discussing the development of nursing after World War I, it is necessary to consider briefly the professional and social setting in which the adjustments were made. Release of tension, economic prosperity, reaction to the prohibition amendment to the Constitution, and the increasing use of automobiles, which combined to create radical changes in social customs, were among the factors that produced the era of "flaming youth." The rapid psychological change in family relationships was humorously illustrated by a parent who said he had never enjoyed the white meat of chicken; in his youth that had been the privilege of his parents and was now claimed as a right by his children! It was a period in which distinctions between mere exuberance and moral issues were not always clear. For example, bobbed hair, a radical change in style, was merely symptomatic of young people's desire for change and independent action, but some schools of nursing attempted to make a moral issue of it by threatening expulsion of students who adopted the new mode. That furor was relatively short-lived but it helped to show the unwisdom of the sternly authoritarian discipline which was still a pronounced characteristic of many schools. A few progressive civilian schools and the Army school were already encouraging their students to develop some form of student government.

Geared to greater activity than ever before, but without a well-defined common objective, the American people entered an era in which a period of economic uncertainty was followed by the tremendous boom which burst in 1929. The Beards thought that "the fruit of a hundred years of agitation and social development had finally been garnered" when the Nineteenth Amendment became law in 1920.[3] But the immediate results of the suffrage amendment were disappointing to many supporters of Susan B. Anthony. Many women refrained from using the vote, but it added to the influence of those who were already working to protect the health of women and children. Among the social phenomena of the postwar period,

[3] Beard, Charles A. and Beard, Mary R.: *The Rise of American Civilization.* The Macmillan Company, New York, 1927, Vol. II, p. 565.

which were to influence the development of nursing, were the rising standard of living and the changing pattern of American life from a predominantly rural to an urban society. Smaller homes and fewer servants plus advances in medicine increased the use of hospitals. Private duty nurses began restricting their practice to hospital work. By the late twenties professionally sponsored registries were reporting many more calls for special nurses for hospitals than for private duty nurses to care for patients in their homes. Whereas in 1909 there had been 4359 hospitals, in 1928 there were 6852, the highest number ever reported by the American Medical Association. Many of them had opened schools of nursing without benefit of advice from the state boards of nurse examiners, and without estimating the adequacy of their clinical and other resources for teaching nursing. The list of schools accredited by the state boards totaled just under 1500 in 1918 but, as previously noted, almost 40 per cent of them fell below the standards of the ARC nursing service. By 1920, another 200 had been added to the list. Keenly aware that the number of young people being graduated annually from high schools and colleges was rapidly increasing, the ANA had recommended in 1918 that the successful completion of one year of high school be the minimum requirement for admission to nursing schools after January 1, 1919, and that it be increased to four years of high school work after January 1, 1922. But more than ten years passed before that goal was achieved. The generally low level of nursing education (a few schools were making good progress) was in sharp contrast to the types of service expected of nurses. In 1918, 10 per cent of the schools enrolled about 35 per cent of the students. The sound of guns had only just died away when the first steps were taken that led to the Winslow-Goldmark study reported in *Nursing and Nursing Education in the United States.*

The revelations of the draft had shocked the nation. Approximately 29 per cent of the young men called up had been found to be physically unfit for military service. As much of the disability had been caused by preventable conditions, the findings gave a tremendous impetus to the health programs of both official and nonofficial agencies. This in turn created such an unprecedented demand for public health nurses that the whole question of the aims and financing objectives and financing of nursing education was forced into the open.

In 1920 there were 28 states in which a state-wide public health nursing program was either contemplated or in successful operation. Only five states had established separate and distinct divisions or bureaus of public health nursing in state health departments. Two voluntary agencies, the National Tuberculosis Association and the ARC, were extremely active in the immediate postwar years. But the trend toward the assumption of responsibility for the people's health by governmental agencies gained such momentum that the decade of the twenties was later described by Smillie as the one which witnessed the beginning of the nationalization of the public health. However, the functions and relationships of official and nonofficial agencies had not yet been clearly defined. The ARC, ending the war with abundant financial resources and a web of chapters which covered the country, undertook a broad-gauge peacetime health program under the leadership of Dr. Livingston Farrand which, although it fell far short of his aspirations, gave a tremendous impetus to public health nursing. Through state associations, the National Tuberculosis Association intensified its efforts to wipe out that preventable disease through emphasis on health education. The scientific studies of the Children's Bureau provided a stimulating basis for its own program, also for the programs of voluntary agencies for the reduction of infant and maternal mortality and the promotion of child health. Influenced by Herbert Hoover, home from his constructive work for children in Belgium and other European countries, two national child welfare organizations were combined to form the American Child Health Association. The NOPHN served as a nursing division for this association which financed the additional staff workers that were required to carry on the program. For more than a decade, this voluntary agency provided a stimulating program of child care beginning with the prenatal period and continued through the school years to the age of industrial employment. School children up and down the length and breadth of the land learned health habits from Cho-Cho, the health clown, or from the charmingly dramatic "health fairy," and from the attractively illustrated materials which the organization provided. School and other public health nurses used these materials extensively.

The general unrest of the early twenties was a challenge to medical and health leadership. Group after group recognized the need for standards which could be used as guides if not as specific goals. Oldest of them all, the American Medical Association, which had already succeeded in markedly reducing the number of medical schools, now announced that it would welcome new schools only if they were amply endowed. It began to encourage the development of courses for the preparation of specialists. But Sedgwick and other authorities in the field of public health deplored the fact that "hygiene and the public health and even preventive medicine have thus far had scanty recognition in our medical schools."[4] This dichotomy in medicine accounts for some of the problems of nurse educators. Nursing was closely bound to traditional medicine, but nursing leaders were constantly under pressure to broaden the base of nursing education by those nurses who were associated with the leaders in the fields of public health and preventive medicine.

The American College of Surgeons, after several years of careful preparation, released its first list of approved hospitals in 1919. The few clearly stated criteria used in this accreditation program dealt with matters fundamental to surgical practice in hospitals. In time, accreditation of a hospital by the college became one of the criteria for the evaluation of schools of nursing. (At mid-century, a joint hospital accreditation program was undertaken by the American Medical Association, the American Hospital Association, and the American College of Surgeons.) *Hospital Progress,* launched by the Catholic Hospital Association in 1920, was the first official publication in its field. The American Hospital Association established headquarters in Chicago shortly after the close of World War I. The executive secretary urged the association to take advantage of the unusual situation in which there was a general and urgent demand for more and better trained hospital executives in a field unham-

---

[4] Sedgwick, William T.: "Modern Medicine and Public Health," *Pub. Health Rep.,* Part I, **36:**109, 1921.

pered by any established ideas, institutions, or organizations. Some years were to elapse, however, before the principle that hospital administration is a field requiring special preparation was generally accepted in hospital circles. The American College of Hospital Administrators, which fosters institutes and other educational programs, was not organized until 1933. Courses of various types were offered by hospitals and universities, but the one established at the University of Chicago in 1934, with the financial assistance of the Commonwealth Fund, became the acknowledged leader in the movement to professionalize hospital administration by provision for sound academic preparation.

A study of the education of hospital social workers published by the AHA in 1921 revealed a significant trend. Although the pioneer departments at the Massachusetts General and Bellevue Hospitals had been developed by nurses, slightly less than one-half of the workers in the 61 departments studied were nurses. Hospital social workers (medical social workers) were feeling need for preparation "adequately adapted to the special and somewhat complex requirements of hospital social services.[5] Hospital dietitians, too, were coping with problems of preparation, and of relationships to the hospitals and to the nursing schools.

Misunderstandings were inevitable in the midst of so much effervescent activity involving relationships with nursing or the utilization of nursing service. In the aggregate, the programs gave no assurance that the medical and health needs of the nation would be adequately covered. Some representative members of the health and hospital groups recognized the desirability of defining functions and of coordinating programs in the public interest. Two significant projects were undertaken. The first one resulted in the organization of the National Health Council in 1921. With a membership of 14 voluntary health agencies, including the National Organization for Public Health Nursing,[6] it established headquarters in New York. The stated purpose of the council was to make it an integrating force

[5] "Education of Social Workers," Report to Trustees of American Hospital Association, *Public Health Nurse*, **13**:230, 1921.

[6] In 1952 the number of voluntary and governmental member agencies had increased to 42.

among independent autonomous agencies. Its important National Health Library was established by pooling the excellent libraries of such member agencies as the National Tuberculosis Association and the National Committee for Mental Hygiene.

The second coordinating agency, the relatively short-lived American Conference on Hospital Service, was initiated by the American Medical Association in 1919. More than a dozen national organizations, including the three national nursing organizations, appointed representatives to it. The conference was concerned with the improvement and development of hospital service. The one tangible result of the work of the conference was the Hospital Library and Service Bureau which later provided the nucleus of the extensive library of the American Hospital Association. The two coordinating agencies thus provided much needed and relatively accessible sources of information in their respective fields. But most voluntary agencies were still in the stage of rugged individualism. Deep-seated loyalty to an agency was likely to be stronger than intellectual convictions about the desirability of coordinating or amalgamating programs in the interest of society. However, a trend toward the development of cooperative relationships was gaining some momentum.

The Committee on Nursing of the Council of National Defense had correctly foretold an increasing demand for nurses in the postwar period. It was created by (1) the new government nursing services, (2) advances in medicine, (3) increased use of civilian hospital facilities as a result of the maternal and infant welfare program developed by the Children's Bureau after the passage of the Maternity and Infancy Act in 1921, and (4) the public health nursing program of the ARC. The beginning of a new era in nursing coincided with the demobilization of nurses in 1919. It was created by a meteoric increase in demands for public health nurses which forced the profession to come to grips with the fundamental question: How shall public health nurses be prepared for their service to society? The postwar decade was notable for its fact-finding studies, its demonstrations of nursing education on a collegiate basis, of public health nursing as a community service and an integral element in over-all public health programs, and for the organization of nonmilitary federal nursing services. Smillie points out that "beginning in 1925 and extending through the present time is the extraordinary phenomenon of the nationalization of the public health. The public health was, for generations, a community affair, administered under local self-government with some slight degree of state government supervision. Public health has now become a subject of nation-wide interest and importance."[7] The ARC made an impressive and pervasive contribution to the development of nursing in the postwar period. Most nurses were unaware of the influence of the voluntary health agencies or that of the two great forces which would continue to influence its development, viz., philanthropic foundations and the federal government.

BIBLIOGRAPHY

Barck, Oscar Theodore, Jr., and Blake, Nelson Manfred: *Since 1900. A History of the United States in Our Times*, rev. ed. The Macmillan Company, New York, 1952.

Dulles, Foster Rhea: *The American Red Cross, A History*. Harper & Brothers, New York, 1950.

Gunn, Selskar M., and Platt, Philip S.: *Voluntary Health Agencies*. The Ronald Press Co., New York, 1945.

Hollis, Ernest V., and Taylor, Alice L.: *Social Work Education in the United States*. Columbia University Press, New York, 1951.

"Hospital Service in the United States, 1950," *J.A.M.A.*, 143:110, 1950.

Ireland, Merritte W.: "Physical and Hygienic Benefits of Military Training as Demonstrated by the War," *J.A.M.A.*, 74:500, 1920.

"Minimum Requirements for Accredited Schools of Nursing as Approved by the Board of Directors of the A.N.A., May 9, 1918," *Am. J. Nursing*, 18:1086, 1918.

Nurse Training Schools, 1917–1918. Bureau of Education, Government Printing Office, Washington, D. C.

Nursing and Nursing Education in the United States. Report of the Committee for the Study of Nursing Education and Report of a Survey by Josephine Goldmark. The Macmillan Company, New York, 1923.

Smith, John A.: "State Programs of Public Health Nursing," *Public Health Nurse*, 12:730, 1920.

[7] Smillie, Wilson G.: *Preventive Medicine and Public Health*, 2nd ed. The Macmillan Company, New York, 1952, p. 10.

Chapter 18

THE FEDERAL GOVERNMENT AND
NURSING SERVICES

In the Government Service today there are, roughly speaking, four thousand nurses on duty in the various departments. . . . War, Navy, Treasury, Interior, Veterans Bureau. . . . There are almost as many standards as there are services. . . .

LUCY MINNIGERODE[1]

THE FEDERAL GOVERNMENT became a large-scale employer of nurses following the war. It also began to influence the development of public health nursing. Within a few years of the Armistice, nursing services were established in the hospital division of the US Public Health Service (1919), the Veterans Bureau (1922), and in the Indian Bureau (1924). And never again were the Nurse Corps of the Army and Navy to be so small or so remote from the main body of professional nurses as they had been before the war.

While the members of the ANC were fully occupied with war service, the profession had endeavored to secure rank for Army nurses. Early in the war, reports from overseas, especially from nurses who were associated with nurses of Great Britain, Canada, and New Zealand, convinced Miss Nutting's committee of the Council of National Defense that rank facilitated the work of military nurses. A special committee which was organized for the purpose of securing congressional action and Helen Hoy Greeley, the lawyer who represented it, met with stubborn opposition that was partly psychological and partly technical. After the Armistice, the proposed

[1] Minnigerode, Lucy: "Inequalities in Standards, Qualifications and Pay of Nurses under Government Service," *Proceedings of the Twenty-fourth Convention of the American Nurses' Association*, 1924, p. 68.

legislation had the enthusiastic support of the American Hospital Association and the new American Legion. But, as after the Spanish-American War, favorable action was not secured until an Army reorganization bill was under consideration. It included provision for relative rank for nurses, secured favorable congressional action, and was signed by President Wilson (1920). The range was from second lieutenant to major. (Doctors, who were commissioned officers, began as first lieutenants.) Julia C. Stimson, superintendent of the ANC and dean of the Army School of Nursing (succeeding Miss Goodrich), was the first woman to wear the gold leaves of a major.

Relative rank was a compromise. It did not give nurses pay schedules and travel allowances equivalent to those of commissioned officers. But it did give them status and more clearly defined their areas of responsibility. Never again, for example, could a soldier-patient willfully refuse needed medication because "I don't have to mind you. You are not a lieutenant!" Not all members of the regular Corps had approved the effort to secure rank, but it was generally conceded that the status of its members had been improved both professionally and socially.[2] Following the war, both services were made more attractive by opportunities for interested and qualified members to take postgraduate courses in nursing and related subjects without cost to themselves.

Much of the actual nursing service required by the Navy, both on ships and in hospitals, is given by hospital corpsmen. Navy nurses are assigned as instructors to the schools in which preliminary courses are given corpsmen, and members of the Navy Nurse Corps (NNC) are responsible for the teaching and supervision of the men when they are assigned to hospital nursing services. By 1924 the schools for hospital corpsmen at Norfolk, Virginia, and Mare Island, California, had been accredited by the boards of nurse examiners of those states. Nurses were also teaching in schools of nursing for native women established under Navy auspices in the Virgin Islands, Samoa, and Guam.

---

[2] Commissioned rank for the duration of World War II and six months thereafter was granted members of both the Army and Navy Nurse Corps in February, 1944; permanent status was secured in 1947.

The oldest federal hospital service was established on a prepayment basis in 1798 to care for sick and disabled seamen. This Marine Hospital Service is a unit of the USPHS which, in 1918, arranged for Lucy Minnigerode, then on the national staff of the Red Cross, to make a study of the nursing service. With one exception, the hospitals were staffed by men "nurses" who could more accurately have been designated attendants. Miss Minnigerode was a Bellevue graduate, a woman of commanding presence and some administrative experience. Following the study she was appointed superintendent of nurses. Early in the following year the US Public Health Service was authorized to furnish medical service to veterans in addition to its responsibility for the marine hospitals. The nursing service organized by Miss Minnigerode had grown to a total of 1800 nurses by 1922, when the care of veterans was again transferred, this time to the jurisdiction of the new Veterans Bureau (later designated Veterans Administration). This left the nursing service of the hospital division of the US Public Health Service with 310 nurses to care for the patients in 24 marine hospitals having a total capacity of 3000 beds; for service in dispensaries and for participation in studies made under the auspices of the service. Since 1921, the USPHS has also operated the National Leprosarium at Carville, which was purchased from the state of Louisiana. The Sisters of Charity (St. Vincent de Paul), who had operated the institution for the state, accepted transfer and these Sisters, who are graduate nurses, have continued to provide the nursing service. The order also provides dietitians and other trained personnel. In 1930, nurses of the hospital division of the USPHS successfully pioneered in the development of nursing services in federal prisons where drug addiction was a major problem. A school of nursing that attracted unusually well-qualified students was established by Emma L. Nichols (Boston City Hospital) at Ft. McHenry early in 1922. Two classes had been admitted and a third accepted when the school was transferred, along with 57 hospitals, to the Veterans Bureau. It was hoped that the school might be returned to the jurisdiction of the USPHS but it was closed. The students were transferred, with full credit, to the Army School of Nursing in the autumn of 1922.

The nursing service of the Veterans Bureau was organized by Mary A. Hickey, who had been Miss Minnigerode's assistant. It began in 1921 with a nucleus of 300 nurses who were caring for ex-servicemen then receiving training provided by the Federal Board of Vocational Education. With the transfer of hospitals from the USPHS, the service had approximately 1500 nurses doing institutional work, and 400 public health nurses doing follow-up work throughout the country. Legislative efforts to have the new services given status comparable to that of the Army and Navy Nurse Corps failed. They were, therefore, essentially civilian services. No standards for the organization and administration of large all-graduate staffs had ever been set up by the profession. The Veterans Bureau had a high percentage of tuberculosis and neuropsychiatric patients; therefore, it was seriously handicapped by the acute shortage of nurses with experience in those fields. Courses in these specialties were developed in some of the veterans hospitals and at the government's St. Elizabeth's Hospital (for mental patients) in Washington. An advisory committee of ten outstanding nurses, including the presidents of the three national nursing organizations, was organized to work with the Medical Council of the bureau. This committee recommended that a staff education program be inaugurated. A conference of all the chief nurses and the introduction of the staff education program helped to stabilize the service which was made up largely of ex-service nurses.

The Indian Service had established its first hospital in 1885, but there was no supervised nursing service until after the war. Then the ARC, on request, provided three well-qualified public health nurses to study the care provided by the service. One made a survey of a large southwestern area; the others worked for longer periods on selected reservations. One of the three, Elinor Gregg, a sister of Dr. Alan Gregg and a graduate of the Waltham School, developed a constructive program on Rosebud Reservation in South Dakota. She was appointed in 1924 to reorganize and supervise the service of field nurses and field matrons for the Indian Bureau. As trachoma, tuberculosis, and other communicable diseases were prevalent, the service required both institutional and public health nurses.

The organization of the three new services promptly brought the subject of civil-service status for institutional nurses into the foreground of professional thinking. Under the classification act of 1923 nurses were placed in a subprofessional class. More than twenty years elapsed before the ANA could announce that its repeated efforts to have nurses classified as professional persons had been successful.

BIBLIOGRAPHY

Blanchfield, Florence A., and Standlee, Mary W.: *Organized Nursing and the Army in Three Wars.* Unpublished manuscript on file, Historical Division, Office of the Surgeon General of the Army, Washington, D.C.

Bowman, J. Beatrice: "The Navy Nurse Corps and Its Relation to the Advancement of Nursing Education," *Proceedings of the Twenty-fourth Convention of the American Nurses' Association,* 1924.

———: "The History and Development of the Navy Nurse Corps," *Am. J. Nursing,* **25**:356, 1925.

———: "History of Nursing in the Navy," *U.S. Naval M. Bull.,* Jan., 1928, p. 123.

Gregg, Elinor D.: "Nursing Service of the Indian Bureau," *Am. J. Nursing,* **25**:643, 1925.

Handbook of the Hospital Corps. US Navy, US Government Printing Office, Washington, D.C., 1939.

Hickey, Mary A.: "The Present Nursing Service of the U.S. Veterans Bureau and What the Veterans Bureau Is Doing for Disabled Ex-Service Nurses," *Proceedings of the Twenty-fourth Convention of the American Nurses' Association,* 1924, pp. 83–89.

———: "Nursing Service of the U.S. Veterans Bureau," *Am. J. Nursing,* **25**:546, 1925.

———: "Staff Education for Nurses in United States Veterans Bureau Hospitals,*" Am. J. Nursing,* **29**:1420, 1929.

Holcomb, Richmond C.: *A Century with the Norfolk Navy Hospital, 1830–1930.* Printcraft Publishing Co., Portsmouth, Va., 1930.

Kline, I. Grace DeWitt: "Hospital Corpsmen of the Navy," *Am. J. Nursing,* **21**:226, 1921.

McCrady, Anna Grace: "National Soldiers' Homes," *Proceedings of the Twenty-fourth Convention of the American Nurses' Association,* 1924, pp. 71–73.

Minnigerode, Lucy: "Classification of Nurses in Government Service," *Am. J. Nursing,* **24**:835, 1924.

———: "The United States Public Health Service," *Am. J. Nursing,* **25**:454, 1925.

———: "Nursing in Federal Prisons," *Am. J. Nursing,* **31**:1056, 1931.

Noyes, Clara D.: "Red Cross Nursing Assistance to Indian Bureau," *Am. J. Nursing,* **23**:207, 1923.

———: "The Relation of the Red Cross Nursing Service to the Government Nursing Services," *Proceedings of the Twenty-fourth Convention of the American Nurses' Association,* 1924, pp. 73–78.

"Nurse Positions Now Classified in the Professional Service by U.S. Civil Service Commission," *Am. J. Nursing,* **46**:561, 1946.

Nursing and Nursing Education in the United States. Report of the Committee for the Study of Nursing Education and Report of a Survey by Josephine Goldmark. The Macmillan Company, New York, 1923.

"Rank for Nurses Achieved," *Am. J. Nursing,* **20**:867, 1920.

Read, Katharine S.: "Nursing in the United States Public Health Service," Supplement 176, *Pub. Health Rep.,* 1944, p. 200.

Sister Martha and Sister Catherine, "The National Leper Home," *Am. J. Nursing,* **24**:795, 1924.

Stimson, Julia C.: "The Army Nursing Service as One of the Educational Functions of the Medical Department," *Proceedings of the Twenty-fourth Convention of the American Nurses' Association,* 1924, pp. 89–95.

———: "Concerning the Army Nurse Corps," *Am. J. Nursing,* **25**:280, 1925.

Stimson, Julia C., and associates: *History and Manual of the Army Nurse Corps.* Medical Field Service School, Carlisle Barracks, Pa., Oct. 1, 1937.

Williams, Ralph Chester: *The United States Public Health Service 1798–1950.* Published by the Commissioned Officers Association of the United States Public Health Service, Box 5874, Bethesda, Md., 1951.

Chapter 19

FACT-FINDING STUDIES OF NURSING
AND NURSING EDUCATION

They [the hospital schools of nursing] share that spirit of devotion and service which has for half a century been the distinction and the legitimate pride of the training schools for nurses; they share also in varying degree the lack of standards and of independent organization, the inadequacy of teaching and equipment, and the exploitation of students, which has been too often accepted in lieu of education.[1]

THE INDIFFERENCE of young people to nursing as a career, the sudden demand for an enormously increased number of public health nurses, and the new government services created a serious shortage of nurses in the immediate postwar period. They were not at first recognized as three parts of one problem because in public health nursing the service of students could not be substituted for that of graduate nurses. The first part of the problem drew attention to the authoritarian discipline and other undesirable conditions in the schools; the second and third focused attention on preparation for practice as graduate nurses in relation to community and federal needs. Thoughtful people began making determined efforts to secure facts about nursing. Concurrently with the studies which are discussed in this chapter, the functions and relationships of public health nurses which were being assessed in a variety of health demonstrations are left to a later chapter for a fuller discussion. Two significant local studies of nursing preceded the two national studies with which we are here concerned.

Cleveland, long noted for cooperative action in the fields of nursing and health, led off with a comprehensive hospital and health

[1] "Nursing," Part IX, *Cleveland Hospital and Health Survey.* Cleveland Hospital Council, 1920, p. 709.

survey which was made by Josephine Goldmark under the direction of Dr. Haven Emerson and published in 1920. Among other weaknesses this study pointed out the serious inadequacy of housing facilities provided for student nurses, a problem by no means limited to Cleveland. It was one against which the state boards of nurse examiners had been able to make little headway. General recognition of inadequate housing and lack of instructional facilities, which were serious handicaps to the recruitment of students, resulted in a wave of building across the country. The decade is notable for the construction of nurses' residences by a considerable number of well-known schools. The inclusion of libraries and classroom suites in these dormitories was a significant step in the evolution of nursing education. The handsome buildings were tangible evidence of the prosperous state of the nation and of a growing recognition of the importance of the schools. Improved living conditions helped to attract desirable candidates.

In 1922, the New York Academy of Medicine published a preliminary report of its nursing section's survey of New York hospitals.[2] This study is significant because it included the first recorded time study of institutional nursing. It uncovered the deeply entrenched but generally unacknowledged hospital practice of permitting far more orders to be written for nursing procedures than could be executed properly by the available nursing staffs. This habitual failure of the administrators of nursing services and of hospitals to bring this anomaly to the attention of the boards of trustees has undoubtedly been responsible for more poor nursing and lowered nursing morale than any other weakness in American nursing. The study also discloses the fact that not one of the 52 schools in greater New York could produce figures to show whether the school was an economic asset or a liability to the hospital which operated it. This failure to distinguish between nursing school and nursing service was by no means unique. A committee of the NLNE found it to be true also of 100 schools carefully selected for study on the basis of geographic location and other criteria.

[2] Lewinski-Corwin, E. H.: "The Hospital Nursing Situation," *Am. J. Nursing,* **22**:603, 1922.

As demands for public health nurses increased, two questions were hotly debated: Should public health nurses give bedside care? If not, why should they be required to take the full undergraduate course before preparing for public health nursing? The Rockefeller Foundation, which had been giving some financial assistance to NOPHN, called a conference for discussion of these questions late in 1918. A committee to study public health nursing education was appointed with Dr. C.-E. A. Winslow, professor of public health at Yale, as chairman. This committee quickly discovered that the problems of nursing and nursing education relating to the care of the sick, and to the prevention of disease, formed one essential whole and must be so considered if sound conclusions were to be reached. The committee was expanded and renamed the Committee for the Study of Nursing Education. The report of the committee, with the study on which it is based,[3] still stands as a beacon in the field of nursing education. At mid-century it was still the only broad-scale study based on *firsthand observation* of nurses at work as public health nurses and as teachers and administrators of nursing schools. The list of 23 schools and 49 public health nursing agencies selected for intensive study was believed to include representative examples of all types in each field. A small study of private duty nursing was included to round out the report. The methodology of the superb Cleveland survey was adapted for use in the larger study.

Public health nurses should first be nurses, that is, graduates of a basic course in nursing, before securing the special preparation in both the classroom and field work that is necessary for the practice of public health nursing. This was the decisive answer to the original question which had brought the committee into being. It was generally accepted by all interested groups; not so, the other recommendations of the committee. They are still, at mid-century, a challenge to the profession and to the nurse-employing public. (See Appendix II.)

The structure and objectives of most nursing schools bore no

---

[3] *Nursing and Nursing Education in the United States,* Report of the Committee for the Study of Nursing Education and Report of a Survey by Josephine Goldmark. The Macmillan Company, New York, 1923.

resemblance to educational institutions. This, the committee found, was the chief reason for the lack of adequate numbers of desirable candidates. The basic problem was stated as follows:

Until the general public by taxation for public institutions, by endowments and gifts for those privately supported, makes the hospital independent of the school for its permanent nursing staff, the hospital must continue its paradoxical attempt to maintain a school without means; the school in its turn must remain in part at least crippled by work in excess of any possible educational program.[4]

And so the committee and Miss Goldmark, who made the study, were confronted by the problem of finance on which Miss Nutting had been speaking and writing for at least a decade. The financing of hospital nursing services is one thing; the financing of nursing schools, as the report makes clear, should be quite another. The committee concluded that endowments for schools of nursing operated under boards or committees, organized especially for that purpose, and the shortening of the course from three years to 28 months by the elimination of noneducational and repetitive services, were measures which must be taken if schools were to attract adequate numbers of desirable students. The committee advocated the preparation and licensure of subsidiary workers for the care of specified types of patients. Emphasis was placed on special preparation, beyond the basic course, for administrators and teachers in nursing schools, and for public health nurses. The development and strengthening of university schools of nursing were considered to be of fundamental importance to the upgrading of nursing with special reference to the preparation of those who might become leaders in the field. But the traditions and fiscal policies of hospitals were not easily changed. Therein lay the crux of the problem. Assuming that the schools reported on in the New York study were typical, hospitals generally had no useful data on the financing of their schools. When the report was published, the AHA was on the eve of publishing its first manual on hospital accounting. But almost twenty years elapsed before that association and the NLNE began collaborating on the development of a method for ascertaining the

[4] *Ibid.*, p. 34.

costs of nursing education and nursing service, but, at mid-century, no generally acceptable method had been developed.

The conclusions, or recommendations, of the committee were presented in advance of publication at a meeting of the NLNE in 1922. They were subsequently well publicized in the magazines of the profession and other publications. Members of the committee were much in demand as speakers at nursing and hospital meetings. But the functions and influence of public relations programs were not then generally understood. Neither broad-scale preliminary publicity nor an organized follow-up was planned in connection with the publication of the report. Hospitals were disaffected by the emphasis on university affiliations and the recommendations for shortening the basic course. The report, therefore, was not as effectively used as had been anticipated. There were, however, some important and immediate results.

The Rockefeller Foundation financed a five-year experiment in methods of educating nurses at Yale University. It was so successful that an endowment of $1,000,000 was provided at the end of the experimental period to ensure the permanency of the school. It required the broad experience, the dynamic leadership, the profound convictions, the flashing personality, and the courage of Annie W. Goodrich to establish a school of nursing on a campus where, for over two hundred years, the undergraduate education of men had been the sole prerogative. The student body did not hesitate to express its disdain of the feminine invasion. But President Angell stood staunchly behind the experiment. Dean Milton C. Winternitz of the medical school was so cooperatively and constructively interested in the development of the school that Miss Goodrich, a quarter of a century later, said that he "opened wide to the nurse the doors of knowledge, so that she might go forth, scientifically and culturally prepared, to take her place in the health program."[5] Dr. Winslow, as a member of the Yale faculty, was a wise counselor and stalwart friend. The New Haven Hospital provided most of the

[5] Goodrich, Annie W.: "An Attempt to Interpret a Great Scientist's Contribution to Humanity Through Medicine and Nursing," *Yale J. Biol. Med.*, **22**:605, 1950.

clinical services required by the new school. The Connecticut Training School, which had pioneered there in 1873, made way for it. Members of the last class received their diplomas at the same ceremony in 1926 at which Yale granted the degree of bachelor of nursing to two graduates of the school which had succeeded it.[6]

To complete that story, it may be said the Yale School of Nursing has long since demonstrated that comprehensive preparation for nursing can be given to mature, well-educated students in less than three years, provided the school exists as a school and not as a service agency. By 1950 Yale had graduated more than 1000 nurses. Their records disprove the rather widely held opinion that the graduates of collegiate schools are interested in leadership positions to the exclusion of the practice of nursing. One-fourth of those in active practice were doing "bedside nursing" as staff or private duty nurses. Many were holding strategic positions throughout the US and in other countries. At the end of its first quarter century, the school was demonstrably fulfilling its mission to prepare nurses who were "scientifically informed, socially experienced and technically expert."

To return to the postwar period of World War I. The Rockefeller Foundation had a long-standing interest in community health in the Southern states which had begun with a campaign in the early part of the century to eradicate hookworm disease. The reorganization of the Vanderbilt University Medical School and the construction of a new hospital in connection with it made Vanderbilt at Nashville, Tennessee, a logical choice for a second experiment (announced in 1925) in nursing education. Here again the success of the experimental period begun in 1930 under the brilliant direction of Shirley C. Titus was rewarded by a million-dollar endowment.

The endowed Western Reserve University School of Nursing (1923) has a quite different history. The "university idea" was germinating in Cleveland before either the report of the Cleveland survey or that of the Committee for the Study of Nursing Education had been published. The survey strongly urged that a university school of nursing be established at the earliest possible date. Western Reserve had become interested in nursing education when plans

[6] Yale has awarded the degree of master of nursing since 1937.

for the Vassar camp were announced. As previously noted, it provided a preliminary course for the students of local schools in the summer of 1918. The report of the survey caused interested lay women to press for further action, and Mrs. Frances Payne Bolton notified the university of her readiness to contribute one-half of the million dollars required by the university for the establishment of a school on a parity with other professional schools. Carolyn E. Gray, widely known for her revision of Kimber's *Anatomy,* was the first dean. The nursing schools of the Maternity and Lakeside hospitals were absorbed in the larger program. These hospitals, plus the Babies' and Children's, provided the clinical practice fields. By 1928, when the "probationary" period was over, the school of nursing had become firmly entrenched in the university, and Mrs. Bolton's endowment had increased to $1,500,000. In honor of her unflagging interest and her munificent contributions to it, the school was named the Frances Payne Bolton School of Nursing.

While these three endowed schools were undertaking a complete integration of the social and health aspects of nursing in the basic course, it must not be forgotten that other universities had begun to open their doors more or less widely to nursing. Miss Goldmark reported 18 colleges and universities which were offering the combined academic and professional course of four or, more frequently, five years. Ten of them were state or municipal universities. They had not, however, discontinued their three-year programs, and a majority of their students were enrolled in them.

Progress was also being made in the field of education for graduate nurses. By the end of the decade, the NOPHN had approved 11 collegiate programs in public health nursing. The board of directors of the proudly independent Illinois Training School (ITS) was finding it increasingly difficult to meet advancing standards of nursing education without a large endowment. It was decided that "the I.T.S. could best fulfill its ideals and aspirations by close affiliation with a university of first rank."[7] The undergraduate school was dis-

---

[7] Schryver, Grace Fay: *A History of the Illinois Training School for Nurses, 1880–1929.* Published by the board of directors of the Illinois Training School for Nurses, Chicago, 1930, Chap. X, p. 152.

continued and students transferred to the new Cook County School of Nursing. The assets of the ITS, valued at one-half million dollars, were transferred to the University of Chicago (1926). The program developed there under the leadership of Nellie X. Hawkinson, first professor of nursing education on the Illinois Training School for Nurses Foundation, quickly achieved high rank as a center for preparation for faculty and administrative positions in nursing schools and nursing services.

In the far West, to meet the need for better prepared faculty personnel, the professional organizations of California (1925) persuaded the state legislature to take the steps necessary to free surplus funds in the Bureau of Registration of Nurses and to establish a Foundation in Nursing Education at the University of California. Mary May Pickering became assistant professor of nursing education January 1, 1927. This program and one previously established in public health nursing were later combined under one director. In Virginia the state nurses' association took the initiative and raised the funds necessary to provide a center for the preparation of graduate nurses for faculty positions. The Sadie Heath Cabaniss Department of Nursing, named in honor of one of the state's pioneer nurses, was established at the University of Virginia in 1927.

Following Miss Nutting's report of its education committee in 1911, the NLNE had unavailingly endeavored to secure foundation interest in a comprehensive study of nursing education. As has been shown, committees of the AHA and the national nursing organizations had spent considerable time, without adopting a course of action, on the general subject of grading nursing schools. Following World War I, the League began working persistently on ways and means for sorting out meritorious schools from the heterogenous mass of over 2000 "training schools." It was agreed, however, that such efforts should be held in abeyance while the Winslow-Goldmark study was under way. In the meantime participants in the postwar national recruitment program, which was sponsored by the nursing organizations and the ARC, were seriously handicapped by lack of information about the schools. Intelligent candidates quite naturally wanted more information than the meager fact that a

school was on the approved list of a state board of examiners, or
that its graduates were eligible for Red Cross enrollment. Following
the publication of the Winslow-Goldmark report, the League committee again set to work to secure the interest and financial support
of other organizations in a program for grading schools of nursing.

Finally in 1925 a program was approved by the three national
nursing organizations, and funds were allocated for the initial stage
of a study. The next step was to secure the interest of other organizations assumed to be concerned with the quality and availability of
nursing service. It was found that a committee of the American
Medical Association had a somewhat similar plan under advisement.
After a series of preliminary conferences, the Committee on the
Grading of Nursing Schools was organized as an antonomous body
early in 1926. Of its 21 members, 14 represented national organizations, including the three nursing organizations, the American Medical Association, American College of Surgeons, American Hospital
Association, and the American Public Health Association. Of seven
members at large, four were educators who made substantial contributions to the thinking of the committee. Despite their devotion
to tradition, nurses generally responded wholeheartedly to the proposal for a searching nationwide analysis of nursing. The non-nurse
members of the committee were amazed by the generous spirit in
which individual nurses and nursing organizations contributed to
the financial support of the program. Chancellor Capen (University
of Buffalo) stated that: "Equally self-sacrificing devotion to a great
public cause has perhaps never been shown by any other profession."[8] When the work was completed, it was found that the profession had provided almost one-half of a budget that approximated
$300,000. The remainder had come from foundations and from Mrs.
Bolton and other friends of nursing.

Dr. William Darrach, a representative of the American Medical
Association, was elected chairman of the committee. When the
AMA withdrew from the study (the reason for withdrawal was not

---

[8] Bachmeyer, A. C., and Hartman, Gerhard (eds.): *The Hospital in Modern
Society;* Capen, Samuel P., "Who is Concerned with the Reform of Nursing
Education?" The Commonwealth Fund, New York, 1943, Chap. VII, p. 156.

made clear) Dr. Darrach was re-elected. May Ayres Burgess, a statistician who had been generously helpful with a study of private duty nursing in New York State, was chosen to direct the study. The purpose of the five-year program adopted by the committee, which ultimately covered an eight-year period, was far broader than anything previously proposed by those desirous of securing a classified list of schools. The committee conceived its function to be "the study of ways and means for insuring an ample supply of nursing service, of whatever type and quality is needed for adequate care of the patient, at a price within his reach."[9] On the basis of this broad platform of purpose, the committee planned three major projects: (1) a study of supply and demand for nursing service, (2) a job analysis, and (3) the grading of nursing schools.

It was agreed that decisive action toward grading the schools could not be taken until the committee had the answers to two questions. Was the country still suffering from a nursing shortage? Was the kind of nurse the hospitals wanted also the kind of nurse the public wanted? Questionnaires were used to secure information from doctors, hospitals, registries, patients, and from nurses in the three major categories, namely, institutional, public health, and private duty nursing.

The replies to those questions, based on data obtained from thousands of questionnaires, astounded many people including some of the members of the committee. At the very height of national prosperity, many private duty nurses were unemployed! That first study, reported in *Nurses, Patients, and Pocketbooks*,[10] presented incontrovertible proof that there were "too many but too few" nurses to meet the nation's needs. There were far more nurses than could be employed under existing conditions; there were too few of all types who could adequately meet the requirements of employers.

All schools were invited to participate in the grading studies. The response was overwhelming. To the astonishment of the staff, 74 per

[9] Burgess, May Ayres: *A Five-Year Program for the Committee on the Grading of Nursing Schools*. Committee on the Grading of Nursing Schools, New York, 1926, p. 10.

[10] Burgess, May Ayres: *Nurses, Patients, and Pocketbooks*. Committee on the Grading of Nursing Schools, New York, 1928, pp. 54–55.

cent of the schools accredited by the state boards (approximately 1500) participated in the first grading and 81 per cent in the second. No other profession had ever tried to cope with an accreditation program of such magnitude.

Two methods for making the surveys were considered: by visitation or by the statistical method. The cost of the first, for such a large number of schools, was believed to be far beyond the resources of the committee. The statistical method of collecting and interpreting information was therefore adopted. The items selected for study were, however, of varying degrees of importance. It has often been said that the Grading Committee did not grade the schools. Each school was graded on each item, in relation to all other schools, in 1929 and again in 1932. Every participating school received, therefore, two reports which showed its standing, item by item, in relation to all other schools, but *they were not classified.* The reports were superb examples of the graphic technics then coming into use by statisticians. But study and interpretation of them called for far more time and thought than many recipients cared to give. Many principals of schools found themselves in possession of three reports, viz., those addressed to the president of the board of trustees, to the administrator of the hospital, and her own. However, some schools made effective use of the reports, and many state boards of nurse examiners welcomed the summarized data they received about the schools under their jurisdiction.

A classified list of schools, so greatly desired by vocational and other advisors, was not made. The committee decided that, on the basis of the data available, any possible list would be unjust to some schools regardless of their quality. In the light of the reaction to the publication of the "School Data Analysis" at mid-century the decision of the Grading Committee seems to have been the height of wisdom. It was announced in the AJN, but through an oversight, under a caption which was not sufficiently descriptive of the content of the article. It failed to attract the widespread attention it merited.[11]

[11] Capen, S. P.: "A Member of the Grading Committee Speaks," *Am. J. Nursing,* 32:307, 1932.

There were marked but not spectacular evidences of improvement between the first and second gradings. Lacking a classified list, it had not been possible to bring the full weight of public opinion to bear on the evidence of a need for improvement. Then, too, the economic depression was dealing a staggering blow to hospitals and nursing schools. It is impossible to single out the specific influence of the Grading Committee's work or to apportion credit to the two phases of its program. It seems probable that the continuous release of vivid, well-illustrated, and informative material, through professional and other media, month after month throughout the life of the committee, did more to raise the general level of nursing education than the carefully detailed reports to the schools. The nursing organizations and the state boards based programs on data provided by the committee. The ANA, for example, immediately followed up the first report on ineffective methods of distributing nursing service by making a field study of the organization of professionally sponsored registries. For many nurses the fact that remained in memory after the stock market crash was the committee's revelation of the paradox that there were "too many but too few" nurses when the nation was at the peak of prospertity, i.e., a plethora of nurses but too few who were adequately prepared for the work required of them. The program of the committee was terminated with the publication in 1934 of *An Activity Analysis of Nursing* and a final report *Nursing Schools Today and Tomorrow*. The recommendations of the committee included the following:

In order to uphold and strengthen the National League of Nursing Education in its work, which is of basic importance to all scientific, social, and economic groups having need of nursing service, it is recommended by the Grading Committee that the National League of Nursing Education press its project of developing a permanent Advisory Council in Nursing Education on which would be represented the groups most closely concerned with nursing education, viz., nursing, medicine, public health, representatives of institutions of higher education, hospitals, and the public.

Since the relation of economic and social change to the development of nursing is daily becoming more apparent, it is further suggested that consideration be given to representation from the fields of economics and sociology. The function of such a Council would be advisory and not administrative.[12]

The NLNE undertook the implementation of the other recommendations of the committee but it did not organize an advisory council.

BIBLIOGRAPHY

Baumann, Elaine A.: "What Yale Graduates Are Doing," *Am. J. Nursing*, **51**:167, 1951.

Burgess, May Ayres: *Nurses, Patients, and Pocketbooks*. Report of a Study of the Economics of Nursing Conducted by the Committee on the Grading of Nursing Schools, New York, 1928.

Faddis, Margene O.: *The History of the Frances Payne Bolton School of Nursing*. Western Reserve University Press, Cleveland, Ohio, 1948.

Geister, Janet M.: "Hearsay and Facts in Private Duty," *Am. J. Nursing*, **26**:515, 1926.

Goodrich, Annie W.: "A Description of the Yale University School of Nursing," *The Social and Ethical Significance of Nursing*. The Macmillan Company, New York, 1932, p. 335.

———: "Yale University School of Nursing," *Methods and Problems of Medical Education* (Twenty-first Series). The Rockefeller Foundation, New York, 1932, p. 1.

Guyot, Sister Henrietta: *A Preliminary Study of the Status of Nursing Education in the State University*. Catholic University of America, Washington, D.C., 1937.

Hawkinson, Nellie X.: "Western Reserve School of Nursing," *Methods and Problems of Medical Education* (Twenty-first Series). The Rockefeller Foundation, New York, 1932, p. 55.

The Hospital Situation in Greater New York, a study made for the Public Relations Committee of the New York Academy of Medicine. G. P. Putnam's Sons, New York, 1924.

Jammé, Anna C.: "A Foundation in Nursing Education at the University of California," *Am. J. Nursing*, **26**:965, 1926.

Johns, Ethel, and Pfefferkorn, Blanche: *An Activity Analysis of Nursing*. Committee on the Grading of Nursing Schools, New York, 1934.

Logan, Laura R.: "Distinguished Alliance and Gift for Nursing Education," *Am. J. Nursing*, **26**:635, 1926.

Nursing and Nursing Education in the United States, Report of the Com-

[12] *Nursing Schools—Today and Tomorrow*. Committee on the Grading of Nursing Schools, New York, 1934, p. 252.

mittee for the Study of Nursing Education and Report of a Survey by Josephine Goldmark. The Macmillan Company, New York, 1923.

Nursing Schools Today and Tomorrow. Final Report of the Committee on the Grading of Nursing Schools, New York, 1934, p. 17.

Pfefferkorn, Blanche, and Rovetta, Charles A. (directors of study sponsored by the American Hospital Association, Chicago, and the National League of Nursing Education, New York): *Administrative Cost Analysis for Nursing Service and Nursing Education,* 1940.

Randolph, Agnes D.: "Virginia's Chair of Nursing," *Am. J. Nursing,* 27:33, 1927.

"Sub-Committee Report on the Cost of Nursing Education," *Twenty-eighth Annual Report of the National League of Nursing Education,* 1922, p. 93.

Titus, Shirley C.: "Factors Determining the Development of Nursing and Schools of Nursing" (with special reference to Vanderbilt University School of Nursing, Nashville, Tennessee), *Methods and Problems of Medical Education* (Twenty-first Series). The Rockefeller Foundation, New York, 1932, p. 63.

Chapter 20

CHANGING EMPHASIS IN
PUBLIC HEALTH NURSING

Public Health is the science and the art of preventing disease, prolonging life and promoting physical and mental health and efficiency through organized community efforts for the sanitation of the environment, the control of community infections, the education of the individual in principles of personal hygiene, the organization of medical and nursing service for the early diagnosis and treatment of disease and the development of the social machinery which will ensure to every individual in the community a standard of living adequate for the maintenance of health.

C.-E. A. WINSLOW[1]

UNLIKE the nursing schools which were introduced into unrelated institutions with long-standing traditions, public health nursing had been in on the ground floor of the public health movement that gained tremendous momentum in the decade following World War I. So important had its contributions been that the following statement, attributed to Dr. William H. Welch, was widely quoted: "America has made two unique contributions to medicine—the Panama Canal and the public health nurse."[2] The US Public Health Service and voluntary agencies such as the American Public Health Association, the American Child Health Association, and the National Tuberculosis Association[3] participated in surveys and in health demonstrations which were financed by the Metropolitan Life Insurance Company and a number of philanthropic foundations. The pioneer health demonstration which was launched at

[1] Winslow, C.-E. A.: *The Evolution and Significance of the Modern Public Health Campaign.* Yale University Press, New Haven, 1923.
[2] *Recent Social Trends in the United States* (Report of the President's Research Committee in Social Trends). McGraw-Hill Book Co., New York, 1933, p. 1090.
[3] Then the National Association for the Study and Prevention of Tuberculosis.

190

Framingham, Massachusetts, just before the US entered World War I, was financed by the MLI and conducted by the NTA.

Those responsible for the earlier studies found it difficult to appraise public health nursing because of what one of the studies described as its helter-skelter development. A study made for the APHA and the USPHS (1920) states that the usually accepted estimate of a reasonably adequate public health nursing service calls for 50 nurses per 100,000 population. It was found that 80 of the largest cities averaged only 16.5 public health nurses to each 100,000 population. The activities of public and private agencies overlapped to an extraordinary degree, and there were wide divergencies of opinion as to the functions of public health nurses. The study made under the auspices of a committee of which Dr. C.-E. A. Winslow was chairman, reported: ". . . a growing tendency to concentrate public health nursing more completely in the hands of the official health agencies of the community and this is a sound and wise tendency . . . the ideal type of public health nursing is that which combines instruction and bedside care in the generalized district plan. . . ."[4]

At the time, the major nonofficial agencies which were promoting the use of public health nursing services were the visiting nurse associations, the ARC, state tuberculosis associations which specialized in their own field but sometimes provided generalized nursing or school nursing, and the MLI. The development of county health departments, in which the USPHS and the International Health Board of the Rockefeller Foundation were interested, stimulated the employment of nurses by these official agencies.

Records of the rapid expansion of public health nursing following World War I convey a sense of sustained drive and enthusiasm which had repercussions in the field of nursing education. It sharpened the awareness of both public health nurses and nurse educators to the need for sound basic programs on which courses in pub-

[4] Winslow, C.-E. A., and Burkhardt, Margaret: "Report of the Committee on Municipal Health Department Practice of the American Public Health Association in Cooperation with the U.S. Public Health Service," *Public Health Nursing*, US Public Health Bulletin, No. 136. US Government Printing Office, Washington, D.C., 1923, p. 153.

lic health nursing for graduate nurses could be superimposed. Three postwar programs had a lasting influence on the development of public health nursing. They were: (1) the extensive peacetime health program of the ARC at home and abroad which made that agency for a time the largest employer of nurses in the world, (2) the Children's Bureau Maternal and Infancy Program of 1921–1929, and (3) the several health demonstrations which were sponsored by foundations and other agencies. How the NOPHN, in the midst of so much activity, became firmly established in a position of leadership is described in the next chapter.

When the ARC launched its peacetime health program, fearless and statesmanlike Elizabeth G. Fox had succeeded Mary S. Gardner as director of the Bureau of Public Health Nursing. The *Public Health Nurse* magazine promptly agreed to a suggestion that a Department of Red Cross Public Health Nursing would be helpful. This was a strategic move. In a period when the areas of responsibility of official and nonofficial agencies were being defined and standards of work were being formulated it was important, as Miss Fox pointed out, for all public health nurses to be informed of the extensive activities of the Red Cross. The policies were clearly stated. The Red Cross would supplement but not supplant the work of legitimate health agencies and it looked toward the time when public health nursing would be conducted as a public service by municipalities, counties, or states. This involved many complicated relationships. "The object everywhere," wrote Miss Fox, "was to obtain the best possible coordination of state activities for the purpose of developing public health nursing in the state according to a single plan; . . ."[5] In some states, the ARC arranged for the supervisors of public health nursing in the state departments of health to function also as state supervisors of Red Cross public health nursing, the ARC financing the position. In 1921 state tuberculosis associations had supervisory nurses in 28 states, the ARC in 31. In 29 states the state board of health had a director or supervisor of public health nursing or of the division of child hygiene.

[5] "The Development of the Red Cross Bureau of Public Health Nursing," *The Public Health Nurse*, 12:180, 1920.

At the beginning of 1919 less than 100 nursing services were under the direction of the ARC. At the height of the boom in Red Cross public health nursing in 1922 there were over 1200. This amazing expansion was due to the existence of the nationwide network of ARC chapters with abruptly terminated wartime programs, the generosity with which the American people had poured money into the treasury of the ARC, and the demonstrable need for public health services in smaller cities and rural areas. It was made possible by the enthusiasm and driving force with which Miss Fox worked with Red Cross and health officials on the one hand and with the directors of public health nursing in the regional divisions of the ARC on the other.

Many ex-service nurses were interested in the service but few of them were qualified for it by either education or experience. Extensive use of scholarships was a partial answer to that problem. In 1919 and 1920 the national Red Cross allocated $100,000 each year, with lesser amounts in successive years, for this purpose. The 250 scholarships made possible by the first grant were supplemented by 150 made available by chapters. A number of institutions of higher education were subsidized by the national Red Cross or by ARC chapters to provide the needed postgraduate courses.

The Town and Country nursing service had been essentially a visiting nurse service with bedside nursing occupying first place on the list of activities reported. No phase of public health nursing was excluded from the new program. Nurses might engage in bedside nursing, prenatal and maternity nursing, infant and child welfare work, school nursing, tuberculosis nursing, communicable disease control, and health education of various sorts. But most of the programs were necessarily restricted to one or two activities. Some of the nurses found that the teaching of classes in "Home Hygiene and Care of the Sick" could be fitted into their programs very effectively. School nursing was most often the entering wedge that aroused an initial interest in broader community health programs.

A guide, *Rural School Nursing*, first published in 1921, was revised at intervals. The preface to the 1925 edition indicates the pioneer nature of the work. Miss Fox wrote:

These procedures are adapted to the circumstances peculiar to rural districts, which confront American Red Cross public health nurses; namely, school nursing as one phase of a general public health nursing problem, school nursing over a large county, school nursing without a medical inspector, school nursing where there are several thousand pupils to one nurse.[6]

The number of services had been reduced to approximately 600 in 1930. This sharp drop was due to a variety of factors. Many nurses, ill-equipped for work calling for initiative, adaptability, and special preparation, had resigned and often could not be replaced. Some chapters had not planned for a continuing service. Some of the services had already been absorbed in broader programs under official agencies. Nurses were giving people in rural areas and small towns a service which won the gratitude of many people as well as the admiration of influential health authorities who had been skeptical about the program in its initial inflationary stages. Some of the nurses working in rugged and isolated areas displayed extraordinary courage and ingenuity in getting to the families in urgent need of their services. Administrative policies in relation to the use of automobiles by nurses became a subject of such local importance that it was freely discussed in *The Public Health Nurse*. Some twenty years later, when the ARC completed its withdrawal from the field of public nursing, it could be said of the ARC public health nurses, "They showed the way."[7]

The passage of the Maternity and Infancy Act (Sheppard-Towner, 1921) is a historic milestone in the evolution of the public health movement and public health nursing. Three years of effort had been required to secure the passage of the act. During that time the findings of studies by the Children's Bureau had been given the widest possible publicity. The significance of the fact that the United States lost over 16,000 mothers in childbirth in 1916 had been driven home by effective use of graphic charts which showed that the United States had a higher maternal death rate than any other principal country except Spain and Switzerland. The program ad-

[6] *Rural School Nursing*, The American Red Cross, Washington, D.C., 1931, p. 5.
[7] *The Red Cross Magazine*, December, 1951, p. 27.

ministered by the Children's Bureau was based on the principle of grants-in-aid from the federal government to the states. Only 33 state agencies had secured legislation that permitted the use of such funds in 1921. By 1929 all but Vermont, the District of Columbia, and Hawaii had secured legislation which included provision, directly or indirectly, for the employment of public health nurses. Marie T. Phelan, an experienced public health nurse who had given distinguished service with the ARC Children's Bureau in France, was appointed consultant nurse in 1923. She was the first nurse to hold a position as consultant under the federal government in peacetime. At the request of state health departments and divisions of child hygiene, she conducted many institutes on maternal and infant care. Miss Phelan was assisted by three field nurses in a program that included participation in studies, nursing demonstrations, and the release of members of her small staff to assist with the development of state programs.

The program created an immediate demand in the states for nurses and other trained workers. Only 5 states were able to establish the requirement that nurses participating in the program should be "fully trained public health nurses," but by 1931, 30 states had devised some method for giving in-service training to employed nurses. Miss Gardner wrote a few years later: "Perhaps the most unique contribution of the United States to public health nursing education is the development of the many forms of continuous staff education carried on by the agencies employing nurses. . . ."[8] All participants in state programs (representatives of private organizations and specialists—pediatricians, nutrition workers, and the like) had attended annual conferences. Nurses, paid in full or in part from maternity and infancy funds, had been assigned to specified areas to work with an established county or other official agency, or to conduct nursing demonstrations. The results of the program in which nurses had such an active part were difficult to measure, but the average maternal death rate, which had been 7.1 maternal deaths per 1000 births in 1915, was reduced to 6.7 for the years between

[8] Gardner, Mary S.: *Public Health Nursing*, 3rd ed. The Macmillan Company, New York, 1936, p. 62.

1925 and 1929. In a final report on the program, the chief of the Children's Bureau noted that *a nurse working alone* had frequently afforded a starting point for the development of a full-time health department.

The demonstration method of forwarding public health was effectively used in the decade 1919–1929. The Community Health and Tuberculosis Demonstration at Framingham, Massachusetts (1917–1923) was already well under way. The Child Health Demonstration sponsored by the ARC and the American Child Health Association at Mansfield, Ohio, was launched in 1922. These and the demonstrations sponsored by the Commonwealth and Milbank funds and other agencies had a far-reaching influence on the development of public health nursing. Nursing was an integral part of the programs, and, because of the volume of service required, a substantial part of each budget was allocated to it. The geographic distribution of the demonstrations is of interest, as health work in every part of the country was influenced by them. The four demonstrations sponsored by the Commonwealth Fund were located in Fargo, North Dakota; Marion County, Oregon; Rutherford County, Tennessee; and in Clarke County, Georgia.

The aim of the Commonwealth demonstrations was "to build up a strong and well-staffed health department functioning in close cooperation with the work of private physicians. From the beginning the nursing program was considered an integral part of the health department organization. All nursing service was completely generalized with each field nurse carrying full responsibility for health center, school and home-visiting activities in a district with about 5000 population and with varying amounts of volunteer assistance."[9] As no two areas had identical resources or health problems, there was necessarily a degree of flexibility in the programs. The report of the Rutherford County demonstration is of special nursing interest. When it began, the city of Murfreesboro and the county covering 600 square miles had only part-time health officers. A single nurse, financed largely by the Red Cross chapter, "was

[9] Winslow, Emma A.: "Service Norms and Their Variations," *Pub. Health Nursing,* **22**:68, 1930.

waging a most admirable, single-handed fight. . . ."[10] She was appointed director of the demonstration nursing service. At the end of the five-year period, Rutherford County had a rural health department with an ample budget provided locally. In cooperation with Vanderbilt University, the health department and the new hospital of Rutherford County became a center for the teaching of nurses and other public health personnel which won an enviable reputation.

The three demonstrations sponsored by the Milbank Memorial Fund were all in the state of New York: in Cattaraugus County, Syracuse, and in the Bellevue-Yorkville section of New York City. The purpose of these demonstrations was to determine whether by the intensive application of known health measures sickness and mortality rates could be substantially reduced at a per capita cost which communities would willingly bear. Here again nursing was an integral part of each program. This was in sharp contrast to the prevailing attitude toward institutional nursing in a period when many hospitals were built without careful preliminary planning for the type of service best suited to their individual needs. Hospitals had antedated modern nursing whereas public health nursing (as visiting nursing) was established before the public health movement began gaining momentum. Each of the health demonstrations added to the sum total of information about the growing field of public health nursing.

The East Harlem Nursing and Health Demonstration has a unique and honored place in the history of nursing. It was launched in 1922 in connection with, but virtually independent of, the East Harlem Health Center which had been established a year earlier through the initiative of the ARC. It was the outgrowth of many experiments in the coordination of health and social services. It was unique in that funds were pooled by four participating service agencies for a common program. The demonstration was so successful that it was reorganized as the East Harlem Nursing and Health Service in 1928. From that time until it was discontinued in 1941, the service

---

[10] Mustard, Harry S.: *Cross-Sections of Rural Health Progress.* The Commonwealth Fund, New York, 1930, pp. 6–7.

provided a field training program for staff workers and public health nursing students. The field teaching service was established in close cooperation with the Department of Nursing Education of Teachers College. The Rockefeller Foundation and other agencies also sent graduate nurse students. The names of Grace L. Anderson and her associate, Mabelle S. Welsh, are imperishably associated with that of the service which gained international renown under their leadership.

The spirit and evolutionary processes which gave the service its unique quality were well illustrated by the nutrition and mental hygiene elements in the program. In the early years correction of defects loomed large as a goal in accomplishment, and intensive work was done in the families of undernourished children by a staff of nutritionists. Year by year the percentage of malnutrition dropped, and the emphasis in health teaching changed from corrective to preventive measures. Nutrition was discontinued as a special service; instead, two nutritionists served as teaching consultants working with and through the nurses and serving as leaders in group work and parent education. The mental hygiene movement had not recognized in the nurse an agent qualified to serve directly in the campaign for the control and prevention of mental disease. The function of mental hygiene supervisors in public health nursing agencies was being studied by the NOPHN and the American Association of Psychiatric Social Workers. Here again, the specialist, the mental hygiene consultant, working through the nurse supervisor, endeavored to help the individual nurse. She also helped the nurse herself with individual families, if the nurse supervisors requested such assistance.

During the demonstration period, many reports and monographs were contributed to the literature of the profession. One of the earliest was based on a comparative study of generalized and specialized nursing in health services.[11] This was one of the most controversial subjects of the period, and the report was widely used. It

[11] *A Comparative Study of Generalized and Specialized Nursing and Health Services,* The East Harlem Nursing and Health Demonstration, New York, 1926.

indicated that there was no demonstrable difference in the quality between the two types of service but there was marked increase in the volume of service that could be given by a generalized staff.

What came out of the study, in addition to the accepted evidence of the greater efficiency of generalization, was a growing appreciation of the essential unity of all health services; a realization that by far the most effective basis for work with younger or older children is that afforded by the maternity service with its beginnings in the prenatal life of the individual; that the nurse's preparation for any type of health work should be grounded on family health service with special emphasis on subject matter pertaining to family life and experience in working with parents.[12]

The literature has been enriched not only by the final reports of the several health demonstrations, the monographs and reports of special studies made during their periods of activity, but also by appraisals, after the lapse of several years, of the permanent values of some of the demonstrations. The phenomenon of the decade 1919–1929, according to Dr. Smillie, "was the beginning of the nationalization of the public health." The voluntary agencies which had pioneered in practically every field of public health beginning with the visiting nurse services, he points out, reached the flood tide of their influence about 1925. Since then, public health has increasingly become a governmental responsibility.[13] As state after state secured enabling legislation which provided for the employment of public health nurses in a variety of capacities, it was clear that in nursing the official agencies were moving toward a position of leadership in public health nursing.

BIBLIOGRAPHY

Anderson, Grace L.: "The Scope and Aim of a Mental Hygiene Program in a Public Health Nursing Association," *Public Health Nurse*, **22**:377, 1930.

[12] *Learning Through Experience in Family Health Work—A Report of Student Participation in the East Harlem Nursing and Health Service Program, 1928–1941.* East Harlem Nursing and Health Service, New York, 1941, p. 15.
[13] Smillie, Wilson G.: *Preventive Medicine and Public Health*, 2nd ed. The Macmillan Company, New York, 1952, p. 10.

A Chapter of Child Health, Report of the Commonwealth Fund Child
   Health Demonstration in Clarke County and Athens, Georgia, 1924–
   1928. The Commonwealth Fund, New York, 1930.
Dublin, Louis I.: *A Forty-Year Campaign against Tuberculosis*. Metro-
   politan Life Insurance Co., New York, 1952.
Dublin, Louis I., and Lotka, Alfred J.: *Twenty-five Years of Health
   Progress*. Metropolitan Life Insurance Co., New York, 1937, p. 350.
Dulles, Foster Rhea: *The American Red Cross, A History*. Harper &
   Brothers New York, 1950, p. 252.
East Harlem Nursing and Health Service, A Progress Report, 1934. New
   York, p. 19.
Five Years in Fargo, Report of the Commonwealth Fund Child Health
   Demonstration in Fargo, North Dakota, 1923–1927. The Common-
   wealth Fund, New York, 1929.
Flagg, Maurice: "They Showed the Way" [Forty Years of the A.R.C.
   public health nursing service which was terminated in 1952], *The Red
   Cross Magazine*, 1:27, 1951.
Fosdick, Raymond B.: *The Story of the Rockefeller Foundation*. Harper
   & Brothers, New York, 1952.
"Health Demonstrations in the United States," Supplement, *Am. J. Pub.
   Health*, Feb., 1927.
Health Survey of 86 Cities. Research Division, American Child Health
   Association, New York, 1925.
Hiscock, Ira V. (ed.): *Community Health Organizations*. The Common-
   wealth Fund, New York, 1932, p. 16.
Kernodle, Portia B.: *The Red Cross Nurse in Action, 1882–1948*. Harper
   & Brothers, New York, 1949, pp. 256–305.
"List of State Supervising Nurses," *The Public Health Nurse*, 14:36, 1922.
McIver, Pearl: "Rural Public Health Nursing Teaching Centers," *The
   Public Health Nurse*, 21:72, 1929.
——: "Public Health Nursing Legislation," *The Public Health Nurse*,
   22:372, 1930.
Municipal Health Department Practice for the Year 1923. Based upon
   surveys of the 100 largest cities in the United States, Committee on
   Administrative Practice of the American Public Health Association,
   in cooperation with the US Public Health Service. Public Health
   Bulletin 164, US Government Printing Office, Washington, D.C., July,
   1926.
Mustard, Harry S.: *Government in Public Health* [Development of State
   Relations]. The Commonwealth Fund, New York, 1945, p. 59.
Noyes, Clara D.: "The Delano Red Cross Nurses," *Am. J. Nursing*,
   24:1113, 1924.

Public Health Organization, White House Conference on Child Health and Protection. The Century Co., New York, 1932.

"Red Cross Public Health Nursing," *The Public Health Nurse*, **12**:92, 1920.

Vanderbilt University School of Nursing Catalog. Nashville, Tennessee, 1951–1952.

Walker, W. Frank, and Randolph, Caroline R.: *Influence of a Public Health Program on a Rural Community, Fifteen Years in Rutherford County, Tennessee, 1924–1938*. The Commonwealth Fund, New York, 1940.

Warner, Estella Ford, and Smith, Geddes: *Children of the Covered Wagon*, Report of the Commonwealth Fund Child Health Demonstration in Marion County, Oregon, 1925–1929. The Commonwealth Fund, New York, 1930.

"When Will the Thermometer Fall?" *The Pubic Health Nurse*, **12**:101, 1920.

Winslow, C.-E. A.: *Health on the Farm and in the Village*. The Macmillan Company, New York, 1931.

———: *A City Set on a Hill*, The Significance of the Health Demonstration at Syracuse, New York. Doubleday, Doran and Co., Garden City, N.Y., 1934.

Winslow, C.-E. A., and Zimand, Savel: *Health Under the El*, Story of the Bellevue-Yorkville Health Demonstration in Midtown New York (Milbank Fund). Harper & Brothers, New York, 1937.

Chapter 21

THE NATIONAL NURSING ORGANIZATIONS
ESTABLISH HEADQUARTERS

. . . the spirit of unity in the nursing profession, the implied and definitely recognized interdependence of all, was the greatest contribution of the 1920 convention. As never before it was acknowledged that the interests of one group in the nursing profession are really not separate from those of any other.

KATHARINE TUCKER[1]

MODERN NURSING in the United States was approaching the half-century mark when the three national nursing organizations established "National Nursing Headquarters." From its earliest meetings the leading spirits in the ANA dreamed of a national headquarters which would provide a focal point for all organizational activities related to nursing. When the NOPHN was establishing its first office in New York, a small committee had been appointed to consider the possibility of developing such a center, but no action was taken because war-related activities began pushing all other projects aside. The progress of both the ANA and the NLNE had been due to the generous contribution of an extraordinary volume of voluntary service by zealous officers, chairmen of committees, and other members. The *Journal* office in Rochester (New York) had provided a base for the interstate secretary, and, for some years, Katharine DeWitt had divided her time between secretarial work for the ANA and that required of her as assistant editor of the *Journal*. The Education Committee of the League, of which Miss Nutting was chairman, carried the major portion of the program of that organization

[1] Tucker, Katharine: "A New Spirit of Unity," *Public Health Nurse,* **12**:449, 1920.

until after the war. An impressive volume of work in connection with the *Standard Curriculum* and other publications had been conducted from her office at Teachers College (TC) in New York. Because of this generous concession to expediency, nurses sometimes mistakenly thought of the League as an adjunct of the Department of Nursing Education of "TC." Both the ANA and the NLNE were urgently in need of well-staffed and well-equipped offices.

The profession had attained a position of considerable distinction during the war. Recognition of the usefulness of nurses in widely varying circumstances began immediately to create an importunate demand for more nursing service than the country had ever had. Following the Armistice, Miss Noyes, then president of the ANA, promptly suggested to Miss Delano that since the Red Cross had helped to get nurses into service it might also help them to readjust to civilian life. Approximately five-sixths of the 24,000 nurses who served during World War I were enrolled Red Cross nurses. Red Cross officials acted promptly and favorably. Early in 1919 a service was organized which was to become the nucleus of national nursing headquarters. This was the ARC Bureau of Information, established in New York, the port of debarkation of most of the overseas nurses. As some of the returning nurses were badly in need of rest or convalescent care, it also established a convalescent home at Bayshore, Long Island. When it had fulfilled its immediate purpose of caring for ex-service nurses, the New York chapter of the ARC and the Association for Improving the Condition of the Poor (which had a large staff of nurses) joined forces to provide a continuing rest and convalescent service for nurses. "Nurses' House," established under the joint auspices of the two services at Babylon, Long Island, continued the tradition of gracious hospitality until 1948. The property was then transferred to an auxiliary which was organized as a nonprofit organization and named "Nurses' House, Inc." Nurses from many states and many countries have enjoyed the hospitality of the spacious house with its beach and delightful garden.

Two broad divisions of work were established in the bureau. Ysabella G. Waters, well known and loved for her contribution of statistical service to the NOPHN, gave several months of volunteer service to the public health nursing division. This unit was soon transferred to the Vocational Bureau of the NOPHN which in turn was combined a few years later with a corresponding service of the American Association of Social Workers to form the Joint Vocational Service. R. Inde Albaugh, who had been a member of the ARC staff in Washington, an experienced administrator with a wide knowledge of nursing school requirements and the provisions of the nurse practice acts, was made responsible for guidance in all other types of nursing service. She also took over the residue of the Student Nurse Reserve which had been transferred to the Red Cross by the Committee on Nursing of the Council of National Defense. The information service was a stabilizing force in the period following World War I. By means of it, nearly 5000 nurses were referred to various positions. It was a boon to the hundreds of nurses who sought advice about opportunities for employment in public health and industrial nursing services, in the federal nursing services, and other fields. Many of them were interested in loans and scholarships for postgraduate work. The ARC's liberal provision for such aids to the advancement of nursing was one of the most constructive outcomes of World War I. Employers, who were avidly awaiting the opportunity to fill vacancies and newly created positions, used the service extensively.

As the bureau had been established on a temporary basis, the ANA and the NLNE arranged to take it over from the Red Cross, the ANA raising its dues from 15 to 50 cents for that purpose.[2] The Red Cross contributed files and equipment and continued to finance the bureau until July 1, 1921. Miss Albaugh carried on the work under the joint auspices of the two organizations for two years. Agnes G. Deans, also a former member of the ARC staff, who had been an elected secretary of the ANA, was then appointed to direct the work of that organization. The NLNE appointed Effie J. Taylor as executive secretary. Miss Taylor had not long been in the position when Miss Goodrich invited her to participate in the great

[2] Inclusive dues for membership in the alumnae, district, or state associations and the ANA were collected at the local level and apportioned on a predetermined basis to the several organizations. Out of its allocation of 50 cents, the ANA paid dues to the International Council of Nurses.

experiment at Yale where, ten years later, she succeeded Miss Goodrich as dean. She was succeeded in 1924 by Blanche Pfefferkorn
(Johns Hopkins), who then began her long period of administrative and technical service for the League. The AJN office remained
in Rochester. Miss Palmer, the magazine's editor-in-chief, had died
in 1920. Miss DeWitt had carried the staggering burden of editorial
work for the magazine and part-time secretarial work for the ANA
until Mary M. Roberts was appointed coeditor in 1921. After a year
in the Rochester office, Miss Roberts was established at national
headquarters in order to facilitate the work of the magazine for the
ANA and the NLNE, and to keep the magazine in touch with the
main stream of professional life.

Many ex-service nurses who had thought they wanted nothing
in the world so much as to get back to their previous way of life
discovered that they no longer fitted the old grooves. Some of them
acknowledged that they missed the stimulating privilege, accompanied though it had been by discomforts and dangers, of caring
for "the best patients in the world." Many such nurses became members of the new government services, but there was continued need
for a center of information for graduate nurses in which the work
of the organizations could be concentrated. In 1921 the three organizations, through the NOPHN's membership in the National Health
Council, were established in New York under the same roof as the
council. The practical advantages of the arrangement, which was
continued until mid-century, lay in the common services provided
by the council and its excellent library facilities. Among the professional advantages was the relative ease with which both formal
and informal conferences could be arranged.

The enormously increased demand for nursing service, which
created a serious shortage of graduate nurses, was accompanied by
a sharp drop in enrollment in the schools of nursing in the immediate years after World War I. A nationwide program to recruit
student nurses was the first major activity directed from the new
offices of the ANA and the NLNE. Frustrations, due to lack of available and qualified nurses, often led to acerbity. The "shortage of
nurses" and of candidates for schools of nursing was widely dis-

cussed in medical and nursing journals as well as in the public press. A popular woman's magazine published a series of four articles[3] which attracted the editorial attention of many other publications. In the leading article, "White Cap Famine," the nursing profession was held responsible for the serious loss of life during the influenza pandemic and likewise for much of the infant and maternal mortality which had been widely publicized in connection with efforts to secure the passage of the Maternity and Infancy Act. The author made no reference whatsoever to the responsibility of society for the development and maintenance of essential health services.

The views of a world-famous surgeon, Dr. Charles H. Mayo, were presented under the misleading caption, "Wanted, 100,000 Girls for Sub-Nurses." The article was motivated by the unmet needs of patients of moderate means. As preparation for general nursing, he recommended a two-year course in hospital nursing based on two years of high school education. It was assumed that such a program would attract large numbers of young women, especially from rural areas. This advocacy of a mediocre standard created a tidal wave of shocked reaction within the profession. A later and more specific article in the *American Journal of Nursing* was more modern in tone. In it Dr. Mayo recommended a two-year program with an optional third year for specialization.

Professional nursing service was indeed beyond the means of many patients of moderate means, but that economic problem could not be solved by self-supporting nurses alone. The controversy served a useful purpose by clarifying and publicizing the basic issue. This was simply stated by the physician who contributed the concluding article. Young women had an increasingly wide range of vocational choices. Unless nursing in preparation and practice could be made attractive to them, there was little hope of enrolling the desired numbers of qualified students in nursing schools, and so of increasing the volume of nursing service required to meet accept-

[3] Parkhurst, Genevieve: "The White Cap Famine," Sept. 1921; Mayo, Charles H.: "Wanted, 100,000 Girls for Sub-Nurses," Oct. 1921; Noyes, Clara D.: "Sub-Nurses? Why not Sub-Doctors?" Dec. 1921; Beard, Richard Olding; "Fair Play for the Trained Nurse," Feb. 1922; *Pictorial Review.*

ably the changing needs of society. Therein lay the challenge of this period to the hospitals which operated nursing schools, to nurse educators, and to the leadership of the nursing organizations. The ANA and the NLNE intensified their efforts to secure reasonable hours, adequate housing, and substantial basic courses for student nurses.

No reliable data were available for use in setting up a national goal or quotas for the recruitment program. Unfortunately a survey of nursing, which the ARC had undertaken on request of the Surgeon General of the Army, had not been completed when the Armistice put a stop to war-related programs. The Red Cross financed the production of liberal quantities of informative leaflets and a beautiful poster "I Lead to Worldwide Opportunity," which was the first poster ever used in a national program for the recruitment of student nurses. It encouraged the chapters to take an active part in filling the schools of nursing with desirable candidates. A few regional programs were developed by nursing councils. At least one hospital association took an active part in recruitment. The schools were filled with students in order to supply the hospitals with nursing service. Since there had been no estimate of opportunities for employment, it is not surprising that by 1925 newly graduated nurses were dismayed to find that there seemed to be no place for them. This unfortunate result of overenthusiastic recruitment re-emphasized the weakness in the educational system which had been revealed by the Winslow-Goldmark report. It aroused new interest in the long-standing need for a national method for making a clear distinction between schools which could prepare students for practice as graduate nurses and those which were nothing more than "diploma mills." As a result the Committee on the Grading of Nursing Schools was organized in 1926.

Having established headquarters, the next step in the adaptation of the national nursing organizations to the rapidly changing social order was an analysis of their structure and relationships. The report of a Joint Committee on Self-Analysis opened with the statement:

The existence of three national organizations in the United States, all concerned with nursing, has for some years occupied the attention of nurses and others and proved a fertile subject of discussion. The questions of duplication in membership; possibilities of weakening professional solidarity, as well as effort and result; economic considerations incident to maintenance of three associations have quite generally been raised.[4]

Individually and collectively the associations decided that the time was not ripe for an amalgamation but that the door should not be closed to further discussion. On request of the NOPHN, Mary S. Gardner made a study of that organization. Critics (what organization does not have them?) believed that the organization was "trying to drive in double harness a team that was never intended to go together, namely, professional interests and community service." After making an exhaustive study to determine the value of the organization (a) to public health nursing as a whole and (b) to local organizations and to individual nurses, Miss Gardner reported that she found no reason for radical changes. Of the nine recommendations, one of the most significant indicates that the program of NOPHN should be limited "to the amount that can be extremely well and properly done . . . and should set a standard for methods employed."[5]

The possibility of amalgamating the two professional journals, the *American Journal of Nursing* and the *Public Health Nurse,* was later studied over a three-year period by a special committee representing the three organizations. It was finally agreed that one magazine could not serve all the purposes of the two publications. The joint effort, however, had pleasantly stimulated rapport and more effective working relationships between the editorial offices.

The facile use of the phrase, "the three national nursing organizations," quite unintentionally conveyed an erroneous concept of the organizations to persons unfamiliar with their structure and functions. They had always had two basic purposes in common; both up-

[4] Report of Joint Committee on Self-Analysis" (Adda Eldredge, chairman), *Proceedings of the Twenty-fifth Convention of the American Nurses' Association,* 1926, p. 22.

[5] Gardner, Mary S.: "Report of Six Months Study of the N.O.P.H.N.," *The Public Health Nurse,* 18:374–386, 1926.

grading and adaptation of nursing to current and anticipated needs, and the promotion of the welfare of nurses. But their memberships as well as their methods of contributing to the development of nursing as a personal, community, and national service were quite unlike, as a summary of the principal elements in their programs in the postwar decade showed.

I

The membership of the ANA consisted exclusively of graduate nurses. Its program was recognized as basic to those of the other two organizations. In 1922, when its reorganization had been completed, it became a federation of state nurses' associations with voting power vested in a house of delegates, in which each delegate represented fifty members. (Representation was later changed to one delegate for each hundred members of a state association.) Through the reorganization, it was anticipated that the national organization would assume responsibility for policies and program planning, and that the state associations would become administrative units responsible for putting into effect such policies and programs as they accepted. But, as a hard-working chairman put it, "the revision committee does not eat the bread of idleness." Many of the state associations continued to require considerable amounts of assistance with matters pertaining to their structure, and to the provisions of the state nurse practice acts.

Participation in the uncompleted national survey had brought home to many of the associations the need for state offices. Some of them began working toward that goal while World War I was still raging. The production of a bulletin or some other type of publication was considered essential to the development of state programs. The Ohio State Nurses' Association had established a central office, chiefly as a repository for records, as early as 1916.[6] It was the first state association to announce the opening of an administrative headquarters. By the end of the decade most of the larger states had well-established offices. Sixteen enthusiastic state executive

[6] August, Elizabeth P.: "Headquarters Ohio State Association of Graduate Nurses," *Am. J. Nursing,* 24:959, 1924.

secretaries attended a five-day institute, the first of its kind, planned for them by the ANA (1930). The organization of registries, the distribution of nursing service, relationships with the state boards of nurse examiners, and program planning were the subjects of primary concern to that group.

Between 1925 and 1929 five groups of states "with analogous interests and problems" organized to form divisions of the ANA. They were the Middle Atlantic, Mid-West, Northwestern, New England, and the Southern divisions. Divisions were expected to function chiefly as discussion groups. But the regional planning of the Mid-West division resulted in the organization of a placement service in Chicago in 1931, which later became an important element in the counseling and placement service developed by the ANA. At mid-century only the New England and Southern divisions were still in existence.

Observers sometimes thought the ANA was more concerned with the details of its structure than with the purposes for which it was created. Its primary purpose was to mobilize the interest of professional nurses everywhere in a program of activities planned to be mutually helpful to nurses and to the nurse-employing public. Therefore, the provision of mechanisms, which would ensure a two-way channel between the grass roots—the district association—and the state association, and for similar mechanisms between the state association and the national office, was a necessary first step in securing the interest of nurses and the development of an *esprit de corps* among them. The record is clear that assistance with such fundamentals as the organization of the structural units of the association, improvement and administration of nurse practice acts, the civil-service status of nurses, the organization and administration of registries, the distribution of nursing service, and the formulation of a code of ethics were major concerns of the ANA in the twenties.

An extremely interesting program was arranged around the report of the ANA's mental hygiene section (Effie J. Taylor, chairman) at the 1928 convention of the three national organizations. "Modern psychiatry and education," says the report, "are pointing the way to the development and care of the total human being, particularly through the formative years of childhood and on through the adolescent period. With this new thought in education, nursing must change its viewpoint and embrace the idea that good nursing care of the physically ill patient involves a knowledge and an appreciation of the influences which the emotional and intellectual life bear on the physical well-being of the patient and *vice versa*."[7] There was unanimity of opinion as to the fundamental importance of including theory and practice in psychiatric nursing in the preparation for any type of service by graduate nurses. But again, as in 1916 (p. 94), the report of a questionnaire study revealed a serious lack of facilities for teaching mental hygiene and psychiatric nursing.

Two field secretaries were appointed to interpret the policies and programs of the ANA to state and local groups. The report of a study of the organization and administration of registries, made by a nurse familiar with nursing in its community relationships, provided a substantial base for further studies leading to the development of standards for registries. None of the registries studied in 1929 had identical aims or methods, but some of them were well aware of the potentialities of registries as focal points for community service. The report urged, for every community large enough to require registry service, the organization of a joint council or coordinating agency on community nursing service. Concern for the welfare of nurses was expressed in the Relief Fund; also by approval, after careful study, of the Harmon Plan for annuities which had been proposed by Mr. William E. Harmon as a means of assisting nurses, especially those with irregular incomes such as private duty nurses, to provide for their own futures. Despite difficulties that had tried the souls of pioneers in securing state legislation, 47 state associations had secured nurse practice acts by 1924. Many of them had been amended; 17 provided for inspection of the schools, and 2 for educational directors.[8]

Nurses were extremely generous contributors to special projects

[7] "Report of the Mental Hygiene Section 1926–1928," *Proceedings of the Twenty-sixth Convention of the American Nurses Association,* 1928, p. 71.
[8] "Round Table Meetings: Legislation" (Janet Geister, chairman), *The Public Health Nurse,* **16:**464, 1924.

in this period. A considerable amount of the time of the clerical staff of the ANA was devoted, in the years after World War I, to collecting and safeguarding the very considerable sums which were contributed for the Delano Memorial in Washington, the American Nurses' Memorial at Bordeaux, France, and to the Relief Fund, all of which are discussed in later chapters. The NLNE accepted responsibility for the funds collected for the work of the Committee on the Grading of Nursing Schools.

II

The membership of the NLNE, like that of the ANA, was limited to graduate nurses and was further restricted to those who were engaged in specified types of activity in the field of nursing education. Although there was a growing number of state and local leagues, membership was on an individual basis. The budget of the NLNE, based on membership dues, bore no realistic relationship to its opportunities, accomplishments, or its aspirations. The League had achieved a position of authority in the field of nursing education because some of the ablest members contributed extraordinary amounts of time to its work. Participation in committee work helped to forge fraternal bonds within the League while strengthening the structure of the whole. This was especially true of the education committee which was constantly spurred on by the inspiring and unconquerable spirit of its chairman, Miss Nutting, aided by the generous and indefatigable efforts of the secretary, Isabel M. Stewart, who succeeded her as chairman in 1922.

Time is required to set in motion the machinery of a national office. By mutual agreement, the placement service, inherited from the ARC, was administered by the NLNE with financial aid from the ANA. But the operation of a placement service calls for special time-consuming skills and is, therefore, costly. As the postwar restlessness began to subside, it appeared that local services could be more useful to institutional nurses than a single service at national headquarters. Because some registries were already placing institutional nurses, representative registrars were asked if the placement service might properly be decentralized to registries. The importance of vocational guidance was recognized both nationally and locally, but it was beyond the resources of the NLNE which discontinued the national service. The NOPHN, on the other hand, strengthened its vocational service as a part of its effort to stabilize public health nursing.

The outstanding contribution of the League in this period was the revision of the *Standard Curriculum,* published in 1927, after more than two years of work by the education committee working with 22 professionally and geographically representative subcommittees. The pages of the *Journal* were freely used in order that the outlines might be tested before they were put in final form. The revision was based on the principle that the basic course should provide a general as opposed to a specialized training, and that it must supply the foundations on which all additional training and experience could be built. This, it may be noted, was in line with the recommendations of the Winslow-Goldmark committee.

In connection with its recommendations for more effective utilization of community resources for nursing education, the League's first study of the service and instructional resources of outpatient departments was published in 1925.[9] This was followed by a three-year demonstration.[10] These studies were conducted under the auspices of a League committee working with the Committee on Dispensary Development of the United Hospital Fund of New York. It is noteworthy that the alumnae association of the Presbyterian Hospital School of Nursing shared financial responsibility for the demonstration with the Committee on Dispensary Development.

The history of nursing education in the United States has been recorded, year by year, in the annual reports of the NLNE. Those for the postwar decade show that the Committee on Education was

[9] *The Pupil Nurse in the Out-Patient Department.* National League of Nursing Education, New York, 1925.
[10] Knapp, Louise: *The Out-Patient Department in the Education of the Nurse.* National League of Nursing Education, New York, 1932.

studying university affiliations before the Winslow-Goldmark study, advocating such affiliation, was published.[11] The *Standard Curriculum* of 1917 had contained a brief statement on university affiliation, but the committee found an extraordinary variety of such relationships. Some of the issues were clarified in 1928 at a five-day conference sponsored by the committee and the Department of Nursing Education at Teachers College. Forty-five universities and colleges were then concerned in some way with the education of nurses, undergraduate or graduate.

The report of a committee on budgets was also an important milestone in the decade following World War I. It is significant that out of 80 carefully selected schools only six returned budgets in a form which could be used for comparative study. The cost of nursing service, in the institutions conducting the six schools, was found to be greater than graduate nursing services would have been. A study, believed to be the first of its kind, was made by financial experts of the school of the Massachusetts General Hospital in 1930.[12] The figures indicated that the elimination of the school would result in financial loss to the hospital. It was assumed that the loss to the community in terms of graduate nursing service would be serious if the school were discontinued. The most important argument presented for continuing a hospital school was that "in a hospital where nursing education exists, just as in a hospital where medical education is carried on, the patient receives better care."

The programs of the League's carefully planned annual meetings in the twenties were centered progressively on educational facilities, preparation of faculty, teaching methods with special emphasis on "the project plan" and on case studies, and on the use of "new-type" examination questions and psychometric tests. The League programs provide abundant evidence that principles and method were replacing empiricism in the teaching of nursing. Further evidence may be found in some of the textbooks of the period and in a bud-

[11] "Preliminary Report on University Schools of Nursing," *Am. J. Nursing,* 21:620–29, 711–16, 799, 1921.
[12] Patterson, Teale, and Dennis: "The Study of the Yearly Expenses for the Training School for Nurses at the Massachusetts General Hospital," *Bull. Am. Hosp. A.,* 6:41–58, 1932.

ding interest in research. Bertha Harmer's *Textbook of the Principles and Practice of Nursing,* her *Methods and Principles of Teaching the Principles and Practice of Nursing,* and Maude Muse's *Psychology for Nurses* mark an important change in the literature of nursing education. The AJN published its first important article on research in nursing in 1927. The Department of Nursing Education at Teachers College, Columbia University, which spearheaded the new movement, began in 1928 the publication of a bulletin devoted chiefly to research in nursing. But more than twenty years were to go by before the profession would have a publication devoted to stimulating and reporting researches in nursing.

III

The NOPHN, from an organizational point of view, had little more than a family resemblance to the two organizations which admitted only nurses to membership. The service that it had been organized to promote was described as follows: "Public health nursing is an organized community service not for profit, rendered by graduate nurses to the individual, family and community. The service includes the interpretation and application of medical, sanitary and social procedures for the correction of defects, prevention of disease and the promotion of health, and may include skilled care of the sick in their homes."[13] The NOPHN had three types of membership: professional, lay, and agency, whereas the others had only one. As has been shown, it started life with an office, a publication, and, thanks to Miss Waters, a statistical service. As a service agency it could contract to provide service in its special field for other agencies. Because of the nature of its membership and programs, it was less concerned with the development of state and local units than the other organizations. The state organizations, or branches, were not an integral part of the parent body. NOPHN's interest in developing relationships with other social and health agencies was in striking contrast to the tendency to self-containment of the older organizations. By 1918 it had become affiliated, through corporate

[13] *Public Health Nursing,* **21**:551, 1929.

membership, with the American Public Health Association, the National Tuberculosis Association, and eight other social and health agencies. After a trial year a public health nursing section was established in the APHA in 1923. The NTA appointed a nurse to its staff in 1920. At its annual meetings the sessions on nursing attracted a representative cross section of all those in attendance.

The NOPHN converted its Standing Committee on Tuberculosis Nursing into a section in 1919. Sections on school nursing and industrial nursing were organized the following year. Their programs and related materials filled many pages of the organization's official magazine. In the midst of the enormously increased postwar demand for public health nursing service, the NOPHN took a firm stand against any lowering of the standards toward which it had been working. The organization's prewar program had stimulated increased use of public health nursing service. The postwar program emphasized standardization of preparation and of service. Minimum requirements for collegiate programs in public health nursing were set up by the education committee in the early twenties, thus making the NOPHN the first nursing organization to develop any type of accreditation. By 1929, 11 programs were on the approved list.

The first census of public health nurses was made in 1924. In 1925, the organization published its *Minimum Qualifications for Public Health Nursing Positions,* a standard which was to be reviewed and revised if necessary at five-year intervals. Annual salary studies were begun that year also. Time schedules never presented so serious a problem to public health nurses as to institutional and private duty nurses. This was due in part to the nature of the work, most of which must be done during the day, but also in part to the fact that agency representatives participating in the work of the NOPHN acquired first-hand information about the problems and conditions of work of public health nurses. The organization's lay members are credited with facilitating the development of good personnel practices in public health nursing agencies.

Industrial nursing was included in the term, public health nursing. The first book on the subject (1919) was written by Florence S.

Wright, chairman of the industrial section of the NOPHN. It was received with such enthusiasm that the first printing was quickly exhausted. In it the likenesses and the differences between industrial nursing and other types of public health nursing as then practiced were clearly defined. Because of the differences, industrial nurses were not included in the census of public health nurses, and a special study, "Nurses in Commerce and Industry," was made by the organization and published in successive issues of the organization's magazine in 1930. The first edition of the *Manual of Public Health Nursing* was published in 1926, and that of the *Board Members' Manual* in 1930. At that time these two volumes were considered the key publications of the NOPHN.

When national nursing headquarters was established, the outstanding achievements of the profession had been largely due to the leadership of a few nurses who possessed the social vision, courage, and energy to blaze new trails. They possessed the capacity for sustained enthusiasm which incited others to follow them. But nursing was on the threshold of a new era in its development in which the momentum of the public health movement would help to carry it forward. It was in the initial stages of a transition from personal to collective or composite leadership. This was due to the more democratic climate of the postwar years, the inevitable loss of some of those who had been acknowledged leaders at the turn of the century, and to the increasing influence of the professional organizations.

When Jane A. Delano, creator of the nursing service of the ARC, died at Savenay, France, on April 15, 1919, it was written of her that: "To help win the war and to give adequate care to the sick and wounded was her religion from the day that war was declared."[14] The thousands of nurses who had followed her leadership felt that she had given her life to her country as truly as had any soldier on the field of battle. Just a year later, when Sophia F. Palmer, the first editor of the AJN, laid down her pen, she was said to have achieved her goal by making the magazine "a medium of communication between nurses, a history of nursing progress, a guide and leader in

[14] Palmer, Sophia F.: "Jane A. Delano As Known by Her Friends," *Am. J. Nursing,* **19**:698, 1919.

nursing thought."[15] Anna C. Maxwell, founder of the Presbyterian
Hospital School of Nursing (New York), a trail blazer in the Spanish-American War and an influential member of many a committee,
retired in 1921. Lavinia L. Dock, whose clear thinking and writing
had done so much to ensure sound foundations for the older professional organizations, retired in 1923. As secretary of the International Council of Nurses she had kept its life blood flowing when
the organization was seriously enfeebled by the restrictive circumstances of war. Through the contents of the *Journal's* foreign department, which she had provided from the magazine's first issue
in 1900, she had encouraged American nurses to become citizens of
the world through nursing. Miss Nutting, who had succeeded Mrs.
Robb as chairman of the NLNE's education committee and had
made it one of the most powerful forces in the profession, resigned
in 1922. Three years later she also relinquished the position at
Teachers College through which she had made that institution both
a national and an international center of nursing education. At that
time Miss Wald said of her: "I do not think that Adelaide Nutting,
intellectual and teacher that she is, has ever believed that education,
through university, lecture, literature or organization, is of conse-
quence to the nurse, except as a guide to the development of her
relationship to the patient, to the institution, to the pupil and to
the community."[16] No higher tribute could have been paid by one
great nurse to another.

Miss Wald was to continue as the internationally known and
nationally beloved head of the Henry Street Settlement and its
nursing service until her retirement in the early thirties. She was no
longer active in national nursing affairs by that time. For her it had
been "most logical that interest in one family should have developed
into interest in a group, a neighborhood, a nation and the brotherhood of likeminded people in all nations. It is a little difficult to
comprehend the many interests that have developed from the Set-

[15] Riddle, Mary M.: "Twenty Years of the *Journal,*" *Am. J. Nursing,* 21:6,
1921.
[16] Wald, Lillian D.: "M. Adelaide Nutting, As Known by Friends, Students
and Co-Workers," *Am. J. Nursing,* 25:449, 1925.

tlement, but they complete a cycle of interest in and responsibility for the world in which we live."[17]

It was in the early postwar period that Ella Phillips Crandall, who as executive secretary of the NOPHN had persuasively and enthusiastically preached the gospel of public health nursing in every part of the country, resigned, and withdrew from the field of nursing. Miss Goodrich, however, was just embarking on the culminating work of her life at Yale. Mary S. Gardner, whose searching analysis of NOPHN's structure and program has been noted, was also to remain a graciously powerful influence in the evolution of nursing for many years. Miss Noyes, who succeeded Miss Delano, and Elizabeth G. Fox, director of the Bureau of Public Health Nursing of the American Red Cross, were respectively the presidents of the ANA and the NOPHN. Isabel M. Stewart, who had succeeded Miss Nutting as chairman of the NLNE's education committee in 1922 also succeeded her as administrator of the Department of Nursing Education at Teachers College. It was in this period the Rockefeller Foundation developed its program of fellowships for nurses, after sending Miss Goodrich and S. Lillian Clayton (principal of the school of the Philadelphia General Hospital) to visit nursing centers in Europe.

The age of the great nurse pioneers was passing into history. Their disciples would carry on. The organizations they had conceived had grown strong and were gaining some degree of maturity. Their continuing success would depend on the skill with which nurses gifted with the characteristics of leadership could subordinate personal opinion to group thinking and action in relation to program. Their usefulness was soon to be tested, and their growth stimulated, by the great depression.

BIBLIOGRAPHY

American Nurses' Association Handbook. American Nurses' Association, New York, 1935.

[17] Duffus, R. L.: *Lillian Wald—Neighbor and Crusader.* The Macmillan Company, New York, 1938, p. 288.

220   *American Nursing: History and Interpretation*

"Anna Caroline Maxwell, R.N.," *Am. J. Nursing*, **21**:688, 1921.

Best, Ella: *Brief Historical Review and Information about Current Activities of the American Nurses' Association, including Certain Facts Relative to the National League of Nursing Education.* American Nurses' Association, New York, 1940, p. 27.

Board Members' Manual. Prepared by the NOPHN. The Macmillan Company, New York, 1930.

Brief and Specifications for Civilian Service in the Federal Government, Foreword by C.-E. A. Winslow. American Nurses' Association, New York, 1930.

Crandall, Ella Phillips: "An Historical Sketch of Public Health Nursing," *Am. J. Nursing*, **22**:641, 1922.

Curriculum for Schools of Nursing. National League of Nursing Education, New York, 1927.

"Death of the Journal Editor" [Sophia F. Palmer], *Am. J. Nursing*, **20**:604, 1920.

Goodrich, Annie W.: "Jane A. Delano," *The Social and Ethical Significance of Nursing.* The Macmillan Company, New York, 1932, pp. 371–80.

———: "Anna C. Maxwell," *The Social and Ethical Significance of Nursing.* The Macmillan Company, New York, 1932, pp. 381–83.

Greener, Elizabeth A.: "Budgets for Schools of Nursing," *Am. J. Nursing*, **24**:970, 1924.

Harmer, Bertha: *Textbook of the Principles and Practice of Nursing.* The Macmillan Company, New York, 1926.

———: *Methods and Principles of Teaching the Principles and Practice of Nursing.* The Macmillan Company, New York, 1926.

"Harmon Plan for Annuities," *Am. J. Nursing*, **29**:346, 1929.

"How Should States Organize for Public Health Nursing?" Report of State Organization Committee of the National Organization for Public Health Nursing [Katherine Tucker, chairman], *Public Health Nurse*, **14**:40, 1922.

Kernodle, Portia B.: *The Red Cross Nurse in Action, 1882–1948.* Harper & Brothers, New York, 1949, p. 253.

"Magazines Not to Be Combined," *Am. J. Nursing*, **30**:314, 1930.

Manual of Public Health Nursing. Prepared by the NOPHN. The Macmillan Company, New York, 1926.

Marvin, Mary M.: "Research in Nursing—The Place of Research and Experimentation in Improving the Nursing Care of the Patient," *Am. J. Nursing*, **27**:331, 1927.

Mayo, Charles H.: "Do You Covet Distinction?" *Am. J. Nursing*, **22**:251, 1922.

Munson, Helen W.: *The Story of the National League of Nursing Education.* W. B. Saunders Co., Philadelphia, 1934.

Muse, Maude B.: *Psychology for Nurses.* W. B. Saunders Co., Philadelphia, 1925.

National Organization for Public Health Nursing—History, Objectives and Present Program (mimeographed). National Organization for Public Health Nursing, New York, 1948.

Noyes, Clara D.: "The Red Cross Bureau of Information for Nurses," *Am. J. Nursing,* **20:**223, 1919.

The Nursing Education Bulletin, Vol. 1, No. 1, Jan., 1928, published twice yearly through 1929 and at irregular intervals thereafter. Department of Nursing Education, Teachers College, Columbia University, New York.

"Nurses' House, Inc.," *Am. J. Nursing,* **48:**410, 1948.

Proceedings of Conference on Nursing Schools Connected with Colleges and Universities. Teachers College, Columbia University, New York, Jan., 1928.

"Report of the Ideal Magazine Committee," *Public Health Nurse,* **22:**153, 1930.

"Representation of National Organization for Public Health Nursing to Other National Health Organizations," *Public Health Nurse,* **10:**342, (Oct.) 1918.

Russell, James E.; Nevins, Georgia M.; Wald, Lillian D.; and Stewart, Isabel M.: "M. Adelaide Nutting, As Known by Friends, Students and Co-Workers," *Am. J. Nursing,* **25:**445, 1925.

The Story of the American Journal of Nursing, 1900–1950. American Journal of Nursing Co., New York, 1950.

"A Suggested Code—A Code of Ethics Presented for the Consideration of the A.N.A.," *Am. J. Nursing,* **26:**599, 621, 1926.

Tattershall, Louise M.: "Nurses in Commerce and Industry," *Public Health Nurse,* **22:**147, 194, 572, 633, 1930.

Tittman, Anna L.: "A Joint Vocational Service," *Am. J. Nursing,* **27:**110, 1927.

Wilkinson, Julia P.: *Report of the Field Study of Registries* (mimeographed). American Nurses' Association, New York, 1930.

Wood, Evelyn: "The Nurse Placement Service," *Am. J. Nursing,* **32:**50, 1932.

Wright, Florence Swift: *Industrial Nursing.* The Macmillan Company, New York, 1919 (reissued, 1928).

SECTION VI. THE YEARS OF
THE BLACK DEPRESSION   1929 – 1935

Chapter 22

SHARING

The depression of the early 1930's was like the explosion of a bomb dropped in the midst of society. All the major social institutions, such as the government, family, church, and school, obviously were profoundly affected and the repercussions were so far reaching that scarcely any type of human activity was untouched.[1]

AFTER the stock market crash (October, 1929) Americans went from panic and business recession to the black depression of the winter of 1932–1933. In the following spring 15,000,000 persons, nearly one-third of the country's workers, were unemployed. Almost 6,000,000 were on state and municipal relief rolls. Apples sold on street corners had become the symbol of personal financial disaster. Less evident to the more fortunate city dwellers, but more poignantly characteristic, were the bread lines, the soup kitchens, and the homeless men who spent winter nights on sidewalk gratings which permitted the escape of warm but polluted air from underground installations.

Some sociologists divide the depression into three segments: prefederal, federal, and postfederal. The federal period lasted from the passage of the Federal Emergency Relief Act (FERA) in May, 1933, to the liquidation of its program in 1935. For many nurses, a depression had begun well in advance of the Wall Street debacle. The profession and the hospitals had been warned against "overproduction" of nurses by the Grading Committee shortly after it began its studies in 1926; but the schools had continued to graduate large

[1] Foreword by the Committee on Studies in Social Aspects of the Depression, *Research Memorandum on Social Aspects of Health in the Depression.* Social Science Research Council, New York, Bulletin #36, 1937, p. v.

classes. Early in 1930, Dr. Burgess repeated the warning at the biennial convention, stating that there were thousands of unemployed nurses eagerly seeking opportunities to become self-supporting.

Private duty nurses are extremely vulnerable to changes in either the economic status or the health of a community. News of the stock market crash was not many hours old when registrars began receiving messages from hospitals canceling previous requests for special duty nurses. Annual visitations of influenza following the epidemic of 1918 had subjected them to seasonal cries of "shortage" of nurses. But the public, mercifully spared an epidemic in 1929, gave no thought to the plight of the nurses who, on the basis of past community needs, had anticipated a period of assured employment. Unlike firemen, private duty nurses are not salaried to ensure their availability when needed. As the depression deepened, clinics became overcrowded and public tax-supported hospitals overflowed with patients. Public health nursing agencies were under heartbreaking pressure to provide care for more and more patients who had less and less food and fuel in their homes. But the occupancy of voluntary hospitals whose patients in normal times employed considerable numbers of special duty nurses fell off abruptly. A sympathetic participant in an early job-finding program noted that a surprising number of the nurses who were frantically searching for employment had one or more dependents. When employment was found, it was necessary to equip many of them with shoes and uniforms before they could go on duty. In the prefederal period, many registries and other state and local organizations developed useful share-the-work programs. The pages of the *Journal* of the period are replete with evidence of the altruism of nurses. But something more was needed. The three national nursing organizations responded to the challenge of the Grading Committee, and to the swift rise in unemployment by establishing a Joint Committee on the Distribution of Nursing Service. This was later made a committee of the American Nurses' Association with representation from the three organizations.

Ella Best (St. Luke's, Chicago), who, before mid-century, had become the executive secretary of the ANA, was then field secretary of the organization and secretary of its important registry committee. She had worked with the committee on a revision of the minimum standards for professionally sponsored registries. Early distrust of central registries was being dissipated by coordinated efforts within the profession. In 1929 there were 35 such registries. Three years later, Miss Best reported that many professional registries were virtually nursing bureaus working closely with other nursing and health agencies in meeting the nursing needs of their communities. Years later, an editorial writer in Grand Rapids neatly summarized the objective for which this committee was aiming when he wrote: "What started out chiefly as a service for nurses has become a vital convenience for the entire community. The Nurses' Bureau should be so regarded." Important though they were, the registries could deal with only a segment of the total problem. The function of the joint committee was "to advise methods for better distribution of nursing service and to stimulate nurses and the public to select and put into practice that which is applicable to their own community needs."

The work of the committee was apportioned to five subcommittees with the ANA's very active registry committee functioning as one of them. When the National Recovery Act (NRA) was passed in 1933, the committee had produced materials "to guide local communities along the following lines:

"1. How to form a council on community nursing,

"2. How to change from student to graduate nursing staff,

"3. First steps in transforming the nurses' registry into a community service,

"4. What hourly nursing is and how to establish it,

"5. Why organized nursing should find a way to secure nursing in poverty-stricken rural and urban areas where the sick are now unnursed."[2]

At an early date the committee sought the cooperation of hospital trustees, hospital administrators, and directors of nursing service in

---

[2] Sargent, Emilie G.: "The Nursing Profession Works for Recovery," *Am. J. Nursing,* 33:1165, 1172, 1933.

a concerted effort to check the overcrowding of the profession by poorly prepared nurses. A letter to them signed by the presidents of the three organizations and the chairman of the committee was widely publicized. The AHA at its next convention agreed in principle with the suggestions of the committee, which had supported its argument for the closing of weak schools, by citing the excellent report of a comparative study of nursing costs in *small* hospitals with and without schools that had been released by the Duke Endowment in 1931. State and district associations, which organized committees on the distribution of nursing service, collected comprehensive data on current conditions in nursing within their jurisdictions as a preliminary to adapting nationally sponsored suggestions to their immediate situations.

Hourly nursing, which had never been practiced extensively, appealed to unemployed nurses as a possible means of earning a livelihood. The Rosenwald Fund, concerned with the provision of medical care for patients of moderate means, thought it might provide a partial answer to that problem also. The fund, therefore, provided partial subsidy for a study planned by the Joint Committee on Hourly Nursing of Chicago which had been promoting such services for several years. An 18-months' experiment was conducted under favorable auspices with cordial cooperation from the American Medical Association, the local medical society, and the hospitals, in addition to that of the central registry and other nursing agencies. The program which included extensive publicity, was directed by a highly qualified nurse. The results were disappointing. The service was used more extensively by well-to-do patients than by those of moderate means. Whether this was due to failure of the carefully planned publicity to reach the families for which the service was primarily intended or to their inability to pay for any nursing service is not clear. The total volume of hourly service made possible by the program could not be estimated because nurses not associated with the project capitalized on the publicity to secure employment for themselves. It was concluded that there is a place, but probably not a large one, for hourly nursing as a part of a total community service.

On the basis of the experiment, a representative of the Rosenwald

Fund announced that there were two reasons why hourly nursing service cannot be successfully carried on either by an organization maintained for that purpose or in conjunction with a nurses' registry. The administrative cost of maintaining and publicizing a limited service was found to be too high to be met from earnings based on reasonable fees. The second reason stated was that, since visiting nursing services can provide hourly appointment service, the organization of a second part-time service would violate a principle advocated by authorities in the field of public health; namely, communities should not only refrain from developing specialized nursing services but they should, on the other hand, promote the development of a single agency offering a generalized public health nursing service. This analyst's final decision was that hourly nursing should be developed "as an integral part of a general public health, or district nursing organization."[3]

Some of the relief agencies that were organized in the prefederal period were helpful to nurses. Among them was the Emergency Work Bureau of New York City which, in a three-year period, found employment for some 900 nurses. The service owed its existence largely to the persuasive powers and organizing ability of Mrs. August Belmont, an ardent worker in the ARC, a member of its central committee, and a long-time friend of nurses and the distressed. The New York State legislature passed a Temporary Emergency Relief Act (TERA) in 1931 under which medical and nursing care along with food, clothing, and shelter were designated "necessities of life." The state health department, in which Marion W. Sheahan was director of nursing, promptly developed a practical program for the employment of nurses under public health nursing agencies, which seems to have provided a pattern for programs subsequently developed under federal auspices. The needs of relief clients for nursing care and of nurses for employment were estimated by means of surveys. The professionally sponsored registries and the Nurses' Service Committee (previously the Relief Fund Committee, which is discussed later) of the New York State Nurses'

[3] Davis, Michael M.: "The Meaning of the Hourly Nursing Experiment in Chicago," *Am. J. Nursing*, 33:111, 1933.

Association cooperated in locating unemployed nurses. The program was developed on the basis of established standards of public health nursing service. This meant that only registered nurses in good standing could be employed and only under the supervision of established public health nursing agencies. The state department of health provided a brief manual for their guidance as most of the unemployed nurses had not had any public health nursing experience.

In the tense days of the depression, the executive officers of the three national nursing organizations, and the editors of their official publications, for the first time arranged monthly conferences on matters of mutual and immediate interest. (For convenience, the group was self-styled "The Headquarters Cabinet.") However, in relation to federal projects, following the passage of the National Recovery Act and the development of a medical care program under the Federal Emergency Relief Administration in the summer of 1933, major responsibility for assisting nurses was carried by the ANA and the NOPHN. The ANA was primarily concerned with the welfare of nurses; the NOPHN with the administrative problems of the public health nursing agencies which were called upon to expand their programs and to supervise the work of nurses without previous experience in that type of nursing. The NOPHN provided a special manual for agency use. Many state nurses' associations acted on an ANA recommendation and set up committees composed of nurses qualified to assist state relief agencies in the assignment of nurses on the basis of the nurses' needs and their qualifications for work to be done. Nurses, as professional workers, did not come under the "blanket code of fair practice" of the National Recovery Act. When informed of this fact, the ANA was also told by the National Recovery Administration that, "to a large extent we shall have to rely on you to see that the spirit of the NRA is complied with."[4] The spirit of the NRA emanated from the basic principle that the opportunity to be self-supporting should be shared. This was not a new concept to nurses. Some of the special duty nurses had already voluntarily reduced their incomes by accepting the eight-hour-day

[4] "A Letter from the NRA to the A.N.A.," *Am. J. Nursing*, 33:1206, 1933.

schedule at rates which divided the amount paid by the patient for twenty-four-hour service with three nurses instead of two. The programs of the various "alphabetical" relief agencies developed under the Federal Emergency Relief Administration were much too complex for detailed consideration here. But the ANA seized the opportunity to break the tradition of long hours for nurses. It distributed widely a leaflet, *The NRA and Nursing,* from which the following excerpt was extensively quoted:

An arbitrary limitation of hours controlled by law violates the whole spirit of nursing, as the comfort of the patient is the nurse's first consideration. Again, no nurse could be expected to hold to a specific hour schedule when engaged in emergency or disaster relief.

However, an attempt should be made to approach reasonable working conditions by encouraging, where possible, in the interest of the patient as well as the nurse, an eight-hour day for those employed on a daily basis, and a forty-eight-hour week for those employed on a weekly or monthly schedule. It is undoubtedly desirable to shorten the hours of duty so that the individual nurse may have a reasonable working day and also that there may be a spreading of work.[5]

Nursing service on a part-time basis was included in the program of medical care for recipients of relief in their homes. The principle, strongly advocated by the two nursing organizations, that nurses employed through the medium of relief should work under the supervision of an existing organization was generally adhered to. For the first time, tax-supported agencies were authorized to utilize and pay for the services of private or voluntary agencies. This was hailed by the NOPHN as one of the most important milestones in the history of public health nursing. The manual prepared by the NOPHN was widely used. At the depth of the depression, through the initiative of the US Children's Bureau, more than 2000 nurses were employed on child health conservation projects. Usually the state departments of health were the agencies responsible for developing a program in cooperation with the state relief administration. The programs varied widely. One state, for example, did a notable piece of work in finding crippled children and securing care

[5] "Notes from Headquarters, American Nurses Association," *Am. J. Nursing,* **33**:1001, 1933.

for them. In many states, school nurses cooperated with nutrition workers in providing hot luncheons for the undernourished children of families on relief.

The Works Progress Administration (WPA) was authorized in 1935. As there was considerable confusion about the classification and functions of nurses in the early stages of this program, the ANA swung into action and succeeded in having graduate nurses placed in the "professional and technical" category. At the peak of this program in 1936 over 2600 nurses were employed on public health projects in 31 states, and 1800 were assigned to other types of work including bedside nursing.[6]

No two state relief agencies utilized the nursing services made available to them under the emergency programs in identical fashion. Nurses were given employment in many ways; in public hospitals, sanatoria, and other institutions, in clinics as well as on public health nursing staffs. They did bedside nursing; they participated in immunization programs and in surveys. Interest in a child health study program was especially keen in some states. The whole FERA program, uneven though it was, had a tremendous influence on the subsequent development of medical care programs. Evidence of its continuing influence may be found in programs developed by the Children's Bureau and the US Public Health Service after the passage of the Social Security Act. During the depression, as during wars, it was sometimes difficult to believe that clouds could have a silver lining. But, as a convention speaker reminded his all-nurse audience:

It is just your good luck that the things you have always wanted to do for improving the health and happiness of the people happen to be the things that must be done in order to make the economic system operate.[7]

The profession had risen superbly to the opportunities for service. "I know of no national organization," said Mrs. Ellen S. Woodward to an ANA audience, "which has made a greater contribution to the

[6] "The WPA and Nursing," *Am. J. Nursing*, **38**:733, 1938.
[7] Coyle, David Cushman: "The Changing Order of Today," *Pub. Health Nursing*, **26**:365, 1934.

public welfare."[8] The effect on the health and morale of the American people of nursing participation in the emergency health and welfare programs of the depression cannot readily be assayed. Nor need it be attempted. The best evidence of desirable results may be found in the opportunities provided for the expansion of nursing services under the Social Security Act of 1935.

The ANA's Relief Fund was decentralized to the the state associations in the midst of the depression. The participation of a state committee in an unemployment relief project has been noted in connection with the early program in New York. Other state committees found it helpful to have direct control of funds provided for the assistance of sick and disabled nurses in the bleak days of the depression. Therefore, a brief description of that fund may be considered at this point.

A plan for a relief fund to give assistance to sick and disabled nurses, in lieu of a pension plan which had been under informal consideration, was enthusiastically adopted by the ANA in 1911. Eight years later, when the association had some 40,000 members, a fund of $25,000 had been built up. It continued to grow through the efforts of the national and state committees. But by 1929 the fund was in serious straits. The planners had not foreseen the menace of tuberculosis to young nurses, or the impossibility of evaluating at a national level either the needs of individual nurses or the local resources available to them. The national committee had ingenuously set up only two requirements for eligibility for benefits. Candidates for assistance from the fund must have been active members of their state associations for two years, and they must have been in the active practice of nursing for at least two years immediately preceding the onset of the illness or handicap for which relief was requested. By 1928 the fund was averaging 175 beneficiaries a month; the benefits averaged $15.00 per month. One half of the nurses then receiving benefits had been graduated five years or less and almost one-half of them had tuberculosis! Relief Fund checks sometimes represented the only income of nurses receiving care in public in-

[8] Woodward, Ellen S.: "Federal Aspects of Unemployment Among Professional Women," *Am. J. Nursing*, 34:534, 1934.

stitutions. The ANA was confronted with a serious humanitarian, financial, and administrative problem. Also, the association had come to realize that its efforts to give long-range relief seriously violated the principles of sound social work practice. Fortunately, the high incidence of tuberculosis among young nurses had already become a matter of concern and constructive action among tuberculosis specialists in this and other countries. The reports of studies of tuberculosis among students in a few schools were stimulating the development of health programs in many schools.

The ANA voted to allocate the fund to the state associations on the basis of their 1932 memberships, with the proviso that the funds would be used in accordance with the ANA's articles of incorporation which permitted the association "to distribute relief to such nurses as may become ill, disabled or destitute."[9] By 1935 allocations of more than $94,000 had been made to the state associations. Due to a policy of holding securities until they could be sold without loss, final distribution of a sum approximating $20,000 was not made until 1950.

Inevitably the painful experiences of the depression left their scars. Fear of a repetition of "overproduction" of nurses caused distrust of the broad-scale plans adopted to meet the nation's need in World War II. But the effect of the depression on the profession as a whole was salutary. It helped to bring nursing out of its inhibiting professional isolationism. As never before, the national nursing organizations worked together and with other agencies, both official and voluntary. It pointed up the need of the professional organizations for continuous research in relation to the education of nurses, the distribution of nursing service, and the welfare of nurses.

Many nurses became aware of their need for a sounder preparation for the practice of their profession. The NLNE, in informal collaboration with the committee on the distribution of nursing service, developed outlines for postgraduate courses in clinical nursing which encouraged institutions to provide part-time employment for nurses eager to take advantage of the offerings of conveniently located universities. The necessity for making work available to the

[9] *Handbook*, American Nurses' Association, New York, 1935, p. 18.

largest possible number of nurses had hastened the adoption of reasonable time schedules. This, and the employment of graduate nurses on a staff basis, started an overdue reform in the administrative practices and personnel policies of many institutions. Adversity seems to bring out the best, or the worst, in people. Some nurse participants in relief programs were recipients of work relief and nothing more. But they were far outnumbered by those who rose to challenging situations by doing excellent work and making constructive plans for their own further development as professional persons. By 1935 the functions of the national and state organizations, which had previously seemed remote to many nurses, were better understood than ever before, and the organizations had been stimulated to develop coordinated programs.

BIBLIOGRAPHY

Ames, Miriam, "Hourly Nursing Service," *Am. J. Nursing,* **33**:113, 215, 1933.
Beard, Charles A., and Beard, Mary R.: *America in Midpassage.* The Macmillan Company, New York, 1939, Vol. II, pp. 834–39.
Burgess, May Ayres: "The Distribution of Nursing Service," *Nurses, Patients, and Pocketbooks.* Committee on the Grading of Nursing Schools, New York, 1928, Chap. 25, pp. 500–520.
———: "The Distribution of Nursing Service," *Am. J. Nursing,* **30**:857, 1930.
Collins, Selwyn D., and Tibbetts, Clark: *Research Memorandum on Social Aspects of Health in the Depression.* Social Science Research Council, New York, 1937, Bulletin #6, p. 130.
Davis, Graham Lee: "$33,000 Loss in 12 Hospitals Due to Nursing Schools," *Hospital Management,* Aug., 1931.
Dines, Alta E.: "Community Resources and Immediate Relief," *Proceedings of the Twenty-ninth Convention of the American Nurses' Association,* 1934, pp. 402–6.
Eliot, Martha M.: "Child Health Recovery Program," *Pub. Health Nursing,* **26**:178, 1934.
"Hourly Appointment Nursing Service, Some Tentative Statements Prepared by the Joint Committee on Distribution of Nursing Service," *Am. J. Nursing,* **31**:567, 1931.

"Institutional Nursing," as defined by the Subcommittee of the Joint Distribution Committee (includes "special nursing" and "group nursing"), *Am. J. Nursing,* 31:689, 1931.

McCormick, Virginia: "The Joint Committee on the Distribution of Nursing Service," *Am. J. Nursing,* 31:444, 1931.

————: "The Registry and the Public," *Am. J. Nursing,* 31:1027, 1931.

The NRA and Nursing. American Nurses' Association, New York, 1933.

"The Nurses' Relief Fund," *Am. J. Nursing,* 19:417, 1919.

"Participation in Federal Projects," *Proceedings of the Thirtieth Convention of the American Nurses' Association,* 1936, pp. 135–36.

Parran, Thomas, Jr.: "Public Medical Care in New York State," *J.A.M.A.,* 101:342, 1933.

Proceedings of the Conference on Emergency Needs of Women, Nov., 1933. The White House, Federal Emergency Relief Administration, Washington, D.C.

"Report of the A.N.A. Committee on Relief Fund," *Proceedings of the Thirty-seventh Conference of the American Nurses' Association,* May, 1950, pp. 193–95.

Schwitalla, Alphonse M.: "The Present Economic Objectives of the Nursing Profession," *Am. J. Nursing,* 33:1135, 1933.

Scott, Alma H.: "A.N.A. Program," *Proceedings of the Twenty-ninth Convention of the American Nurses' Association,* 1934, pp. 147–51.

Sheahan, Marion W.: "An Experiment in Double Relief," *Pub. Health Nursing,* 25:378, 1933.

Swope, Ethel: "The C.W.S. [Civil Works Service] Program and the American Nurses' Association," *Am. J. Nursing,* 34:356, 1934.

————: "The Eight-Hour Day Makes Progress," *Am. J. Nursing,* 35: 1147, 1935.

Terris, Milton: "Medical Care for the Needy and the Medically Needy," *Ann. Am. Acad. Polit. & Soc. Sc.,* 273:84, 1951.

Tucker, Katharine: "Biennial Report of N.O.P.H.N. Activities," *Pub. Health Nursing,* 26:307, 1934.

Wecter, Dixon: *The Age of the Great Depression, 1929–1941.* The Macmillan Company, New York, 1948.

"What Patients Think of the Eight-Hour Schedule," *Am. J. Nursing,* 33:1153, 1933.

Whitney, Jessamine S.: "Tuberculosis among Young Women—with Special Reference to Tuberculosis among Nurses," *Am. J. Nursing,* 28: 766, 1928.

"The WPA and Nursing," *Am. J. Nursing,* 38:733, 1938.

Chapter 23

SOME SIGNIFICANT REPORTS

Life is our only real possession. It is because of this that its preservation is constantly before us.

RAY LYMAN WILBUR[1]

BENEATH the emergency plans for coping with the turbulent seas of the depression there ran a tide of long-range plans for the improvement of health and medical care programs. The reports of three studies begun in the prosperous twenties provided an extraordinary volume of factual information and of stimulating recommendations for the use of policy-making professional organizations, institutions, and other planning agencies. In the main, they re-emphasized facts and trends with which well-informed nurses were already familiar. The one wholly new proposal in relation to nursing (the idea was far from new) dealt with the status, preparation, and functions of nurse-midwives. The reports were those of the Committee on the Grading of Nursing Schools, the very extensive reports of the Committee on Costs of Medical Care, and the White House Conference of 1930.

The Grading Committee, as previously noted, did not publish its final report until 1934 although the second grading of schools had been completed two years earlier. However, results of successive studies had been published and were influencing the thinking of nurses, doctors, hospital administrators, and state boards of nurse examiners. The report of the economic study[2] published in 1928 stressed two major weaknesses; the overproduction of nurses inade-

[1] "A Survey and a Challenge," Address by Ray Lyman Wilbur, *The White House Conference*, 1930. The Century Company, New York, 1931, p. 16.

[2] Burgess, May Ayres: *Nurses, Patients, and Pocketbooks*, The Committee on the Grading of Nursing Schools, New York, 1928.

quately prepared for the practice of nursing and the faulty distribution of nursing services. It pointed out nurses' need for:

> Reasonable hours
> Adequate income
> Opportunity for growth
> Constructive leadership

Between 1930 and 1940 more than 400 hospitals were closed. The total number of schools was decreased by almost 600. But many weak schools continued, among them some which had ten or fewer students! The total enrollment of students had been reduced by 20 per cent (17,000) during the most acute period of the depression. The decrease was due in part to the closing of hospitals and in part to the admonitions of the Grading Committee. In the spirit of the times, hospitals were encouraged to employ graduate nurses on a staff basis at minimum salaries to keep them out of the bread lines. By 1939, when the threat of war had caused the economic pendulum to swing the other way, the profession was often criticized for its activities in relation to the restriction of enrollment. However, by 1940, the enrollment exceeded that of 1935. (The long-range effects of the depression on nursing were discussed in the previous chapter.) The immediate effect on the schools was wholesome.

An education, which could be obtained at little or no financial outlay in the hospital schools, attracted such large numbers of applicants that the schools were able to make a more careful selection of students than had been possible for many years. Through the leadership of the NLNE and some of the state boards of nurse examiners, many of the schools began using psychometric tests during this period. Tragic though it was in its immediate effect on the lives of many nurses, there is evidence that the long-range effect of the depression on nursing was constructive. Efforts to improve the preparation of nurses were intensified. The development of wholesome personnel policies continued to be a major concern of the American Nurses' Association.

The conclusions of the Grading Committee in relation to the functions of nurses were amplified and discussed in the "activity analysis" prepared for the committee.[3] This analysis provided material which was useful in curriculum planning. It should be noted that the unwholesome conditions in nursing which brought the Grading Committee into being were not limited to the United States. Studies of nursing were published in Canada in 1932, and in England in 1932 and 1938. The usefulness of the report of the excellent and comprehensive Canadian survey was in no way limited by the boundaries of that country. All these reports focused attention on the importance of improving the status of nursing because the profession provides a service essential to national welfare.

Eight foundations contributed approximately $1,000,000 for the work of the Committee on the Costs of Medical Care. So searching were its inquiries that the name of the committee became practically synonymous in medical circles with "controversy." "Between the physician, dentist, nurse, or hospital—able and willing to provide service—and the persons who need it stands a barrier compounded of ignorance and of inability to pay."[4] This was the core of the massive and complex problem to which the committee tried to find an answer. Members of a highly qualified research staff produced an impressive series of illuminating factual reports. In the field of nursing, studies were made only to supplement the concurrent work of the Grading Committee. The development of sickness insurance and the extension of group practice of medicine—the major recommendations of the committee (which was not unanimous in support of them)—were not acceptable to organized medicine. One-half of the 48 members of the committee were physicians about equally divided among those engaged in private practice and those in medical education, public health, and other fields. In addition to representatives from nursing and the other health and related professions, there were a number of distinguished economists and social scientists. Medical critics of the report felt that the committee and staff were overweighted with social scientists who were not sufficiently in-

[3] Johns, Ethel, and Pfefferkorn, Blanche: *An Activity Analysis of Nursing.* Committee on the Grading of Nursing Schools, New York, 1934.

[4] Falk, I. S.; Rorem, C. Rufus; and Ring, Martha D.: *The Costs of Medical Care, A Summary.* Vol. 28, The University of Chicago Press, Chicago, 1932, p. vi. (Foreword.)

formed about the private practice of medicine. Factual data, compiled for the committee, have, however, been used effectively in many subsequent efforts to make medical care available to all the people of the United States.

The recommendations on nursing are of continuing interest. It was recommended that: (1) nursing education be thoroughly remolded to provide well-educated and well-qualified registered nurses, and (2) provision be made for the preparation of (a) nursing aides and attendants and (b) nurse-midwives.[5] The Grading Committee had not made a comprehensive study of auxiliary services but had recommended that a study be made to determine whether "all workers who charge money for nursing sick patients should be licensed by the state."[6]

The recommendation that nurse-midwives be trained was in line with a recommendation from the White House Conference of 1930. A confidential report, prepared in advance of that meeting by a research staff, provided a substantial basis for discussion at the conference. Much progress had been made in the care of babies in the 20-year period since the first White House conference and the subsequent organization of the Children's Bureau. It was estimated that due to the combined efforts of the Children's Bureau and many public and private agencies 122,000 babies survived in 1929 who would have died had the conditions of 1909 prevailed. Maternal care presented a less encouraging picture, but the mortality rate had been started downward. Much remained to be done in both fields. The challenging, and oft-quoted, Children's Charter was a sublimation of the recommendations of that conference.

Some of the subcommittee reports have significance in relation to the development of nursing. The findings and recommendations of the Committee on Nursing paralleled those of the Grading Committee. The very inclusive recommendations for the improvement of preparation for pediatric nursing emphasized the fundamental im-

[5] *Medical Care for the American People*, Final Report, No. 28 of the Publications of the Committee on the Costs of Medical Care. The University of Chicago Press, Chicago, 1932, p. 138.

[6] *Nursing Schools—Today and Tomorrow.* Final Report of the Committee on the Grading of Nursing Schools, New York, 1934, p. 247.

portance of knowledge of the normal child. Pediatric nurses who took the report of that conference to heart were instrumental in securing the organization, a few years later, of a committee on "the child in nursing education" in the NLNE. In preparation for the conference and with the cooperation of registrars, state boards of examiners, and directors of postgraduate courses in public health nursing, the subcommittee on obstetrical nursing had asked hundreds of nurses to answer two carefully phrased noncontroversial questions. They were: (1) "State what you consider constitutes complete care for a mother from the beginning of pregnancy until the baby is six weeks old. (2) How can maternal mortality be prevented?"[7] Experienced private duty nurses were found to be better informed than recently graduated nurses. Public health nurses enrolled in university postgraduate courses were better informed than either of the other groups. But in almost every instance, the replies were incomplete. The committee regretfully reported: "There seems to be no escape from the conclusion that nurses do not know what adequate maternity care is."[8] Because most nurses thought of maternity nursing only in terms of the technics used in relation to parturition, the *American Journal of Nursing* asked Hazel Corbin, the dynamic and farseeing director of the Maternity Center Association (New York City), to provide correct answers to the two questions for publication in the magazine.

The committee's investigation of hospital postgraduate courses corroborated the findings of a study which had been made for the *Journal* by Carolyn E. Gray a year or two earlier. Both studies indicated that such courses were offered to augment the nursing personnel of hospitals and provided little more than added experience on the level of undergraduate programs. Shortly thereafter the NLNE undertook the promotion of more comprehensive postgraduate clinical programs.

The Maternity Center Association intensified its efforts to promote

[7] "Method of Securing Information," *Obstetric Education*, Report of the Subcommittee on Obstetrical Teaching and Education, White House Conference on Child Health and Protection. The Century Company, New York, 1932, p. 125.

[8] *Ibid.*, p. 127.

patient-centered nursing service. Many nurses were keenly aware of the limitation of their preparation. Far more were asking for experience under the direction of the association than could be accommodated. It, therefore, expanded the base of its operations to provide for national and international relationships. Between 1929 and 1935, a member of the staff conducted institutes in most of the states under the auspices of state nurses' associations, local nursing and health agencies, and universities. Since the days of World War I, when Anne A. Stevens, skilled nurse and inspired crusader, had knocked on tenement doors to offer guidance and assistance to those in need of maternal care, nursing had been practiced as a fine art, "one of the finest of the fine arts," by nurses on the staff of that association under the dynamic leadership of her successor, Hazel Corbin. In order to ensure such practice, the association, at an early date, accepted responsibility for teaching its own staff and some other nurses. The institutes were conducted with missionary zeal. Demonstrations of the art of obstetrical nursing were exciting experiences for the nurses who attended. As they looked and listened, their concepts of maternity nursing gained depth and breadth. They acquired a new respect for their calling when they recognized the importance of good maternal care to the patient, her family, and the race. They returned to their tasks equipped with new knowledge, supplemented by lists of the publications and other teaching aids for which the association has acquired a world-wide reputation.

The report of the Committee on Midwives presented at the White House conference is prefaced by an interesting historical sketch of the striking contrast between the development of midwifery in Europe and in our own country. In its recommendations, the committee pointed out that the ultimate solution for good obstetric care rests with the medical schools but that under then existing conditions the midwife was a necessity. For economic reasons, the need was especially urgent in communities having large industrial and Negro populations. There was need for nurse-midwives in departments of health to assist in the development of standards of preparation and in the supervision and control of midwives. Negro nurses with midwifery training, it was suggested, would find an expanded field of opportunity. The first school for nurse-midwives in the United States was established in New York City the following year.

The report of a study of maternal deaths in New York City also advocated the preparation of nurse-midwives. This committee concluded that "two-thirds of all the deaths studied could have been prevented if the care of the woman had been proper in all respects. Contrary to the generally accepted opinion," says this report, "the midwife is an acceptable attendant for properly selected cases . . . the midwife should have a position in the scheme for providing maternity care. It remains for the medical profession to define what that position should be."[9] This committee advocated schools for midwives and schools which would prepare nurse-midwives for supervisory positions under medical direction.

The recommendations of the three committees which favored the preparation of nurse-midwives were based on knowledge of unmet needs. Physicians generally, however, were strongly opposed to the idea because they believed it to be an intrusion on the field of medical practice. There were, however, a few notable exceptions, men whose social vision matched their unchallenged professional competence. The Association for the Promotion and Standardization of Midwifery was incorporated in the state of New York in 1931 with Dr. George Kosmak as chairman. A training school for nurse-midwives was set up and financed for a three-year period. It was named in memoriam for Dr. Ralph W. Lobenstine who had inspiringly favored its inception.[10] At the end of the demonstration period, the Lobenstine Clinic and School were amalgamated with the Maternity Center Association. When the School of Nurse-Midwifery had rounded out 20 years of teaching, 205 experienced nurses had completed the course and, under a charter granted by the state of New York, were entitled to be known as certified nurse-midwives.

[9] *Maternal Mortality in New York City*, A Study of All Puerperal Deaths 1930–2, New York Academy of Medicine Committee on Public Health Relations (Ransom S. Hooker, director of the study). The Commonwealth Fund, New York, 1933.
[10] Report of The Committee to Study the Relation of Nursing to Maternal Care, *Thirty-eighth Annual Report of NLNE*, 1932, pp. 38–39.

Many of them became consultants in federal, state, or local health departments; supervisors of obstetric departments in hospitals; or professors of nursing education in university schools. Others pioneered in areas where such services had previously been unknown. For the 13 years ending in 1950 the maternal death rate for Maternity Center's delivery service was zero! And this occurred on New York's East Side where nurses worked in an overcrowded, polyglot community of low income families.

The general medical resistance to the concept of the nurse as midwife has been such that these specialists rarely use the title nurse-midwife. However, they believe that preparation in nurse-midwifery qualifies them to function as specialists in "the team of professional and other workers concerned with the care of child-bearing women, and after licensure and with medical guidance, to manage antepartal, intrapartal and postpartal phases of childbearing and to give and supervise care to newborn babies."[11]

Prior to the organization of the Maternity Center School, nurse-midwives on the staff of the Frontier Nursing Service, who had been working in a sparsely settled mountain area of Kentucky since 1925, had humanely (and statistically!) demonstrated the usefulness of such service where doctors were not readily available, and where there were few families which could pay for medical care. Mary Breckinridge, founder of that unique midwifery and health service, had secured her midwifery training and her "CMB"[12] in England, where the nurse-midwife is so respected that many more nurses secure their CMB's than expect to practice midwifery. The nurse-midwives on her staff were also British trained. One of them was loaned to Maternity Center to help establish its midwifery program.

When World War II broke out, nurses of British birth quite naturally wanted to care for their own people. To replace them a Graduate School of Midwifery, which had been under consideration for some time, was established by the Frontier Nursing Service at

[11] Announcement, School of Nurse-Midwifery, Maternity Center Association, New York, 1950.
[12] Certificate of the Central Midwives' Board.

Hyden, Kentucky (1939). Many of the one hundred and fifty or more graduates of the school are now at work in faraway primitive areas. To complete discussion of the nurse-midwife, it should be noted that a short-lived school for Negro nurse-midwives was established at the Tuskegee Institute in Alabama and was assisted by federal funds during the war period. The third school of nurse-midwives in existence at mid-century was established in Santa Fe in 1944 by Medical Mission Sisters, who are nurse-midwives trained by Maternity Center and who hold degrees from Catholic University with which the school is affiliated. Plans were carefully laid for the school by the Archbishop of Santa Fe, the state department of health, and the Children's Bureau. The state medical society approved the plan for patients who could not afford to pay for medical care. The work of the Sisters was immediately successful. It has been said to have opened up a new era in the lives of mothers and fathers in the Santa Fe area. Not until 1944, when the NOPHN established its Nurse-Midwifery Section, did the national nursing organizations take formal cognizance of this cautious movement for improvement of care for the nation's mothers. The section defined its purpose as clarification and interpretation to public health administrators and other co-workers of the position, functions, and qualification requirements of nurse-midwives in public health agencies. Standards set up by the section were made the basis for the licensure of nurse-midwives in New Mexico.

The complete reports of the 1930 White House Conference, and those of the Committee on the Costs of Medical Care, occupy something in the neighborhood of fifty volumes. Their findings and recommendations have had an extremely important influence on the evolution of health and medical care programs. For example, the continuing influence of the Committee on Costs' recommendation for "the development of suitable hospitals into comprehensive community medical centers with branches and medical stations where needed,"[13] can be found in the report of the Commission on Hospital Care and the mid-century hospital program of the USPHS,

[13] "Medical Care of the American People," Final Report of the Committee on Medical Care, #28. University of Chicago Press, Chicago, 1932, p. 110.

which are discussed in later chapters. In the nursing profession's continuing effort to improve the preparation of nurses for the practice of nursing there are few sharp dividing lines from which to measure the influence of new stimuli. It was fortunate that a nursing organization, the Maternity Center Association, was in existence which could take decisive and courageous action. By mid-century, when the USPHS reported that 95 per cent of all births were attended by physicians, it seemed that the practice of midwifery might never become a major field of service for nurses. But, through the efforts of the Maternity Center Association and the Children's Bureau, more and more nurses were being adequately equipped for a place on "the team of professional and other workers concerned with the care of childbearing women." The next chapter continues the discussion of evolutionary processes which were at work in the thirties.

BIBLIOGRAPHY

Breckinridge, Mary: *Wide Neighborhoods*. Harper & Brothers, New York, 1952.

Briefs, Maternity Center Association, Winter 1950–1951, Vol. XIV, No. 6.

Buck, Dorothy F.: "The Nurses on Horseback Ride On," *Am. J. Nursing*, **40**:993, 1940.

Burgess, Elizabeth C.: "Eight Years of the Grading Committee," *Am. J. Nursing*, **34**:937, 1934.

Corbin, Hazel: "Modern Obstetric Nursing," *Am. J. Nursing*, **46**:535, 1946.

Gray, Carolyn E.: "Postgraduate Courses," *Am. J. Nursing*, **29**:709, 1929.

Hemschemeyer, Hattie: "Midwifery in the United States—How Shall We Care for the Million Mothers Whose Babies Are Born at Home?" *Am. J. Nursing*, **39**:1181, 1939.

"How Would You Have Answered?" *Am. J. Nursing*, **31**:450, 1931.

Interim Report, Inter-Departmental Committee on Nursing Services. His Majesty's Stationery Office, London, England, 1939.

Johns, Ethel, and Pfefferkorn, Blanche: *An Activity Analysis of Nursing*. Committee on the Grading of Nursing Schools, New York, 1934.

Kosmak, George W.: "The Trained Nurse and the Midwife," *Am. J. Nursing*, **34**:421, 1934.

Maternity Center Association, 1918–1943. The Association, New York.

Nursing Schools—Today and Tomorrow. Final Report of the Committee on the Grading of Nursing Schools, New York, 1934.

Obstetric Education, Report of the Subcommittee on Obstetric Teaching and Education, White House Conference on Child Health and Protection. The Century Co., New York, 1932, Part II, "Obstetric Education of Nurses and Nursing Attendants," pp. 123–66; Part III, "Obstetric Education of Midwives," pp. 169–226.

Peebles, Allon, and McDermott, Valeria D.: *Nursing Services and Insurance for Medical Care in Brattleboro, Vermont,* #17, Publications of Committee on the Costs of Medical Care. University of Chicago Press, Chicago, 1932.

Quarterly Bulletin, US Public Health Service, Washington, D.C., Spring 1951, p. 42.

Reed, Louis S.: *Midwives, Chiropodists and Optometrists: Their Place in Medical Care,* #15, Publications of the Committee on the Costs of Medical Care. University of Chicago Press, Chicago, 1932.

Rochstroh, Edna C.: "Enter, the Nurse-Midwife," Foreword by Mary Breckinridge, *Am. J. Nursing,* 27:198, 1927.

"Schools of Nurse-Midwifery," *Pub. Health Nursing,* 35:477, 1943.

Stewart, Isabel M.: "Postgraduate Education—Old and New," *Am. J. Nursing,* 33:361, 1933.

Viney, Hester: "The English Midwifery Service," *Am. J. Nursing,* 30:408, 1930.

Weir, G. M.: *Survey of Nursing Education in Canada.* University of Toronto Press, Toronto, 1932.

"The White House Conference on Child Health and Protection," *Am. J. Nursing,* 31:452–55, 581–86, 1931.

Chapter 24

CROSS CURRENTS—AND ADVANCES IN
COLLABORATIVE RELATIONSHIPS

The committee believes that fundamental improvement in nursing edu-
cation is a vital essential for the health of the American people and pre-
sents perhaps the most important opportunity in the whole field of Ameri-
can education. We are confident that the evidence of the need for reform
is unassailable and that the general lines of progress have been ade-
quately outlined.

COMMITTEE ON THE GRADING OF NURSING SCHOOLS[1]

NURSING, in little more than half a century, had become an essential
and many-sided social service but was still in a state of professional
adolescence. It was sometimes awkward in its interprofessional relationships and tended to be unduly sensitive to criticism. There
were, however, significant evidences of growing maturity in the
fields of nursing education and of public health nursing. Nursing
education and the administration of institutional nursing services
were controversial subjects. They had become so closely interwoven
that the concept of an independent existence for the schools was at
once anathema to many hospital administrators and the hope of
salvation to an increasing number of nurse educators.

The earlier development of nursing, as we have seen, had been
conditioned by the rapid development of surgery and the concurrent
increase in the number of hospitals. Scientific advances in medicine,
resulting in increasing specialization in medical practice, and the
public health movement were major factors in the conditioning of
nursing in the twenties and thirties. Increasing numbers of internists

[1] *Nursing Schools—Today and Tomorrow*, Final Report. Committee on the
Grading of Nursing Schools, New York, 1934, p. 253.

245

and pediatricians using the newly discovered insulin for diabetes, liver therapy for pernicious anemia, vitamins for rachitic children, and, in general, making use of the "newer knowledge of nutrition," wanted nurses who could give intelligent care to their patients. They wanted nurses who could also help to teach patients and their families not only how to follow instructions but why they should do so. Members of each group of medical specialists had their own concepts of what constituted good nursing; such concepts were often divergent.

The remarkable increase in opportunities for public health nurses in the twenties had put a new emphasis on the importance of including the sociological and psychological implications of poverty and disease in the basic curriculum. Institutions wanted an abundance of low cost nursing service but made almost no distinction between skilled nursing and the sum total of skilled and less skilled services required in a total nursing service. Change was difficult to achieve because there was no coordinating agency through which conflicting concepts of the functions of nurses and, therefore, of the education of nurses could be reconciled. There are, however, some important evidences of progress in the evolution of nursing, and in the field of interprofessional relations in the period when the nation, and nursing with it, was struggling through the depression.

The Grading Committee recognized the National League of Nursing Education, historically and strategically, as the organization best qualified to carry forward the programs it had outlined. Without loss of autonomy, the League had been made the department of education of the American Nurses' Association in 1932. This gave it the professional, if not financial, support of a membership of over 100,000 registered nurses. It opened the way for the development of cooperative relationships between the League and the state boards of nurse examiners. It strengthened in other ways the programs of the two organizations. The Grading Committee recommended that the League "press its project of developing a permanent Advisory Council in Nursing Education on which could be represented the groups most closely concerned with nursing education, namely, nursing, medicine, public health representatives of institutions of higher education, hospitals, and the public."[2] But not until the late forties, when the National Committee for the Improvement of Nursing Service was organized (Chap. 46), was a method devised for such a pooling of interest.

There are, however, significant evidences of progress in cooperative planning during and after the black depression. About 2000 hospitals, out of approximately 7000 listed by the *Journal of the American Medical Association* in 1927, were then operating state-accredited schools of nursing. Preparation of students for practice as graduate nurses was a stated aim of very few of them. Beginning with its first volume in 1900, the AJN frequently carried articles on nursing in mental and other state institutions which were struggling with nursing service problems. But nowhere in the periodical literature of the first quarter century is there evidence of a clearly defined and vigorously promoted sponsorship by the nursing organizations of any system of institutional nursing service other than that provided chiefly by student nurses. Nor had the professional organizations provided leadership in relation to postdiploma education, except in the field of public health nursing. Most of the "postgraduate" courses offered by hospitals existed primarily for the same purpose as the undergraduate schools, namely, to provide on-the-spot nursing service.

The general concept of apprenticeship, of learning to do by doing, had persisted into an era in which the relationship between the learner and the "master craftsman" had become exceedingly tenuous. The load of nursing service required by hospitals had grown by accretion rather than by any orderly process. But there had been little change in administrative policies. The Grading Committee noted that, regardless of fluctuations in need for nursing service, the superintendents of nurses were expected to perform the administrative miracle of having all work handled by existing staffs in periods of high hospital occupancy.

As medicine became increasingly scientific, physicians required more and more service in connection with diagnostic procedures. The treatments they ordered increased in both number and com-

[2] *Ibid.*, p. 252.

plexity. The educational programs for medical students also absorbed considerable amounts of the time of nurses in "teaching" hospitals. Ward order books frequently contained more orders than could be properly executed by the available nursing personnel. Many physicians seemed to evaluate nursing on the basis of the personal service they received rather than on the nursing care provided for their patients. This problem of nurse educators had been well stated by Isabel McIsaac at the turn of the century when she asked, "*Are we preparing nurses, or assistants to surgeons?*" More years would go by before the basic problem could be stated explicitly and unmistakably as, "How many nurses are required who have had a professional preparation for nursing, and how many who have been trained for technical services only?"

"Loyalty to the physician," as taught in many classes in ethics had quite generally resulted in subservience instead of an intelligent response to instructions which would have created a natural tendency to confer on methods of accomplishing desired results. As their needs for service grew, many physicians expressed exasperation or frustration by criticising nursing education. The oft-repeated statements, "nurses are being overeducated," and "the students are always at class," may occasionally have been based on the curriculum (as they understood it), but such comments were far more often due to the fact that some specific desired service was delayed or not available because of a shortage of personnel. The League's *Curriculum* (1927) called for only 230 more hours of theoretical instruction than the earlier edition,[3] but the wholesome change from evening to daytime classes was often the underlying source of medical dissatisfaction. Nurse educators were concerned about the health of students while striving to keep pace with advances in medicine, therapeutic and preventive, and in public health. This could be accomplished only by enriching and adapting the curriculum as well as improving the teaching of nursing in connection with nursing practice on the wards. Nursing is under lasting obligation to many physicians who have given time and thought to the instruction of

[3] The *Curriculum* of 1917 called for a total, for a three-year program, of only 585 to 595 hours.

nurses. Too many lectures, however, were merely abridged and simplified reproductions of material prepared for medical students. The fundamental distinction between medicine and nursing had not been generally recognized. Nursing is neither a dilution of medicine nor an accretion of the functions medicine has transferred to it. It is an art related to, but different from, the practice of medicine. It was in this period that nurse instructors, following the brilliant lead of the Yale school, endeavored to transform the case-study technic which had tended to become routinized on the basis of medical orders into patient-centered nursing care studies. Teaching, based on study of the psychological and physical needs of the patients, has been one of the Yale school's most important contributions to nursing. But routines and technical procedures were so demanding that there was little time in most schools for ward teaching and for the practice of the more subtle arts of nursing through which nurses make a constructive contribution to the recovery of the sick and to the peace of mind of their families. As the director of nursing in a busy teaching (university) hospital put it, "We don't *nurse* patients any more. We have time only to follow doctors' orders." That nurse and Miss McIsaac, separated as they were by more than a quarter of a century, would have understood each other perfectly.

Relatively few nurses or hospital administrators had as yet comprehended the urgent necessity for making a clear distinction between the functions of a nursing school and those of a nursing service. The most notable exceptions to this generalization were to be found in the endowed university schools with their emphasis on patient-centered teaching. The profession has been slow to recognize the importance of the position of the director of nursing service. It honors Effie J. Taylor for the lifetime of effort that made her the second dean of the Yale school and president of the ICN. It forgets that, working in connection with Miss Goodrich as director of nursing service at the New Haven Hospital, she pioneered in a field of primary importance, viz., the administration of institutional nursing service as distinct from the administration of a nursing school with which it might (or might not) be expected to cooperate. The care of the sick is the primary function of nursing. Education is a means to that end but kudos, in nursing, had always been accorded the educator rather than practitioner. All honor to Laura M. Grant[4] and the others who pioneered in the same field. While cooperating with nursing schools they devoted their efforts to the improvement of nursing practice through enlightened administration of nursing services.

Many medical societies appointed committees on nursing during this period, but none of them probed so deeply into the causes of dissatisfaction as had the committee of the New York Academy of Medicine a few years earlier. (Page 177.) A committee of the AMA brought out a comprehensive report on nursing in the association's journal in 1927 which was widely publicized. The statistical report on nursing schools was especially useful to boards of nurse examiners because it called attention to schools operated by hospitals which were not approved by the AMA. In more recent years, the AMA's annual statistical reports have become increasingly useful to nursing and other members of the health family. Although positive in tone, the AMA committee's report did not get to the heart of the problem of nursing and nursing education. It advocated encouragement of the use of visiting nurse services and a trial of hourly or part-time nursing. (As noted, the association later participated in a study of hourly service in Chicago.). This committee advocated a two-year program for nursing schools, following a four-month preliminary course. It recommended continued support of the Grading Committee. The AMA, however, as noted elsewhere, withdrew from the Grading Committee shortly thereafter.

The report of a committee on nursing of the Association of American Medical Colleges gave encouraging educational and moral support but no direct assistance to the advocates of nursing education on a collegiate level. This association was interested in nursing education because of the influence of nursing on medical education. Significantly, it recommended that in all university schools there should be (1) a sound form of administrative organization on a uni-

---

[4] Director of nursing service at the University Hospitals of Cleveland; successor to Miss Taylor as director of nursing service, New Haven Unit, Grace-New Haven Community Hospital.

versity level, (2) one of the many forms of faculty organizations which have proven satisfactory to other schools of the university, (3) independence of budgetary control to the same extent as obtains in other schools or colleges of the same university, and (4) curricular control of both theoretical and practical courses coordinate with the curricular control in other divisions of the same institution. The report of a study of medical education made under the auspices of this association, and published at about the time the Grading Committee was completing its work, contains a brief section on nursing from which we quote. Nursing is recognized as "an essential factor in the health program of the country, and its fundamental foundations are in the medical sciences. No one can dispute the exploitation of nurses in the past as a means of cheap labor for hospitals and the failure of hospitals and universities to develop a real educational training for the profession. . . . A sound educational plan is an essential contribution which universities can make. It would seem logical that the content and methods of training should be guided in large part by medical faculties, leaders of which are familiar with the fundamental sciences upon which it is dependent, and with the medical, public health, hospital and community needs to meet which nurses are trained and directed."[5] Unfortunately, the admitted lack of "interest or knowledge on the part of many clinical teachers of the preventive aspects of their own subject"[6] vitiated the argument for medical guidance of nursing education by medical schools. Through its committee on education and its council of course directors, the NOPHN was then actively promoting its program of endorsement of university courses in public health nursing.

The desire of nurse educators for a list of accredited schools, thwarted by the Grading Committee's decision not to publish a classified list, brought forth the Association of Collegiate Schools of Nursing. Professional and academic institutions had been stimulated to attain good standards by membership in organizations. Why should the principle not work equally well in an organization

[5] *Final Report of the Commission on Medical Education*, New York, 1932, pp. 218–220.
[6] *Ibid.*, p. 220.

of collegiate schools of nursing? The report of the Committee on Nursing of the Association of American Medical Colleges may have given impetus to plans for a new organization which had been discussed in a series of informal conferences. The assumption that subsidy could be found for an association of collegiate schools proved to be wishful thinking. With almost no funds, but sustained by the aspirations of its founders, and encouraged by the eagerness of collegiate schools to secure membership, the durable old pattern of arduous committee work by zealous unpaid workers was again started under the leadership of Miss Goodrich, first president of the association. By 1935, standards had been developed, and 20 collegiate schools, fortunately well distributed throughout the country, had acquired active or associate membership.

The Catholic Hospital Association organized a council on nursing education after the first Grading Committee reports had been sent to the schools. Approximately 20 per cent of all nursing schools in 1930 were under Catholic auspices; and all of them were "the offspring of hospitals." The council used a questionnaire of such excellence that the Grading Committee secured permission to publish it for use by any schools which might wish to utilize it as a self-testing device.

One of the postwar phenomena had been the appearance of Sisters on the campuses of universities which offered postgraduate work in nursing. The Grading Committee had noted the extremely uneven range of preparation for faculty positions in schools of nursing. It is therefore noteworthy that one-fourth of the directors of Catholic schools had achieved a bachelor's degree by 1930. The council and the association aimed to have all of them attain that level of academic education by 1937. Some of the state boards of nurse examiners noted that the Catholic schools were securing well-prepared directors much more rapidly than other schools but seem not to have associated the fact with the need for scholarships.

When the NLNE broadened the base of its service to the profession by establishing a Department of Studies in 1932, high priority was given to studies of various aspects of the administration of institutional nursing services. "Measuring Nursing, Quantitatively and

Qualitatively" was the significant title of the first article released by
Blanche Pfefferkorn, director of the new department. It was the first
of a series in which the importance of research in relation to patient
care was stressed. Hospitals were endeavoring to ameliorate the
effects of the depression on nursing by employing more graduate
nurses than ever before. The first major study made by the new
department was concerned with the utilization of the services of
graduate nurses. When committees of the American Hospital Association began working with nurses on problems of mutual interest,
the services of the department were made available for special
studies. A small study of personnel policies was made in 1935. A
manual on the administration of hospital nursing services published
the following year marked the beginning of a new era in collaborative planning. Here, for the first time, authoritative data on the average hours of bedside nursing service required by the several categories of patients—adults (medical and surgical), mothers and
babies, and pediatric patients—were sponsored by the two organizations.

The League by this time had also begun working with the American Psychiatric Association which had instituted a program for
the standardization of schools in mental hospitals early in the
century. A survey of nursing schools in psychiatric hospitals was
made by a special worker under the joint auspices of committees of
the two organizations. It was an important cooperative gesture, but
the recommendations lacked specificity. The education committee
of the NLNE produced two important manuals in this period. *The
Nursing School Faculty* was published in 1930, and the first edition
of the *Essentials of a Good School of Nursing* came out almost simultaneously with the *Manual of the Essentials of a Good Hospital
Service,* sponsored by the AHA and the League, in 1936.

The Grading Committee had adopted the following principles at
an early date. But neither that committee, nor any of the others
which had made studies of nursing education, came to grips with
the fundamental problem: How shall nursing education be financed?
"(1) No hospital should be expected to bear the cost of nursing education out of funds collected for the care of the sick. The education

of nurses is a public responsibility. (2) The fact that a hospital is faced with serious financial difficulties should have no bearing upon whether or not it will be connected with a school of nursing. The decision should be based solely upon the kinds and amounts of educational experience which the hospital is prepared to offer."[7] The Grading Committee did not stimulate the construction of "lighthouses" along the path of nursing education comparable to the endowed university schools which are attributed to the influence of the Winslow-Goldmark report. But its more pervasive influence helped to raise the general level of nursing education. The results of the second grading, according to the Curriculum Committee of the NLNE, showed that "many of the schools in the upper quartile had practically caught up with the 1927 recommendations of the committee and, in some cases, had gone well beyond them.[8] Its reports had also, as we have endeavored to show, provided the basis for collaborative planning by hospital and nursing organizations.

BIBLIOGRAPHY

Bailey, Harriet: "Nursing Schools in Psychiatric Hospitals," Report of a Survey, *Am. J. Nursing*, **36**:495, 1936.

Beck, Sister M. Berenice: "Hospital or Collegiate Schools of Nursing?" *Am. J. Nursing*, **36**:716–25, 1936.

Bibliography on basic professional curricula in nursing leading to degrees, *Am. J. Nursing*, **37**:297, 1937.

"Can Your School Pass?" *Am. J. Nursing*, **31**:1243, 1931.

"Catholic Schools of Nursing in the United States," excerpts from Report of the Council on Nursing Education of the Catholic Hospital Association, *Hospital Progress*, April, 1934.

Capen, Samuel P.: "Who Is Concerned with the Reform of Nursing Education?" *Mod. Hosp.*, **43**:67–70, 1934. Reprinted in Part III, Chap. VII, *The Hospital in Modern Society*, edited by Arthur C. Bachmeyer and Gerhard Hartman. The Commonwealth Fund, New York, 1943, pp. 156–61.

A Compilation of Students' Records Required for the Course in Medical

[7] Burgess, May Ayres: *Nurses, Patients, and Pocketbooks.* The Committee on the Grading of Nursing Schools, New York, 1928, p. 450.

[8] *A Curriculum Guide for Schools of Nursing,* prepared by the Curriculum Committee of the NLNE, New York, 1937, p. 5.

Nursing, Bulletin 3. Yale University School of Nursing, New Haven, Conn., 1931.

Corbin, Hazel: "Community Responsibility for Adequate Maternity Care," *Thirty-ninth Annual Report of the National League of Nursing Education*, 1933, pp. 139–45.

Davis, Michael M.: "Public Responsibility for the Education of Nurses," *Thirty-ninth Annual Report of the National League of Nursing Education*, 1933, pp. 166–74.

Deferrari, Roy J.: "Schools of Nursing—A Part of the Educational System of the Country," *Forty-fifth Annual Report of the National League of Nursing Education*, 1939, pp. 109–19.

Essentials of a Good School of Nursing. National League of Nursing Education, New York, 1936.

Gilbert, Ruth: *The Public Health Nurse and Her Patient.* The Commonwealth Fund, New York, 1940.

Gray, Carolyn E.: "Postgraduate Courses," *Am. J. Nursing*, 29:709, 1929.

Hospital Number, *J.A.M.A.*, March 12, 1927.

Jones, Anita M.: "The Nurse's Responsibility for Adequate Maternity Care," *Thirty-ninth Annual Report of the National League of Nursing Education*, 1933, pp. 145–52.

Kilpatrick, William H.: "The Educational Challenge," *Forty-first Annual Report of the National League of Nursing Education*, 1935, p. 99.

Kosmak, George W.: "The Place of the Trained Nurse in Obstetric Practice," *Thirty-ninth Annual Report of the National League of Nursing Education*, 1933, pp. 126–39.

Lyon, E. P.: "The Concern of the Medical School in Nursing Education," *Thirty-ninth Annual Report of the National League of Nursing Education*, 1933, pp. 159–65.

McGrath, Earl J.: "Public Support of Nursing Education," *Forty-fifth Annual Report of the National League of Nursing Education*, 1939, pp. 119–30.

Mahan, P. J.: "Relation of the School of Nursing to the Hospital," reprinted from *Hospital Progress*, 1930, in *Nursing Education*, Bulletin #6, Catholic Hospital Association, 1930–1931.

Manual of the Essentials of a Good Hospital Nursing Service. Prepared by the Division on Nursing of the Council of the American Hospital Association and a committee of the National League of Nursing Education, 1936.

Nursing Education and Schools of Nursing—Methods and Problems of Medical Education (Twenty-first Series). The Rockefeller Foundation, New York, 1932.

The Nursing School Faculty—Duties, Qualifications and Preparation. National League of Nursing Education, New York, 1930.

The Nursing School Faculty. National League of Nursing Education, New York, 1933.

Pfefferkorn, Blanche: "Measuring Nursing, Quantitatively and Qualitatively," *Am. J. Nursing,* **32**:80, 1932.

———: "Nursing and Medical Education," *Am. J. Nursing,* **33**:1188, 1933.

Principles and Practices in Public Health Nursing, including Cost Analysis. Prepared by the National Organization for Public Health Nursing. The Macmillan Company, New York, 1932.

Report of the Committee on Nursing Education, Bulletin #10. The Catholic Hospital Association of the United States and Canada, 1931-1932.

"Report of the Committee on Nursing Education," *J. A. Am. M. Coll.,* Jan., 1933, pp. 28–39.

"Report of a Study of Salaries, Physical Examinations, Illness, Vacations, and Leaves of Absence" (mimeographed). Made by a committee of the American Hospital Association and the National League of Nursing Education, 1935.

Stewart, Isabel M.: *The Educational Programme of the School of Nursing.* The International Council of Nurses, Geneva, 1934.

———: *The Education of Nurses.* The Macmillan Company, New York, 1943.

A Study of the Use of the Graduate Nurse for Bedside Nursing in the Hospital. National League of Nursing Education, New York, 1933.

Survey of Public Health Nursing, Administration and Practice, by the National Organization for Public Health Nursing. The Commonwealth Fund, New York, 1932.

Wayland, Mary M.: *The Hospital Head Nurse.* The Macmillan Company, New York, 1938.

Works, George A.: "The Bases of Accreditment of Higher Institutions," *Forty-first Annual Report of the National League of Nursing Education,* 1935, pp. 105–11.

Chapter 25

A PERIOD OF RAPID SOCIAL CHANGE

*. . . 1935 saw the passage of more social legislation than any other year
in the nation's history, including the national labor-relations act, the social-
security act, the wealth-tax act, the public-utility act and the most liberal
relief program ever undertaken by any government, the Works Progress
Administration.*

DIXON WECTER[1]

THE SOCIAL LEGISLATION of 1935, by effecting a sharp turn away
from the rugged individualism which had continued to be a national
characteristic throughout the twenties, had a powerful influence on
the American way of life and on nursing. The Social Security Act
opened wide the door of opportunity for public health nurses and
expedited the evolutionary process which goes on continuously—
sometimes rapidly, often slowly—within the whole field of nursing.
The extraordinary opportunities for the expansion of nursing services made possible by that legislation are discussed in the next chapter. This one is chiefly concerned with fundamental changes in nursing and the emergence of concepts of interprofessional relationships
which was one of the most important characteristics of the period.

Prosperity did not return to the United States until industries began speeding up production to meet the requirements of the national
defense program. The reluctance of medicine to adapt to social
change tended to create crosscurrents of interest within the nursing
profession. But scientific advances in medicine and social trends

[1] Wecter, Dixon: *The Age of the Great Depression, 1929–1941.* Vol. XIII,
A History of American Life, Schlesinger, Arthur M., and Fox, Dixon Ryan, eds.
The Macmillan Company, New York, 1948, p. 96.

which had been expedited by the depression had combined to stimulate the employment of nurses and the adaptation of nursing to medical, economic, and social changes.

In addition to the discovery of the potency of liver extract, and the introduction of the first of the sulfa drugs, to which reference has already been made, the identification and use of one vitamin after another had made headline news throughout the period of the depression. Nutritionists converted the findings of the laboratories together with the language of science into everyday terms of family market baskets and reduced budgets. As consultants to public health nursing agencies, they secured the enthusiastic interest of nurses in teaching elementary lessons in nutrition to the mothers in the homes they visited. Through their assistance with school health programs, undernourished children and their families were encouraged to change faulty food habits. Nutritionists participated in the revision of the *Curriculum Guide,* and hospital dietitians became increasingly interested in teaching the elements of sound nutrition and diet therapy to student nurses. The depression revolutionized social work, placing it among the primary functions of government. Recognition of the distinction between the social components of nursing and the functions of professional social workers became increasingly important to the planners of curriculums in both groups as well as to the administrators of services requiring the participation of both types of workers. Physiologists and anesthesiologists worked tirelessly to produce safe anesthetic agents which would have minimal aftereffects. Cyclopropane was introduced in this period as were the barbiturates for intravenous use. The employment by hospitals of nurse anesthetists had become standard administrative practice in many parts of this country.

The introduction of the Wangensteen and other methods of applying the principles of suction and siphonage to the care of surgical and cord-injury patients called for radical changes, psychological and technical, in the practice of nursing. Cardiac surgery, previously considered impossible, required the highly developed powers of observation as well as the deft sureness of nurses who were well grounded in the psychological and scientific principles on which good nursing is based. Pneumonia, which had been the supreme test of nursing through the first three decades of the century, was giving way to sera which were later outmoded by the sulfa drugs and antibiotics. The greatly extended use of oxygen therapy added another technic to be mastered by nurses for use in a wider range of circumstances.

As medicine became increasingly scientific, without any appreciable increase in the number of doctors graduated each year, more and more responsibility was placed on nurses for the management of equipment, for the collection and transmission to the laboratories of a considerable variety of specimens, and for routines which previously had been classified as medical rather than nursing procedures. Some of the analysts of medical education and practice observed that the necessarily standardized routines of medical care in hospitals tended to depersonalize the medical attention given to patients.[2] When this happened, it had a seriously inhibiting influence on nurses if, as so often happened, the nursing services were understaffed. The delicate art of nursing, in which a sympathetic relationship with patients is of supreme importance, was in grave danger of being lost as nurses raced to keep up with the technical demands of scientific, and often impersonal, medicine. That trend, as we shall see, was later halted by a new emphasis on specialization in nursing practice comparable to that inaugurated by the Maternity Center Association which was discussed in Chapter 23.

Advances in medicine were paralleled by a phenomenal increase in the use of hospital facilities. Between 1935 and 1943 the number of births in hospitals increased by 96 per cent. Concomitantly the number of puerperal deaths per 10,000 live births declined from 62 in 1933 to 25 in 1943. Better antenatal care, due in part to the work of public health nurses, and better asepsis in hospitals were contributing factors. Both institutional and public health nurses undoubtedly played an important part in this same period in securing

[2] Curran, Alonzo Jean: *New Steps in Public Health—Provision for Better Medical Care.* Milbank Memorial Fund, New York, 1945, pp. 47–59.

a 45 per cent reduction in infant deaths from dysentery, diarrhea, and enteritis.[3]

Prepayment plans for hospital care were making a strong appeal to the people of moderate means to whom hospital bills had previously spelled hardship or even tragedy. By 1940 approximately four and one-half million persons were enrolled in plans approved by the Blue Cross Commission of the American Hospital Association. A joint committee of the ANA and NOPHN encouraged continuous study of prepayment plans for health services by state and local nursing organizations in anticipation of the inclusion of nursing in them.

The registry reports for 1940 indicated an encouraging increase in the employment of private duty nurses. There was no indication that the nation might soon be faced with a shortage of nurses. In addition to the external forces which were molding nursing in this period, there were fundamental issues at work within the profession itself which were gaining force and influence.

The major programs of the nursing organizations had been based on conceptions of nursing service in relation to community needs, although these needs were less clearly defined by the two older organizations than by the NOPHN. The ANA's continuous assistance to the state associations in their effort, through state registration, to protect the nurse-employing public, illustrates the point. The programs of the NLNE and the new (1932) Association of Collegiate Schools of Nursing (ACSN) vigorously and courageously adhered to the principle stated in the *Curriculum Guide* that education for practice as graduate nurses in relation to the varied needs of communities should be the goal of all schools of nursing.

With community needs in mind, the NLNE, which had voted against such action in 1919, broadened the base of its membership in 1943 by providing for lay members. In that year too, along with the ACSN, it became a constituent member of the American Council on Education in which it had previously had only the status of as-

---

[3] Gooch, Marjorie: "Ten Years of Progress in Reducing Maternal and Infant Mortality," *The Child*, Nov., 1945, Division of Statistical Research, Children's Bureau, Washington, D.C.

sociate member. It was in 1935 also that the ANA, recognizing the value of NOPHN's experience in promoting community relationships, requested its assistance in promoting community interest in the development of nursing. A joint committee on community nursing service with strong representation from the three older organizations was set up with a full-time executive secretary. Efforts were concentrated on the development of community nursing councils and the preparation of a manual for use in surveying the nursing resources of a community.

Health and hospital councils had already demonstrated their usefulness as coordinating agencies. Several well-established nursing councils were already in existence when Dr. Winslow presented the idea of community nursing councils to an enthusiastic convention audience in 1928. Cleveland, for example, had for a long time had a council which effectively coordinated the work of public health nursing agencies, and which had successfully recruited student nurses. It had also secured some community-wide improvement in the personnel policies of hospitals. The Central Council in Chicago, and an eastern one patterned after it following World War I, had recruited students for their member schools. The Detroit Council had a broad program which included experiments in methods of teaching and supervising practical nurses. By 1940, this council could report no less than 38 cooperating agencies. The Community Nursing Council of Boston published a handbook of nursing services in 1940. A few new councils had been organized when the national preparedness program caused the joint committee to declare its program in abeyance for the period of the emergency.

The social climate of the depression and recovery years stimulated the development of cooperative relationships between the nursing organizations and those of the other health professions. Shared poverty had stimulated both altruism and interest in constructive planning. Despite the hazards of the depression, all had made some progress with their basic long-range programs. The pioneer university course in hospital administration and the educational programs of the American College of Hospital Administrators, which were launched in the midst of the depression, promoted the growing professionalization of hospital administration. The ANA reported that one-third of the programs planned for the national nursing organizations for 1936 provided for the joint participation of two or more associations. It was anticipated that the number of joint projects would be increased.

Patients, doctors, hospital administrators, nurses, and educators had participated in the studies of the Grading Committee. The reports of that committee gave a real impetus to cooperative planning, but they stopped short of providing data on costs which could be used in securing financial support of nursing schools or a system of nursing education. The American Hospital Association went on record in 1936 as believing that "a plan of cooperative action of all interested organizations" should be adopted in relation to nursing education.[4] But a joint committee, comprised of representatives of the AHA and the NLNE, agreed that excellent material was already available for the evaluation of nursing schools. Conversely, although opinions had been freely expressed by various groups, there was no nationally sponsored guide for use in evaluating hospital nursing services. The NLNE had published two manuals, *The Nursing School Faculty* (1932) and the *Essentials of a Good School of Nursing* (1936). The *Curriculum Guide* was in preparation for publication in 1937. Both the NLNE and the Nursing Council of the Catholic Hospital Association, which had published the first report of its Committee on Nursing Education in 1930, launched accreditation programs in the late thirties. The *Fundamentals of Administration of Schools of Nursing*, based on a two-year study anonymously financed through the Research Foundation of the Children's Hospital of Cincinnati, was published by the NLNE in 1940.

Fortunately the NLNE, in its Department of Studies, was well equipped to participate in cooperative studies. The purpose of the *Manual of the Essentials of Good Hospital Nursing Service*, prepared and published by the joint action of the AHA and NLNE (1936), was to set up the principles by which a nursing service could be operated *without* dependence on a nursing school. When

[4] Report of the Committee on Resolutions, 1936 Annual Convention, *Hospitals*, 10:28, 1936.

the manual was revised in 1942, representatives of the American Medical Association, the American College of Surgeons, and the American Nurses' Association also sat on the joint committee responsible for the publication. The five organizations were also represented on the committee which guided the production of the 1950 successor of this publication, *Hospital Nursing Service Manual.* The AHA and the NLNE, however, bore the major responsibility for the mid-century edition. It is much more comprehensive than the earlier manuals.

In the interval between the publication of the first and second editions of the *Manual,* the AHA and NLNE collaborated on the preparation and publication of *Administrative Cost Analysis of Nursing Service and Nursing Education.* Prior to this study of the cost of nursing education and nursing service, a special study of the illness of institutional nurses, student and graduate, was published in 1938. Although the principles of administration advocated in the *Manual* were believed to be applicable to any type of institution, it was conceded that the primary interest of the committee was in providing assistance for general hospitals with active services. The importance of nursing in hospitals for psychiatric and tuberculosis patients, however, was not overlooked in this period of budding collaborative relationships.

Few men have striven more persistently to provide good nursing for the mentally ill than Dr. William L. Russell. In his view, the training of nurses was established in mental hospitals by the governors of the hospitals and physicians because the Nightingale movement passed by on the other side of those institutions. Before 1900, the Royal Medico-Psychological Association of Great Britain began setting standards for the training of "mental nurses" with emphasis on the administrative needs of the hospitals rather than on the education and professional growth of nurses. The American Psychiatric Association adopted a similar policy shortly after the turn of the century when the nursing organizations were just beginning their work for the standardization of nursing through state legislation. As previously noted, the National Committee for Mental Hygiene and the ANA had collaborated in a study of the care of the insane in 1915 but we find no significant evidence of cooperation between the APA and the nursing organizations until the early thirties. At the NLNE convention of 1933, a full session was devoted to psychiatric nursing at which Dr. Arthur P. Noyes painted a bright future for psychiatric nursing. Standards for care and for teaching varied widely in the institutions which operated schools.

Among nurse educators, opinions varied as to the potential value of mental hospital facilities for the development of basic courses or for affiliations. Harriet Bailey, the first nurse to write a textbook on psychiatric nursing, made a small study of seven schools in six states under the auspices of the APA and the NLNE. Her recommendations were based on the assumption that mental hospitals, provided they have funds, facilities, and interest in the education of nurses—as contrasted with the immediate provision of nursing service—could properly operate nursing schools. The study marks the beginning of cooperative efforts to adapt nursing to the need of the mentally sick and to incorporate the principles of psychiatric nursing and mental health in the basic curriculum.

The National Tuberculosis Association cooperated with the three national nursing organizations in a study of the institutional nursing care of tuberculosis patients in 1938. On the basis of observations and time studies, made by Esta H. McNett, a schedule of the time required to give adequate care to patients in each of four categories was set up. Although this was in the period when many nurses were unemployed, or engaged on relief projects, tuberculosis hospitals were generally understaffed. Additional studies were needed to determine, among other things, the availability of qualified nurses for the care of tuberculosis patients and the extent to which subsidiary workers could be safely used. Some years earlier, the NTA had financed the preparation of a *Handbook on Tuberculosis Nursing for Public Health Nurses* by Violet H. Hodgson, then a member of the NOPHN staff. When it became outdated, Mrs. Hodgson prepared a second book (1939) which was published, with the approval of the NOPHN, by the NTA.

Since public health nurses were more immediately affected by the

Social Security Act than other groups, it is interesting to find that NOPHN was well equipped to assist administrators of public health nursing services in their adjustments to an enormously expanded opportunity for service. Three publications produced between 1930 and 1940 tell a story of long-range planning and cooperative relationships. A practical handbook based on careful studies was made possible by the cooperation and generosity of the Metropolitan Life Insurance Company and the John Hancock Mutual Life Insurance Company. The original suggestion for the studies, on which the book was based, had been made by the MLI. Dr. Livingston Farrand, who had been director of the National Tuberculosis Association and of the American Red Cross, before he became president of Cornell University, pointed out in a foreword to *The Survey of Public Health Nursing* (1934) the special significance of that study. He commended it for its emphasis on public health nursing "as simply one part of a unified community program."[5] He noted that progress was being made in many places in the direction of better mutual understanding between official and nonofficial agencies. The most important of the conclusions, he pointed out, was the emphasis on the immediate need for improvement in the preparation of public health nursing personnel.

A timely study of *Personnel Policies in Public Health Nursing*, although it was restricted to official agencies, was regarded as a major adventure in fact finding in the field of public health nursing. It was made possible by the Milbank Fund and was carried through with some assistance from the MLI. About 36 per cent of all nurses working with official agencies were employed under civil-service rulings, but "civil service regulations as such are not necessarily a factor in promoting higher standards for appointment to public health nursing positions."[6] The recommendations were based on need

[5] *Survey of Public Health Nursing, Administration and Practice,* by the NOPHN, (Katharine Tucker, general director; Hortense Hilbert, assistant director). The Commonwealth Fund, New York, 1934.

[6] Randall, Marion G.; *Personnel Policies in Public Health Nursing,* A Report of Current Practice in a Sample of Official Health Agencies in the United States, prepared for the NOPHN. The Macmillan Company, New York, 1937, p. 21.

for well-defined standards and, since the supply of public health nurses was increasing, on higher standards of selection and practice. The book was timely since the 1939 amendments to the Social Security Act made it obligatory for state employees who were engaged in administering the various phases of the federal security program to be employed under a merit system of personnel administration. In this period the school nurse found that, as the accepted pattern of school health programs changed to a concept of "health in the school programs," she had two parents, namely, the NOPHN and the National Education Association.[7]

As the Winslow-Goldmark report had pointed out, ". . . subsidiary service is an existing fact, whether we like it or not."[8] Difficulty in finding a descriptive name for a secondary type of worker, which would be satisfactory to both groups, had been the outward evidence of a serious psychological block to the development of a wholesome attitude toward a second group since the early eighties. While the professional organizations were promoting both the "share the work" principle and endeavoring to maintain good standards in all branches of nursing during the depression, the problem became acute. The Winslow-Goldmark report had advocated the preparation and registration of a "subsidiary" worker, although it pointed out that such service could probably not be provided at a cost much below that of graduate nurses. The Grading Committee advocated wider use of methods of distributing graduate nurse service, such as hourly and group nursing rather than the development of a secondary type of worker. The Committee on the Costs of Medical Care, as we have seen, recommended the training of "nursing attendants who are competent to furnish simple nursing service under the supervision of visiting graduate nurses, who are willing to do housework when necessary, and who accept somewhat lower rates of pay." That committee recommended that "their status, like that

[7] Chayer, Mary Ella; "New Concepts in School Nursing," *Pub. Health Nursing*, 29:495, 1937.

[8] *Nursing and Nursing Education in the United States*, Report of the Committee for the Study of Nursing Education, C.-E. A. Winslow, chairman, and Report of a Survey by Josephine Goldmark. The Macmillan Company, New York, 1923, pp. 14–16, 26.

of all persons who nurse for pay, should be defined by law, and state registration or licensure should be compulsory."[9]

The ANA, in connection with its continuous registry studies, began collecting data about the nature and extent of calls for subsidiary services. Registry reports indicated that economic conditions, coupled with lack of public information about available professional services, influenced requests for subsidiary workers. The joint boards of the three national organizations faced the issue squarely (1936) and went on record as believing that responsibility for outlining principles and policies for the control of subsidiary workers in the care of the sick rested with the nursing profession. By 1939 the ANA board had adopted a policy previously voted by the joint board that "all who nurse for hire should be licensed." The implementation of this seemingly simple and direct policy was, of course, far from simple since licensure is based on legal enactment. It presupposes the establishment of state standards and the development of courses which will make it possible for aspirants to meet the legal requirements. The first of a series of brochures in which principles and nationally approved policies were defined was prepared by a joint committee of the three national nursing organizations and published in 1940.[10] The subject was highly controversial. Many nurses, still suffering from bitter experiences during the depression, feared competition. It may be assumed that "practical nurses," since they were then unorganized, had suffered at least as much as registered nurses. Many advocates of the preparation of a second type of nurse seemed to be more interested in reducing the cost of nursing service than in the functions or welfare of such workers. Doctors reporting on the subject to the Grading Committee seemed to be especially concerned with that aspect of the problem. But nursing, through the national organizations, was at last firmly on record as having assumed responsibility for guiding the development of nursing on all levels. It had demonstrated its growing maturity

[9] *Medical Care for the American People*, Publication #28, Final Report of the Committee on the Costs of Medical Care. The University of Chicago Press, Chicago, 1931, p. 143.

[10] *Subsidiary Workers in the Care of the Sick*. American Nurses' Association, 1940 (revised, 1941).

as a profession by the development of cooperative relationships with other groups in the congeries of health professions.

BIBLIOGRAPHY

"Accrediting Plan for Catholic Schools of Nursing," *Am. J. Nursing,* 37:1210, 1937.

Bailey, Harriet: "Nursing Schools in Psychiatric Hospitals," *Am. J. Nursing,* 36:495, 1936.

Beard, Charles A., and Beard, Mary R.: *America in Midpassage,* Vols. I and II. The Macmillan Company, New York, 1939.

Bruno, Frank J.: *Trends in Social Work as Reflected in the Proceedings of the National Conference of Social Work, 1874–1946.* Columbia University Press, New York, 1948.

"Detroit Council on Community Nursing," *Am. J. Nursing,* 41:310, 1941.

Education and Training, Nursing Reconstruction Committee, Report, sec. II. The Royal College of Nursing, London, England, 1943, p. 26.

Friley, Charles E.: "Standardizing Agencies in the Field of Education," *Thirty-eighth Annual Report of the National League of Nursing Education,* 1932, pp. 210–21.

The Fundamentals of Administration of Schools of Nursing. National League of Nursing Education, New York, 1940.

Goodrich, Annie W.: "Association of Collegiate Schools of Nursing," *Am. J. Nursing,* 33:239, 1933.

Hampton, Isabel A., and others: *Nursing of the Sick, 1893;* Kinney, D. H.: "Association for the Training of Attendants." McGraw-Hill Book Co., New York, 1949, p. 204.

Health Insurance. A brief study guide prepared jointly by the American Nurses' Association and the National Organization for Public Health Nursing, New York, 1938.

Hollis, Ernest V., and Taylor, Alice L.: *Social Work Education in the United States.* Columbia University Press, New York, 1951.

Hodgson, Violet H.: *Handbook on Tuberculosis for Public Health Nurses.* National Tuberculosis Association, New York, 1939.

Hospital Nursing Service Manual. Prepared by a committee of the American Hospital Association and the National League of Nursing Education, 1950.

Manual of the Essentials of Good Hospital Nursing Service. American Hospital Association and the National League of Nursing Education, 1936.

Noyes, Arthur P.: "Nursing Needs in State Mental Hospitals," *Am. J. Nursing,* **33**:787, 1933.

"Nursing Care of the Insane in the United States," *Am. J. Nursing,* **16**:198, 1915.

"Nursing Your Community," Suggestions from the Joint Committee on Community Nursing Service, *Am. J. Nursing,* **41**:427–30, 1941.

Pfefferkorn, Blanche, and Rovetta, Charles A.: *Administrative Cost Analysis of Nursing Service and Nursing Education.* Published by the American Hospital Association and the National League of Nursing Education, 1940.

Principles and Practice in Public Health Nursing, including Cost Analysis. Prepared by the National Organization for Public Health Nursing. The Macmillan Company, New York, 1932.

Proceedings of the Thirtieth Convention of the American Nurses' Association, 1936, p. 141.

Reed, Louis S.: *Blue Cross and Medical Service Plans.* Federal Security Agency, US Public Health Service, Washington, D.C., 1947, p. 12.

Reid, Grace L.: "Councils on Community Nursing," *Am. J. Nursing,* **38**:49–54, 1938.

Report of the Committee on Nursing Education, Bulletin #10. Catholic Hospital Association of the United States and Canada, St. Louis, Mo., 1931–1932.

Robinson, G. Canby: *The Patient as a Person—A Study of the Social Aspects of Illness.* The Commonwealth Fund, New York, 1939.

Russell, William Logie: *The New York Hospital—A History of the Psychiatric Service, 1771–1936.* Columbia University Press, New York, 1945.

Sargent, Emilie: "The Nursing Profession Works for Recovery," *Am. J. Nursing,* **33**:1165–72, 1933.

Schedule for a Survey of Community Nursing Service, rev. By the Joint Committee on Community Nursing Service of the National Organization for Public Health Nursing, American Nurses' Association, and the National League of Nursing Education, New York, 1944.

A Study of the Incidence and Costs of Illness among Nurses. American Hospital Association, National League of Nursing Education, and American Nurses' Association, 1938.

"A Study of the Nursing Care of Tuberculosis Patients," *Am. J. Nursing,* **38**:1021–37, 1938.

"What Registries Are Doing," *Am. J. Nursing,* **41**:904, 1941.

Chapter 26

THE SOCIAL SECURITY ACT—AND EXPANSION
OF NURSING SERVICES

. . . to provide for the general welfare by establishing a system of Federal old-age benefits, and by enabling the several states to make more adequate provision for aged persons, blind persons, dependent and crippled children, maternal and child welfare, public health, and the administration of their unemployment compensation laws; to establish a Social Security Board; to raise revenue; and for other purposes.[1]

SUCH WAS THE PURPOSE of the Social Security Act passed by Congress in 1935 and amended in 1939, 1946, 1948, and 1950. Through its provisions for expanded health programs to be administered by the USPHS and the Children's Bureau, the act exerted an immediate and continuing influence on the education and practice of nurses. Its influence on the lives of nurses as citizens was less immediate but, with the amendments of 1950, practically all nurses, including "self-employed" private duty nurses, became eligible for "old age security."

The studies of the Committee on the Costs of Medical Care had shown that, for large segments of the population, it was difficult or impossible to secure adequate medical care for "between the physician, dentist, nurse, or hospital—able and willing to provide service —and the persons who need it stands a barrier compounded of ignorance and of inability to pay."[2]

[1] Public Law No. 271, 74th Congress, H.R. 7260.
[2] Falk, I. S.; Rorem, C. Rufus; and Ring, Martha D.: *The Costs of Medical Care—A Summary of Investigations on the Economic Aspects of the Prevention and Care of Illness.* Publication of the Committee on the Costs of Medical Care, #27. University of Chicago Press, Chicago, 1933, p. vi.

The report of the National Health Survey, a house-to-house study made with WPA funds in 1935–1936, augmented the findings of the Committee on Costs and provided data for the formulation of a national health program which was discussed at a National Health Conference in 1938 in preparation for congressional action. The program was based on recommendations for: (1) expansion of public health and maternal and child welfare services, (2) expansion of hospital facilities, (3) medical care for the medically needy, (4) a general program of medical care, and (5) insurance against loss of wages during sickness. Following the conference, the program was widely discussed throughout the nation. "The objective of a National Health Program," said President Roosevelt in a message to Congress the following January, "is to make available in all parts of our country and for all groups of our people the scientific knowledge and skill at our command to prevent, and care for, sickness and disability."

One of the most important amendments of 1939 required the establishment and maintenance of personnel standards on a merit basis for personnel employed in federal and state programs administered under the act. The ANA for some years had diligently endeavored to stimulate the interest of the US Civil Service Commission in nursing and the interest of nurses in civil service. The association had been especially concerned to secure the appointment of a qualified nurse in the US Civil Service Commission. Not until 1944, however, was Ruth A. Heintzelman, well equipped by education and experience, appointed to the medical division. The NOPHN, as discussed in the preceding chapter, had already published a study of personnel practices in official agencies. The most important action taken by a voluntary agency, however, was that of the American Public Health Association. With the approval of the USPHS and the Children's Bureau, it set up an administrative unit called the Merit System Study (1942). Dorothy Deming, who had been editor of *Public Health Nursing* and director of NOPHN, was appointed to the technical staff and served as subject consultant on public health nursing for ten years. Within that period the service was enormously expanded with more than 40 states making use of its materials. Its usefulness in the broad field of health services might be compared to that of the NLNE's Department of Measurement and Guidance in the field of nursing education.

The policies relating to the national health program adopted by the AMA, the AHA, and other hospital associations, and by the three national nursing organizations, which were of primary concern to nurses, were summarized in the AJN.[3] The hospital associations, which had been opposed to the insurance provisions of the Social Security Act, announced their decision to work for "proper enabling legislation . . . so that hospital employees will come under that part of the Social Security Act relating to old-age assistance. . . ." The opposition of the AMA to sickness insurance had been bluntly stated before the act was passed. When the act became the law of the land, the House of Delegates of the AMA reaffirmed its opposition to all forms of compulsory sickness insurance. It also reaffirmed its policy of encouraging local medical organizations to establish plans for the provision of adequate medical service for all the people by voluntary budgeting to meet the costs of illness. On the basis of their own studies, the three nursing organizations pledged their "best cooperative efforts in planning for the coordination and utilization of the experience and services offered by all official and voluntary agencies."[4]

Medicine, hospitals, and nursing in this country owe their origins and early development to the imagination, courage, and initiative of individuals and voluntary agencies. Such agencies have been the standard bearers. Their methods were often adopted by or adapted to the needs of official agencies. The nursing organizations were equipped to assist in setting up standards of education and of nursing service. Public health nursing was generally conceded to have provided a spearhead for the public health programs. Public health nurses made up approximately one-half the roster of all health agency employees. They received approximately one-third of the total sum expended for public health services.

[3] "Federal Legislation and The World We Live In," *Am. J. Nursing,* **40:**176, 1940.
[4] "The National Health Program," *Am. J. Nursing,* **39:**233, 1939.

The programs outlined under two of the titles of the Social Security Act could not be put into effect without greatly increased numbers of public health nurses. The Children's Bureau received a substantial annual appropriation for the care of mothers and children, especially in rural areas and in areas suffering from severe economic distress. It also received funds for locating and securing care for crippled children. Both allocations were increased later. The USPHS received funds for the purpose of assisting states, counties, health districts, and other political subdivisions of the states in establishing and maintaining adequate public health services, and for the training of personnel. The standard for public health nurses was based on NOPHN's *Minimum Qualifications for Those Appointed to Positions in Public Health Nursing*. The provision for the training of personnel has had a far-reaching influence on all nursing.

The allocation of funds by a federal agency by means of a grants-in-aid program was not an innovation. The program, which had been so ably administered by the Children's Bureau under the Sheppard-Towner Act in the twenties, paved the way for the nursing programs of the USPHS and the Children's Bureau that were made possible by the Social Security Act. The immediate effects, in relation to nursing, of the allocation of funds to the two agencies were the appointment of Naomi Deutsch, who had been closely associated with Miss Wald at Henry Street, as director of public health nursing in the Children's Bureau, and the expansion of the nurse consultant service of the USPHS, which had been established in 1934 as a direct result of the depression. The Surgeon General, Dr. Hugh S. Cummings, had been aware that the two voluntary agencies, the APHA and the NOPHN, believed that nurse-consultant service should be provided by the federal agency. He had borrowed farsighted and statesmanlike Sophie C. Nelson from the John Hancock Life Insurance Company to make a survey of the service, in relation to nursing, in 1932. Her crystal-clear recommendations were as valid at mid-century as when they were made. They had not, however, been put into effect when the need of state health departments for consultant service, in connection with FERA programs, forced action in 1934.

Fortunately, Pearl McIver, who had been a conspicuously successful state supervising nurse, was then with the USPHS on a temporary assignment. She accepted appointment in what became the
States Relations Division of the USPHS on condition that the position be classified in the professional grade by Civil Service. Although
there was only that one position to be filled, Miss McIver and some
20 other public health nurses passed the first examination in that
grade that was ever offered nurses by the federal Civil Service Commission. This list of experienced and eligible nurses was invaluable
in securing six nurses who were assigned to the service after the
passage of the Social Security Act. Miss McIver was designated
senior public health nursing consultant. An interdepartmental committee which was promptly created prepared a statement on public
health nursing policies and procedures which provided a substantial
basis for cooperative relationships between the USPHS and the Children's Bureau. The states quickly grasped the opportunity to expand their services. By the end of the first year, all 48 states, the
District of Columbia, Alaska, and Hawaii were providing an advisory service of some type for local public health nursing agencies.

In the early stages of the new program a very high percentage of
stipends made available for the preparation of personnel were
awarded to nurses. By 1940 approximately 3000 nurses had been
granted stipends and tuition from Social Security funds for some
type of preparation for public health nursing. No other health profession was able to augment its resources so swiftly. In the search
for suitable candidates, the qualifications of the 6000 nurses, who
were still employed on WPA projects, were carefully screened. Participation in work projects had stimulated the interest of nurses in
public health nursing who might otherwise not have considered entering that field. The assistance of the NOPHN in developing the
new program was generously acknowledged by Surgeon General
Parran who wrote: "The U.S. Public Health Service has drawn
heavily upon the resources of the National Organization for Public
Health Nursing in preparing recommendations with regard to the
public health nursing developments made possible through Social
Security funds. The standards and requirements recommended by

the National Organization for Public Health Nursing have guided the state and territorial health officers in the development of their public health nursing programs and they will continue to look to this professional group for guidance and assistance."[5]

Stimulated by the Children's Bureau program, every state department of health had a division of maternity and child health under the direction of a physician by 1940. More than 4000 nurses were being paid wholly, or in part, from funds allocated by the Children's Bureau, and the states had paid, wholly or in part, for the special preparation of 762 nurses.

Before the passage of the act, a variety of services for the care of crippled children had been developed. Some of the large visiting nurse associations, for example, had well-developed orthopedic services staffed by nurses who were also trained physical therapists. But there were no generally recognized standards for the preparation of nurses who were to practice orthopedic nursing. Relationships with other specialists, such as dentists, nutritionists, social workers, and teachers, were to become increasingly important as the work developed. Realizing that the number of orthopedic nurses was far too small to meet the needs of the new program for crippled children, the Children's Bureau sought information and advice from the profession. There were no postgraduate courses in that field. Replies from the state boards, as to the nature of the orthopedic training included in the basic courses, were not encouraging. The NLNE could say only that the new *Curriculum Guide* was expected to stimulate improvement in them but that it would require time. The problem was then taken to the NOPHN. That organization, which had been receiving requests for assistance from various quarters, acted promptly. A new orthopedic council proceeded to set up tentative standards for courses for graduate nurses. Universities were encouraged to offer advanced courses in orthopedic nursing, and also basic courses for public health nursing supervisors who had not had good undergraduate preparation for that field. Within a short time plans were under way for courses at Harvard, Western Reserve, and Teachers College.

[5] "Encouraging Words from a Friend," *Pub. Health Nursing*, **29**:290, 1937.

A little later, NOPHN received a subsidy from the National Foundation for Infantile Paralysis (NFIP) to provide for the employment of a consultant in orthopedic nursing. The arrival of modest little Jessie L. Stevenson (Mrs. Harry R. West) at national nursing headquarters in October, 1939, was not recognized at the time as an epochal event. In retrospect, it signalizes a revitalization of the concept of nursing as a fine art. Miss Stevenson was both a public health nurse and a physical therapist. She had been supervisor of the widely known orthopedic unit of the Chicago Visiting Nurse Association, a part-time instructor at Northwestern University Medical School, and associate editor of the *Physical Therapy Review.* Within a year she wrote *The Care of Poliomyelitis,* and had begun the conferences and institutes which were to do for orthopedic nursing what Maternity Center's Anita Jones and others had done for maternal care a few years earlier.

"Every nurse," said Miss Stevenson, "institutional, private duty or public health, who gives bedside care or teaches the art of nursing to student nurses or to families, is responsible for making or preventing crippling. . . . Orthopedic nursing must be a part of all good nursing but the reverse is equally true, all good nursing is a part of orthopedic nursing."[6] How the NOPHN and NLNE joined forces to promote the development of orthopedic nursing will be discussed in Chapter 40.

As the profession rose to grasp these opportunities, nurses quite generally became aware of the serious inequalities in the basic preparation of nurses. Ambitious graduates of schools that had ignored state board recommendations in relation to high school prerequisites, or provision by affiliation for experience in obstetrics, pediatrics, and other clinical fields in which they were deficient, found themselves seriously handicapped. They were required to take courses to supplement their inadequate basic education as a preliminary to admission to programs in public health nursing. Leaders in public health nursing joined nurse educators in urging wider use by the schools of the NLNE's *Curriculum Guide.*

[6] Stevenson, Jessie L.: "What Is Orthopedic Nursing?" *Am. J. Nursing,* **39**:11, 1939.

The NOPHN had been approving (accrediting) courses in public health nursing for graduate nurses since 1920. Rapidly changing medical, health, and social conditions, and the sudden influx of students, were creating both problems and opportunities for the institutions of higher education which were offering programs in public health nursing. The NOPHN asked the USPHS to participate in a public health nursing curriculum study. In response, Mary J. Dunn, a nursing consultant on the USPHS staff who was especially well equipped for the task, was designated to give the major part of her time to the work. The resultant *Public Health Nursing Curriculum Guide* was published in 1942. Emphasis was placed throughout on the preparation of the *practitioner* of public health nursing, not on the advanced preparation for supervisory, administrative, or teaching positions. Consideration of the 16 functional areas—maternal health, infant health, tuberculosis, and the like—into which public health nursing was subdivided provide the body of the *Guide*. Its usefulness was greatly enhanced by special sections devoted to the development of sound relationships.

By January 1, 1940, more than 23,000 public health nurses were on duty in the United States and the territories of Hawaii and Alaska. They were touching the lives of more than a quarter of our population. The number employed in rural health departments had increased by 57 per cent as compared with an over-all increase of 19 per cent in a three-year period. Even so, more than 800 counties were still without any type of public health nursing as were 20 cities with populations of 10,000 or more. Up to this time nonofficial agencies, such as the visiting nurse services, had been the major factor in public health nursing. The period marked a sharp upturn in a trend which had begun in the twenties. Whereas the nonofficial agencies had employed about 40 per cent of all public health nurses in 1931, they employed only 29 per cent in 1940. (By 1950, official agencies were employing over 90 per cent of all public health nurses.)

Industrial nursing was believed to be an unstandardized field. More closely related to management than to organized nursing, the standards of work, of interplant relationships, and effective use of community agencies in promoting the health and welfare of the workers were believed to be extremely variable. The findings of a comprehensive study in the Pittsburgh area (1939) confirmed that opinion. Under the provisions of the Social Security Act, state and local health departments had begun to develop industrial hygiene units. Indiana was the first state to employ a consultant industrial nurse. Others quickly followed. When industries began speeding up production in the preparedness program, they employed more and more nurses to help maintain the health of the workers. Whereas in 1941 there were over 5000 graduate registered nurses employed as industrial nurses, the National Survey of 1943 secured returns from over 11,000 such nurses.

Industrial nursing had become so important that a national study was undertaken by the public health nursing section of the APHA (1940). It was conducted with the assistance of the Division of Industrial Hygiene of the National Institute of Health. The report, *Nursing Practices in Industry*, a major addition to the fundamental studies of nursing, indicates the need for standards of industrial nursing practice and includes "Recommendations for Acceptable Practices."[7] Olive M. Whitlock, one of the authors of the report, was the nursing consultant of the Industrial Hygiene Division of the USPHS. Data from the study were used as a basis for the chapter she contributed to the *Manual of Industrial Hygiene*.

The NOPHN, which had organized its industrial nurse section in 1920, seems not to have met the felt needs of a considerable number of industrial nurses. This may have been due to the fact that industrial nursing is a combination of the activities of hospital and public health nurses practiced in a variety of settings which are quite unlike those of either of the other groups.

The Social Security Act was the result of a sharp change in public opinion about the ability of individuals to provide for their own needs throughout life. This chapter, however, has been concerned only with the effect of its liberal provisions, in relation to public

---

[7] Whitlock, Olive M.; Trasko, Victoria M.; and Kahl, F. Ruth: *Nursing Practices in Industry*. Public Health Bulletin #283, USPHS, US Government Printing Office, Washington, D.C., 1944, p. 70.

health, on nursing. Because of it the trend toward the nationalization of the public health, which began in the twenties, took a sharp
turn upward. After 1935, the federal government was to have an
increasingly potent influence on the evolution of American nursing.

BIBLIOGRAPHY

American Medical Association Bulletin, June, 1935, p. 91.

Belsley, G. Lyle: "Nursing and the Merit System," *Am. J. Nursing,* **37:**387, 1937.

Better Government Personnel. Published for the Commission of Inquiry on Public Service Personnel. McGraw-Hill Book Co., New York, 1935.

Daily, Edwin F.: "Maternal and Child Health Programs under the Social Security Act," *Am. J. Pub. Health,* **31:**117, 1941.

Deming, Dorothy: "Testing Program of the Merit System Service," *Am. J. Nursing,* **51:**569, 1951.

Deming, Dorothy, and Heintzelman, Ruth A.: "How Federal Civil Service Works in Relation to Nurses," *Am. J. Nursing,* **46:**319, 1946.

Douglas, Paul H.: *Social Security in the United States* (An Analysis and Appraisal of the Federal Social Security Act). McGraw-Hill Book Co., New York, 1936.

Draper, Warren F.: "The National Health Program and the Nurse," *Am. J. Nursing,* **39:**471, 1939.

Falk, I. S.: "Voluntary or Compulsory Group Payment of Sickness Costs in the United States?" *Security Against Sickness—A Study of Health Insurance.* Doubleday, Doran and Co., Garden City, N.Y., 1936, Chap. XV.

Gafafer, William M. (ed.): *Manual of Industrial Hygiene and Medical Service in War Industries.* W. B. Saunders Co., Philadelphia, 1943.

Goldmann, Franz: *Public Medical Care—Principles and Problems.* Columbia University Press, New York, 1945.

Heintzelman, Ruth A.: "Preparation for Orthopedic Nursing," *Pub. Health Nursing,* **30:**302–7, 1938.

Hilbert, Hortense: "A Nurse and the Merit System," *Am. J. Nursing,* **41:**1397, 1941.

Klein, Alice Campbell: *Civil Service in Public Welfare.* Russell Sage Foundation, New York, 1940.

Kruesi, Walter: "The Social Security Act and the Nurse," *Am. J. Nursing,* **42:**524, 1942.

McIver, Pearl: "Public Health Nursing in the United States Public Health Service," *Am. J. Nursing,* **40:**996–1000, 1940.

————: "How Many Public Health Nurses?" *Pub. Health Nursing*, **33:**21, 1941.

Mountin, Joseph W., and Greve, Clifford H.: *The Role of Grants-in-Aid in Financing Public Health Programs*. Public Health Bulletin #303, Federal Security Agency, Washington, D.C.

National Health Conference, July 18–20, 1938. Called by the Interdepartmental Committee to Coordinate Health and Welfare Activities, Washington, D.C.

Parran, Thomas: "Public Health Nursing Marches On," *Pub. Health Nursing*, **29:**617–22, 1937.

Perrott, George St. J.; Tibbetts, Clark; and Britten, Rollo H.: "The National Health Survey—Scope and Method of the Nationwide Canvass of Sickness in Relation to Its Social and Economic Setting" (financed as a WPA project, p. 1668), *Pub. Health Rep.*, **54:**1663–87, 1939.

The Public Health Nursing Curriculum Guide. Prepared by a joint committee of the National Organization for Public Health Nursing and the U.S. Public Health Service, 1942.

Public Health Reports, **54:**815–16, 1939.

"The Platform of the American Medical Association," *J.A.M.A.*, **113:**2322, 1939.

Sheahan, Marion W.: "The Merit System Applied to Nursing," *Pub. Health Nursing*, **32:**248–54, 1940.

Sinai, Nathan; Anderson, Odin W.; and Dollar, Melvin L.: *Health Insurance in the United States*. The Commonwealth Fund, New York, 1946, p. 110.

Smillie, Wilson G.: *Public Health Administration in the United States*, 3rd ed. The Macmillan Company, New York, 1947, p. 558 (The Social Security Act of 1935).

Social Security Legislation Throughout the World, Bureau Report #16. US Social Security Administration, Federal Security Agency, US Government Printing Office, Washington, D.C., 1949.

"Standards [Merit System] Recommended by the Children's Bureau," *Am. J. Nursing*, **40:**289, 1940.

Stern, Bernhard J.: *Medical Services by Government—Local, State and Federal*. The Commonwealth Fund, New York, 1946.

Stevenson, Jessie L.: *The Care of Poliomyelitis*. The Macmillan Company, New York, 1940.

"A Study of Industrial Nursing Services" [by a committee selected from the membership of the Public Health Nursing Section of the American Public Health Association], *Pub. Health Nursing*, **32:**631–36, 1940.

"W.P.A. and Nursing," *Am. J. Nursing*, **35:**1154, 1935; **37:**994, 1937.

Chapter 27

THE CURRICULUM GUIDE

... *"health" nursing is just as fundamental as "sick" nursing and the prevention of disease at least as important a function of the nurse as the care and treatment of the sick. Indeed, these functions cannot be separated though they are undoubtedly represented in different proportions in the different fields of nursing. Moreover, the nurse is essentially a teacher and an agent of health in whatever field she may be working, though here again the emphasis varies. All nurses must be concerned with the social conditions which so directly affect the condition of the patients and their prospects of cure. The subordination of the "human element" in our work to the physical and technical is one of the severest criticisms we have to meet in nursing today, and it seems strange that there should be any question that a much stronger emphasis on these human and social factors is needed, whether we are dealing primarily with sick nursing or health nursing.*[1]

A CURRICULUM in nursing has one thing in common with a nurse practice act: neither can be set up once and for all time since nursing is continuously in a state of adaptation to medical advances and changes in the social order. The League's *Curriculum for Schools of Nursing* (1917) and the revised edition, the *Standard Curriculum* (1927), had been widely used. They had placed the League in a strong position of leadership in the field of undergraduate, or basic, nursing education. The studies of the Grading Committee indicated that the time was ripe for a new, rather than merely a revised, curriculum, and the Committee on the Costs of Medical Care had stated that:

There should be a rearrangement of curricula and a revision of the fundamental purposes of many nursing schools, so that they will produce

[1] *A Curriculum Guide for Schools of Nursing.* National League of Nursing Education, New York, 1937, p. 21.

socially-minded nurses with a preparation basic to all types of nursing service. The care of hospital patients is not, in and of itself, sufficient preparation for professional nursing. Nurses should be prepared not only for the practice of a profession, but for life and its manifold home and community duties as well.[2]

The Survey of Public Health Nursing (1934) substantiated the "inescapable and disconcerting facts" revealed by the two reports. This important study indicated that "the health approach for relating nursing to the public health field as well as scientific knowledge and the techniques of nursing need to be infiltrated through the whole curriculum."[3]

A League committee was ready to work toward reconstruction of the *Curriculum* the moment the final report of the Grading Committee could be made available to it. Isabel M. Stewart, chairman of the committee and director of the Division of Nursing Education at Teachers College, had worked with Miss Nutting on the first two editions of the curriculum. Probably she alone realized the Herculean nature of the task delegated to the committee. Few, if any, nurses have contributed as much voluntary selfless service to the advancement of nursing education. Under her dauntless and energetic leadership a large central curriculum committee was set up with an executive committee and 22 production committees. Fortunately, a generous anonymous gift eased the burden by providing a full-time secretary, some expert assistance from the field of education, funds for travel, and some scholarships for participating nurses. Teachers College donated office space.

In the statement on the educational philosophy and aims of the new curriculum, the committee broke away from the authoritarian concept of nursing with its emphasis on the subordination of the individual, stating that:

The changes in modern life are largely the results of science and technology. Nurses must be able to adjust to these rapidly changing con-

[2] *Medical Care for the American People*, Publication #28, Final Report of the Committee on Costs of Medical Care. University of Chicago Press, Chicago, 1931, p. 142.

[3] *Survey of Public Health Nursing Administration and Practice*, by the National Organization for Public Health Nursing. The Commonwealth Fund, New York, 1934, p. 18.

ditions, and this means that they require a different type of preparation than would be needed for a relatively static society.[4]

On the basis of this premise, the committee selected the "adjustment aim" and subjected it to careful analysis by committee members, educators, and all interested readers of the *Journal*. "Adjustments," said the committee, "between people or groups, should not be one-sided nor result in sacrificing one individual or one group to the other. . . . The emphasis in the nursing school as in all professional schools must be on fitting its students for actual professional practice. . . ."[5]

Curriculum construction is a highly technical process. To orient the profession to the initial thinking of the committee and to pave the way for democratic action, a series of six articles was published in the *American Journal of Nursing*. Much effort was concentrated on securing the participation of experts from the field of education, representatives of nursing school faculties, members of state boards of nurse examiners, and other persons interested in the project. In a three-year period, between 200 and 300 persons took part in the work. Stimulated usually by state leagues, study committees were organized in 35 states, the District of Columbia, and Hawaii. On them sat, in varying combinations, educators, doctors, nurses, hospital administrators, social workers, nutritionists, and other interested persons. A group of cooperating schools tested tentative course outlines, prepared by the production committees, while the work was in progress.

Resistance to change is a characteristic of human nature. Inevitably the *Guide* aroused fear with concomitant resentment in some quarters. The new curriculum was planned for use, as its title indicated, as a guide and not as a program to be slavishly followed. Like its predecessors, it was intended to serve as a pace-setter for the upper 25 per cent of the schools. It was not intended to salvage feeble schools with poor prospects. The sale of the book exceeded all expectations. A questionnaire a year after its publication revealed

[4] *A Curriculum Guide for Schools of Nursing*, prepared by the Committee on Curriculum of the National League of Nursing Education. National League of Nursing Education, New York, 1937, p. 17.

[5] *Ibid.*, p. 19.

marked diversity of opinion as to the most helpful and most controversial sections, but progress was being made, especially in those
parts of the country where there had been participating committees.
Many schools could not make effective use of the *Guide* without
larger and better prepared faculties, increased instructional facilities, and shorter hours. As one experienced principal put it, the most
difficult problem might be the financing of the additional graduate
staff nurses required by the shortened hours recommended for students. Higher admission requirements (one or more years of college
work), more careful selection of students, more effective use of community resources to secure greater breadth of experience for student
nurses, expansion of the basic clinical requirements to include psychiatric nursing, suggestions for experimentation with alternative
units of experience—these were among the objectives of the *Guide*.
They were not, however, stated so compactly that they can readily
be quoted.

The hours of regular ward teaching, it was planned, were to be
included in the hours of organized instruction allocated to the
various clinical fields. The recommended hours of instruction were
increased to somewhere between 1200 and 1300 hours in a three-
year program, with the hours of practice (too often thought of as
time on duty rather than as *supervised practice*) reduced to an
average of 38 to 42 hours weekly during the clinical part of the
program.

The *Guide* was sometimes criticized as too diffuse. A consultant
service to the schools, which would have ensured better understanding and more effective use of the *Guide*, was then beyond the resources of the League. Most nursing schools accelerated their
courses as required by the US Cadet Nurse Corps during World
War II, but the *Guide* continued to provide a sound foundation for
adjusted wartime programs.

BIBLIOGRAPHY

Caswell, Hollis L., and Campbell, D. S.: *Readings in Curriculum Development.* American Book Co., New York, 1937.

"Curriculum Revision," *Am. J. Nursing*, Vol. 35, 1935.

1. Taylor, Effie J.: "The Next Step Forward," p. 57.
2. Stewart, Isabel M.: "A Tentative Program for Curriculum Reconstruction," p. 153.
3. Stewart, Isabel M.: "What Educational Philosophy Shall We Accept for the New Curriculum?" p. 259.
4. Stewart, Isabel M.: "What Standards Shall We Accept for the New Curriculum?" p. 359.
5. Smith, C. Mabel: "What Sources and Technics Shall We Use in Revising the Curriculum?" p. 459.
6. Stewart, Isabel M.: "How Shall We Plan the Program of Study?" p. 568.

"Curriculum Revision—A Symposium," *Forty-fourth Annual Report of the National League of Nursing Education*, 1938, pp. 181–99.

Johnson, Sally: "Discussion Relative to the Installation of the Curriculum Guide," *Forty-third Annual Report of the National League of Nursing Education*, 1937, p. 153.

Methods and Problems of Medical Education—Nursing Education and Schools of Nursing (Twenty-first Series). The Rockefeller Foundation, New York, 1932.

Nursing Schools—Today and Tomorrow. Final Report of the Committee on the Grading of Nursing Schools, New York, 1934.

Stewart, Isabel M.: "Curriculum Revision—An Essential Step to the Reconstruction of Nursing Education, *Am. J. Nursing*, 35:58, 1935.

———: "Report of the Committee on Curriculum," *Forty-first Annual Report of the National League of Nursing Education*, 1935, pp. 67–71.

———: *The Education of Nurses*. The Macmillan Company, New York, 1943.

Chapter 28

THE INSTITUTIONAL STAFF NURSE
TAKES THE STAGE

The widespread interest in the question [graduate staff nursing] would seem indicative of a growing consciousness on the part of nursing and hospital administrators that the graduate nurse, by virtue of her complete training and more mature experience, is superior as a worker to the student, and that her employment is basic to consistently good nursing service.[1]

THE LONG-RANGE INFLUENCE of the depression on nursing, like that of war, was constructive. There is no more striking evidence of this fact than the rapid rise in the employment of graduate staff nurses by hospitals which were operating schools of nursing. Employed in many instances at minimum salaries in order that they might "share the work," they stabilized the services and improved the care of patients. They also helped to ensure better balanced programs of clinical experience for student nurses. The number of "floor" or "general duty" nurses rose from 4000 in 1929 to over 28,000 in 1937.[2] By 1941 it was estimated that over 100,000[3] nurses were regularly employed as hospital staff nurses in institutions with and without schools. They far outnumbered both the private duty nurses, who had previously constituted the largest group in the profession, and the total student enrollment.

Studies of the Grading Committee had shown that, although gen-

[1] *A Study on the Use of the Graduate Nurse for Bedside Nursing in the Hospital.* National League of Nursing Education, New York, 1933, p. 26.
[2] "Did You Ever See a Nurse Nursing?" *Am. J. Nursing,* 38:27, 1938.
[3] "Is There a Shortage of Nurses?" *Am. J. Nursing,* 41:747, 1941.

erally better paid than private duty nurses (they received maintenance if regularly employed) general duty was least popular of all
types of nursing in the late twenties. They were less well paid and
had less freedom than staff nurses in public health agencies. Causes
of unpopularity were administrative and psychological. Broken
hours and insistence on acceptance of accommodations in nurses'
dormitories were among the administrative policies which disaffected mature women who wanted to live normal lives unrestricted
by hospital discipline when off duty. The causes were deep-seated,
and stemmed from the weaknesses in the American system of nursing. The plan for the Nightingale School in London had been
projected against a background of nursing service in which carefully
selected head nurses (ward sisters) and graduate staff nurses, as
soon as they were available, had a very important place. Not so in
the American adaptation of the Nightingale system. In the beginning, undergraduates served as head nurses because there was no
source of supply of prepared nurses on this side of the Atlantic. But,
according to Louise Darche, "what was at first regarded as a misfortune came to be considered a part of the system."[4] The course was
extended from one year to two in order that the service of pupils
who had completed the year of "training" could be retained and
utilized as head nurses. The extramural demand for nurses was then
so great that it was believed that no hospital or school could com-
pete with the compensation offered by "outside" employers. After
World War I, when there were not enough students to provide the
required volume of service, hospitals that operated schools began
employing graduate nurses, but merely to supplement the service of
students. In other words, the services of graduates were utilized as
an expedient rather than as a part of planned programs of patient
care. Under the pressure of hospital routines there was little opportunity for them to develop genuine competence in the care of individual patients. This fact and lack of status for these nurses caused
a psychological trauma from which the profession is still suffering.
The heads of the schools and nursing services were themselves

[4] Hampton, Isabel A., and others: *Nursing of the Sick, 1893.* McGraw-Hill
Book Co., New York, 1949, p. 96.

products of "the system." They had inherited the authoritarian philosophy of their Victorian predecessors. The 50-year-old concept of students as a primary source of service was still strongly entrenched in the minds of most of the nursing and hospital administrators. But the *Journal* and contemporary nursing and hospital publications are prolific sources of material on many aspects of institutional staff nursing in the late twenties and through the following decade.

Nurses *like* to nurse. But the concept of hospital nursing as student service tended to inhibit imaginative thinking or constructive planning by either administrators or nurses. Conversely, in both visiting and private duty nursing, the care of patients was not only the function but the privilege of graduate nurses. It is significant that nursing was then so sharply compartmentalized in the minds of nurses that the experiences of one group were rarely considered applicable to those of another. Had there been a closer liaison between the administrators of public health nursing services and those responsible for institutional services, the results of the accumulated experience of the public health nursing agencies with graduate staff nurses might have been more readily available to the administrators of institutional nursing. Dealing constantly with all-graduate staffs, the more highly organized public health nursing agencies had learned that the development of *esprit de corps* calls for respect of nurses as individuals, efficient staff organization, and well-developed staff education programs. The administrators of institutional nursing services also learned these things through experience, but more slowly because, in most institutions operating schools of nursing, the schools were granted a prior claim on the time and interest of administrative personnel.

Some small hospitals, however, had reason to be proud of the service rendered by graduate nurses. When many small institutions were closing their schools, the *Journal* sought for information which might be helpful to them, and which might also solve the riddle of the general reluctance of well-qualified graduate nurses to accept institutional staff positions. The ten-year experience of the director

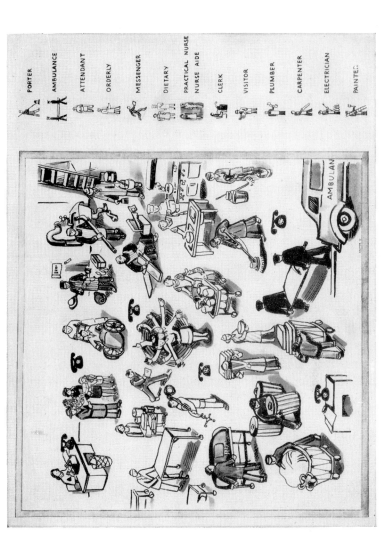

PORTER

AMBULANCE

ATTENDANT

ORDERLY

MESSENGER

DIETARY

PRACTICAL NURSE

NURSE AIDE

CLERK

VISITOR

PLUMBER

CARPENTER

ELECTRICIAN

PAINTER

Plate IX. The mid-century head nurse. Nurse, teacher, administrator, or traffic manager? (*Courtesy of Frances Reiter Kreuter.*)

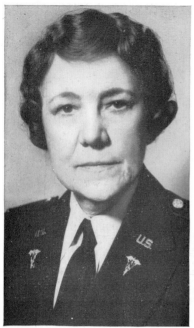

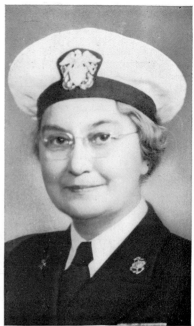

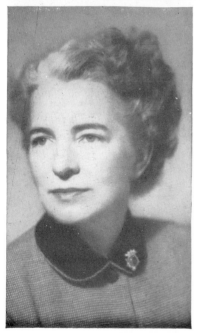

Plate X. Throughout most of World War II, the military nursing services were directed by Colonel Florence A. Blanchfield (*upper left*), Superintendent, Army Nurse Corps, 1943–1947 (*US Army photo*), and Captain Sue S. Dauser (*upper right*), Superintendent, Navy Nurse Corps, 1942–1945 (*Bachrach*). Lucile Petry Leone (*lower left*), now Assistant Surgeon General, USPHS, director of the Division of Nurse Education, 1943–1946, was administrator of the US Cadet Nurse Corps (*Blackstone Studio*).

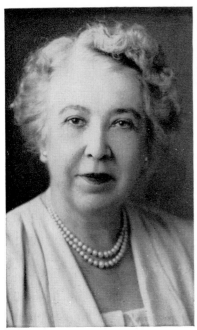

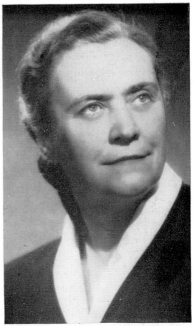

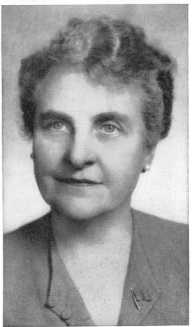

Plate XI. Alma C. Haupt (*upper left*) was executive secretary of "the Government's Subcommittee," 1941–1943. L. Louise Baker (*upper right*) was director of the Nursing Division, Procurement and Assignment Service, War Manpower Commission, 1943–1945 (*Amos Carr, Hollywood*). The name of the Honorable Frances Payne Bolton (*lower right*) was imperishably associated with nursing before she sponsored the act which provided for the US Cadet Nurse Corps in 1943 (*Harris & Ewing*).

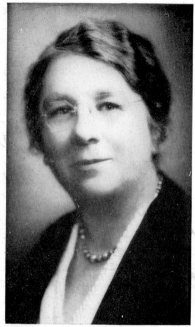
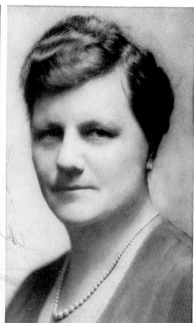
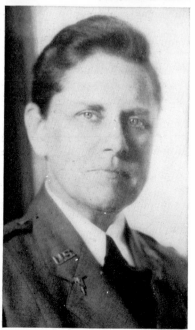

Plate XII. The onerous duties of chairman of the National Nursing Council were carried successively by Colonel Julia C. Stimson (ret.) (*lower left*), president of the ANA, 1940–1942; Stella Goostray (*upper left*), president, NLNE, 1942–1946; and Sophie C. Nelson (*upper right*), a former president of the NOPHN, 1946–1948. (*Photos by Underwood & Underwood, Bachrach, and Bachrach, respectively.*)

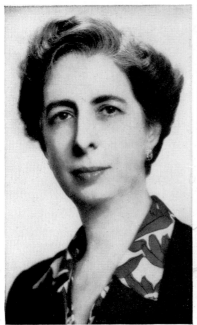

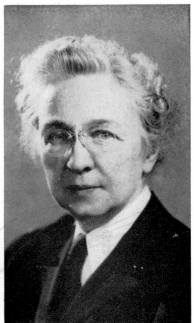

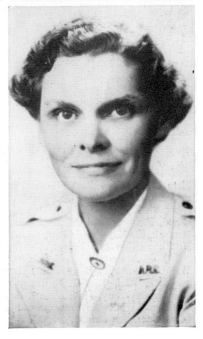

Plate XIII. As wartime pressures for more and more military and civilian nursing service increased, the National Nursing Council became a natural target for criticism. Mrs. Elmira Bears Wickenden (*upper left*) bore that heavy burden and served courageously as executive secretary from 1942–1947. Sensitive and none-too-robust Mary Beard (*upper right*) broke under the terrific pressure to which the ARC Nursing Service was subjected, and was succeeded in 1944 by Virginia M. Dunbar (*lower right*) (*photos by Harris & Ewing*).

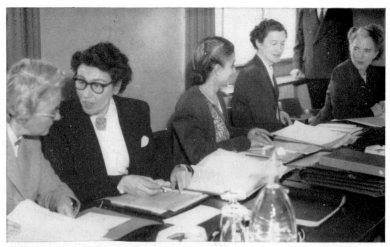

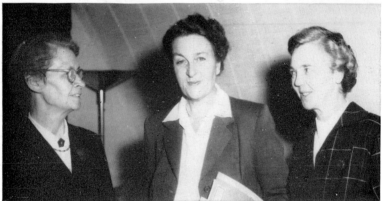

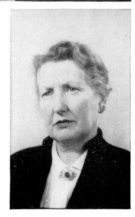

Plate XIV. (*Top*) First meeting, Expert Committee on Nursing, WHO, 1950. (*Left to right*) Elizabeth Brackett, USA, nursing adviser; M. L. David, France; T. K. Adranvala, India; Yvonne Hentsch, LORCS; Lucile Petry Leone, US Public Health Service (*J. Cadoux, Geneva*). (*Lower right*) Olive Baggallay, chief, Nursing Section, WHO. (*Center, left to right*) Gerda Höjer, president, ICN, 1947–1953; Daisy C. Bridges, executive secretary, ICN; Ellen J. Broe, director, Florence Nightingale International Foundation (*Goncalnes, San Paulo*).

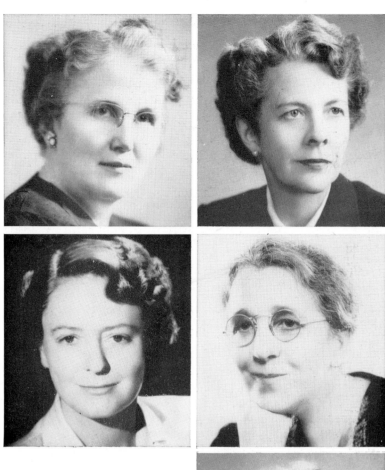

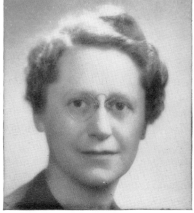

Plate XV. These nurses are internationally known for their educational statesmanship. They are (*left, top to bottom*) R. Louise McManus (*White Studio, N.Y.*); Mildred L. Tuttle (*M. Lillie Studio, Battle Creek Mich.*). (*Right, top to bottom*) Virginia Arnold (*Harris & Ewing*); Isabel M. Stewart; Mary Elizabeth Tennant (*Bradford Bachrach*).

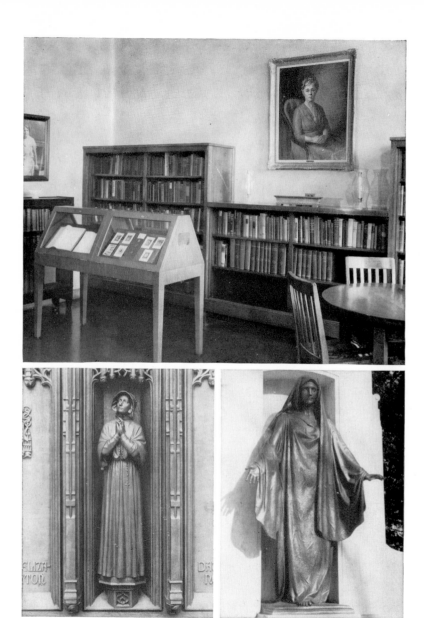

Plate XVI. (*Top*) Phoebe M. Kandel Section of the Solomon W. Levi Memorial Library, College of Nursing and Health, University of Cincinnati. (*Lower left*) Mother Seton, as memorialized on the bronze main door of St. Patrick's Cathedral, New York (*courtesy of the Cathedral*). (*Lower right*) The Delano Memorial, Washington, D.C. (*American Red Cross*).

of one of three small county hospitals, which had been established
in Missouri in the early nineteen twenties, provided a valuable
clue. Following the general pattern of the times, it had been assumed that each hospital would secure nursing service by setting up
a school of nursing. Fortunately, the administrator of the first institution to be built was a socially minded and farsighted nurse, whose
example was followed by the other two. Beginning with a graduate
staff, she spent a year in studying the community, its needs, and its
social resources. By that time she had learned that the resources for
the development of a good school were not available. She had also
learned that, in order to attract a good type of graduate nurse, a
hospital "must build on a sound business basis, render a high type
of service to the community, and see to it that a proper atmosphere
is maintained not only in the hospital but in the nurses' home."[5]
This nurse administrator was well ahead of the times in arranging
for staff nurses to attend professional meetings and for leaves of
absence for postgraduate work. During the twenties, both the ANA
and the NLNE endeavored to secure shorter hours for nurses, but
they took no other formal action in relation to the adaptation of
institutional personnel practices to the needs, psychological or other,
of graduate nurses.

Shortly after the three county hospitals—previously mentioned—
were built, the Commonwealth Fund began a rural hospital program
which, in the course of 20 years, developed more than a dozen
permanent demonstration centers in 13 states. All of these community hospitals were staffed with graduate nurses supplemented
by nurse's aides or attendants and, in some instances, by volunteer
workers. In the compactly lucid summary of the fund's experience,
we find an excellent statement on a nursing setup for the small
community hospital which is as germane to a discussion of nursing
education as to a consideration of staff nursing. The fund found that
". . . the fifty-bed hospital cannot run a satisfactory nurse training
school and must therefore be staffed with graduate nurses. . . .

[5] Keely, L. Eleanor: "Graduate Nursing in Rural Hospitals," *Am. J. Nursing,*
32:960–62, 1140–42, 1932.

There is plenty of room for debate over the question whether student nursing is cheap nursing; it certainly is not so in this type of hospital."[6]

In the summer of 1940 approximately 400 small hospitals (less than 100 beds) provided the ANA with data which were used as the basis for a series of *Journal* articles. Most of these institutions were in towns of 10,000 or less population. Two-thirds of them relied entirely on graduate nurses. There were wide variations in the degree of satisfaction in their work expressed by the nurse hospital superintendents, the supervisors, and by the staff nurses themselves. The most marked characteristic of the replies received from 3000 staff nurses was their lack of clearly defined objectives. Their responses verified the need, which had already been recognized by some nurse educators, for guidance programs in the schools of nursing as well as for well-planned staff education programs in the employing institutions.

Until the *Manual of the Essentials of Good Hospital Nursing Service* was published in 1936,[7] there were no established standards for the guidance of administrators of nursing services in hospitals without schools of nursing. Here, for the first time, administrators of all types of hospital nursing services could find, in compact form, practical suggestions on such matters as (1) the time required for the performance of nursing service for patients in the several commonly accepted categories, (2) qualifications of personnel, and (3) personnel practices covering hours, salaries, maintenance, and health services. The section on "Staff Education" is especially pertinent to this discussion of graduate staff nurses. Herein lay the hope of developing among the staff nurses of an institution an *esprit de corps* which would at one and the same time improve the service and help nurses to achieve a reasonable degree of satisfaction in their work. However, *"the greatest menace to a good nursing service,"* says the

[6] Southmayd, Henry J., and Smith, Geddes: *Small Community Hospitals.* The Commonwealth Fund, New York, 1944.

[7] *Manual of the Essentials of Good Hospital Nursing Service,* prepared by the Division of Nursing of the Council of the American Hospital Association and a committee of the National League of Nursing Education, 1936 (revised 1942) (revised 1950; renamed *Hospital Nursing Service Manual*).

manual, *"undoubtedly is placing more work upon the shoulders of nurses than they are able to do and do well."*[8]

A resolution of the ANA House of Delegates in the mid-thirties called for:

. . . provision of working conditions which make it possible for the nurse to give good care to the patient; a salary schedule which gives consideration to the nurse's need for a reasonable degree of security; living conditions conducive to good health; and opportunities for development.[9]

Publication of the manual was followed by recommendations based on the ANA's study of *Income, Salaries and Employment Conditions.* This was a stellar event of 1938. More than 2000 staff nurses participated in the study, but the findings were grouped under the general heading of institutional nurses. As previously noted, the ANA recognized the importance of this type of nursing practice by providing for the organization of a General Staff Nurses Section in 1940.

The depression had created conditions conducive to the employment of graduate nurses on a staff basis in hospitals. When it was over, general duty nurses (as they prefer to be called) had achieved an important and permanent, but not wholly satisfactory, place for themselves. The institutional staff nurse had moved to the center of the stage of professional nursing service when the United States entered World War II.

BIBLIOGRAPHY

Annual Salaries and Salary Increases and Allowances Paid to General Staff Nurses. American Nurses' Association, New York, 1943.
Beck, Sister M. Berenice: "General Staff Nursing," *Am. J. Nursing,* 37:57, 1937.
Bogardus, Mary I.: "The Graduate Nurse in Hospital Service," *Am. J. Nursing,* 35:112–16, 1935.
Burgess, May Ayres: *Nurses, Patients, and Pocketbooks.* Report of a study of the economics of nursing, conducted by the Committee on the Grading of Nursing Schools, New York, 1928, pp. 96, 353–57, 395.

[8] *Ibid.,* p. 11.
[9] "Resolutions on the General Staff Nurse and Employment Conditions on Which Good Nursing Service Depends," *Am. J. Nursing,* 36:817, 1936.

Densford, Katharine J.: "Selection of General Staff Nurses," *Forty-second Annual Report of the National League of Nursing Education,* 1936, p. 126.

Faddis, Helen W.: "Experiments in Solving the Staffing Problem," *Am. J. Nursing,* **37**:991, 1937.

Graduate Nurse Service. Some practical points for consideration by hospitals contemplating the use of graduate nurse service. American Nurses' Association, New York, 1933.

"Hospital Staff Nurse Recommendations Concerning Her Status and Problems," *Am. J. Nursing,* **41**:55, 1941.

Jones, Virginia A.: "What Pattern Staff Education?" *Pub. Health Nursing,* **29**:212, 1937.

Mosiman, Margaret A.: "Graduate Staff Education," *Am. J. Nursing,* **30**:201, 1930.

"Professional Drifts and Shifts," *Am. J. Nursing,* **41**:1, 1941.

Reeve, Irma E.: "Staff Education," *Am. J. Nursing,* **36**:819–24, 1936.

Sister John of the Cross: "Securing and Keeping Satisfactory Graduate Staff Nurses," *Forty-second Annual Report of the National League of Nursing Education,* 1936, p. 134.

"Small Hospitals," *Am. J. Nursing,* Vols. 40–41, 1940–1941.
  1. "Nursing in Small Hospitals in Small Towns," **40**:1370, 1940.
  2. "She Administers a Small Hospital," **41**:167, 1941.
  3. "The Small Hospital Supervisor," **41**:315, 1941.
  4. "3000 General Staff Nurses," **41**:422, 1941.

Study of Incomes, Salaries and Employment Conditions Affecting Nurses (exclusive of those engaged in public health nursing). American Nurses' Association, New York, 1938.

Taylor, Anna M.: "A Staff Nurse Program," *Am. J. Nursing,* **40**:137–45, 1940.

Wolf, Anna D.: "How Can General Duty Be Made More Attractive to Graduate Nurses?" *Am. J. Nursing,* **28**:903, 1928.

Chapter 29

PUBLIC INFORMATION—AND THE
NURSING INFORMATION BUREAU

The profession of nursing must, if it is to take and retain its fitting place in the economy and society of today, speak out for itself. This is not only that it might be heard, but, what is even more important, so that it might properly think out its own problems.

IAGO GALDSTON[1]

AT THE NADIR of the depression the American Nurses' Association took stock of its functions and resources. In the interest of economy, and to coordinate its public information program more closely with the work of the AJN, the board of directors asked the *Journal* to assume responsibility for all information "through the written word." Thanks to Walter Lippmann's postwar *Public Opinion,* and a few other works, members of the *Journal* staff had some appreciation of the psychological principles which provide the basis for public information programs. But they were as uninformed about the technics employed by experts in that field as had been the founders of the *Journal* about the technics of editing and publishing. Advice was sought from Dr. Iago Galdston, well known for his administration of public information programs for health and medical organizations. With his assistance, after many conferences, the Nursing Information Bureau (NIB) was established in 1934 as an administrative unit under the aegis of the *Journal.* Representatives of the three national associations sat on the advisory committee. The new unit was officially named "The Nursing Information Bureau of the American Nurses' Association cooperating with the National League of Nursing Education and the National Organization of Public

[1] Galdston, Iago: "Making Nursing Articulate," *Am. J. Nursing,* 34:839, 1934.

Health Nursing." That unwieldy baptismal name was promptly reduced for everyday use to "the NIB." Its stated purpose was "to disseminate, through appropriate channels, such information about nursing as may lead the public to demand a sounder preparation for and a wider and more discriminating use of nursing service."[2]

Imaginative and hard-working Ernestine Wiedenbach, a Johns Hopkins graduate with a background of institutional and public health nursing experience, but none in the field of public relations, became executive secretary. Any success the NIB achieved was due to her idealism and tenacious loyalty to good standards in nursing, and to the generous support of the board of directors of the AJN. The profession's need for a program which would promote understanding of its aims and its services had long been recognized. Miss Dock had discussed it at an early date. Miss Palmer had made it the subject of editorials as early as 1910, when she discussed the need for a systematic plan for informing the better educated young women of the country about the opportunities in nursing. The NLNE attempted to develop such a program soon thereafter. The pamphlet *Opportunities in the Field of Nursing* had been prepared by Isabel M. Stewart in the early teens when vocational guidance was beginning to take on the characteristics of a profession. It had undergone many revisions as the *pièce de résistance* of the wartime recruitment program developed under the aegis of Miss Nutting's committee of the Council of National Defense. It had also been used in the postwar program spearheaded by the ARC in cooperation with the new headquarters staffs of the ANA and NLNE.

The ANA's early efforts toward developing a public information program had been made in connection with the first published list of schools accredited by the state board of nurse examiners (1916). But nothing of importance was accomplished until national nursing headquarters had been established and a publicity secretary employed (1925). The ANA offered to share the services of the profession's first worker in the field of public information with the other two organizations. But they then had no well-defined common pur-

[2] "Some Facts About Nursing and Nursing Information," *Am. J. Nursing,* **35:**820, 1935.

pose, and each organization was absorbed in promoting its own program. Until it transferred the responsibility for a larger program to the AJN, the ANA directed its program to its component state nurses' associations.

In the meantime, the NOPHN (1929) employed a non-nurse secretary to work with its board and committee members' section. The first fruit of that effort was the production of a *Board Members' Manual* (1930) which was used as a basis for study programs. Consultant service and the preparation of informative materials then became the two aims of the NOPHN's public information program. That organization, already well served by the *Public Health Nurse,* added a bulletin, *The PHN,* to its services for its membership in 1940. Since it was well equipped to do public relations work in its special field, the NOPHN had little more than a fraternal interest in the NIB, but its representatives served faithfully on the advisory committee. On the other hand, the ANA and the NLNE had a broad base of common interest.

Under Dr. Galdston's tutelage, the principles on which the NIB was established were those fundamental to the development of nursing as a profession rather than to the specific development of the organizations. Upon that broad base, a spacious program could have been developed had available resources permitted. It was necessary, because of the limited resources, to select those units of a total program which would make the most important contribution to the fulfillment of the aims of the profession. The ANA was handling its immediate problems, chiefly those related to the depression, extremely well and was in closer touch with its component state associations than ever before. It was agreed, therefore, that a long-range program should be developed by the NIB.

Sound public relations programs are based on the results of analytical studies, that is, on research, not on yearning hopes for recognition. On the basis of its evaluation of an enormous mass of data, the Grading Committee had formulated 12 recommendations. The NIB based its program on the first one which reads as follows: "There are various reasons why patients are unnursed or poorly nursed. One is that nurses have been inadequately trained. Measures to be immediately undertaken to make good nursing available to those who need it would be to close many of the present schools. . . ."[3] Schools could not be closed by fiat, but the flow of students into the poor ones might be checked and enrollment in the better ones increased.

The NIB was advised to develop a program which would help potential students to analyze the offerings of the schools. The careful selection and guidance of students were matters of primary concern to both the ANA and the NLNE. A vocational guidance program was implicit in the over-all program of the NLNE, but this organization lacked the resources for an active program in that area of interest. The NIB, therefore, embarked on a modest program which included the preparation and distribution of pamphlets. Their availability was made known by press and radio. They were widely distributed by the public information committees which the state nurses' associations were encouraged to develop and by nursing schools. Some of the state associations provided all high school counselors with NIB pamphlets or with comparable materials adapted to the conditions within their own jurisdictions. Pamphlet titles were reminiscent of the World War I program. Among them were: *How to Choose a Nursing School; Nursing and How to Prepare for It; Nursing, a Profession for College Women*. Many schools revamped their catalogs to state their aims and their offerings more specifically and attractively than they had ever done. By 1940, almost a million of the pamphlets had been distributed and had been supplemented by the distribution of thousands of state and other publications of a similar type. The NIB had established excellent cooperative relationships with the state public information committees. Representatives of the press and radio expressed appreciation of a central source of general information about nursing. The handbook *Facts about Nursing*, a collection of statistical data on nursing from authoritative sources, was first published in 1935. It provided dependable information and, by revealing gaps in the profession's knowledge of itself, stimulated research.

[3] *Nursing Schools—Today and Tomorrow.* Final Report of the Committee on the Grading of Nursing Schools, New York, 1934, p. 246.

When the National Nursing Council was organized it set up its own public relations program. The NIB program was thereafter subordinated to it but it maintained a liberal emergency supply of vocational pamphlets for use by the council when needed. The *Bulletin of the NIB,* a continuation of the earlier *ANA Bulletin,* became an important channel of communication between the council and national nursing organizations and the state and local organizations. Miss Wiedenbach's graphic summaries and correlations of basic information made a valuable contribution to the profession's war effort and its postwar readjustment. Despite the financial stringencies of the thirties, the ANA doubled its membership in that decade and ended it (1940) with a membership of over 167,000 registered nurses. The limited NIB budget, provided almost wholly by the AJN, did not permit the greatly desired distribution of the *Bulletin* to all members. But the mailing list was carefully planned to reach those who could share information, viz., the key nurses in organizational, administrative, or educational positions. Mailing lists were also built up for special groups such as hospital administrators, related professional publications, and the like.

The NIB was discontinued in 1948.[4] The national organizations were not ready, as its founders had hoped, to make it the nucleus of a unified central information service for the profession. The *Journal,* which had almost doubled its circulation during the war, was due for a radical reorganization and expansion, and could not continue to finance it. The NIB's legacies to the profession are *Facts about Nursing,* which the ANA has enlarged and published annually since the demise of the NIB, and an appreciation of the importance of organized public information programs as a factor in the evolution of nursing.

BIBLIOGRAPHY

Dewey, John: *The Public and Its Problems.* Henry Holt & Co., New York, 1927.

[4] "The N I.B Dissolved," *Am. J. Nursing,* 48:139, 1948.

Lippmann, Walter: *Public Opinion*. Harcourt, Brace & Co., New York, 1922.

Lynd, Robert S., and Lynd, Helen Merrell: "Getting Information," Chap. XXVII; and "Group Solidarity," Chap. XXVIII; *Middletown*. Harcourt, Brace & Co., New York, 1929.

Wiedenbach, Ernestine: "Toward Educating 130,000,000 People—a History of the Nursing Information Bureau," *Am. J. Nursing*, **40**:13, 1940.

Chapter 30

PREPAREDNESS

The grim logic of events rather than ardor steadily drew the nation closer to war.

DIXON WECTER[1]

THE ARMY NURSE CORPS announced at the biennial convention of the three national nursing organizations in 1938 that its authorized strength had been increased from 600 to 675 nurses and that, for the first time, nurses were to be assigned to Army Air Corps stations.[2] So, without fanfare, a movement began which reached its peak only at the close of World War II. (Forty-two per cent of all active nurses had volunteered for services with the armed forces; American nurses had been distributed over the face of the globe.) War clouds were gathering,. but there was nothing in that cautious announcement to forewarn the profession that military requirements would provide the pivotal point around which nursing would revolve for almost a decade. National sentiment toward the political problems of other nations had been expressed in the Neutrality Act (1938). But President Roosevelt had succeeded in securing authorization from a reluctant Congress for substantial increases in the armed forces. Well before Pearl Harbor, the profession was informed through the *Journal* and other media that the ANC would require an additional 4000 nurses before July 1, 1941.

The United States, and nursing with it, was emerging from the great depression. The profession could count some measurable gains.

[1] Wecter, Dixon: *The Age of the Great Depression,* Vol. XIII of *History of American Life,* edited by Arthur M. Schlesinger and Dixon R. Fox. The Macmillan Company, New York, 1948, p. 308.

[2] ANA *Proceedings,* 1938, p. 425.

The 3000 or more nurses who had received stipends under the Social Security Act were an impressive addition to the nation's public health nursing resources. In five years the number of nursing schools meeting the minimum legal requirements of the states had decreased by 11 per cent whereas the average number of students enrolled in schools had increased from 48 to 65. The number graduated annually had risen until the classes of 1940 totaled 4000 more than those of 1935.[3] The trend toward affiliation with institutions of higher education was definitely upward. New programs for graduate nurses were being developed at Catholic University and other universities. But the period of relative balance between supply and demand for nursing service was short-lived. With the return of prosperity, which had been stimulated by the preparedness program, there came a mounting demand for hospital and health services. More nurses were required. Enrollment in approved hospital care plans, which began in 1933 and was an increasingly important factor in the changing situation, had risen to nearly four and a half million in 1940.

The ANA's summaries of reports from professionally sponsored registries indicated a high level of employment for private duty nurses, especially in the larger cities. These reports also showed serious difficulty in filling requests for temporary graduate staff (general duty) nurses for hospitals. This condition was described by some of the administrators who were inconvenienced as a "flight from the bedside care of patients." The flight, if such it was, was not from the care of patients but from the personnel policies of institutions. Many hospitals had gone to considerable lengths to provide employment for nurses during the depression. But nurses who had accepted minimum salaries sought other opportunities, especially in the rapidly expanding field of industrial nursing, when institutions were laggard about improving salary schedules and other personnel policies as their circumstances improved. One of the astonishing phenomena of the period was the effort of many institutions to employ staff nurses on a temporary basis at a per diem rate equivalent to one-thirtieth of the monthly salary for permanent service.

[3] "Fewer Schools—More Students," *Am. J. Nursing*, 40:1148, 1940.

Under such circumstances, nurses had neither status nor adequate incomes, and the routine services usually required of them provided little opportunity for the exercise of nursing skills. This was the type of problem that had led the ANA to make its extensive study of employment conditions, published in 1938. The reaction of nurses to the stubborn resistance of some institutions to the need for adjustment of personnel policies left painful scars in both groups. However, the most serious problem of the profession, as the preparedness program got under way, was not quantitative. This was the perennial shortage of qualified teachers, principals for nursing schools, and of administrators for hospital and public health nursing services. It was intensified by the growing importance of nursing in all health and medical care programs after the National Preparedness Program called for the addition of 1,500,000 men to the armed forces.

To assist the profession in its adaptation to the nation's needs, two organizations swung into action. Long before the first cantonment was built, the Red Cross nursing service launched an enrollment program based on quotas assigned to the states. This was in accordance with its traditional functional responsibility for providing a reserve for the military services. The second agency was the Nursing Council of National Defense, to be discussed later. The ARC nursing service had, however, been caught somewhat "off base." A study designed to provide a basis for reorganization had been made by Alta E. Dines following the death of Miss Noyes and the retirement of Ida F. Butler. But circumstances forced the stepping up of enrollment before plans for the reorganization of the service and clarification of its relationships could be completed. In 1938 Mary Beard and Virginia M. Dunbar became director and associate director of the ARC Nursing Service. Miss Beard was a distinguished public health nurse. She had been president of the NOPHN throughout World War I and was keenly aware of some of the problems involved in making wise use of the nation's nursing resources. As a member of the staff of the Rockefeller Foundation she had, for a ten-year period, been more directly concerned with international than with national nursing affairs. A sensitively idealistic and sympathetic person who had never enjoyed robust health, Miss Beard was forced by ill health to resign (1944) at the height of wartime pressure. (Her death occurred two years later.) She was succeeded by Miss Dunbar, now dean of the Cornell University–New York Hospital School of Nursing. Miss Dunbar, a Johns Hopkins graduate, brought to the Red Cross a broad background of preparation in nursing education and experience in teaching in schools of nursing on both coasts, plus a year of study under the aegis of the Florence Nightingale International Foundation (FNIF) in London. Her experience in working with the professional organizations had been relatively limited. With superb courage and unshakeable integrity they undertook the reorganization of a far-flung service that had no known counterpart.

Due to a variety of evolutionary developments, the ARC nursing service no longer enjoyed quite the prestige that had made the wearing of its badge a proud privilege during and after World War I. In the interval between wars, important nonmilitary federal nursing services had been established, and the national nursing organizations and many of their component units had become influential. The Army and Navy Nurse Corps had become well-developed administrative units in their respective branches of the armed forces. Equally important changes had taken place within the ARC. When Miss Beard took office, the chapters, the basic units of the Red Cross structure, had greatly increased in both number and efficiency. A considerable number of them had promoted the development of public health nursing services. Many of them provided courses in home nursing (Home Hygiene and Care of the Sick). They were soon to accept responsibility for the preparation of nurse's aides. But chapters had no part in the program for the enrollment of reserve nurses. That major unit of the nursing service continued to maintain its liaison with the ANA and the state nurses' associations that had been initiated in 1909. This dichotomy caused many Red Cross workers to believe that the nursing service was badly organized, and that the influence of the professional organizations overshadowed that of the Red Cross itself.

The services which had been subdivided after World War I were consolidated under Miss Beard's direction. The traditional method for increasing the First Reserve of enrolled nurses (nurses eligible for military service) remained practically unchanged. Well before destruction fell from the sky at Pearl Harbor to change the face of the world, it had become apparent that many nurses long enrolled in the First Reserve would not be available for military service. They were in positions essential to the maintenance of nursing schools and nursing services. In due course it was found that a pool of five enrolled nurses would be required to provide one nurse for military service. The National Red Cross nursing committee was reorganized. A small advisory committee, which was also appointed, outlined a farsighted program of cooperation with the national nursing organizations which included recommendations for federal aid for nursing education. Little had been accomplished, however, when it became apparent that the program should be synthesized with those of other national agencies.

When the ANA, NLNE, and NOPHN met in convention in Philadelphia the week of May 12, 1940, the lowlands of Western Europe had just been invaded as a prelude to the projected Battle of Britain. Hamburg was in flames, and newspaper headlines blazoned a story of ruthless destructiveness. Telegrams were transmitted to President Roosevelt offering the support and strength of the organizations in any nursing activity in which they could be of service to the country. But some of the nurses who vividly recalled the stresses and strains of World War I left the convention with an uneasy sense of unfinished business. They wanted answers to such questions as: "If the US should enter the war, is the profession ready to meet its obligations?" Isabel M. Stewart, who had done so much arduous spade work for Miss Nutting's committee and the NLNE in World War I, set the ball rolling that resulted in the organization of the Nursing Council of National Defense. Late in July, Julia C. Stimson, president of the ANA, called together a group of nurses who represented five national nursing organizations, the ARC nursing service, and the federal agencies most immediately concerned with the extension and use of nursing resources. They were deeply stirred by Miss Beard's response to a key question: "I have no words to tell you how serious I believe this thing is going to be." Before the end of that anxious July day, the nucleus of the Nursing Council of National

Defense was organized and its functions broadly outlined.[4] That act epitomized the evolutionary development of the profession between the two world wars. The dynamic leadership of a few outstanding women had been a marked characteristic of World War I. In the interval, the five national organizations and many of their state and local components had become influential. The complexities of the situation and the democratic spirit of the times called for group action.

In general, the functions of the council were to determine the role of nurses and nursing in the program of national defense, and to unify all nursing activities directly or indirectly related to it. This involved making a study of actual and potential nursing resources and planning for the most effective use of them. It was agreed that the council should endeavor to maintain existing standards of nursing education and nursing service; that it would act as a clearing house in relation to nursing and national defense; and that it would cooperate with other agencies having related activities and functions. This meeting occurred three months before compulsory peacetime military service was inaugurated (for the first time in American history), when the Secretary of War drew the first of 16,000,000 numbers from a glass bowl in Washington.

The new council was organized to meet a recognized need, but it had no means of support except such modest sums as could be squeezed out of the budgets of the national nursing organizations.

[4] The agencies originally represented on the council were:

Nursing Membership Agencies	*Nursing Service Agencies*
American Nurses' Association	Nursing Service of the American Red Cross
National League of Nursing Education	Federal Children's Bureau
National Organization for Public Health Nursing	United States Army Nurse Corps
Association of Collegiate Schools of Nursing	United States Navy Nurse Corps
National Association of Colored Graduate Nurses	United States Public Health Service
	a) Division of States Relations
	b) Division of Hospitals
	Nursing Service of United States Veterans Administration
	Nursing Service of Department of Indian Affairs

Newell, Hope: *The History of the National Nursing Council.* NOPHN distributor, 1951, p. 2.

The ANA shared its office and secured the temporary service of Ida F. Butler to carry the work in the initial stage. The state nurses' associations responded generously to an appeal for financial assistance. Mrs. Elmira Bears Wickenden, a former member of the NOPHN staff, who had come out of the retirement of matrimony to work in Washington with the Red Cross, was appointed executive secretary some two months before Pearl Harbor. Shortly thereafter, Louise Kieninger of Colorado was appointed to assist her, and Susan C. Francis, ex-president of the ANA, became a full-time volunteer member of the staff.

The council burgeoned under Mrs. Wickenden's energetic leadership. New quarters were found in the same building as the national organizations. It promptly began working on two main projects: A survey of national nursing resources and a plan to secure federal funds to expand the nation's resources for nursing education. The ANA, long aware of the need for comprehensive information about the nursing resources of the country, had urged the US Census Bureau to provide specific data on nursing. As a result, in the census of 1940, registered nurses were classified, for the first time, as professional. Census data could not, however, be used by planning agencies because students had been included with graduate nurses in the tabulations. Nor, for two reasons, could data from the state boards of nurse examiners be cumulated. Many nurses were registered in more than one state. Some of the state boards did not require periodical re-registration; therefore, they carried unknown numbers of out-of-date records in their files.

With the approval of the nursing organizations, the council requested advice and assistance from the US Public Health Service which not only agreed to sponsor the survey but also outlined a cooperative plan which it largely financed. Questionnaires were tried out by the Graduate Nurses' Association of the District of Columbia. The work was then carried out through the well-established channels of the ANA, namely, with the state nurses' association assuming responsibility for the collection of data within their own jurisdictions. A designated officer of each state association was appointed as a special agent of the US Public Health Service. The

Red Cross provided funds for special statistical service because the objectives of the proposed survey were closely identified with some parts of the ARC service. Nurses responded with enthusiasm by returning 75 per cent of the questionnaires. When these replies from almost 300,000 active nurses were analyzed, it was found that, if professionally qualified, almost 100,000 nurses were eligible for military duty (unmarried and under forty) provided they could pass the physical examinations. Of the inactive nurses, 25,000 could be available for full-time services.[5]

The ARC and the National Nursing Council were making progress with mutually agreed upon programs for nursing in national defense, when a third agency was organized. The government's Subcommittee on Nursing,[6] as it was commonly known, was one of six subcommittees of the Health and Medical Committee of the Council of National Defense. Mary Beard was the first chairman of the subcommittee, and Alma C. Haupt, the intellectually energetic and administratively experienced director of the Bureau of Nursing Service of the Metropolitan Life Insurance Company, was released by that organization to serve as executive secretary with an office in Washington. As a preliminary to formulating a program for the subcommittee, Miss Beard called a meeting of some 80 persons. Included in this group were nurse leaders representing all phases of nursing, representatives of nurse-employing agencies and of such offices as that of Civilian Defense and the still existent "depression agencies," the National Youth Administration (NYA) and WPA. It is noteworthy that this important meeting, arranged by a federal agency concerned with over-all planning for nursing service, was held almost a year later than the conference sponsored by the ANA and other professional nursing organizations[7] which had brought the council into existence.

The function of these two national agencies was to coordinate all

[5] McIver, Pearl: "Registered Nurses in the U.S.A.," *Am. J. Nursing,* **42**:769, 1942.
[6] The Subcommittee on Nursing of the Health and Medical Committee of the Office of Defense Health and Medical Services. Hereafter referred to as the government's Subcommittee on Nursing.
[7] "An Epochal Meeting," *Pub. Health Nursing,* **33**:448, 1941.

nursing programs in their respective areas, namely, federal and voluntary, and to work cooperatively through appropriate channels to devise the most effective methods for expanding and utilizing the nation's nursing resources. The council was primarily a planning agency although it took on some administrative responsibilities. Its functions were stated as:

1. To determine the role of nurses and nursing in the program of national defense;

2. To unify all nursing activities which are directly or indirectly related to national defense;

3. To study nursing resources; to plan the most effective use of these nursing resources; to provide for necessary increases; and to set up the machinery which will insure the quickest possible functioning in case of need;

4. To insure the continuance of the high quality of nursing schools and services in order that effective nursing may be maintained in a national emergency;

5. To act as a clearing house regarding nursing and national defense, and to cooperate with other agencies having related activities and functions.

The functions of the subcommittee were investigative and advisory. They were (1) to analyze the country's need for professional nursing services in both military and civilian situations, (2) to make plans for meeting that need, and (3) to cooperate as might be necessary with the nursing services of the allied nations. The council and subcommittee worked harmoniously to provide a two-way channel for the interchange of information essential to comprehensive planning. The subcommittee's major contribution had been made by July, 1943.[8] The council voted to remain active "for the duration and six months thereafter." It did not, however, go out of existence until 1948. The position of the ARC nursing service, which functioned midway between the voluntary and governmental agencies, was not always clearly understood. Together they formed a two-way channel between the nursing profession and the federal agencies concerned with the immediate emergency. As in World War I, nurse

[8] Congressional appropriations for the Health and Medical Committee and its subcommittees were discontinued as of June 30, 1943.

planners were frequently accused of being more concerned with the maintenance of professional standards than with the provision of nursing service. But they were unshakeably convinced, as had been their predecessors, that both emergency and long-range needs of the nation could best be met on the foundation of established principles.

Consideration of the preparation and assignment of nurse's aides by the ARC had aroused one of the bitterest controversies of World War I. Such aides were to become an extremely important national resource in World War II. After a year of careful study and experimentation, the Red Cross outlined a new course for nurse's aides and encouraged chapters to set up training programs. This was fortunate. When the Office of Civilian Defense (OCD) was established it also made plans for preparing aides. To avoid complications, the ARC agreed to step up its program in order to prepare the 100,000 aides the Office of Civilian Defense believed would be needed. That organization agreed to assign only aides who had been approved on completion of the eighty-hour ARC course. Insignia bearing the symbols of both the ARC and the OCD were devised for the aides. The OCD urged nurses to take the ARC courses in first aid.

The number of nurses available through the professionally sponsored registries for private duty and other types of nursing was greater in 1941 than in preceding years. An exhibit at the APHA convention emphasized the need for an additional 10,000 public health nurses. That figure, however, represented both theoretical needs and unfilled positions. In April of that year, the NLNE made a quick survey of institutional nursing. Well over half of the hospitals that replied had no vacancies in graduate nurse positions. Of 5000 vacancies reported, more than half had been caused by the release of nurses "for defense" in response to military needs, and the calls of new and expanding industries for industrial nurses. Institutions on the Atlantic Coast felt the loss of nurses most keenly, those on the Pacific Coast the least.

Still another study indicated that nursing schools could not be expected to increase their enrollments appreciably without assistance. Few had adequate and well-prepared faculties. They had no financial resources with which to increase instructional or housing facilities. Isabel M. Stewart prepared for the US Office of Education suggestions for federal aid for nursing education, which came to be known in the council and other planning groups as "The Proposal." When this plan for a $12,000,000 program was rejected, the Nursing Council revamped it and secured the endorsement of the Health and Medical Committee of the Council of National Defense and of the Subcommittee on Nursing. This time the request for assistance was channeled through the US Public Health Service. It was largely due to the alertness of Congresswoman Frances P. Bolton, who had championed the Army school in World War I, that an Appropriations Act for 1942 included funds for nursing education. This act, effective July 1, 1941, provided $1,200,000 plus $50,000 for administration under the supervision of the Surgeon General of the USPHS.[9] A new administrative unit was set up in the States Relations Division, USPHS, under Pearl McIver, the senior nurse consultant. Margaret Arnstein, of the New York Department of Health; Lucile Petry, of the faculty of the University of Minnesota; and Eugenia Kennedy Spalding, of the faculty of Catholic University, accepted provisional appointments as consultants to assist in developing the new program. The Subcommittee on Nursing and other agencies provided advisory service.

The plans for refresher courses for married and other graduate nurses, who had been professionally inactive, had been of special interest to the Bureau of the Budget and to some members of Congress. Not realizing that student nurses provide very considerable amounts of hospital nursing service, they had not easily been persuaded that increasing the number of student nurses would be a practical method for meeting an emergency situation. However, the program was so successful in achieving its stated aims that a second and larger appropriation was secured. The two-year federal aid program (July 1, 1941, to June 30, 1943) aimed to (1) increase enrollment in nursing schools, (2) prepare additional teachers and other nurse personnel for positions requiring advanced education,

[9] "Public Law 146, 77th Congress," *Am. J. Nursing,* **41**:933, 1941.

and (3) provide refresher courses for inactive nurses willing to return to active practice.

The total amount expended in the two years was slightly less than $4,500,000. Basic schools had been assisted by the provision of scholarships, funds for maintenance of additional students, and salaries for the teachers who had been added to their faculties because of increased enrollments. Enrollments were increased by almost 13,000 students, for whom maintenance was provided. Almost 2000 students received scholarships, and 240 institutions received aid under this part of the program. Of the 4200 graduate nurses who secured advanced work, about one-half were public health nurses. Most of the others were preparing for teaching or some other type of position in nursing education. The response to the offer of refresher courses was interesting. Whereas more than 2000 took advantage of the opportunity in the first year, less than a thousand did so in the second. It was believed that, as need for their services became more acute, inactive nurses returned to active practice without being "refreshed."

Following the declaration of war, the base of the council's structure was broadened. It was incorporated as the National Nursing Council for War Service. Its two major projects, the recruitment of student nurses and the attempt to balance military and civilian needs, were referred to the subcommittee and through it to governmental agencies. The further work of the council, the spectacular program of the US Cadet Nurse Corps, and the Procurement and Assignment Service of the War Manpower Commission are discussed in Section VIII. The sequence is interrupted at this point to consider the status of men nurses and their contribution to the nation's need for nursing service.

BIBLIOGRAPHY

"A National Inventory of Nurses," *Am. J. Nursing,* **40**:1246, 1940.
"Federal Funds to Increase the Nurse Power of the Nation," *Am. J. Nursing,* **41**:931, 1941.

Gregg, Alan: "Mary Beard, Humanist," *Am. J. Nursing,* **47**:103, 1947.

Haupt, Alma C.: "The Government's Subcommittee on Nursing," *Am. J. Nursing,* **42**:257, 899, 1942.

———: "The Program of the Government's Subcommittee on Nursing," *Proceedings of the Thirty-third Convention of the American Nurses' Association,* 1942, p. 147.

Kernodle, Portia B.: *The Red Cross Nurse in Action, 1888–1948.* Harper & Brothers, New York, 1949, pp. 371–76.

Lippmann, Helen Byrne: "100,000 Volunteer Nurse's Aides for Civilian Defense," *Am. J. Nursing,* **41**:1393, 1941.

Manual; Volunteers in Health, Medical Care and Nursing. US Office of Civilian Defense, Washington, D.C., January, 1942.

Newell, Hope: *The History of the National Nursing Council.* National Organization for Public Health Nursing (distributor), New York, 1951.

"Nursing Council for National Defense," *Am. J. Nursing,* **40**:1013, 1940.

"Nursing Preparedness," *Am. J. Nursing,* **40**:1014, 1940.

"Opportunity in the A.N.C.," *Am. J. Nursing,* **40**:1366, 1940.

"The Organization of Nursing in Defense" (with diagram), *Am. J. Nursing,* **41**:1414, 1941.

Reed, Louis S.: *Blue Cross and Medical Service Plans.* Federal Security Agency, US Public Health Service, Washington, D.C., 1947, p. 12.

Study of Incomes, Salary and Employment Conditions Affecting Nurses (exclusive of those engaged in public health nursing). American Nurses' Association, New York, 1938.

Trott, Lona L.: "It's Good of You to Want to Help! The Red Cross Volunteer Nurse's Aide Corps," *Am. J. Nursing,* **40**:1355, 1940.

The United States Cadet Nurse Corps and Other Federal Nurse Training Programs. US Public Service Publication #38, US Government Printing Office, Washington, D.C., 1950.

Chapter 31

MEN NURSES

. . . in the early Christian period, and for centuries thereafter, men of the priestly class, or belonging to military or religious orders, have been responsible for at least one half of the nursing service through mediaeval times up to a very recent period.[1]

THE FIRST Nightingale schools had been in existence little more than a decade when the first schools for the training of men nurses were established. By 1910, according to the US Census, about 7 per cent of all student and graduate nurses were men. For the next thirty years, the percentage steadily decreased and relatively few of those who graduated remained in nursing. Many of those who did so were individualists. A few believed and acted on the belief that their professional status and opportunities could be improved by organized effort. The national preparedness program provided an opportunity for them to press their claim to professional equality with women. The organization of the Men Nurses' Section of the ANA in 1940 was the culmination of persistent effort which had been started almost twenty years earlier. Since this is the first reference to men nurses in this volume, a synopsis of their history is in order.

The status of men in nursing had been comparable to that of women in medicine, i.e., they were a neglected minority, but with an additional complicating factor. Until well into the present century, the majority of men nurses were graduates of schools connected with psychiatric institutions in the Eastern part of the country, although a few schools connected with general hospitals in the

[1] Nutting, M. Adelaide, and Dock, Lavinia L.: *A History of Nursing.* G. P. Putnam's Sons, New York, 1907, Vol. I, p. 101.

Middle West and on the Pacific coast were organized on a coeducational basis. The Grace Hospital Training School (Detroit) admitted men from its opening until 1906, but, in a 17-year period, only 27 men were graduated and one-third of them entered other professions. It is of interest that men were admitted to this school at 19 but the entrance age for women was 22. Seventh-day Adventist schools in Michigan and California admitted men before the turn of the century, and the school of the Los Angeles County General Hospital began admitting men in 1903. The first school in the state of Washington was established on a coeducational basis in connection with what is now the Tacoma General Hospital, but the only man ever graduated was a member of the first class (1897)!

The standards of the schools in mental hospitals derived from those of the long-established Medico-Psychological (later named the American Psychiatric) Association which had followed the example of its British prototype. The standards of the organized nursing profession, in the earlier development, were based on needs of patients in general hospitals and experience in caring for them. Few affiliations had been provided by means of which students in either group could acquire a background of experience in the other field. Psychiatric nursing was quite outside the experience of the majority of nurses who participated in the early development of the professional nursing organizations. There was, therefore, no common bond of interest between most of the men and the majority of women nurses. In addition, there was a considerable degree of possessiveness on the part of women toward the calling which was opening doors of opportunity for them and which they were making peculiarly their own.

The first woman to secure a degree in medicine, Dr. Elizabeth Blackwell, was a crusader for the right of her sex to an education in medicine. There is no evidence that men entered nursing as crusaders for either the "rights" of their sex or for the advancement of nursing.

What is believed to have been the first American school for men was the School for Male Nurses established in connection with the New York City Training School for Nurses on Blackwell's (Welfare)

Island. The City Training School was operated in connection with the City Hospital and provided nursing service for it and for four hospitals in Manhattan which were also operated by the city. The School for Male Nurses was operated by the City Training School on the same principles. Mrs. Cadwalader Jones, a staunch supporter of these schools (and author of the Modified Hippocratic Oath for Nurses) reported that "in 1895 the Male Training School which has existed since 1886 took on new life."[2] But that renaissance was short-lived.

The following year the school was made responsible for the nursing service at Fordham Hospital. Apparently, the men traveled daily by ferry and other transportation from the central school on Blackwell's Island, as did the women students, to the hospitals in the city. It was a rugged life. The nursing time schedule required a 10-hour day and a 14-hour night on duty with classes at the end of the day.

The school was closed in 1903 for lack of suitable applicants and because additional accommodations were required for the steadily increasing number of women students the hospitals were requesting for their nursing services. The following year the principal of the City Training School gave high praise in her annual report to the men nurses. One hundred and forty men had graduated but most of them had become doctors. Nursing was so often considered a stepping stone to medicine for both women and men that at least one of the well-known early schools made it a rule to decline applicants with that intention.

In 1886 men were admitted to the school which Dr. Edward Cowles had established at McLean Hospital (Waverly, Massachusetts) in 1882. Dr. Cowles had previously been superintendent of the Boston City Hospital where he had engaged Linda Richards to establish the school of nursing. His interest in the nursing care of patients was very far in advance of that of most physicians and hospital administrators of the time. The school offered a two-year

---

[2] Jones, Mrs. Cadwalader: "Looking Back Through Fifty Years," *The Alumnae Journal of New York City Hospital School of Nursing*, Golden Anniversary Number, 1875–1925, July, 1925, p. 11.

course in the care of the mentally ill and in general nursing. In addition provision was made for women graduates, who wished to do so, to take a year of work at the Massachusetts General Hospital and to receive the diploma of that school also.[3] (The two institutions were and still are under the direction of one board of directors.) Through the years, although the arrangement has not been continuous, students in each school have profited from some type of affiliation with the other. Four men were graduated, with 20 women, in 1888. This was the first formally organized nursing school in a hospital for the mentally ill in the world. Its example was followed by a considerable number of both voluntary and state mental hospitals in the Eastern part of the country. This was notably true of the state hospitals in New York where the first school was established at the Buffalo State Hospital (1883).

The Mills Training School for Male Nurses, established in connection with Bellevue Hospital in New York City (1888), was made possible by a substantial gift to the city by the philanthropist Darius Ogden Mills. In a letter of presentation, Mr. Mills wrote: "The training school for female nurses was a great gain. Personal observation of the good it has done has led me to think that an equal service might be rendered by an institution for the training of male nurses."[4] A building, one of the earliest to be erected in the US for the sole use of a nursing school, stood for 50 years as a monument to the man whose name it bore and as a mute reminder of the concept of a school of nursing as an institution with a purpose and a personality all its own. The building still stands, but the school has been transferred to two floors of one of Bellevue's spacious buildings.

Despite its auspicious beginnings, the progress of the Mills school has twice been interrupted. For a 10-year period it was replaced by a course for the preparation of orderlies or attendants presumably because it was difficult to secure adequate numbers of desirable candidates. Nursing, as a vocation for men, had no prestige. When reopened, the school was again (1922) placed on the approved list

[3] Washburn, Frederic A.: *The Massachusetts General Hospital, Its Development, 1900–1935.* Houghton Mifflin Company, Boston, 1939.

[4] O'Hanlon, George: "Men Nurses in General Hospital," *Am. J. Nursing,* **34**:16, 1934.

of the New York State Examining Board. Since 1929 the Mills and the Bellevue schools have retained their separate identities, but under the direction of one faculty. These schools make no distinction of race, creed, or color. The first Negro to be graduated from the Mills school was Lawrence A. Sumler of the class of 1942. The school was closed a second time during World War II and was not reopened until 1948. The two Bellevue schools became identified with New York University in 1942 as the Division of Nursing of the College of Medicine.

In the Middle West two schools for men nurses were established by the oldest religious nursing order of men in existence. The Congregation of the Alexian Brothers established schools of nursing in their hospitals in Chicago and St. Louis, which provide all types of care for men and boys, in 1898 and 1928, respectively. The Chicago school, however, did not begin admitting lay students until 1929 and not in any considerable numbers for ten years after that. This school has never been closed although it did not admit classes for two years during World War II. Following the war it had a maximum enrollment, many of the students being ex-servicemen whose experiences as hospital corpsmen interested them in nursing as a profession. Members of the alumni association take an active part in the work of the state nurses's association. They stood solidly with other representatives of the association in working for legislation to secure legal status for qualified practical nurses because ex-hospital corpsmen were swelling the number of unlicensed persons offering costly and unregulated service as "nurses" to the public. The school is affiliated with De Paul University which provides instruction in ethics and the biological, physical, and social sciences. Students interested in working for a degree matriculate in the university.

The Alexian Brothers school in St. Louis was temporarily closed in the summer of 1951. In anticipation of its reopening, members of the alumni began preparing for faculty positions. This school is an affiliate of the school of nursing of St. Louis University. Proposed changes in the hospital will provide excellent experience in psychiatric nursing. The alumni are active in the Missouri State Nurses'

Association. It is believed that most of the graduates of the Alexian Brothers schools remain in nursing. Nurse-fashion, they are widely scattered. They hold an interesting variety of positions and are greatly in demand, especially in the fields of industrial nursing, anesthesia, psychiatric nursing, and private duty.

The fifth school founded for the preparation of men nurses was established in 1914 in connection with the Department of Mental and Nervous Diseases of the famous Pennsylvania Hospital which owes its origin to Benjamin Franklin. From the beginning, this school has operated in harmony with the older Pennsylvania Hospital School for Nurses. Faculty members have made important contributions to the periodical literature on men in nursing. The director of the school, LeRoy N. Craig, a graduate of the pioneering McLean school, was the farseeing chairman of the Men Nurses' Section of the ANA during the earlier part of World War II. He has selflessly and persistently continued the crusade for military rank for men nurses which was then launched by the national organization. He is, of course, not alone in this effort. His successors in office were equally convinced that recognition of the professional equality of men and women nurses by the armed forces would stimulate the enrollment of men in schools of nursing and thus augment the nursing resources of the nation.

Information about the number of coeducational schools was not systematically collected before 1941. In that year there were 64. Ten years later the number had increased by more than one hundred. However, that statement should not be construed to indicate that all have men enrolled as students. According to the US Census, the number of men in nursing in 1940 was approximately 2 per cent[5] of the total number of graduate and student nurses.

The leaders in this minority group, well aware that many institutions were providing poor nursing service for men patients, and concerned with their own lack of professional status, were determined to do something about it. Improvement in their status, they believed, would provide a practical approach to the problem of recruiting and educating more men. References to an American As-

[5] *Facts about Nursing*, 1942, ANA, p. 6.

sociation of Male Nurses appear occasionally in the literature between 1915 and 1935, but the initiative for the integration of men in the professional nursing organizations seems to have come chiefly from men in New York City and Philadelphia. The alumni of the Mills School had made an excellent start on organizational relationships early in the century. Mills men had been as active as Bellevue nurses in early activities in connection with the development of professional organizations in New York. The name of a Mills graduate, L. Bissell Sanford, appears in the membership of the first New York Board of Nurse Examiners, of which Sophia F. Palmer, editor of the AJN, was president. Mr. Sanford, who was secretary of his alumni association and registrar of the Mills registry, died before his term of office on the state board expired. Due to some misunderstanding about the appointment of his successor, the alumni withdrew from membership in the professional organization.[6] And thus was the course of history deflected. Had that one association remained in the Associated Alumnae, provision for the membership of men nurses could not have been ignored when the organization, which had been renamed the American Nurses' Association in 1911, was reorganized between 1916 and 1922. Unfortunately at that time, it will be recalled, the Mills school was closed. When it was reopened, members of the alumni association were affronted by the discovery that the membership requirements of the ANA made no provision for men nurses. This was not a feminist gesture. Apparently the existence of men nurses was simply overlooked. Through the persistent effort of a few men, the ANA bylaws were revised in 1930 in order that properly qualified men nurses might be admitted to membership.

The Grading Committee found 54 schools were prepared to admit men and that less than 1 per cent of all students were men. Although insistently repetitious about the necessity for reducing the number of nurses, the Grading Committee advocated the preparation of more men nurses. It was assumed that many men patients

[6] Nash, Herbert J.: "Men Nurses in New York State," Historical Sketch with Notes on Present Problems, *Trained Nurse and Hospital Review*, August, 1936. p. 123.

needed better care than they were receiving because procedures requiring the skill of nurses were being entrusted to unskilled attendants and orderlies. Esther Lucile Brown made a similar observation 16 years later in *Nursing for the Future*. At the time of the Grading Committee's report, the New York State Nurses' Association had begun to take an active interest in men nurses. A session of the association's 1933 convention program was devoted to the several aspects of their preparation and employment. It was reported that only four of the universities in the US then offering courses for graduate nurses would accept men nurses. One hospital school offering postgraduate courses would accept men but only for work in hospital administration. Despite the limited opportunities for advanced work, a few men were then holding positions on nursing school faculties. The Men Nurses' Section of the state association antedated the organization of the Men Nurses' Section of the ANA by four years. At the end of 12 years, during which several other state associations also organized sections, the Men Nurses' Section of the New York association was discontinued because it had served its purpose. The interests of men members had been integrated in the total program of the association. For the same reason the ANA section was disbanded in 1952.

Women nurses dislike the appellation "female" quite as much as men dislike being called male nurses. But the law which brought the ANC into being in 1902 designated it as the "Army Nurse Corps, Female." The word "female" was also included in the law which created the Navy Nurse Corps in 1908. Immediately after the Men Nurses' Section of the ANA was organized, it began working for legislation which would provide opportunities, equal to those for women nurses in the medical departments of the armed forces. The problem was laid before the board of directors of the ANA early in 1941. ANA correspondence, based on a request from the Men Nurses' Section, with the offices of the Surgeons General of the Army and the Navy indicated that no changes in military procedures in relation to men nurses could be made.

The ARC was already well aware of the problem of men nurses and of the several types of medical technologists whose skills were also badly needed by the medical departments of the Army and the Navy. It arranged to enroll qualified men nurses as medical technologists.[7] The Medical Department of the Army agreed that men nurses holding the registration card of the Red Cross should, after the initial four-months' service as trainees, be promoted to the grade of technical sergeant providing a vacancy in that grade was available. This was far from satisfactory to the men. When the ANA met in convention in 1942, the US had entered the war. An increasing need for nurses and for wise use of the nation's nursing resources was everywhere apparent. The membership of the ANA, as represented by the House of Delegates, approved the principle of "equal rights" for men nurses in a resolution which was transmitted to the two surgeons general. It requested that registered professional men nurses who were members of the ANA be given opportunity to serve as professional nurses as soon as possible after enlistment or induction into the armed forces. This principle was later endorsed by the board of trustees of the American Hospital Association. Acknowledgments of receipt of the ANA resolution again indicated that no change would be made in the administrative practices of either the Army or the Navy. The office of the Surgeon General of the Army gave assurances of its effort to have honored the ARC cards which indicated enrollment as medical technologists.

By this time, the National Nursing Council had become much concerned with the over-all problem of effective use of all nursing resources. It did not, however, take action in relation to the military status of men nurses. In the opinion of the council, that question would be decided outside the medical departments of the two services and, under then current selective service rulings, little could be done to change the status of men. From the standpoint of the War Manpower Commission, concerned with millions of men, the number of men involved was infinitesimal. From the standpoint of the nursing profession, men nurses were equipped to render a service for which the Army was insistently begging, especially in relation to the care of psychiatric patients. Vigorous protests were received by the nursing organizations from men who had been as-

[7] *Am. J. Nursing,* **40**:453, 1414, 1940.

signed to rugged non-nursing duties and who were well aware of the Army's need for their special skills.

The ANA received more than 1000 returns in a survey of men nurses conducted in 1943. The number of replies received from men already in military service was small but significant. A high percentage of those in the Army were in departments where it might be assumed that their professional nursing experience could be used. In rank, they ranged from private to first lieutenant; this range was true also of the smaller percentage in departments where it seemed obvious there would be no opportunity for nurses. Base pay ranged from the private soldier's $50.00 per month to $166.67 received by the first lieutenants. The men in the Navy who answered the ANA's questionnaire had all been assigned to the Hospital Corps with ratings from Pharmacist's Mate, third class, to Chief Pharmacist's Mate (permanent). Base pay in this group ranged from $78.00 to $138.00 per month.[8] But, to the men, "a nurse is a nurse, is a nurse," and the beginning base pay of nurses was that of second lieutenants.

The ANA tried to secure the deferment of men student nurses by suggesting to the state associations that they take such steps as might seem appropriate in connection with the local draft boards. This, too, proved ineffective. The schools were practically denuded of men students and of masculine faculty members of military age. The percentage of men who completed their interrupted education in nursing when the war was over is not known.

In 1944 a member of the House of Representatives introduced a bill[9] to give men nurses the temporary commissioned rank of second lieutenant in the Army and of ensign in the Navy which had been granted to members of the Nurse Corps. This bill had the active support of the ANA but was never brought out of committee. Efforts were renewed in 1950, without results, to secure status for men in the armed forces comparable to that of women nurses who by this time had been granted commissioned rank in the Nurse Corps of the Army, Navy, and the new Air Force. Men nurses were encouraged, however, by a memorandum sent to local draft boards

[8] "Men Nurses and the Armed Forces," *Am. J. Nursing,* 43:1066, 1943.
[9] H.R. 68—79th Congress, First Session.

early in 1951 by the director of the Selective Service System.[10] It calls attention to "the dire shortage of male nurses . . . especially in our state mental institutions. This communication points out that, although no blanket deferment is possible under existing law, . . . it would be advisable that male student nurses continue their training so that upon graduation they can help fill the large number of vacancies resulting from the critical shortage."

The ANA's source book, *Facts about Nursing,* provides data which support the argument for permitting men student nurses to complete their training. From 1945 through 1948, the largest number of men nurses graduated in any one year was 42.[11] The number enrolled in schools of nursing in January, 1939, was only 725, and by 1945 the figure had dropped to 169,[12] and there were no new enrollments that year. As previously noted, at least one of the schools for men was closed for several years and another admitted no classes for two war years.

The picture of nursing as a profession for men is changing. This is partially revealed by the enrollment for January, 1951. There were then more than 1000 men in 181 nursing schools, only three of which restricted enrollment to men. In a 10-year period the number of schools admitting men had almost trebled. Men nurses are licensed by the state boards of nurse examiners, as are all other nurses, as general practitioners, not as specialists in psychiatric or other branches of nursing. Therefore, according to the NLNE, there should be no differentiation in the basic curriculum for men and women nurses.[13] This is a fundamental step toward full equality of opportunity. Men have already demonstrated their usefulness in pediatric nursing. They are now asking for periods of observation, but not yet of practice, in obstetrics.

Statistics are useful milestones but they cannot tell the whole story of an evolutionary process such as that which, by mid-century,

[10] Hershey, Lewis B. (director, Selective Service System): *Male Student Nurses,* Local Board Memorandum #33, May 8, 1951. US Government Printing Office, Washington, D.C., 1951.
[11] *Facts about Nursing,* 1951, ANA, p. 44.
[12] *Facts about Nursing,* 1946, ANA, p. 35.
[13] *Fifty-sixth Annual Report of the NLNE,* 1950, p. 165.

had brought the interests, problems, and achievements of men nurses into wholesome integration with those of the main body of the profession. The soundness of the judgment of the men who believed that integration with the ANA would improve their status and advance the cause of good nursing more rapidly than a national organization of men nurses had been demonstrated by improvement in organizational and professional relationships. The premise that the sound preparation of more men nurses would ensure improvement in the care of patients and in health services is no longer debatable.

Membership in the Men Nurses' Section of the ANA and in the sections organized by five state nurses' associations stimulated the interest of men in the work of other organizations also. Some of them became active in the NLNE and indicated growing interest in the work of the NOPHN. So many men are industrial nurses that some of them became members of the American Association of Industrial Nurses (AAIN) (1942) as a matter of course. (The ANA then had no industrial nurses' section.) The American Association of Nurse Anesthetists (AANA), which is not affiliated with the professional nursing organizations, made provision for the membership of men in 1947. This is one of the many fields in which there is an urgent demand for more nurses and in which men are very acceptable. Twenty-six of the 88 schools recognized by the AANA accept men. One school for nurse anesthetists is directed by a man nurse.

There is perhaps no more fundamental evidence of mid-century rapport between men and women nurses than the readiness of the professional organizations, both national and state, to promote the recruitment of men for schools of nursing. New York has far more men nurses than any other state. The New York State Nurses' Association made an interesting survey of the education and employment of men nurses in 1948 in preparation for a recruitment program. Eighteen of the 22 New York schools then admitting men were in state mental hospitals. All could admit more students. The chief barrier to the admission of men to general hospital schools of nursing was found to be the problem of housing in more than half of the reporting schools. This alibi, men nurses point out, has some-times been used to camouflage prejudice or indifference toward men nurses. The mid-century shortage of feminine candidates for nurs-ing schools has been an important factor in creating a more hos-pitable attitude toward men students. The survey showed that:

> The existing barriers to the employment of men nurses appear to be due . . . to sentiment and tradition. . . . There are more positions for men nurses than there are applicants. . . . The men nurses who are equipped to advance in nursing education may matriculate at any one of the six universities offering postgraduate nursing education.[14]

A special folder prepared by the state nurses' association for the recruitment of men in New York bore convincing evidence that women nurses were overcoming the tendency to possessiveness in relation to the profession. It bears the title, "Nursing Is a 'Man-size' Job!"

The mid-century shortage of nurses—due to the long-continued period of national prosperity, the shortening of time on duty to en-sure a relatively normal life for nurses, the steadily increasing awareness of Americans of the importance of health, and the in-creasing use of hospitals—has been favorable to the develop-ment of expanding opportunities for men nurses. Quite as important has been the steadily increasing emphasis, in all the professional or-ganizations, on over-all planning to meet community needs for nursing service. Men nurses have been alert to opportunities, partly because they have had strong leadership within the group, and partly because many of them used the educational opportunities provided for veterans of World War II under the "GI Bill of Rights"[15] to prepare themselves for responsible positions. The di-rector of at least one school for men believes that many veterans of World War II, as a result of their war experiences, felt im-pelled to dedicate themselves wholly or partly to the service of their fellow men and that this motivation accounted for much of

[14] *Survey of Men Nurses, Education and Employment.* New York State Nurses' Association, Albany, New York, April, 1948. (Mimeographed.)
[15] The Servicemen's Readjustment Act of 1944.

the increase in enrollment of men in schools of nursing following the war.

In a period of rapid expansion there are many "firsts." A recently appointed man nurse now heads a school of nursing which, to date, has enrolled only women. Another is dean of a collegiate school of nursing. A Mills man is an editor in an important publishing house. One is employed by the Sister Kenny Foundation. An Alexian graduate has established a leper colony in an area where he observed the need while on military duty. Another has been commissioned in the US Public Health Nursing Service. Hospital administration is not a new field for men nurses, but it is significant that one of them is now executive secretary of a state hospital association. Two men are chief nurses in Veterans Administration (VA) hospitals. Two and one-half per cent of all the nurses in the VA are men. Their position assignments run the entire gamut of the service.

And what of the future of men in nursing? Like that of women, it will be what they make it. The 1949 Inventory of Nurses[16] showed that only 0.8 of 1 per cent of all active registered professional nurses were men. Only six states then had more than 100 men nurses. They range, in the following order, from New York with 883, California 360, Pennsylvania 233, Illinois 172, Massachusetts 133, to New Jersey with 102. The numbers are small, but the zeal of the leaders in this minority group which stretches from coast to coast is remindful of that of the pioneers who established the ANA and the NLNE. Opportunities to participate in programs for improvement of the nation's health—physical, mental and spiritual—lie all about us. Of the potential opportunities for men nurses, LeRoy Craig, who is sensitively aware of the possibilities for improving nursing service, especially in the developing field of psychiatric nursing, has written, "We are still doing only a token job."

BIBLIOGRAPHY

Brief History of the Mills School, "My Oath." Fiftieth anniversary publication of the Mills School of Nursing, New York, 1937.

[16] *Inventory of Professional Registered Nurses,* 1949, ANA.

Brown, Esther Lucile: *Nursing for the Future*. Russell Sage Foundation, New York, 1948, p. 188.

Course of Study and Syllabus for Guidance of Nurse Training Schools. Higher Education Bulletin 28, New York State Education Department, Albany, New York, 1907.

Craig, LeRoy N.: "Opportunities for Men Nurses," *Am. J. Nursing*, **40**:666, 1940.

Crummer, Kenneth T.: "Men Nurses—A Survey of the Present-Day Situation of Graduate Men Nurses," *Am. J. Nursing*, **28**:467, 1928.

Giles, Dorothy: *A Candle in Her Hand*. A story of the nursing schools of Bellevue Hospital. G. P. Putnam's Sons, New York, 1949.

Hartnett, William: "Men Nurses in the Veterans Administration," *Am. J. Nursing*, **52**:586, 1952.

Henry, George W.: "The Care and Treatment of Mental Disease—Yesterday and Today," *Mod. Hosp.*, Nov., 1929.

Mannino, Anthony J.: "Men in Nursing," *Am. J. Nursing*, **51**:198, 1951.

May, Mary Elizabeth: "Nurse Training Schools of New York State Hospitals," *Am. J. Nursing*, **8**:18, 1907.

Monteith, Mary Colby: "Seventh Day Adventist Schools of Nursing," *Am. J. Nursing*, **51**:113, 1951.

Nash, Herbert H.: "Men Nurses in New York State, Historical Sketch with Notes on Present Problems," *Trained Nurse and Hospital Review*, Aug., 1936, p. 123.

The New York City Training School for Nurses: *Twenty-ninth Annual Report*. The School, New York, December 31, 1904, p. 10

Newell, Hope: *The History of the National Nursing Council*. National Organization for Public Health Nursing (distributor), New York, 1951, p. 45.

O'Hanlon, George: "Men Nurses in General Hospitals," *Am. J. Nursing*, **34**:16, 1934.

Parsons, Sara E.: *History of the Massachusetts General Hospital Training School of Nursing*. Whitcomb & Barrows, Boston, 1922, p. 187.

Perreault, Edward F.: "Evaluating the Status of Men Nurses," *Nursing World*, **125**:148, 1951.

Riddle, Mary M.: *Boston City Hospital Training School for Nurses—Historical Sketch*. Boston, Massachusetts, 1928.

Russell, William L.: "Men Nurses in Psychiatric Hospitals," *Am. J. Nursing*, **34**:19, 1934.

———: "Nurse Training: Advances in Scientific and Clinical Study and Practice," Chapter XXIX of *The New York Hospital—A History of the Psychiatric Service, 1771–1936*. Columbia University Press, New York, 1945.

The Second Grading of Nursing Schools. Committee on the Grading of Nursing Schools, New York, 1932, p. 13.

Walton, Harold M., and Nelson, Kathryn Jensen: *Historical Sketch of the Medical Work of Seventh Day Adventists from 1866 to 1896.* Review & Herald Publishing Association, Washington, D.C., 1948.

Washburn, Frederic A.: "The McLean Hospital Training School for Nurses," *The Massachusetts General Hospital—Its Development, 1900–1935.* Houghton Mifflin Co., Boston, 1939, pp. 285–87.

Witte, Frances W.: "Opportunities in Graduate Education for Men Nurses," *Am. J. Nursing,* **34:**133, 1934.

SECTION VIII.   AMERICAN NURSES
IN WORLD WAR II

Chapter 32

WARTIME NURSING ON THE HOME FRONT

We are in the line of the pilgrims and of the pioneers, in the line with those who founded the country and in the line with those who preserved it. We are not tenants in the house that they built and users of what they left us. We shall make history ourselves, and hand down to those who come after us the story of what men and women did in these days in which we live.

WALTER LIPPMANN[1]

As THE NATION moved toward war, manufacturers stopped making automobiles and other widely used products and retooled their plants for the production of munitions. Nursing had no such choice. While America's output of war materials was astonishing the world, one out of every four active nurses entered service with the armed forces. They went without the mandate of a draft or the lure, as in industry, of exceptional financial rewards. The absence of millions of men did not lessen the calls for nursing service at home. Quite the contrary. The use of hospital facilities increased so rapidly that the number of admissions in 1945 was 6,000,000 greater than the number in 1940.[2] To help safeguard the health of workers in the fast-paced wartime industries 10,000 more nurses were required than had ever before been so employed.

Based on experience in World War I, the NOPHN began at an early date to urge public health nurses to remain in the field of their special competence. Despite this effort, a study indicated that

[1] Lippmann, Walter: "The American Cause," *Am. J. Nursing,* **42:**725, 1942.
[2] "Hospital Service in the United States," *J.A.M.A.,* **49:**149, 1952.

328

approximately 10 per cent may have entered military services which had little need for their special skills. The staffs of well-established public health nursing agencies were also depleted by calls for nurses to develop new services in overcrowed industrial areas and the like.

"In the earlier part of the war," an experienced hospital administrator told an AHA convention audience, "nurses approached their war problems more resolutely and more consistently than hospital administrators."[3] The tardiness of many hospital administrators to grasp the import of the abrupt change from a plethora to a shortage of nurses, and of the effect of the rapidly rising cost of living on the incomes of nurses, resulted in a lack of rapport between the groups, which had unfortunate repercussions. At the time that the National Nursing Council was organized (1940), hospitals still tended to be highly individualistic. The AHA, however, had participated in the preparation of two editions of the *Manual of the Essentials of Good Hospital Nursing Service*. It had also published its first manual on job specifications.[4] The association became an active participant in the council when it was reorganized after war was declared. In hospitals which operated schools of nursing, the transition from student to student plus graduate service had been greatly accelerated during the depression, but marked unevenness and inconsistencies in personnel policies tended to make general duty nurses restless. Student enrollments were being increased but services had not been stabilized, following the depression, when the government began calling for nurses for military service.

As noted in Chapter 30, "Preparedness," the necessity for expansion of nursing services and the development of additional nursing resources had been foreseen by alert nursing leaders. They could not, however, have anticipated the full magnitude of the task ahead any more than Selective Service could know, when it was organized, how many millions of men would be under arms by 1945. Nurses could not have guessed, for example, that the number of new hos-

[3] Munger, Claude B.: "Convention Digest," *Mod. Hosp.*, **61**:6, 1943.
[4] *Job Specifications for a Hospital Organization*, Bulletin #202, Personnel Management in Hospitals Series. American Hospital Association, Chicago, 1940.

pital beds made available for the care of the sick in a single war year (1944) would be equivalent to a new 220-bed hospital for each day in the year. But thoughtful nurses were keenly aware that adaptations would have to be made. They were convinced that the quality of nursing service on the home front would have a more lasting influence on the evolution of nursing than the military experiences of nurses, heroic though they might be. Therefore expediency, as a criterion, was suspect just as it had been in World War I. Nurses were confronted with a condition which had been stressed in the manual on hospital nursing service, namely, "A fact to be faced by hospital and nursing administrators is the impossibility of doing two hours of work in one hour of time and maintaining good standards."[5]

Psychological and other difficulties were encountered as nurse administrators endeavored to replace patterns of "service as usual" with concepts of "essential service." As one result of that conflict in ideologies we shall find a new emphasis on patient-centered care in the postwar period. During the war many nurses, whose thinking and practice had been conditioned by years of administrative emphasis on technics and routines in relation to the physical care of patients, were resistant to changes which required continuous exercise of judgment in relation to the basic needs of patients. So, too, some doctors could not be convinced that special duty nurses should not be assigned to the care of well-to-do patients solely on the basis of their ability to pay for luxuries. Obduracy on this point by patients and nurses, as well as doctors, created problems for both hospital administrators and nurses.

When war was declared, many nurses had already been withdrawn from institutional and other civilian services. Army and Navy nurses were poised and ready to move "swiftly, secretly, and silently," to stations around the world. By means of surveys the US Public Health Service was endeavoring to forestall hazardous health conditions, similar to those in the extra-cantonment zones in World War I, in areas where Army camps and new or expanded industries

---

[5] *Manual of the Essentials of Good Hospital Nursing Service.* AHA, Chicago, and NLNE, New York, rev. 1942, p. 36.

would attract large numbers of civilians. One hundred and sixty-three public health nurses, recruited chiefly from large voluntary agencies, had been given an orientation course at the National Health Institute, Bethesda, Maryland. These nurses had been assigned to official agencies in 34 states, the District of Columbia, Hawaii, Alaska, and Puerto Rico. Many of them were assigned to local defense areas where "trailer towns" sprang up almost overnight. Others went to special "rapid treatment" veneral disease projects, and to supervisory positions.

As previously noted, the number of industrial nurses increased by more than 10,000 between 1938 and 1943.[6] Doubtless it was the withdrawal of this large number of nurses from other civilian services that gave rise to the rumor, never authenticated but highly detrimental to the morale of the profession, that very considerable numbers of nurses were deserting their profession (as a few were known to have done) to earn large wages on the assembly lines of industry. The lure of higher earnings in industrial plants seriously depleted the supply of practical nurses in some areas. Year by year the American Medical Association reported phenomenal increases in the use of hospital facilities. The mounting birth rate and the Emergency Maternity and Infant Care (EMIC) program of the Children's Bureau also put an unanticipated strain on many hospital nursing services. Three-quarters of a million more babies were born in hospitals in 1945 than in 1940.[7]

The EMIC program (1943) was devised within the framework of the Social Security Act, and decentralized to the state health departments, to provide care throughout the maternity cycle for the wives of servicemen in the four lowest pay grades. Lack of resources for the care of their wives and children, in the early months of the war, had seriously lowered the morale of the servicemen. Red Cross social workers in the training camp areas had reported many calls for assistance. Newspaper accounts of proposed Congressional appropriations brought clamorous demands for the service. The

[6] *Facts about Nursing*, The Nursing Information Bureau, New York, 1939, p. 9; and 1943, p. 7.
[7] "Hospital Service in the United States," *J.A.M.A.*, **116**:1066, (Mar. 15) 1941; and **130**:1082, (Apr. 20) 1946.

need of these young women was indeed urgent. Many of them were huddled together in unsanitary surroundings near camps located far from their own homes. Administrative machinery was set up with the utmost speed. The provision of continuous supervision of young women, who moved from place to place when their soldier husbands were transferred, taxed the ingenuity of social workers and public health nurses. The overcrowded hospitals in which their babies were born were often far from the place at which they first sought assistance. The Children's Bureau urged that as a matter of routine policy, in all communities where public health nurses were employed by official health agencies, the nursing service provide postpartal bedside nursing care for women delivered at home or discharged from the hospitals very early in the postpartal period. So great was the pressure for hospital beds in some areas that maternity patients were permitted to remain only two or three days after delivery. Provision was made for the purchase of nursing service on a "case basis" when official public health services were not available.[8] Although there was some dissatisfaction about the method of payment for medical and hospital care, there was wide participation in the program. When it was terminated (1949) well over one million mothers and almost a half million sick children had received care. Nearly one-half of the doctors, and 90 per cent of the hospitals in the US, had participated in the program. The usefulness of qualified nurse specialists, as consultants, was especially noteworthy when they could bring nurses from hospitals and public health agencies together for consideration of common problems. The recommended standards of nursing care were practical, specific, and notably timesaving. In this, as in other types of nursing, it was often difficult to persuade nurses that established methods should be replaced by simpler technics that had been tested for safety, efficiency, and economy of time and materials. To bathe or not to bathe the baby was, for example, a frequently discussed topic. In the hospitals, especially those in military and new industrial areas, such as those surrounding the new shipbuilding plants and airplane factories, the crowding of beds in wards and corridors in

---

[8] "Help for Military Families," *Pub. Health Nursing*, **35**:59, 1943.

order to give care to the largest possible number of young mothers was a serious obstacle to good care, a situation which was increasingly complicated by inadequate numbers of nurses.

Nursing services suffer from their "fatal availability" since, in many institutions, it is the only service in continuous operation around the clock. Furthermore, it is the only service which is always in evidence. As more and more doctors departed for military service, many medical routines and procedures were delegated to the depleted nursing services. The high wages of industry had a catastrophic effect on all types of nonprofessional service since hospital salaries were low, by tradition and practice, even in normal times. Nurses found themselves required to take on some medical responsibilities, also housekeeping and other functions which were necessary to the continuing care of patients. They were handicapped by shortages of medical and surgical supplies, of linens due to short supply and irregular laundry service, of dishes due to lack of maid service, and of equipment due to lack of maintenance service and replacements. That enumeration is significant because every hour of nursing time devoted to a non-nursing activity was irrevocably subtracted from time for care of patients. Lack of time to do good nursing is a frustrating experience for nurses at any time. During the war it took on a nightmarish quality in many places. Nursing on the home front called for perception of the distinction between the essential and nonessential elements in nursing procedures and in programs of nursing care, coupled with the ingenuity and strength of character to make the necessary adjustments. When institutions and agencies failed to adjust their routines in accordance with that fundamental principle, a chronic sense of frustration tended to lower morale with a resultant restlessness that caused some nurses to make frequent changes. A few hospitals found it necessary to close departments for lack of nurses and other personnel. In retrospect, however, it seems incredible that so many beds were kept in use, and that so many thousands of patients were given essential care, if not always the comfort which is one of the primary aims of good nursing. There were many unsung heroines on the home front among the nurse practitioners who stayed on the job and the administrators who developed methods for utilizing the services of an extraordinary variety of persons who came to them with and without preparation for the tasks required of them. Had this not been the case, there would have been many more closed wards and departments.

In its consideration of nursing personnel the *Manual of the Essentials of Good Hospital Nursing Service* included (1) orderlies and ward helpers, (2) ward clerks, and (3) volunteer nurse's aides. In the period of preparedness many nurses had been resistant to the general introduction of nurse's aides into hospital nursing services. There were two principal reasons for their initial lack of cordiality. With depression experiences fresh in memory, many nurses feared competition. Administrators of nursing services, especially those who were also responsible for nursing schools, were reluctant to assume responsibility for a type of worker unfamiliar to most of them. Relatively few nurse administrators had then learned to make distinctions between the essential elements of nursing care and the nexus of services we call nursing service. The technics of job description and job analysis were not in general use. Throughout the war experienced administrators and their staffs contributed many articles on the results of experiments in the simplification of administrative routines and of nursing technics to the professional publications and to convention programs. Clare Dennison discussed the subject in a classic paper before a large biennial convention audience in 1942. "There is," she said, "a vast difference between the services rendered by nurses and the nursing care of patients given by nurses."[9] She concluded with a statement to the effect that "there is no substitute for the well-trained nurse in the administration of nursing care; but subsidiary workers on different levels and volunteers may provide an important part of nursing service." The following excerpt from that paper is included, with the author's permission, for historic interest, since it had a marked influence on nursing thought:

[9] Dennison, Clare: "Maintaining the Quality of Nursing Service in the Emergency," *Am. J. Nursing*, **42**:774, 1942.

How simple *is* the care which goes on day and night in the hospitals? Let us look at the record. During the latter part of 1940 and the first of 1941 our nursing office did a spot study on the treatments and procedures which could not be given to subsidiary workers. We did this three times at two-month intervals for twenty-four hours, and while we know the findings are not conclusive, since so many head nurses, assistant head nurses, and night nurses collected the data, they are rather interesting. Outside of the operating room, the labor and delivery rooms, the out-patient department, and the emergency department, and excluding all diagnostic and research tests, we found about one hundred items covering periods of time ranging from approximately two minutes as in taking the apex pulse to twenty-four hours of constant attendance as in watching patients in respirators. From an average of 473 patients, 109 were ordered blood pressures in intervals of every fifteen minutes to once a day. Sixty patients, or one patient in every eight, received parenteral fluids or transfusions, and while these were not done by nurses, they required the help of a nurse and on two of these days patients were receiving continuous intravenous fluid and required constant attendance. The nurses gave gavages, placed fifth leads for electrocardiograms, and applied suction to surgical wounds, tracheotomies, chest cavities and throats.

They managed the apparatus for Wangensteen suction, tidal irrigation, and bladder decompression. They irrigated eyes, cecostomies, colostomies, draining wounds, urethral and ureteral catheters. They gave colonic irrigations. They did artificial respiration in the interval needed to obtain a respirator, and then started the operation of the respirator. They applied sterile compresses and painted lesions. They did approximately 230 dressings in a day, and this does not include the times these dressings were taken down to show the wound to a surgeon. They did catheterizations, sitz baths, and turpentine stupes. They used the Danzer apparatus. They gave insulin and taught the patient or his relatives to give the drug and examine urine. They administered approximately 1,500 medications daily, by mouth or hypodermic. They had an average of seven patients a day under oxygen therapy and specialled patients after craniotomies, tracheotomies, and the usual surgery. They assisted with lumbar punctures, thoracenteses, paracenteses, and phlebotomies.

While all this went on, they met the usual expectations of the staffs. They knew, night or day, without direction, what to watch for and report for the thyroidectomies, the breast amputations, and the prostatectomies. In general, it was not necessary for the surgeon to give specific directions nor to see his patient for several hours after the operation. It was not necessary to tell the head nurse to watch for any toxic symptoms, even after chemotherapy; it was taken for granted that all this would be done. It was understood that the nurses would know how to administer any drug—and pick up any error in writing the order.

They would not be exonerated from responsibility if by error 4 cubic centimeters of belladonna were written instead of .4 cubic centimeter and any nurse followed the written order. The nurses would have been condemned if a patient scheduled for a cataract went to the operating room with even slight symptoms of a cold—or if any patient went there with a premonition that he was going to die. It was not a simple matter to decide on the evidence of symptoms shown whether or not to call the doctor at 2:00 A.M. or to calculate to a nicety the time the doctor should be called in order to appear in the delivery room at the proper moment, but the right decision was usually made. It would have been very inconvenient for all concerned during those days if the nurses had not known a good deal about the apparatus used in orthopedics, the machinery of the respirators, the oxygen tents, and the suction machines, but the fact that they did know was probably never noticed, so long have nurses been considered an extension of all the services in the hospital. In addition to this, each nurse accepted the responsibility for all services rendered her patient by any subsidiary worker, and every minute of every twenty-four hours the nurses were responsible for the prompt observation and reporting of any change in the condition of any patient.

At the same convention, the director of an important public health nursing service pointed out that "withered routine is due for a pruning."[10] This sententious statement was applicable to both institutional and public health services since nursing routines had tended to take on the sanctity of traditions in both, and were almost equally resistant to change. The NOPHN followed up that presidential address by publishing committee reports on practical methods for coordinating, and utilizing with economy, community nursing resources, and for supplementing them by the utilization of auxiliary workers. The reports were timely since the National Nursing Council had secured a wide distribution of its pamphlet, *Priorities for Nurses*, which clearly defined the types of nurses who were essential for the maintenance of minimum nursing services as well as those who could be released for military service.

[10] Ross, Grace: "The Future Commands Our Attention," *Pub. Health Nursing*, 42:293, 1942

A study of nursing service in general hospitals in 1943 showed that the number of hours of bedside nursing provided by hospitals varied from less than one-half hour to over five hours! Well over one-third of such care in hospitals without schools was given by paid auxiliary workers. The average number of hours was well below that of those with schools. In general, patients in hospitals with schools of nursing received one hour more of nursing care per 24-hour day than did patients in hospitals without schools.[11]

The wartime issues of the nursing and hospital publications bear eloquent testimony to the enormous contribution of previously inactive nurses and of non-nurses, both volunteer and paid, to both hospital and public health nursing services. The concept of volunteer service was not new. The number of social agencies which operated registers of volunteers increased enormously, and a considerable variety of services was developed. Those of the ARC were the most extensive. A comparison of the ARC programs during the two world wars reveals some striking changes. The elements of the "three-way nursing" program of World War II had all been present in that of World War I but they had not been accepted as parts of a whole. They were: (1) the traditional function of recruitment to provide a reserve for the Nurse Corps of the Army and Navy, (2) the preparation of nurse's aides, and (3) the teaching of home nursing. In the interval between wars, two changes had taken place. The public had become health conscious; it expected and demanded far more nursing service than ever before. The nursing profession had conceded, somewhat reluctantly, that professional nurses could not possibly provide all the nursing services needed by the American people.

Plans of the initially high-powered Office of Civilian Defense, for the preparation of 100,000 volunteer nurse's aides, galvanized the ARC into swifter action than had been thought possible. On the basis of a program which had been carefully tested during the preparedness period, that seemingly impossible goal was reached within a two-year period under the brilliant leadership of Mrs. Walter

[11] Tattershall, Louise M., and Altenderfer, Marion E.: "Hours of Nursing Service in General Hospitals," *Am. J. Nursing*, 44:963, 1944.

Lippmann. The ARC-OCD nurse's aides gave comfort and a sense of security to many hundreds of patients in both civilian and governmental hospitals who would otherwise have had far too little of either. Primarily interested in hospital work, some of them also accepted assignments in school nursing clinics, outpatient departments, and visiting nurse associations where they were greatly appreciated. The ease with which nurse's aides acquired skill in elementary nursing procedures suggested to instructors that schools of nursing might be spending an undue amount of time in repetitious teaching. The aides represented a cross section of intelligent American womanhood. Some were women of leisure; many were homemakers who had to make careful adjustments to secure the time they gave so generously; a surprising number were business and professional women who gave their evenings and week ends. When assigned to institutions or agencies by a chairman appointed by an ARC chapter, they provided an enormous volume of cheerful dependable service which effectively supplemented that of nurses.

Nurses, deeply absorbed in the almost overwhelming demands upon them, sometimes forgot what careful adjustments many of the volunteer nurse's aides had to make in their personal lives in order to fulfill their assignments. Nor did all head nurses, many of whom were young and inexperienced, always know how to use volunteer or other supplementary assistance effectively. In general, however, aides and nurses learned how to work together and, in so doing, to respect each other. The sum total of voluntary aide service during the war cannot be reckoned in hours of service, or in the numbers of patients to whom they cheerfully gave needed service. They helped to keep the hospitals open and functioning. Of that there can be no doubt. The speed with which most of the volunteers dropped out of the picture, when the war was over, must have reassured any nurse who had ever thought of volunteer nurse's aides as competitors. They gave patriotic service on the home front because the nation was at war. But their influence has been far reaching. They helped to teach nurses, quite incidentally, the importance of making a real distinction between skilled nursing care and nursing service.

The ARC home nursing program is a common-sense method of giving homemakers some sense of security in relation to the care of their families in case of illness. A half-million persons had completed the course by the end of 1942. As the war went on, almost twenty thousand nurses participated in the teaching of the many thousands of women who were recruited and organized in nurse's aide or home nursing classes by the chapters of the ARC. Many of them contributed their only "free" hours for that purpose.

Pioneer nurses had often said, "Once a nurse, always a nurse," although marriage automatically removed them from active practice. The validity of that concept was effectively established when the need for the service of inactive nurses was widely publicized, and when refresher courses were offered. Back they came, mothers and grandmothers, with long unused technics but with understanding hearts. "I gave him a toy before I gave him the first hypodermic I'd given in years," said one of them after preparing a child for surgery. "I explained that it would hurt a little and he forgave me." Many of them had to make important family adjustments. Young children were placed in day nurseries or nursery schools, some of which were set up for this particular purpose. Older children took on unaccustomed responsibilities so "Mom" could return to work in a hospital or public health nursing service. Not infrequently those who had to employ household help, in order to devote their time to nursing, found that the remuneration they received did not balance their outlay. The significance of this discrepancy between the social and financial values placed on nursing was not overlooked by the ANA in its postwar planning.

When a second national survey of nurses was made by the USPHS in 1943, it showed that although 36,000 nurses were already in military service, the number of active registered nurses in the United States was only 2500 less than in 1941. There was also a very considerable reservoir of inactive nurses whose services could be utilized by skillful administrators for some type of local nursing service. The widely discussed shortage of nurses was due to the rapidly increasing requirements for nursing service. Since the proposed third survey was not made, there is no way of estimating the total number of nurses who returned to active practice. But it should never be forgotten that they made an extremely important contribution to wartime nursing on the home front. Fortunately, too, since nurses are believed to have the highest marriage rate of all professional women, some of them found that a career in nursing need not be incompatible with marriage. Other outcomes of adaptations of nursing on the home front will be discussed in later chapters.

When Winston Churchill predicted that 1942 would be a "stern and terrible year," the nursing profession, as represented by the National Nursing Council, had already faced that probability and agreed on a program which called for (1) economical and effective utilization of all available professional resources, (2) the use of auxiliary nursing personnel for every function not requiring nursing skill, and (3) the preparation of increasing numbers of student nurses.

BIBLIOGRAPHY

Altenderfer, Marion E.: "Wartime Nursing Care in Representative General Hospitals," *Pub. Health Rep.*, **60**:99, 1945.
Blackburn, Laura: "To Bathe or Not to Bathe the Baby," *Am. J. Nursing*, **40**:767, 1940.
Brackett, Alice F., and Schmidt, William M.: "Nursing in the EMIC Program—A Progress Report," *Pub. Health Nursing*, **37**:234–38, 1945.
Brigh, Sister Mary: "We Cannot Afford to Hurry" (training within industry applied to nursing), *Am. J. Nursing*, **44**:223, 1944.
Christopher, Virginia L.: "Economics of Nursing Service in Wartime," *Am. J. Nursing*, **44**:136, 1944.
"Cooperation with American War Community Services," *Am. J. Nursing*, **45**:666, 1945.
"The Critical Months Ahead," *Am. J. Nursing*, **43**:626, 1943.
Deming, Dorothy: "Mental Hospitals in Wartime," *Am. J. Nursing*, **43**:1013, 1943.
———: "Nursing in Tuberculosis Hospitals," *Am. J. Nursing*, **43**:1101, 1943.
———: "S.O.S. from Norfolk," *Am. J. Nursing*, **43**:619, 1943.
———: "Trailer Town," *Am. J. Nursing*, **43**:524, 1943.
———: "We Couldn't Do without Aides," *Am. J. Nursing*, **43**:889, 1943.
"The Emergency Maternity and Infant Care Program, Minimum Requirements for Participating Hospitals," *Am. J. Nursing*, **44**:242, 1944.

Fuller, Agnes: "More about Wartime Adjustments," *Pub. Health Nursing*, **37**:242, 1945.

Groseclose, Katharine McLaughlin: "They Serve That Men Shall Be Saved—How the Inactive Nurses Mobilized in One District Association," *Am. J. Nursing*, **43**:1071, 1943.

Heisler, Anna: "U.S. Public Health Service Nurses in War Activities Areas," *Am. J. Nursing*, **43**:474, 1943.

"The Hospital and the Community," *Am. J. Nursing*, **42**:1404, 1942.

Jones, Virginia: "Public Health Nursing in Hawaii at War," *Pub. Health Nursing*, **34**:179, 1942.

Kernodle, Portia B.: "The Home Programs" (pp. 396–405) and "Three-Way Nursing" (pp. 414–16) of *The Red Cross Nurse in Action, 1882–1948*. Harper & Brothers, New York, 1949.

Lippmann, Helen Byrne: "The Future of the Red Cross Volunteer Nurse's Aide Corps," *Am. J. Nursing*, **45**:811, 1945.

"Maintaining Mimimum Public Health Nursing in Wartime," *Pub. Health Nursing*, **34**:659, 1942.

Moore, Anna R., and Chard, Marie: "Private Don Jones' Baby, A Co-operative Plan in a Military Area," *Am. J. Nursing*, **43**:46, 1943.

"National Council on Red Cross Home Nursing Meets," *Am. J. Nursing*, **43**:404, 1943.

"Nurses Work with Volunteers," *Am. J. Nursing*, **43**:337, 1943.

"OCD—Red Cross Joint Statement," *Am. J. Nursing*, **42**:768, 1942.

Palmer, Mellie: "Essentiality of School Nursing," *Pub. Health Nursing*, **36**:221, 1944.

"Public Health Nursing Responsibilities in a Community Health Program," *Pub. Health Nursing*, **41**:67, 1949.

Ross, Grace: "We Plan Ahead," *Pub. Health Nursing*, **33**:334, 1941.

Sinai, Nathan, and Anderson, Odin W.: *EMIC, A Study of Administrative Experience*. Bureau of Public Health, University of Michigan, Ann Arbor, 1950.

"Some Experiences in Acceleration," *Am. J. Nursing*, **43**:577, 1943.

Taylor, Ruth G.: "What We Learned from the EMIC Program," *Pub. Health Nursing*, **41**:263, 1949.

"A Three-Point Program for '43" (editorial), *Am. J. Nursing*, **43**:2, 1943.

"Wartime Modifications in Public Health Nursing Services for the Sick," *Pub. Health Nursing*, **35**:79, 1943.

Widmer, Carolyn L.: "The Housewife Re-enters Nursing," *Am. J. Nursing*, **43**:10, 1943.

Ziegler, Mark V.: "Public Health Problems in War Areas," *Forty-eighth Annual Report of the National League of Nursing Education*, 1942, pp. 141–46.

Chapter 33

AGAIN THEY FOLLOW THE FLAG

. . . . Their untiring services, their professional skill, and their ability to sustain the unparalled morale of the wounded in their care, will always reflect the highest credit to the Nurse Corps, U. S. Navy. . . .

W. F. HALSEY, FLEET ADMIRAL, US NAVY[1]

. . . . Your untiring and unselfish efforts have made possible the eminent record of the Medical Department in this war, a record which in scope and achievement is unsurpasssed in military medical annals. . . .

NORMAN T. KIRK, MAJOR GENERAL,
THE SURGEON GENERAL, US ARMY[2]

NAVY NURSES on duty at the Pearl Harbor hospital, and those aboard the hospital ship *Solace,* were catapulted into war service on the morning of December 7, 1941, "a date which will live in infamy" because a Japanese air and submarine force attacked the Navy base while diplomatic representatives of the Land of the Rising Sun were conducting negotiations with the Department of State in Washington. They met the results of the perfidious attack with competence and gallantry. So, too, did the half-dozen Army nurses at nearby Hickham Field. Citations by the commander of the Pacific Fleet of the nurses at the Naval Hospital and the personnel of the *Solace* were first on the list of more than 1900 honors, ranging from Purple Hearts (a few of which were awarded posthumously) to the Distinguished Service medal, accorded Army and Navy nurses in World War II.[3]

[1] *White Task Force,* The Story of the Nurse Corps, US Navy. US Government Printing Office, Washington, D.C., 1945.

[2] "Surgeon General Kirk Congratulates Nurses," *Am. J. Nursing,* **45**:774, 1945.

[3] *Facts about Nursing,* ANA, 1948, p. 28.

"When the first of the Japanese bombers roared over her nurse's cottage," a newspaper man reported, "Miss Arnest resolutely adjusted her peaked white cap banded with the two gold stripes that mark her rank, walked calmly across the shell-furrowed lawn to the hospital . . . a hail of anti-aircraft shells was falling around her, shrapnel whistled close by. Having entered the hospital, she stayed there ten days with her nurses, who worked till they dropped. . . . They came through gallantly . . . those women from all over the United States. . . ."[4] Calls for assistance were swiftly relayed to nurses throughout Hawaii by the Red Cross and the Office of Civilian Defense in Honolulu. Nurses responded promptly, some of them departing on a few hour's notice to care for the wounded who had been placed aboard transports bound for the States. From that day until May, 1945, when the Surgeon General of the Army informed the president of the ANA that no more nurses would be needed, the profession labored unceasingly to meet the stated needs of the military and to provide essential nursing services for the civilian population. When the American Red Cross enrollment for military service was discontinued, over 40 per cent of all active registered nurses had volunteered for service, a matchless record. Over 104,000 nurses had been certified to the Army and Navy by the ARC and over 70,000 were then, or had been, in service with the armed forces.

Before the war ended, a flag-studded map in the office of the ANA indicated that nurses had been stationed on the soil of some fifty nations scattered over the face of the globe. The installations rimmed the North Atlantic, the Caribbean, and the Mediterranean. In the vast spaces of the Pacific they extended from Alaska and the Aleutians to Australia and New Zealand. Nor should the difficult China-India-Burma theater be overlooked where Burmese nurses gave excellent care to some of our sick and wounded soldiers before American nurses could be assigned there. In this country and in the various theaters of military operations, nurses worked and lived in the permanent installations of the Army and the Navy, in hotels and

---

[4] Gertrude B. Arnest was chief nurse, Pearl Harbor Naval Hospital, on December 7, 1941. "Competition in Recruitment," *Am. J. Nursing,* **42**:403, 1942.

other structures adapted to military needs, in cantonment barracks, in tent hospitals, and in quonset and other prefabricated huts. Nurses on the staff of an evacuation hospital gave care to patients in a 200-year-old cathedral in the Philippines.[5] Patients with the ordinary run of illnesses and accidents were given care in static hospitals and dispensaries far from hostilities. But most nurses coveted active service near the front. When not fully occupied, their discontent created a variety of problems, some of which occasionally necessitated recall.

Speed in giving care to the wounded was a primary factor in reducing the Army's death rate from the 8.1 per cent of World War I to 3.3 per cent. The sulfonamides, the advent of penicillin, DDT, new developments in antimalarial therapy, and the ready availability of blood and blood derivatives, plus the heroism and ingenuity of the medical corpsmen, were among the factors which contributed to that favorable result. The War Department reported that "much of the Medical Department's success with new drugs, such as penicillin and the sulfa drugs, has been due to the constant care and watchfulness of the Army nurse. Her ability and resourcefulness and her willingness to serve in all theaters under trying conditions has made a great difference in the recovery of sick and wounded soldiers."[6] That statement could, of course, have been made with equal cogency about the work of Navy nurses. A nurse correspondent who remembered the days of constant irrigations of draining wounds in World War I wrote: "One daily gave thanks to the good God for the new chemotherapy."[7]

Within the first few months, as blow followed blow in the Pacific, nurses endured, with their patients and other personnel, the agonies of Bataan and Corregidor, the most tragic military epic of our times. They cared for patients in the open air hospital they helped to create in the jungle on Bataan, and in the tunnel hospital of beleagured Corregidor. When driven out, a few escaped but more were im-

[5] Forrest, Nola G.: "Army Nurses at Leyte," *Am. J. Nursing*, 45:44, 1945.
[6] "A Proud Profession," War Department Release, May 5, 1944, *Am. J. Nursing*, 44:525, 1944.
[7] Hayes, Teresa M.: "It Was Hot on the Island," *Am. J. Nursing*, 44:1058, 1944.

prisoned. Under the superb leadership of the chief nurses interned with them they gave needed nursing care to fellow internees even when debilitated by inadequate food. Probably those who escaped imprisonment and were taken to Australia by submarine had the most unusual of all wartime nursing experiences. But the point can be disputed. Army nurses went ashore under fire and dug their own foxholes at Anzio. Navy nurses were the first white women ever to set foot on Tinian in the Marianas. The "shooting war" ended after the bombing of Hiroshima and Nagasaki on August 14. Nurses who were aboard hospital ships in Tokyo Bay on Victory in Japan (V-J) Day (Sept. 2, 1945) can never forget the unearthly silence of that great harbor as the world waited for news of the formalities on the mighty battleship USS *Missouri,* which ended the war. One of them wrote: "It seems ironic to be within sight of the focal point of the world today and to know nothing of what is happening." Nor can they ever forget the seemingly endless belt of landing barges which carried thousands of men released from Japanese prisons to our waiting ships.

Installations in some of the primitive areas in the Pacific raised questions as to the wisdom of sending nurses to posts where guards were required for their protection. Some of the Navy's pharmacist's mates, who had pioneered in the jungle, quite naturally were resentful when nurses arrived to replace them in administrative nursing positions. But there was much for both groups to do. In addition to the men who had suffered trauma from explosives, there were those who suffered from the results of submersion and extensive burns from flaming oil and gasoline. All required skilled nursing. Then, too, malaria, the dysenteries, and a wide variety of other tropical diseases called for nursing of a high order.

Over and above their professional contribution to the care of patients, the presence of nurses in all theaters of war had an important influence on the morale of sick and wounded men. This was especially important for those who feared the reaction of mothers, wives, and sweethearts to news of permanently disabling injuries. Nurses who possessed an intuitive or acquired knowledge of mental hygiene helped seriously injured men to face their handicaps with courage. Knowledge of mental hygiene and psychiatric nursing came to be recognized as priceless attributes of military nursing. As a chief nurse, stationed on Guam during the Iwo Jima campaign, put it: "In addition to her nursing duties, the Navy nurse listened to many a heartsick, lonely boy's story. Even the toughest marine, when wounded, was just another home-sick American boy yearning for his home and his loved ones."[8]

On the Atlantic, submarines continued to take dreadful toll of shipping throughout 1942, but the five nurses of the ARC-Harvard Unit who lost their lives in 1941 were the only American nurse victims of that horror. The quiet courage of those who shipped out immediately after that early catastrophe was something of which the profession could be very proud. As transportation became available, more and more nurses were sent out. The Army nurses who went ashore with our invading troops in North Africa, late in 1942, were said to have followed the troops farther and more closely than American nurses in any previous war. And after North Africa they went on into the hardships that preceded the conquest of Italy. The men and women of this theater of war were said to have had more actual battle experience than American military personnel in any other theater. Army nurses who had been longest in the South Pacific and other areas had begun to feel that they had been overlooked for rotation and promotion, before an effective system for replacing and reassigning them was inaugurated in 1943.

In the early months of the war, many nurses were sent overseas without the drill and orientation to military life that were later provided for all nurses entering the service. As large units began crossing the Atlantic, staging (training) areas were established where nurses were prepared for the work to come. By D day (June 6, 1944) 10,000 Army nurses had been assigned to 88 different units and organizations in Great Britain. In addition to the military courses, special courses in anesthesia and in psychiatric nursing were provided for some of the nurses. Despite these activities, waiting was an inescapable factor in the planning which placed an army of

[8] Goudreau, Alice Aurora: "Nursing at an Advanced Naval Base Hospital—During the Iwo Jima Campaign," *Am. J. Nursing*, **45**:886, 1945.

almost 3,000,000 men in Europe for one vast coordinated movement. It tended to have a destructive influence on the morale of nurses. Reports of relative inaction to overbusy friends at home, like those from the earlier period in the South Pacific, had a seriously inhibiting effect on recruitment.

Nurses landed on the Normandy beachhead on D day + 4. Here, as elsewhere, nurses assigned to mobile surgical units and evacuation hospitals were almost aggressively proud of that privilege. One such unit "'flew the same flag over this hospital in the cow pastures of Normandy, during the St. Lo offensive, in a heather field in Belgium, and in Holland when the unit supported the Arnheim-Nijmegen operations of the airborne."[9] Such units had need for nurse anesthetists and skilled surgical nurses. Units of every type, including those assigned to trains, planes, and hospital ships, needed more psychiatrically trained and experienced nurses than were available. And throughout the war the ANC had unfilled needs for nurses with administrative experience.

The monotonous life at static stations, such as those in the Aleutians and the Canal Zone, and in staging areas where little nursing was required and recreational facilities were limited, generated dissatisfaction with which it was extremely difficult to cope. Lack of appropriate uniforms was also a source of dissatisfaction throughout the early years of the war. Nurses adapted GI clothing to their needs as best they could. Here is how General Eisenhower has described the "uniform" of the chief nurse of a hospital so close to the guns in Tunisia that it was planned, at considerable risk to wounded men, to evacuate. "She was dressed in old O.D. jeans and the rest of her uniform conformed with that article. She was covered with mud. . . . But there was something shining in her face. . . . She said, 'The nurses of this hospital are going to stay here with the wounded, . . .' and she didn't ask permission!"[10] The General "was never prouder of American womanhood." Such nurses were not thrilled by the information that Army and Navy nurses, as the

[9] "Army Nurses in the ETO," *Am. J. Nursing,* 45:386, 1945.
[10] Eisenhower, General Dwight D.: *Address to the Graduating Class,* Presbyterian Hospital School of Nursing, New York, 1949.

best dressed women of the year, were awarded the Fashion Academy's gold medal in 1945. Nurses in service had waited overlong for the best of all the wartime uniforms for women.

Determined efforts had been made in 1942 to procure uniforms adapted for use in the extraordinary range of climatic conditions of the several theaters, but two crowded years passed into history before both nurse corps were adequately equipped. Physical discomfort due to inappropriate and inadequate clothing was aggravated psychologically by the knowledge that the Women's Army Corps (WAC) and other newly organized feminine services[11] had been promptly and effectively outfitted. The lure of uniforms had been considered an important factor in recruiting for the new militarized services. It was for this reason their outfits were given priority. The glamour of uniforms was also played up in recruiting for the non-militarized US Cadet Nurse Corps.

The relative rank granted members of the Army Nurse Corps by Congressional Act in 1920 had been considered of doubtful value by some members of the corps. Any remaining doubt was dissolved when plans for the Women's Army Corps (originally the Women's Army Auxiliary Corps [WAAC]) and other uniformed services for women were announced. In December, 1942, after effective support of the desired legislation by the ANA, a new act provided for relative rank for all members of both the Army and Navy Nurse Corps with the same pay and allowances as officers of comparable rank (without dependents) in other branches of the services. Prior to the passage of that bill, the superintendent of the ANC, Julia O. Flikke, had been promoted from major to colonel. The improvement in the pay schedule was an important factor in recruitment as nurses had not been immune to the effect of the swift rise in the cost of living. In 1944, both services were given commissioned rank "for the dura-

[11] Schaffter, Dorothy: "The Women's Military Services in World War II," *What Comes from Training Women for War*, American Council on Education, Washington 6, D.C., 1948, p. 3. (The new women's military services were the Women's Army Corps [WAC], Women's Reserve of the Naval Reserve [WAVES], Women's Reserve of the Coast Guard Reserve [SPAR], Marine Corps Women's Reserve [MCWR], and Women's Air Force Service Pilots [WASP]—not militarized but otherwise similar to the other feminine corps).

tion and six months thereafter." To complete the record, it should be noted that an act signed on April 16, 1947, provides permanent commissioned rank for both Army and Navy nurses.

The speed with which seriously sick and wounded men were transported from the theaters of war to hospitals in the US was one of the marvels of World War II. Hospital ships and trains were again effectively used, and the feasibility of transporting many types of patients by air was demonstrated at an early date. The Naval Air Force and the Flying Marines had moved more than 25,000 patients from Pacific islands before the end of 1943. Navy nurses, however, were not prepared for flying until the Flight Nurse School for Nurses and Corpsmen was established at Alameda, California, late in 1944. The nursing section of the Army Air Force which had been established two years earlier was transferred to the jurisdiction of the commander of the Air Force. (Provision was made for Army nurses to transfer to the Air Corps Nurse Force when it was established in 1949.) Courses in flight nursing were set up at Bowman Field, Kentucky, from which almost 1500 nurses had been graduated by the autumn of 1945.

The experience of nurses at Mitchell Field near New York was fairly typical of that encountered at debarkation hospitals on both coasts. There, after the invasion of Normandy, plane load after plane load of seriously wounded men arrived in swift succession. Some of the men had been wounded so recently that they were still in battle uniforms. Among them were the amputees, the blinded, and the cord cases who would require special treatment. Most of them remained only long enough for preparation for transfer to the hospitals nearest their homes which could provide the orthopedic or other special care needed by each one. Inadequately staffed for the first massive wave of patients, nurses were torn (as had been all nurses close to the lines) between the urgent physical requirements and the deep-seated emotional needs of their patients. A hypodermic for pain could be given quickly, but reassuring a suffering patient and helping him to decide how he would break the news of extensive injury to his family or sweetheart required more time.

They had only fragmentary information to share with the men about the excellent rehabilitation programs which were being developed elsewhere. As they flew from bed to bed, sensitive nurses were keenly aware of their patients' unspoken need for reassurance. They were filled with boundless admiration for the camaraderie of the men. They offered many a silent prayer for those who would need determination and skilled assistance in adapting to a wholly new way of life.

The Army planned to return all transportable patients to the United States, by plane or ship, within 90 days of Victory in Europe (V-E) Day. By July 31, 1945, more than 100,000 sick and wounded men had been returned. The total job was completed well in advance of the deadline. The number who could not be transported promptly was relatively small. There were about 18,000 nurses in Europe.[12] When it became apparent that victory was in sight, the Army's Director of Nursing Service in the European Theater of Operations (ETO), Lt. Col. Ida W. Danielson, set wheels in motion to secure information about the wishes of nurses in relation to discharge or reassignment.

Nurses would be needed for the several hospitals required by the Army of Occupation for the care of military personnel and civilians, including the unfortunates, practically all of whom were patients, who had been in concentration camps. The frugally staffed cantonment and other hospitals in the States were in urgent need of reinforcements. There was also the problem of replacements for nurses who had been longest in the Pacific. The bombing of Hiroshima and Nagasaki, which would end the war, was only three months away. But the planners in Europe could not know that. When Nell V. Beeby of the AJN's editorial staff visited the ETO during that exciting summer she talked with groups of the proud, restless, and worried nurses who were awaiting orders. They were proud of the work of the units with which they had served. They were restless because at least six weeks would be needed for the physical examinations and other routines required to ensure the completion of essential records for immediate and future use and for

[12] "Redeployment of Nurses in the ETO," *Am. J. Nursing*, 45:507, 1945.

securing transportation.[13] Eligibility for discharge was dependent on careful evaluation of a number of factors. Some of the eligibles had been anticipating promotion and wished to remain in service until that had been accomplished. Many nurses feared that the Cadet Nurse Corps had "flooded the market" with nurses. They were worried about the future. In general, military service was more popular than recruitment committees would have believed. The ANC found that about one-half the reserve nurses who were eligible for discharge wanted to remain in service. However, demobilization proceeded apace. More than 25,000 nurses had been released by the Army by the end of 1945. Among them were nurses who freely expressed their unhappiness because they had not been permitted to remain in service. As military requirements for nurses decreased, those of the Veterans Administration increased and provided opportunity for a large number of ex-service nurses to continue caring for sick and wounded men who had served their country.

The adjustment of ex-service and other nurses to postwar conditions is discussed in a later chapter. Collectively, the nurses who responded to the military demands of global war added to the prestige of a maturing profession. Long lists of citations and awards, including the Distinguished Service Medals received by Col. Florence A. Blanchfield, superintendent of the ANC, and Capt. Sue S. Dauser, superintendent of the NNC, are outward evidences of the quality of the service rendered. As in any large group of human beings, there were some who were liabilities rather than assets to the services and to the profession. But the number seems to have been small. Nurses had often been "difficult" when they were not busy. But throughout the war in every theater of operations they responded to the utmost of their ability, as had their predecessors in other wars, when "the best patients in the world" needed their care. The release of so many thousands of nurses from their normal occupations, without a draft, had been due to four factors: (1) the traditions of the profession, (2) the courageous and patriotic decisions of individual nurses, (3) the broad-scale planning of the Na-

[13] Beeby, Nell V.: "My Visit to the Family in the ETO," *Am. J. Nursing.* **45**:880, 1945.

tional Nursing Council and other agencies (which is discussed in the following chapter), and (4) the courage and ingenuity with which nurses "carried on" on the home front.

BIBLIOGRAPHY

Aynes, Edith A.: "This Waiting War," *Am. J. Nursing*, 43:542, 1943.

Blanchfield, Florence A.: "Calling All Nurses," *Am. J. Nursing*, 45:91, 1945.

———: "Report from the ETO and MTO," *Am. J. Nursing*, 45:427, 1945.

Blanchfield, Florence A., and Standlee, Mary W.: *Organized Nursing and the Army in Three Wars.* Unpublished manuscript on file, Historical Division, Office of the Surgeon General of the Army, Washington, D.C.

Bolton, Frances Payne: "Home from ETOUSA" (European Theatre of Operations, United States Army), *Am. J. Nursing*, 45:5, 1945.

Bradley, La Verne: "Women in Uniform," *Insignia and Decorations of the U.S. Armed Forces*, rev. ed. National Geographic Society, Washington, D.C., 1944, pp. 159–98.

Clarke, Alice R.: "Thirty-seven Months as Prisoners of War," *Am. J. Nursing*, 45:342, 1945.

Cooper, Page: *Navy Nurse.* McGraw-Hill Book Co., New York, 1946.

Curtis, Dorothy E.: "The Patients in Car D," *Am. J. Nursing*, 45:804, 1945.

Desmarais, Mary Virginia: "Navy Nursing on D-Day Plus 4," *Am. J. Nursing*, 45:12, 1945.

Evans, Jessie Fant: "Release from Los Banos," *Am. J. Nursing*, 45:462, 1945.

Flikke, Julia O.: *Nurses in Action—The Story of the Army Nurse Corps.* J. B. Lippincott Co., Philadelphia, 1943.

"The Heroic Nurses of Bataan and Corregidor," *Am. J. Nursing*, 42:896, 1942.

Hohf, Josephine: "Somewhere in Australia," *Am. J. Nursing*, 45:42, 1945.

Kernodle, Portia B.: *The Red Cross Nurse in Action, 1882–1948.* Harper & Brothers, New York, 1949.

Newcomb, Ellsworth: *Brave Nurse—True Stories of Heroism.* D. Appleton–Century Co., Inc., New York, 1945.

"The Nurses' Contribution to American Victory—Facts and Figures from Pearl Harbor to VJ Day," *Am. J. Nursing*, 45:683, 1945.

"Nursing in a Debarkation Ward," *Am. J. Nursing*, 45:135, 1945.

O'Toole, Sarah: "They Pioneered on Tinian," *Am. J. Nursing*, 45:1013, 1945.

Peto, Marjorie: *Women Were Not Expected.* An informal story of the nurses of the 2nd General Hospital in the ETO. Published by the author (1293 Sussex Road, West Englewood, N.J., 1947).

"Redeployment of Nurses in the ETO," *Am. J. Nursing,* **45**:507, 1945.

Redmond, Juanita: *I Served on Bataan.* J. B. Lippincott Co., Philadelphia, 1943.

Rodabaugh, James H., and Rodabaugh, Mary Jane: *Nursing in Ohio— A History.* The Ohio State Nurses' Association, Columbus, Ohio, 1951, pp. 221–36.

Schwartz, Doris: "Nursing Aboard a Hospital Ship," *Am. J. Nursing,* **45**:996, 1945.

"Six Navy Nurses Returned from the War Area," *Am. J. Nursing,* **42**:1202, 1942.

"What Army Nurses Do," *Am. J. Nursing,* **45**:436, 1945.

White, Ruth Young: "The 'Solace' Plies the Tasman and Coral Seas," *Am. J. Nursing,* **44**:552, 1944.

Chapter 34

COMPOSITE LEADERSHIP IN WARTIME

We need unity today in our profession as never before; unity which expresses itself in common action which gives proof to our oft-expressed belief that our primary concern is to render the nursing service the country needs at all times. The standards of nursing schools and nursing services are the responsibility of the whole profession and can only be maintained by the constructive thinking and action of all groups.

STELLA GOOSTRAY[1]

FROM PEARL HARBOR until V-J Day the requirements of the armed forces conditioned all nursing plans and programs. The National Nursing Council, reorganized and incorporated (1942) as the National Nursing Council for War Service, shared responsibility for over-all planning with the Government's Subcommittee until congressional appropriations for the committee were discontinued (1943), and two major projects of mutual concern had been taken over by federal agencies. Under the USPHS the US Cadet Nurse Corps (July, 1943) became responsible for increasing the supply of nursing at the source, viz., by the enrollment of greatly increased classes for the nursing schools. The Nursing Division of the Procurement and Assignment Service of the War Manpower Commission had been made responsible for an equitable distribution of nurses for military and civilian services.

In the interval between the wars, nursing and the base of its leadership had undergone a marked transformation. Whereas the personal leadership of a few outstanding nurses was a dominant characteristic of nursing in World War I, a determined effort to fuse the elements of a fragmented profession into an effective agency for

[1] "Address of the President," *Forty-eighth Annual Report of the National League of Nursing Education*, 1942, p. 99.

the service of the nation was its most notable characteristic in World War II. The professional organizations, including many of the constituent state and local organizations, had grown strong. Federal nursing services were beginning to have an important influence on the development of the profession. Considerable numbers of nurses had gained distinction and recognition outside of, as well as within, the profession. Nursing education, for participation in medical and health services of increasing complexity, was developing partnerships with related disciplines as well as with interested laymen.

The National Nursing Council assumed that, through unity of purpose and coordination of the programs of the participating organizations, military needs could be given priority with minimal disruption of civilian nursing services. It was launched with lofty aspirations and an uncertain budget. When war was declared, it had a staff of only four persons, one of them a nurse volunteer. Its voting members represented five national nursing organizations,[2] the ARC nursing service, and the six federal nursing services. The structural units of the ANA, namely the state nurses' associations, it was assumed, would provide a sound foundation for a network of wartime services.

Beginning with the reorganization of the council, and the addition of representatives from the AHA, all agencies with a primary interest in nursing were represented on the council before the end of the war.[3] The participation of the AHA was not, however, limited to membership on the council. At the insistence of that association, a joint committee of the AHA and the council was organized to facilitate cooperative planning. This was logical and important since the nursing services are by far the largest administrative units in any hospital. Few people bore heavier wartime burdens than the administrators of those extremely complex institutions, the hospitals. At the beginning of the war, there was serious lack of rapport between doctors, hospital administrators, and nurses, due largely to outworn

[2] ANA, NLNE, NOPHN, ACSN, NACGN.
[3] Those added were: Division of Nursing Education, USPHS; National Association for Practical Nurse Education; International Council of Nurses; Federal Nursing Council; American Association of Industrial Nurses; and sixteen members at large.

traditions. If nurse administrators felt that they bore the greater burden it was due to two conditions. Nurses on the "firing line" of the civilian front were continuously and unremittingly aware of the needs of patients as individuals. The hospital nursing services, always the coordinating element in the nexus of services to patients, became "buffer" services, which were expected to absorb the shocks created by losses from both the upper and lower eschelons of medical and hospital services while struggling with shortages in its own group.

Because of the prestige of the council's member agencies and of the individuals who held membership on the council and the sub-committee, their representatives secured access to important sources of advice and information pertinent to the nursing program. Working cooperatively, the two wartime agencies carried nursing into the upper levels of national planning. The council's preliminary work was financed by the profession. Later, although it received allocations for special projects from other foundations and from private sources, the W. K. Kellogg Foundation became, from 1942 on, the council's principal source of income. It contributed a total of over $300,000 for the program. Throughout the war, state nurses' associations, which had contributed to the support of the council in its formative months, carried much of the local expense of council-sponsored projects.

The council[4] had three presidents: Julia C. Stimson, ex-superintendent of the ANC and president of the ANA, served throughout the formative period; Stella Goostray, principal of the school of nursing, Children's Hospital, Boston, and president of the NLNE, elected after the reorganization in 1942, was a wise and stabilizing force throughout most of the strenuous period of active warfare. She was succeeded in the postwar period by Sophie C. Nelson, director of visiting nursing of the John Hancock Life Insurance Company and an ex-president of the NOPHN. In its two years of active work, the Government's Subcommittee had three chair-

[4] The National Nursing Council was organized July, 1940, as the Nursing Council for National Defense; reorganized 1942 as the National Nursing Council for War Service, Inc.; in November, 1945, the name was changed to the National Nursing Council, Inc.; it was dissolved in October, 1948.

men: Mary Beard, director of the ARC nursing service; Marion Sheahan, director of the Division of Nursing of the New York State Department of Health; and Marion C. Howell, dean of the Frances Payne Bolton School of Nursing, Western Reserve University, with Alma C. Haupt, on leave from the Metropolitan Life Insurance Company, serving as executive secretary. Mrs. Wickenden carried administrative responsibility for the council through the tempestuous war years and well into the postwar period. After her resignation (1947), Surg. Gen. Parran of the USPHS, at the direction of President Truman, awarded her the Medal of Merit. This medal was awarded to civilians for "exceptionally meritorious conduct in the performance of outstanding service in the war effort." It was accepted by Mrs. Wickenden as recognition of the wartime service of the profession.

At the time the council was organized, it must be remembered that many of the state nurses' associations, state leagues of nursing education, and some of the state organizations for public health nursing had vigorous programs based on those of the national organizations and related to local needs. Some of the state associations were already participating in the programs of state defense councils. But the joint boards of the three national nursing organizations had not developed a coordinated defense program in relation to them. The ARC nursing service was pressing more and more urgently for increased enrollment in its First Reserve for military service. Some hospitals were already having serious difficulty in filling positions vacated by the departure of nurses for military service or accepting opportunities for promotion. Marion G. Randall, then assistant director of the Henry Street Nursing Service of New York City, was appointed nursing consultant to the medical division of the Office of Civilian Defense. Following the declaration of war, the USPHS also loaned a few nurses who served as consultants to the OCD's deputy nurses. They were under pressure to develop emergency nursing programs in state and local civilian defense areas. The need for broad-gauge and coordinated planning was increasingly self-evident.

National plans cannot provide nursing service any more than

blueprints provide shelter. Their usefulness is dependent upon the effectiveness with which they can be adapted by those working in local situations. A manual was prepared and widely distributed by the National Nursing Council through the channels of the ANA for use in organizing state and local councils and in interpreting their functions. At the end of the first war year, 49 state councils had been established under which almost 1000 city and other local councils were at work. Lacking a field staff, the council was dependent on national and regional conferences for keeping this chain of units, and the profession as a whole, oriented to the program. The purpose of this network of councils was to facilitate, state by state, effective use of existing nursing resources, to assist the ARC with its enrollment of nurses, and to "increase the supply [of nursing service] by (a) getting professionally inactive nurses back to work, (b) increasing the enrollment in schools of nursing, and (c) using volunteers and auxiliary workers."[5]

Briefly stated, the National Nursing Council accepted over-all responsibility for developing nursing programs to meet wartime needs on the basis of principles already established by the profession. (1) It reviewed wartime projects in relation to the functions of the member agencies and recommended new projects to appropriate agencies. (2) It administered projects which did not fall within the scope of any one member agency. (3) Under the changing conditions of war, it outlined projects which seemed to be beyond the scope of any voluntary agency and referred them to the Government's Subcommittee. The council was never adequately staffed for such a comprehensive program. It worked under terrific pressures and considerable criticism. Many of its projects were dependent upon securing on loan for brief periods the service of nurses with special qualifications. Its most serious problems were due to misunderstandings about the functions and relationships of existing agencies in terms of over-all planning, and the great difficulty of keeping all participating agencies promptly and fully informed of changes in a fast-moving program.

[5] *Distribution of Nursing Service.* National Nursing Council for War Service, New York, 1942.

Data obtained in the National Survey provided the foundation for council programs. A committee on recruitment of student nurses was the first permanent committee set up by the council,[6] and recruitment, with changes in emphasis, remained a major interest well into the postwar period. Programs were planned on the basic assumption that there are two phases to a recruitment program; namely, an over-all publicity program to create a favorable climate of opinion on national, state, and local levels, and a direct appeal to potential students and groups closely in touch with them, such as high school and college counselors. One of the merits of the inclusive council-type organization was the facility with which cooperative public relations programs could be developed, through its department of public information, with other organizations. The wartime nurse program of the National Federation of Women's Clubs was an outstanding example of broad-gauge planning in cooperation with the council and the ARC. But many other agencies, including the Auxiliary of the American Medical Association, the American Legion Auxiliary, the Women of the Moose, and Rotary Clubs, assisted with recruitment in the early war period, usually by raising funds for scholarships. To care for a flood of inquiries about nursing, the council set up a clearing bureau and established a special postal address for it in New York City. Enrollment in the schools increased rapidly, but not sufficiently to meet the swiftly mounting need.

The subcommittee set the quota of nursing students for 1941 at 50,000 and that for 1942 at 55,000. Three times in 1942 the powerful Office of War Information sponsored extensive use of radio and other media in support of the council's student recruitment program but less than 50,000 students were enrolled. Inquiries received by the clearing bureau clearly indicated that the quotas could not be filled without extensive use of scholarship or other financial aid for students. Throughout the war, the over-all student recruitment programs directed by the National Nursing Council, and after mid-July, 1943, by the US Cadet Nurse Corps, were planned to interest high

---

[6] Katherine Faville, dean of nursing, Wayne University, the chairman, was also consultant on recruitment to the subcommittee on nursing.

school graduates. There were, however, sound reasons for attempting also to interest college women in nursing. Experience had indicated that the more mature college-trained students could be prepared more rapidly than high school graduates for teaching and administrative positions. Then, too, collegiate schools, of which there were 76 in 1940,[7] could not be expected to depend solely on their own recruitment efforts in a highly competitive situation. Recalling the brilliant results of the Vassar camp of 1918, the ARC financed a preclinical course on the Bryn Mawr campus the summer before Pearl Harbor. Hastily planned and lacking the dramatic appeal of war service, the enrollment fell far short of the anticipated goal. However, the course was repeated in the three following summers in cooperation with a few nursing schools and without Red Cross financing. Several times during the war the council attempted to interest college women in nursing. In a 12-week period (1942), Edith H. Smith, dean of nursing at Syracuse University, visited 26 eastern colleges. The reported lack of interest in nursing as a profession for college women provided a basis for the next attempt. In cooperation with the Cadet Nurse Corps (Chap. 36) the council borrowed 35 carefully selected nurses with collegiate backgrounds for a second effort. Within a six-month period they visited some 600 senior and junior colleges, including those for Negro women. The following year, 17 counselors returned to about half of the institutions previously visited. The specific result of these programs is not known. The field workers were cordially received and interviewed a few thousand students. They believed that "long and intensive efforts would be required to recruit large numbers from the college group."[8]

When it became apparent that the student quota of 1942 would not be attained, the subcommittee and council were advised by Dr. George Baehr, medical director of the Office of Civilian Defense, and Dr. Thomas Parran, Surgeon General of the USPHS, that more

[7] *Facts about Nursing*, NIB, 1942, p. 21.
[8] Newell, Hope: *History of the National Nursing Council.* NOPHN, New York, distributor, 1951, p. 61.

aggressive steps should be taken to increase the nurse power of the nation without delay. These should involve "(1) acceleration of nurse-training programs and (2) plans for recruiting and training auxiliary personnel above the custodial level."[9] The subcommittee cooperating with the National Nursing Council spearheaded the movement, in which representatives of interested agencies and appropriate departments of the government participated, which brought the US Cadet Nurse Corps into existence under the aegis of the USPHS. The extraordinarily successful recruitment program of the corps was directed from Washington, but the USPHS contracted with the council for the continuance of its clearing bureau and "Box 88, New York," to which potential students could direct inquiries. This and the procurement of uniforms for the Cadet Corps, also under contract with the USPHS, were the most extensive administrative responsibilities carried by the council.

The NLNE was well established as the source of information and guidance on nursing education. It had recommended the acceleration of nursing school curriculums many months before the Cadet Corps made acceleration of the basic program obligatory for schools wishing to participate in that program. Several of its valuable bulletins, such as *Nursing Education in Wartime,* had already been published. (For the NLNE's wartime program, see Chap. 39.) The Cadet Corps provided limited consultation service for participating schools which were receiving its directives. But the schools were under tremendous pressure to provide increasing volumes of service for hospital patients while readjusting their basic programs to meet Cadet Corps requirements. Since it was necessary to do this within the framework of state board rulings, it is not surprising that some confused, if not resentful, thinking occurred in the schools. The council, as a coordinating agency, provided a special field service. Under the direction of Helen Schwarz, then director of the College of Nursing, University of Cincinnati, it provided 76 two-day institutes for representatives of schools and of state boards of nurse examiners. As some state board rulings were found to be serious

[9] *Ibid.,* p. 28.

obstacles to acceleration, the ANA established the Bureau of State Boards of Nurse Examiners (discussed in Chap. 38) which has proved to be one of the constructive results of wartime experiences.

In the council program, next to the work of the Recruitment Committee in time and importance came that of the Supply and Distribution Committee. Psychologically and practically, it had the most difficult task assigned to any of the many council committees.[10] Its functions were to assist the ARC in enrolling nurses for the military services, and to distribute fairly the remaining nurses. Here again, national planning was effective only insofar as it could be adapted to local situations. A guide, *Distribution of Nursing Service During War*, was prepared to assist state and local committees. When the ARC began calling for 3000 nurses each month for the Army and Navy, the committee distributed thousands of copies of *Nurses to the Colors* (1942). A third widely distributed pamphlet, *Priorities for Nurses* (1943), contained sections prepared by each of the three older national organizations as a means of assuring members that their particular interests and problems were being considered, and to show that the national organizations were actively cooperating in the council program.

In 1943, with the Pacific aflame and the campaign against Italy getting under way, the use of civilian hospitals reached record-breaking heights. It was increasingly difficult to persuade either military or civilian agencies that the profession was putting forth maximum effort to provide the volume of nursing service that each required. Private duty nurses, who had not gone into military or other organized services quite generally, and often unjustly, suffered from the jibe "luxury nurse." Many of those who were not eligible for military service restricted their practice to the care of the acutely ill. Some institutions made a real effort to limit the use of special duty nurses to the care of those in actual need of such service, but others encouraged their employment. The predominance of gray-haired practitioners of private duty and staff nursing was a striking characteristic of many hospital nursing services. But

[10] Katharine Tucker, director, Department of Nursing Education, University of Pennsylvania, chairman.

throughout the war it was difficult to persuade some doctors, hospital administrators, and nurses that need should be the sole criterion in procuring nurses for special duty. The national survey of 1943 showed that the number of active private duty nurses, as compared with 1941, had been decreased by more than 44 per cent.[11] The patriotism of nurses who remained in positions essential to the continuation of nursing schools and nursing services was sometimes impugned by patriotic but uninformed persons. The National Nursing Council decided that the problem of equitable distribution of nurses on the basis of fundamental needs was too complex to be handled by a voluntary agency. It asked the subcommittee to explore the possibility of having the procurement and assignment of nurses taken over by a governmental agency. After months of conferences and investigation by federal agencies, including the Bureau of the Budget, the nursing section of the War Manpower Commission was established on the same date as the US Cadet Nurse Corps, July 1, 1943.[12] (See Chaps. 35 and 36.) By that act, the government of the United States recognized nursing as essential to the successful prosecution of the war.

Having transferred its major responsibilities to the federal government, the council now turned its attention to untapped sources of nursing service. This led to consideration of (1) Negroes in nursing, (2) men nurses, and (3) practical nurses. The council's department of public relations prepared appropriate and attractive folders about the opportunities in nursing for each of these groups for the use of recruitment committees. The effort to secure Negro students was rewarding. The others were not. The draft made no provision for deferring men who were students in schools of nursing. The lag in enrollment in schools of practical nurses was generally attributed to two factors: (1) industry offered more lucrative opportunity and (2) except in a few areas, trained practical nurses had not been accorded an assured vocational status. In the early days of the war, inquiries about Negro nurses and opportunities for Negroes in

[11] *Facts about Nursing*, NIB, 1943, p. 36.
[12] Newell, Hope: *History of the National Nursing Council.* NOPHN, New York, distributor, 1951, pp. 35–37.

schools of nursing were referred by the council to the NACGN. It now appeared that a more positive program would be productive. With financial aid from the General Education Board of the Rockefeller Foundation, the council set up a Negro unit on an experimental basis. Estelle Massey Riddle,[13] a former president of the NACGN and a member of the faculty of New York University, was appointed to direct the unit and to serve as a consultant. The preliminary work was so promising that a second consultant was appointed and the work of the unit integrated with the general program of the council. With support from the General Education Board and the W. K. Kellogg Foundation, this work was carried into the postwar period. The special functions of the consultants were (1) to compile data relative to the status and problems of Negro nurses and (2) to stimulate the progress of Negro nurses through further integration in the major professional organizations. As staff members, Mrs. Riddle and her associates participated in conferences on all aspects of nursing that were of concern to the council.

In 1940 there were approximately 7000 Negro nurses in the United States.[14] In general they professed indifference to enrollment in the ARC because very few Negro nurses had been admitted to the Army Nurse Corps in World War I. None had been accepted by the Navy. A few were accepted by the ANC in the early days of World War II. In connection with its search for untapped resources, the National Nursing Council formally resolved in 1943 that Negro nurses should be appointed to the Nurse Corps of the Army and Navy "on the same basis as any other American nurses who met the professional requirements." Copies of the resolution were sent to the Surgeons General of the Army and the Navy. This action was vigorously followed up by the NACGN which was supported by other Negro organizations and by influential persons, both white and colored, who were working for democratic racial relations. As a result, approximately 600 Negro nurses were in the ANC at the peak of military activity. The Navy accepted its first Negro nurse in 1945.

The unit carried on an extensive program of field work, its rep-

[13] Now Mrs. Osborn.
[14] *Facts about Nursing*, NIB (quoting US Census), 1945, p. 11.

resentatives serving as consultants or resource personnel at conferences on nursing education and related subjects. The pinnacle of success for the unit was reached when Hampton Institute, which had made earlier efforts to develop a school of nursing, established a collegiate school with clinical experience provided by three participating hospitals. The first class was graduated and received degrees in 1946. By the end of the war, there were significant evidences of progress in attaining equality of educational opportunity in nursing for Negroes and of equality of opportunity in employment in institutions and in public health nursing.[15] The council had made an important contribution to the improvement of interracial relationships along with its effort to broaden the base of nursing service for the American people.

At war's end the Veterans Administration was in general disfavor. The number of patients requiring care was mounting rapidly. There were 2000 vacancies in the hospital nursing service. An effort, sponsored by the council and led by the ANA, to secure legislation authorizing a commissioned corps had failed in 1944. The council appointed a small committee to confer with the administrator of the Veterans Administration. An offer of assistance was accepted, after which a limited study of the nursing service in veterans hospitals was made by three nurse consultants appointed by the council. The major recommendation, that an advisory committee be organized, was accepted. History was repeating itself. An advisory committee had given stalwart support to the director of that service in the late twenties under somewhat similar circumstances. The tremendous expansion and the marked improvement in the quality of the nursing service of the Veterans Administration have an important place in our postwar history.

The abrupt termination of World War I had not been anticipated, and left many persons with the strange sensation of being suspended in space. To avoid a possible repetition of that experience, the US had hardly begun to participate in World War II when group after group began planning for the period of reconstruction.

[15] Newell, Hope: "The Council's Negro Unit," *History of the National Nursing Council.* NOPHN, New York, distributor, 1951, pp. 49–51.

Nursing was no exception. By 1944 each of the national nursing organizations had a committee working on postwar plans. The National Nursing Council suggested that such plans might profitably be analyzed and coordinated. A National Nursing Planning Committee functioned, under the chairmanship of Marion W. Sheahan and Pearl McIver successively, from 1944 to 1948. In preparation for the work of this committee, a study of nursing needs and resources was made by a committee of which Miss McIver was chairman. Estimates were projected to 1946.[16] Versatile Marjorie B. Davis was employed as full-time secretary of the committee. By sheer coincidence, the comprehensive program[17] developed by Miss Davis under the aegis of the committee was published in the first issue of the AJN to appear after V-J Day.

The work of the National Nursing Council was rounded out by the publication of a limited edition of its history. Only the major elements in its ambitious and perhaps too diffuse program have been considered here. Despite many stresses and strains it functioned as a coordinator and promoter of nursing education and nursing service throughout the war. It provided the ground work for postwar developments. In its varied activities it was supported by the professional nursing and related publications and by the Nursing Information Bureau. Through its releases, fact sheets, and news bulletins the public was better informed on many facets of nursing than ever before. The council provided a broad base for continued composite leadership, and for the postwar development of nursing, which is discussed in later chapters. The procurement and assignment of nurses, which the council had referred to the subcommittee for action, is discussed in the following chapter.

BIBLIOGRAPHY

Baehr, George: "Mobilization of the Nursing Profession for War," *Proceedings of the Thirty-third Convention of the American Nurses' Association*, 1942, p. 153.

[16] "Nursing Needs and Nursing Resources," *Am. J. Nursing*, **44**:1044, 1944.
[17] "A Comprehensive Program for Nationwide Action," *Am. J. Nursing*, **45**: 707, 1945.

Barck, Oscar Theodore, Jr., and Blake, Nelson Manfred: *Since 1900, A History of the United States in Our Times.* The Macmillan Company, New York, 1952.

"Critical Months Ahead in the Manpower Commission," *Am. J. Nursing,* 43:638, 1943.

Foster, Mary Louise: "For More Information—Write Box 88," *Am. J. Nursing,* 44:226, 1944.

"Government's Nurse Supply Unit," *Am. J. Nursing,* 43:523, 1943.

Haupt, Alma C.: "The Government's Subcommittee on Nursing," *Am. J. Nursing,* 42:257, 1942.

Kernodle, Portia B.: *The Red Cross Nurse in Action, 1882–1948.* Harper & Brothers, New York, 1949.

"National Nursing Council for War Service" (postwar planning), *Am. J. Nursing,* 44:70, 1944.

"National Nursing Planning Committee," *Am. J. Nursing,* 45:513, 1945.

Newell, Hope: *The History of the National Nursing Council.* National Organization for Public Health Nursing, distributor, New York, 1951.

"Nursing in War Manpower Commission" (with organization chart) *Am. J. Nursing,* 43:741, 1943.

"Nursing Needs and Nursing Resources," *Am. J. Nursing,* 44:1044, 1944.

Nursing Participation in the Emergency Medical Service. Medical Division Bulletin #6, US Office of Civilian Defense, Washington, D.C., December, 1942.

"President's Medal of Merit Awarded to Mrs. Wickenden," *Am. J. Nursing,* 47:708, 1947.

Randall, Marian G.: "*Your* Part in Civilian Defense," *Am. J. Nursing,* 42:60, 1942.

Smith, Edith H.: Report of the Student Recruitment Visits to Colleges," *Forty-ninth Annual Report of the National League of Nursing Education,* 1943, p. 175.

"War Manpower Commission; Classification, Clearance, and Appeals Procedures," *Am. J. Nursing,* 43:885, 1943.

"Wartime Nursing Is Different," *Am. J. Nursing,* 43:835, 1943.

"Wickenden, Elmira B.: "The National Nursing Council Reports," *Am. J. Nursing,* 43:807, 1943.

————: "Nurses United for War Services," *Pub. Health Nursing,* 36:340, 1944.

————: "The NNCWS and V-E Day," *Am. J. Nursing,* 45:508, 1945.

Many other articles in the *American Journal of Nursing* and *Public Health Nursing,* 1940–1945.

Chapter 35

VOLUNTARY PROCUREMENT AND ASSIGNMENT—
OR A DRAFT?

. . . I urge that the Selective Service Act be amended to provide for the induction of nurses into the armed forces. . . .

FRANKLIN DELANO ROOSEVELT[1]

IN RESPONSE to the shock of Pearl Harbor there had been a sharp but relatively temporary rise in the ARC enrollment of nurses for military service. The invasion of North Africa almost a year later had a similar effect. The brilliant success of the invasion of Normandy and improved conditions in the Pacific in the summer of 1944 caused the American people, nurses among them, to be unduly optimistic about an early end to the war. Enrollment lagged. In the interval between those invasions, many nurses had entered military service but the pressure for more and more civilian nursing made it increasingly difficult for nurses to turn their backs, as it were, on the self-evident needs of patients in their homes and in hospitals, in order to serve under conditions created by a global war which was wholly outside their experience and about which there were many misunderstandings. This was not due to any lack of confidence in Col. Florence A. Blanchfield, the highly competent superintendent of the ANC, or in Capt. Sue S. Dauser, the equally experienced superintendent of the Navy Nurse Corps. Information about the nursing requirements of the armed forces was conditioned by over-all military policies in relation to national security. The situation was complicated by the involved methods employed to recruit nurses.

At the end of the government's fiscal year in June, 1942, when

[1] Annual Message to Congress, January 6, 1945.

the war effort had begun to gain momentum, there were over 12,-000 nurses in the ANC, almost 11,000 of whom were Reserves. This was almost double the number on duty at the time of Pearl Harbor. The NNC had practically doubled its enrollment with 1777 nurses of whom 950 were Reserves.[2] Despite all difficulties, when the war was over, it could be shown that the ARC had certified 104,500 nurses to the military and 70,500 had been assigned. This is a record of which the profession may well be proud since it had been estimated in 1943 that the total number of professionally active nurses, exclusive of those in military service, was only 170,599.[3] The methods by which that result was achieved can be only briefly discussed here. They are fully set forth in Kernodle's *The Red Cross Nurse in Action.*

The ARC nursing service made a valiant effort to fulfill its traditional obligation to provide reserve nurses for the armed forces. It used established routines in the earlier part of the war, and, in order to avoid any misunderstanding, the Surgeon General of the Army officially reaffirmed this function in 1942. The ARC relationship with the NNC, although it served both corps, had never been as definitive as that with the Army. In 1942 the NNC decided to do its own recruiting, working cooperatively with the local committees of the Procurement and Assignment Service of the War Manpower Commission. Thereafter, the ARC sent all applications to the NNC unprocessed, when a preference for Navy service had been indicated. Month after month, in the latter part of the war, the Navy requirement was stated to be 500 nurses a month with a maximum corps strength of 11,500. When the question of drafting nurses was under consideration by Congress early in 1945, the Navy, having well-trained hospital corpsmen, required only three nurses for each thousand naval and Marine Corps personnel. It turned over approximately 2500 excess applications to the ANC.

Efforts to meet the very much greater needs of the Army were complicated by lack of definite information about the specific ob-

---

[2] *Facts about Nursing,* NIB, 1943, p. 17.
[3] "The National Survey of Registered Nurses, U.S.P.H.S., 1943," *Facts about Nursing,* NIB, 1944, p. 5.

jectives to be attained at various stages of the war. An army of 8,500,000 men had been widely discussed before the maximum strength was set at 7,500,000 in 1943. On the basis of the War Department's ration of 6 nurses to each 1000 troop strength, this meant the difference between 51,000 and 45,000 nurses for the ANC. Mrs. Kernodle, in discussing this problem, points out that, in order to understand what appeared to be fluctuations in the Army's requirements, it is necessary to assume that when the smaller figure was decided upon for the Army "proportionate personnel reductions were allowed to pass unnoticed by several divisions of the Surgeon General's Office."[4] This oversight, if such it was, created a serious problem for the ANC, and for the whole nursing profession as well. As the war progressed, lack of consistently firm figures on the ANC's needs had a seriously deterrent influence on the profession's plans for recruitment at the time of the Army's greatest need for nurses. Before discussing that problem, it is necessary to consider the methods by which the profession, under the general leadership of the National Nursing Council, endeavored to meet military needs without disrupting or destroying the basic structure of the American system of nursing.

When the Supply and Distribution Committee of the National Nursing Council[5] became convinced (1942) that a voluntary agency could not achieve an equitable distribution of nurses, the council referred the problem to the Government's Subcommittee. Later in that year, after many conferences, the War Manpower Commission agreed to set up a new division, Supply and Distribution of Nurses. Novices as they were in matters relating to the authorization and administration of federal services, the representatives of the subcommittee and the council promptly set to work on plans which were to be discussed at a conference of representatives of the state councils. Two days before the scheduled date of that June meeting in Chicago, word was received that the Bureau of the Budget had not approved a separate division for nurses but that a place would

[4] Kernodle, Portia B.: *The Red Cross Nurse in Action, 1882–1948.* Harper & Brothers, New York, 1949, p. 423.
[5] Katharine Tucker, chairman.

be made for them in the Procurement and Assignment Service for Physicians, Dentists, Veterinarians, and Sanitary Engineers. Time did not permit either the cancellation of the conference or the necessary revamping of plans! Three months later, that sterile meeting was followed by an informative and productive conference. But almost a year elapsed, a year of intense wartime activity and seething emotions, between the first effort to secure governmental assistance and the actual initiation of the procurement and assignment program.

The preliminary work for organization of the nursing. division was carried forward on a part-time basis by Miss Haupt, the far-seeing executive secretary of the subcommittee. L. Louise Baker, previously assistant director of the ARC nursing service in the Pacific area, assisted her and was appointed to administer the new service when it was inaugurated July 1, 1943. Miss Haupt then returned to her position with the Metropolitan Life Insurance Company. Miss Tucker, who had been chairman of the council's procurement and assignment committee, was appointed chairman of the advisory committee of the new division. The division's functions were: (1) to procure nurses to meet the needs of the armed forces, having due consideration for civilian nursing needs, and (2) to bring about equitable distribution of nurses in order to maintain the best possible nursing service for the civilian population and non-military governmental services.

The name of the new agency was misleading. Since women were not subject to the provisions of the Selective Service Act, it could neither procure nor assign nurses in the precise meaning of those terms. As an administrative unit it had arrived late on the scene of wartime action, but the staff and its advisory committee attacked the assigned projects with energetic determination. The Procurement and Assignment Service (P&AS) for Nurses lacked the "teeth" of the Procurement and Assignment Service for Physicians but, as compared with the National Nursing Council, it had the advantages of federal prestige and of sufficient federal financing to permit the development of a small headquarters and field staff. It also provided travel funds and limited clerical assistance for the federally appointed, but nonsalaried, chairmen of state committees upon whom devolved the extremely heavy responsibility for securing local action. The nursing division of P&AS undertook the enormous task of locating all professional nurses, of classifying them in accordance with their essentiality in their civilian positions or of their availability, if in nonessential positions, for military service. It was responsible for assigning to the states quotas of nurses to be procured for military service. The new agency accepted the ARC nursing service as the constituted recruitment agency for the military just as the National Nursing Council had done. But it restricted ARC recruitment to nurses classified as 1-A, viz., those who were professionally available for military service. Within a year 300,000 nurses were classified by local committees which were composed of well-qualified nurses, who were holding demanding positions, assisted by capable volunteers recruited from parent-teacher associations and other civic organizations. Those who observed some of these committees at work, often far into the night, declare their service to be one of the unsung sagas of the war. When the service was organized, more than 30,000 nurses were already in the ANC and 5000 in the NNC. Among them were considerable numbers of nurses whose departure had seriously weakened the schools of nursing. One of the primary functions of P&AS was the prevention of further losses to the military of nurses who were essential to the maintenance of nursing schools or to the administration of institutional, public health, or industrial nursing services. No consideration was given to the serious need in the military services for nurses with administrative experience.

Due to the last-minute change in the proposed organization of the nursing division of P&AS, its first productive conference with the chairman of state committees was not held until September, 1943. But a study of nursing in civilian hospitals, which yielded valuable information, had been made in that summer by two statisticians on leave from the USPHS and the ANA, respectively. A series of articles subsequently published in the AJN revealed the extraordinary unevenness of the distribution of nurses among hospitals. Location, personnel policies, and a variety of other factors caused astonishing variations in the provision of nursing care for patients. In the 500 representative hospitals studied, the range was from less than half an hour to over five hours of nursing care per patient per day.[6] In the meantime the staff, using the criterion of essentiality previously developed by the Committee on Procurement and Assignment of the National Nursing Council, set up the forms and directives that were necessary for the collection of data, the classification of nurses, and the administration of the service. Those in attendance at the September meeting were informed by the Surgeon General's office that the Army quota for the fiscal year ending in June, 1944, would be over 51,000 nurses. The figure was accepted without question. It presented the greatest challenge yet offered to all planning committees. State chairmen of councils and P&AS committees returned to their homes determined to do three things: To discover the total nursing assets in their jurisdictions by finding the retired and otherwise "hidden nurses" who might help to save the day by releasing eligible nurses for military service, to encourage local redistribution of nurses when that seemed indicated, and, above all, to meet the quotas for military service assigned to them by P&AS.

The National Nursing Council, the P&AS, and the ARC secured the interest of the Office of War Information and the War Advertising Council in promoting a National Nurse Mobilization Week early in 1944. Through the proposed program it was believed that the true nursing situation could be made known in every part of the country. Preliminary publicity had been given these plans when the War Manpower Commission was informed that the authorized quota for the ANC for 1944 was 40,000 instead of the 51,000 goal toward which all nursing agencies had been striving. This information set off a high emotional charge among the planners who had been preparing for a top-level public information program. Plans for a National Nurse Mobilization Week were dropped and the P&AS turned its attention to civilian needs.

The ARC, in the meantime, was pressing forward with a reorganized recruitment program. The method of handling applications had been revised and expedited. The long-established state and

[6] "Hospital Nursing Service in Wartime," *Am. J. Nursing,* **45:**222, 1945.

local committees[7] were disbanded and replaced by a more extensive chain of chapter recruitment committees, thus breaking the long-standing relationship with the ANA. Recruitment centers were established in cities of 25,000 or over. The ARC did everything possible to show that it was recruiting for the military rather than for the Red Cross itself, a point which had frequently been misunderstood. Nurses unfamiliar with the traditional relationship between the ARC and the ANC were frankly critical of the ARC as a portal to military service. (It had never been an exclusive means of admission since nurses could apply directly to either of the corps.) In the early part of the war, the restrictions imposed on the Army and Navy for security reasons limited the information concerning the activities of nurses already in service that could be released to the ARC. This had been a serious handicap to early recruitment efforts. When the restrictions were eased, the services were more effectively publicized; both corps assigned nurses to participate in recruitment programs, the Navy independently, the Army in cooperation with the ARC.

The requirements for admission to the military services were often criticized by persons to whom a nurse was a nurse regardless of age, physical condition, marital status, or professional preparation. The ANC raised its age limit for reserve nurses from 35 to 45. It dropped the ban on married nurses at a relatively early date. Later the NNC, when it discovered that 80 per cent of its attrition rate was due to matrimony, also conceded that nurses who married while in service might remain in the corps. The ambitions and patriotic aspirations of minority groups were widely publicized in connection with programs for augmenting nursing resources. Little could be done for men nurses since they were subject to Selective Service. The acceptance of Negro nurses by both the ANC and NNC has been discussed elsewhere. Provision was made for Army hospitals in the US to employ civilian nurses ineligible for the ANC and nurse's aides on a salaried basis. The Surgeon General of the USPHS reminded all units of the US Cadet Nurse Corps, late in

[7] Kernodle, Portia B.: *The Red Cross Nurse in Action, 1882–1948.* Harper & Brothers, New York, 1949, p. 413–14.

1944, of the Army's need for senior cadets. During the life of the corps more than 6000 cadets (Chap. 36) were assigned to Army hospitals for their senior experience.

The P&AS was responsible for assigning quotas for recruitment for military service to the states based on the stated needs of the Army and Navy. In 1943 a quota of 28,000 nurses was distributed to the states based on the Army's planning figure of 51,000 nurses by June 30, 1944. Early in December, the Army notified P&AS without explanation that it required only 40,000 instead of 51,000 nurses. By early April, 1944, the Army had secured the 40,000 nurses. The nurses applying for commissions were notified that their services were not required at that time. That news traveled fast! Too fast to be overtaken by the information received by P&AS before the end of the month, that the Army would require 50,000 nurses by April, 1945, and that one-half of the additional 10,000 would be needed within six months. Quotas to the states were revised accordingly. But P&AS had lost its public relations staff when plans for Mobilization Week were dropped. It could influence the profession and public opinion only through its directives to committees and materials published by the nursing and related magazines. From that time until V-E Day the local P&AS committees and ARC recruitment committees worked ceaselessly to overcome the lag created by the catastrophic fluctuation in stated Army requirements.

By September, 1944, 30,000 sick and wounded men were being returned from all theaters each month. Hospitals in the US were seriously understaffed. It was announced that 11 Army hospitals had been sent overseas without nurses. Probably no announcement of the war had a more immediate effect on professionally minded nurses. The fact that the equipment, not the personnel, of those hospitals was needed overseas was not revealed until much later. The Surgeon General of the Army was becoming more and more exigent in his demand for enough nurses to give adequate care to men who had fought for their country. The Army nurse, he believed and stated later, was doing "one of the truly great jobs in this war,"[8]

---

[8] Kirk, Norman T.: Statement before the House Committee on Military Affairs, January 19, 1945.

and he was determined to maintain that standard. Believing that voluntary recruitment had failed, he appealed to the President. The atmosphere was already psychologically supercharged. When the "Battle of the Bulge" was beginning late in 1944, famed columnist Walter Lippmann called the attention of his thousands of readers to the need for more nurses to care for the enormously increased numbers of sick and wounded men. He assumed that the 27,000 nurses classified 1-A by P&AS were readily available but were not responding to the appeals of the recruitment committee. He showed no appreciation of the importunities of civilian agencies for the services of these nurses. The idea of drafting nurses as presented by him was by no means new. It had been considered and set aside by some nursing groups early in the war.

President Roosevelt's message to the Congress on January 6, 1945, galvanized a worn and weary profession. He said in part:

One of the most urgent immediate requirements of the armed forces is more nurses. . . . The present shortage of Army nurses is reflected in undue strain on the existing force. . . . It has been estimated by the War Manpower Commission that 27,000 additional nurses could be made available to the armed forces without interfering too seriously with the needs of the civilian population for nurses. Since volunteering has not produced the number of nurses required, I urge that the Selective Service Act be amended to provide for the induction of nurses into the armed forces. . . . The care and treatment given to our wounded and sick soldiers have been the best known to medical science. Those standards must be maintained at all costs. We cannot tolerate a lowering of them by failure to provide adequate nursing for the brave men who stand desperately in need of it.

The President also recommended, as he had a year earlier, the passage of a National Service Act which would be used only to the extent absolutely required by military necessities. Three days later the chairman of the House Committee on Military Affairs introduced a bill to ensure adequate care for the armed forces. The sole purpose of this bill was to secure nurses by "registration and selection for and induction into the land and naval forces of the United States under the Selective Training and Service Act of 1940. . . ."[9] A sec-

[9] H.R. 1284, 79th Congress, First Session.

ond more detailed bill with the same purpose was introduced a few days later.[10]

Following the President's message, nursing made the headlines all across the nation. Public opinion was thoroughly aroused. Some public relations experts felt that the prestige of the profession had been dealt a serious blow. Nursing opinion of the proposed legislation varied. Some looked upon a draft as the only feasible method for procuring a complete roster of nurses and for ensuring fullest use of the nurse power of the nation. Some considered it an affront to a profession which had already responded valiantly. Either way the profession could have pride in the acknowledged essentiality of its service. Swiftly the ANA, which bears responsibility for the profession's activities in relation to any legislation affecting nursing, and the National Nursing Council went into action. Despite the difficulties of wartime travel, the board of directors and the advisory council of the ANA met in conference in New York City with 34 states represented. Thereafter the board of directors, which alone has legal authority to act for the association between meetings of the House of Delegates, endorsed the principle of a draft of nurses as the first step to Selective Service for all women and endorsed the enactment of a National Service Act as recommended by the President to the Congress.[11] It may be noted in this connection that the WAC and other feminine services had not reached their authorized strength.

The House Committee on Military Affairs held hearings on the two bills in January and February, at which time the ANA and all other interested agencies were given an opportunity to express their views. The ANA Advisory Council, called for a second time, was in session in Washington when the association's local representative, Edith Beatty, brought the news that the House of Representatives had passed by a large majority a bill to conscript nurses, an action for which there was no precedent in American history. The representatives of the state nurses' associations thus had an unrivaled opportunity to discuss the views of their constituencies with the

[10] H.R. 1666, 79th Congress, First Session.
[11] "The Proposed Draft of Nurses," *Am. J. Nursing,* **45**:88, 1945.

members of both houses of Congress. The Senate Committee on Military Affairs also held extensive hearings. The professional organizations and all other interested agencies, federal and voluntary, were again given opportunity to present their views. The Senators were obviously reluctant to vote for the conscription of women.

The NLNE and NOPHN were in agreement with the principle adopted by the ANA, namely, Selective Service for nurses as a first step in a general mobilization of all women. The National Nursing Council approved the principle of Selective Service. It urged the enactment of a national service act to supplement any Selective Service legislation. That point was stressed by the representative of the American Hospital Association in his testimony. Hospital administrators were well aware that nurses were carrying a large volume of non-nursing work due to personnel shortages in other services. The profession has never had a finer tribute than the friendly tone of the Congressional hearings. The records indicate respect for nurses and great admiration of those with the armed forces.

Just as the hearings began, the Army announced that its requirement had been increased from 50,000 to 70,000 nurses. It was this figure, previously unknown to the profession, which had provided the basis for the President's message. It was, however, a planning figure and not a statement of authorized strength. That remained at 50,000. The ANC requested 10,000 nurses at once. The P&AS committees were instructed to continue uninterruptedly with the work of classification of nurses in order to build up a pool of Class I nurses[12] (nurses presumed to be available for military service). The ARC had already put on a "night shift" of workers and streamlined its method of handling applications for enrollment. But the War Department issued an order to the effect that nurses who volunteered, and were otherwise qualified, would be accepted without regard to their procurement and assignment classifications. The Army broke the bottleneck in its own procedure by accepting nurses as they became available instead of on designated dates. The Surgeon General secured the assistance of the Office of War Informa-

[12] "Where We Stand and What We Can Do," *Am. J. Nursing*, **45**:88, 1945.

tion and the War Advertising Council in developing a public information program in which the ANA participated.

Many nurses had been bewildered by the clamor of the conflicting voices of employers and the several agencies concerned with recruitment for the military services. The one clear call from the President of the United States caused them to apply for military service by the thousands. During the first five months of 1945 over 20,000 nurses were certified by the ARC to the Army and Navy.[13] During this period ARC nurse's aide figures also surpassed all previous records. The Navy made no change in its procedures and, as previously noted, referred some hundreds of excess applications to the ANC. On May 30, 1945, the Surgeon General of the Army informed the president of the ANA that the Acting Secretary of War had suggested "that no further action be taken looking to the passage of the act for the draft of nurses."[14]

Through approximately 900 state and local committees, the P&AS had classified about 300,000 nurses. Many of its committees had acquired a comprehensive knowledge of nursing resources in their communities that could be of continuing usefulness. The ARC had certified 104,500 nurses to the military. The military recorded 70,-500 assignments of nurses.[15]

Several factors require consideration in any evaluation of the situation which led President Roosevelt to ask Congress for legislation to draft nurses. Among them were:

1. The fluctuation, without explanation to the profession, in the Army's requirement for nurses at a crucial period of the war.

2. The triangular process of recruitment which required clearance by the P&AS and certification by the ARC to the ANC.

3. The National Nursing Council, functioning as a coordinating agency representative of the nursing profession, lacked the resources for a comprehensive public relations program.

4. The phenomenal rise in demands for civilian nursing services and

[13] Kernodle, Portia B.: *The Red Cross Nurse in Action, 1888–1948.* Harper & Brothers, New York, 1951, p. 451.

[14] "Surgeon General Norman T. Kirk, Major General U.S. Army, to Katharine J. Densford, President, A.N.A.," *Am. J. Nursing,* **45**:505, 1945.

[15] Kernodle, Portia B.: *The Red Cross Nurse in Action, 1888–1948.* Harper & Brothers, New York, 1949, p. 453.

the increasing reluctance of institutions, toward the end of the war, to concede priority to military needs.

World War I left the highly controversial issue of the preparation and employment of nurse's aides dangling in the air. The advent of World War II brought a quick and constructive solution to that problem. In turn, it left dangling the question: "In case of military need, shall nurses be conscripted?" And so it remained until after nurses had again been called to care for sick, wounded, and frost-bitten soldiers, this time the casualties of the battle fronts in Korea. At the convention of 1952 the House of Delegates of the ANA authorized the board of directors to approve legislation for Selective Service for nurses in the event such legislation should be introduced during a national emergency. The proposed draft revealed to the profession and to the world the essentiality of nursing service in our national life. Throughout the war, the majority of nurses conscientiously endeavored to meet both military and civilian needs for nursing service. "Of all sections of the American population," says *The Red Cross Nurse in Action,* "nurses made the greatest response to the war demands in proportion to resources."

BIBLIOGRAPHY

Altenderfer, Marion E.: "Wartime Nursing Care in Representative General Hospitals," *Pub. Health Rep.,* **60**:99, 1945. Quoted in *Am. J. Nursing,* **45**:222, 1945.

"A.N.A. Testimony on Proposed Draft Legislation," *Am. J. Nursing,* **45**:172–74, 1945.

"A.N.C. Testimony on Proposed Draft Legislation," *Am. J. Nursing,* **45**:175–76, 1945.

"The Armed Forces Have Enough Nurses!" *Pub. Health Nursing,* **37**:288, 1945.

Baker, L. Louise: *History of the Nursing Section, Procurement and Assignment Service* (War Manpower Commission). Unpublished manuscript in *American Journal of Nursing* files.

———: "Supply and Distribution of Nurses," *Transactions of the American Hospital Association,* Chicago, 1943, pp. 273–75.

Blanchfield, Florence A.: "The Needs of the Army Nurse Corps," *Pub. Health Nursing,* **35:**546–48, 1943.

————: "Calling All Nurses," *Am. J. Nursing,* **45:**91–93, 1945.

Blanchfield, Florence A., and Standlee, Mary W.: *Organized Nursing and the Army in Three Wars.* Unpublished manuscript on file, Historical Division, Office of the Surgeon General of the Army, Washington, D.C.

"Classification of Nurses in National Services," *Am. J. Nursing,* **45:**150, 1945.

"Criteria of Essentiality for Nurses," *Am. J. Nursing,* **43:**977–79, 1943.

"Criteria of Essentiality for Public Health Nurses and for Nurses in Industry," *Pub. Health Nursing,* **35:**543, 1943.

"Detroit's 'Hidden Nurse' Campaign," *Am. J. Nursing,* **43:**949, 1943.

"Hospital Nursing Personnel," *Am. J. Nursing,* **44:**206, 1944.

Kernodle, Portia B.: *The Red Cross Nurse in Action, 1882–1948.* Harper & Brothers, New York, 1949.

"Mobilize Your Resources: A.N.A. Resolutions and Recommendations Re Cooperative Planning for Maximum Utilization of Nursing Resources," *Am. J. Nursing,* **45:**256, 1945.

"National Classification Committee Has New Chairman" (functions of committee), *Am. J. Nursing,* **44:**1186, 1944.

Newell, Hope: *History of the National Nursing Council.* National Organization for Public Health Nursing, distributors, New York, 1951.

" 'Nurse Draft' Bill Passed by the House," *Am. J. Nursing,* **45:**255, 1945.

Nurses for the Armed Forces: Hearings before the Committee on Military Affairs, U.S. Senate on HR 2277. US Government Printing Office, Washington, D.C., 1945.

"The Nurses' Contribution to American Victory, Facts and Figures from Pearl Harbor to V-J Day," *Am. J. Nursing,* **45:**683–86, 1945.

"Nursing in War Manpower Commission," *Am. J. Nursing,* **43:**741–44, 1943.

"Procurement and Assignment," *Am. J. Nursing,* **44:**596, 1944.

Procurement of Nurses: Hearings before the Committee on Military Affairs, House of Representatives, 79th Congress on HR 1284. US Government Printing Office, Washington, D.C., 1945.

"Recommended Mimimum Wartime Public Health Nursing Service," *Pub. Health Nursing,* **36:**262–64, 1944.

Tattershall, Louise, and West, Margaret D.: "Wartime Nursing Care in 604 General Hospitals," *Am. J. Nursing,* **44:**211–14, 1944.

"Tell Me about Procurement and Assignment," *Am. J. Nursing,* **44:**251–54, 1944.

"The War Manpower Commission," *Am. J. Nursing,* **43:**885–87, 1943.

"War Manpower Commission; Classification, Clearance and Appeals Procedure," *Am. J. Nursing*, **43**:885, 1943.

"Wartime Nursing Is Different—A Statement by the Directing Board of the Procurement and Assignment Service, War Manpower Commission," *Pub. Health Nursing*, **35**:548, 1943.

"Where We Stand and What We Can Do," *Am. J. Nursing*, **45**:88, 1945.

Wickenden, Elmira B.: "The NNCWS and V-E Day," *Am. J. Nursing*, **45**:508–12, 1945.

"W.M.C.'s New Stabilization Order," *Am. J. Nursing*, **44**:95, 1944.

Chapter 36

THE US CADET NURSE CORPS

The nursing profession cannot meet the needs of military and civilian nursing services through numbers alone—quality of preparation must be considered . . . an essential factor in meeting those needs.

NELLIE X. HAWKINSON, Oct., 1942[1]

ALL OF THE AGENCIES whose programs were concerned with the basic education of nurses, the ANA, the NLNE, the ACSN, and the state boards of nurse examiners, were in fundamental agreement with the principle stated by Miss Hawkinson. Through the years one of the major efforts of organized nursing had been concentrated on the upgrading and adaptation of nursing education to changing needs for nursing service. It had been paralleled by efforts to safeguard the professional and economic status of persons legally qualified to practice as registered professional nurses. The principle enunciated by Miss Hawkinson became, therefore, a tenet of the National Nursing Council and of the Government's Subcommittee on Nursing. Through the efforts of these two wartime organizations, two programs for augmenting the nursing resources of the US were developed. Federal aid for nursing education was secured. The first program, which was discussed in Chapter 30, "Preparedness," covered the period from July, 1941, through June, 1943.[2] By means of that program, the schools increased their enrollments by about 13,000 students. The 4000 nurses for whom it provided postgraduate (postdiploma) study were urgently needed by the nursing schools

---

[1] Chairman, National League of Nursing Education Committee on Educational Problems in Wartime.

[2] Federal aid was authorized by Public Law No. 146—77th Congress.

and public health nursing agencies. It provided refresher courses for over 2000 graduate nurses. The need for nurses was so effectively publicized in connection with this and other programs that an unknown number of nurses returned to the practice of their profession without the formality of reorientation through refresher courses. But the sum total of this effort, while gratifying, fell far short of meeting the clamorous demands for more and more nursing service. Confronted by mounting needs, the National Nursing Council and the subcommittee swung into cooperative action with the subcommittee carrying the ball on the federal front.

The Army School of Nursing had been organized in World War I to augment the nation's supply of nurses at the point of most obvious need. But conditions were so unlike those of the earlier war that there were few advocates of a revival of that school in World War II. The Surgeon General of the Army was not interested in a program of nursing education. The status of women was so changed that nursing was no longer the sole portal to service with the armed forces. The structure and curriculums of nursing schools had improved in the interval between the wars. The hospital associations had grown powerful. The public health movement had gained tremendous momentum. The federal government had become an important employer of nurses. Civilian needs were much more clearly defined. The US Public Health Service, which had no nursing service when the US entered World War I, was now providing consultative service for a nationwide network of official public health nursing agencies, and had replaced nonprofessional with professional nursing for its Marine hospitals. The Children's Bureau was also stimulating more extensive use of public health nursing service. The Veterans Administration hospitals had not reached the anticipated peak of admissions resulting from World War I when they began receiving veterans of World War II, and were increasingly understaffed. The employment of many thousands of women in practically every type of war industry and the mobilization of other thousands for the new militarized services placed recruitment of students for nursing schools in a competitive position undreamed of in 1918. Military needs had priority in nursing as in all national affairs, but nonmilitary nursing services—institutional, public health, and industrial—were equally importunate about their need for nursing personnel.

The second federal aid program provided for the organization and development of the US Cadet Nurse Corps. It also made provision for postgraduate preparation for nurses. The new programs were made possible by the Nurse Training Act of 1943,[3] commonly known as the Bolton Act. The preparation of the bill, which was an "administration measure," was preceded by many conferences in which representatives of governmental agencies, the subcommittee, the National Nursing Council, the AHA, and other organizations participated. Honorable Frances Payne Bolton, congresswoman from Ohio, already widely known for her interest in nursing, presented the measure in the House of Representatives. An identical bill was introduced in the Senate. The purpose of the measure was to provide for the training of nurses—for the armed forces, governmental and civilian hospitals, health agencies, and war industries—through grants to institutions providing such training and for other purposes. The bill was passed in both houses without a dissenting vote. Because compromises had been made and a high degree of accord had been reached through preliminary conferences, the president of the AHA, reporting to the membership of that organization, could proclaim—"United we stand."[4] The principle of federal aid for educational projects was already established, but the plan was unique in that financial assistance was given directly to a large number of participating institutions without the intervention of an official state agency.

Through cooperative planning and well-organized advance publicity, the stage was set for quick action after the bill had been signed by President Roosevelt (June, 1943). Lucile Petry, one of the consultants on nursing education in the earlier program, was appointed director of the Division of Nurse Education, which was set up in the USPHS to administer the Cadet Nurse Corps program. The new division had sections on nurse education, consulta-

[3] Public Law No. 74, 78th Congress (June, 1943).
[4] Hamilton, James A.: "United We Stand," *Mod. Hosp.*, **61**:75, 1943.

tion, public relations, and management. Six district offices were staffed with teams of nurse consultants, public relations personnel, and auditors. The following year, under the Public Health Service Act of July 1, 1944, a division of nursing was created in the USPHS which was given "general supervision over all nursing operations carried on by the Public Health Service and professional supervision over all nursing personnel of the Public Health Service, including personnel assigned for duty with other governmental agencies."[5] This order abolished the Division of Nurse Education and placed the direction of the nurse education program in the new unit. Miss Petry, who became Chief Nurse Officer, subsequently (1949) received appointment as Assistant Surgeon General, the Public Health Service equivalent of Brigadier General, the first nurse in the world to achieve a position of such distinction. She was well equipped for it. A graduate of the University of Delaware and the Johns Hopkins Hospital School of Nursing (with the aid of borrowed funds), she had won successive promotions. She participated in the revision of the *Curriculum Guide* of 1937. She was at the University of Minnesota School of Nursing, where she was assistant to the dean, when she was loaned to the USPHS. As director of the Cadet Nurse Corps, she acquired a comprehensive knowledge of nursing and nursing education throughout the country. Endowed with a keen but sympathetic intelligence, by mid-century Miss Petry had become one of the best known nurses in the world.

There were three distinct phases of the program set up in the hectic summer of 1943: administration, assistance to participating schools, and recruitment of student nurses. Through the corps, the profession learned the value of a well-planned public relations program. After the war, the recruitment program, which had been developed around such slogans as "join a proud profession," was rated by the Office of War Information, which had given it strong support, the most successful of all wartime recruitment programs. Of all

[5] *The United States Cadet Nurse Corps and Other Federal Nurse Training Programs,* 1943–1948, Federal Security Agency, USPHS Publication #38. US Government Printing Office, Washington, D.C., 1950, p. 94.

students entering schools approved by state boards of nurse examiners in 1943, 1944, and 1945, 78 per cent, 88.5 per cent, and 70.0 per cent, respectively, were members of the US Cadet Nurse Corps.[6]

The influential War Advertising Council, organized to assist war service programs, in two years secured donated advertising space and radio time valued at thirteen million dollars. Practically every known method of reaching the public was utilized. Programs were carefully timed in relation to the admission dates of the schools. The corps offered prospective students a free education, indoor uniforms, a glamorous and distinctive outdoor uniform, and monthly stipends for a maximum period of 30 months. It offered participating institutions:

1. Maintenance of students for the first nine months,
2. Tuition fees throughout the program,
3. Assistance in securing funds for expansion of residential and educational facilities.

Contracts were made with the American Hospital Association and the National Nursing Council, which permitted transfer to them of funds for services in connection with the recruitment program. The AHA accepted responsibility for establishing nursing information centers in hospitals. The council served as the purchasing agent for the cadet uniforms. Securing uniforms for a large number of non-militarized women in a time of rigid rationing was no easy task. The council also relieved the corps of an enormous amount of detail by continuing the clearing bureau which it had established in 1941. Thousands of inquiries about nursing were addressed to it.

Annual quotas for recruitment were based on the estimated maximum expanded capacity of the schools, and the assumption that 10 per cent of the young women graduating from high school could be interested in nursing as a war service leading to a career. The attractive gray uniform, with its touches of scarlet, was specially designed for the teen-age group. As previously noted, the Cadet Nurse Corps also cooperated with the National Nursing Council in a special program for the recruitment of college women. There was no interdiction to the admission of men to the corps, but,

[6] *Facts about Nursing*, 1946, NIB, p. 35.

as Selective Service made no provision for the deferment of men student nurses, no effort was made to recruit them.

The public relations experts assigned to the regional offices helped the schools and the state and local recruitment committees, which were an integral part of the council structure, to adapt the national program to local situations. Through these personalized local services many inquiries were translated into positive action resulting in enrollment. The quotas of 65,000 for the first year, and 60,000 for the second year of the cadet program were "oversubscribed." Radios were filling the air with the third-year appeal when the surrender of Japan put an abrupt end to recruitment. Between July, 1943, and October 15, 1945, the final date for admissions to the corps, almost 170,000 cadets had entered 1125 of the nation's 1300 schools. Critics of the corps and of the mass method of recruitment pointed to the large number of cadets who did not complete their training. The attrition rate for the two war years was approximately 8 per cent higher than that of the last peacetime class.

The facilities and conditions under which mass recruitment methods were adopted in the two world wars were, in many respects, dissimilar, but the results merit comparison. Army school students, in general, were older. Many had well-developed occupational interests. They had been in the school only about a year when the war was ended. This fact may account for some of the difference in the attrition rates for students recruited during the two wars. It seems probable that the major difference was due to the circumstances in which they gained their earliest impressions of nursing; the temporary cantonment hospitals to which most of the Army students were assigned had no future whereas the civilian institutions to which cadets were assigned were a part of the social structure of their communities. Slightly less than one-third of the wartime class of the Army school was graduated as compared with two-thirds of the two classes of the Cadet Corps. The noteworthy fact is that more than 124,000 cadets had been graduated by 1948, and the nursing resources of the institutions which had participated in the program had been enormously increased.

Participating schools were required by law to adopt an accelerated program. The staff and the advisory committee to the Surgeon General (composed of nationally known representatives of education, nursing education, and hospitals) made use of the NLNE's manual, *The Essentials of a Good School of Nursing,* and also the principles formulated by that organization's Committee on Problems of Nursing Education in Wartime. The ANA and the NLNE arranged a three-day conference of representatives of state boards of nurse examiners for consideration of the problems which would arise in connection with accelerated programs. The ANA set up a clearing bureau on state board problems to facilitate that aspect of the program. Under the plan of acceleration, essential instruction and experience were condensed into 30 months which were divided into two periods: (1) Pre-Cadet, 9 months, and (2) Junior-Cadet, 21 months. Because many state laws required a 36-month training period, an additional six months of supervised experience was provided in military and other federal hospitals, in civilian hospitals, or in public health nursing agencies. This was called the Senior-Cadet period. The students received monthly stipends of $15.00 and $20.00 in the Pre-Cadet and Junior Cadet periods, respectively. These stipends were paid from federal funds. During the Senior-Cadet period the students received $30.00 or more monthly, which was paid by the institutions utilizing their services. In the case of federal hospitals the stipend was set at $60.00, which was paid by the governmental agency operating the hospital.

One of the most difficult administrative problems arose in connection with tuition fees. The educational offerings of the participating schools ran the gamut. Some of them had never offered programs which warranted tuition fees. At the other end of the scale were the schools which offered courses leading to degrees and were operated on the same basis as other schools in a university. Under the terms of the Congressional appropriation for the second year, a graded scale of fees was established. In the Senior-Cadet period, although the students remained under the general jurisdiction of their schools, it was intended that they should be free to apply for assignment to governmental hospitals, both military and nonmilitary, or to civilian institutions needing nurses and offering supervised practice acceptable to the corps and to the state boards of nurse examiners. Many of the schools, naturally, were reluctant to release their senior cadets although they were urged to do so in order that they might admit more students. The corps had also to cope with the formalities of the civil-service requirements of some of the federal services. Approximately one-half of the 35,000 seniors who applied for federal service in the last year of the war were assigned to the Veterans Administration; the others went to the Army, Indian Service, and the Public Health Service hospitals. At the height of the program, cadets supplied 80 per cent of the nursing service in the institutions which operated the participating schools. Such excessive use of student service, often for non-nursing services, and under supervision of extremely varied quality, could be condoned only by the exigencies of war. But the AHA credited the Cadet Corps with saving civilian hospital nursing services from collapse.

The fractionization of the nursing profession into a half-dozen organizations had made it impossible for any one of them to give comprehensive, direct, and practical assistance to the schools of nursing. The Cadet Corps had the resources, not only for initial conferences with hospital and nursing school administrators, but for consultant services in relation to recruitment, nursing school administration, and finance. The nurse consultants helped to solve problems of curriculum adjustments in relation to acceleration and affiliations in an effort to expand the educational offerings of the school. They also advised on the use of scholarship funds to strengthen the administrative and instructional staffs of the schools. Special emphasis was placed on broadening curriculums to include not only the basic services required by all state boards, but also psychiatric nursing and the elements of public health nursing service. Many schools needed and would have welcomed far more consultation service than could be provided for them.

The keeping of accounts is a necessary concomitant to the expenditure of federal funds. But many schools were so embedded in the hospitals that separate accounts for nursing education and nursing service had never been set up. This was one of the most difficult problems confronted by the corps. A manual of cost analysis, methods, and procedure was provided for the use of the schools.[7]

The nurse consultants of the corps worked closely with the boards of nurse examiners in their respective states. The boards, in turn, contributed to the success of the program in many ways, especially in relation to the transfer of senior cadets from one state to another for their period of internship in federal institutions and other agencies. Without doubt, these consultants helped the faculties of some of the schools to acquire a better understanding of the organization and functions of a school of nursing as distinguished from those of a nursing service.

The total cost to the federal government for the five-year program (1944–1948), administered under the provisions of the Nurse Training Act of 1943, "including the expenses of administration, uniforms, maintenance, tuition and fees, and stipends was $160,-326,237."[8] Expenditures for each cadet for three years averaged $1,360. The total expenditures included approximately $3,500,000 expended for concentrated postgraduate work for 10,309 graduate nurses in 57 universities, and for on-the-job courses provided in 70 institutions for 6516 graduate nurses who could not be released for study in a university program.

In addition to expenditures for nursing education, under the provisions of the Bolton Act, the USPHS secured additional expenditures of $25,657,785 under the Lanham (National Defense Housing) Act of 1940.[9] These funds provided new facilities, such as living quarters, library space, and classrooms and demonstration rooms for 239 schools. Schools in all but nine states received this type of assistance. More than 12,000 beds were added to existing

[7] Petry, Lucile, and Block, Louis: *Cost Analysis for Schools of Nursing, A Manual of Methods and Procedures.* USPHS, Federal Security Agency, US Government Printing Office, Washington, D.C., 1946.

[8] *The United States Cadet Nurse Corps and Other Federal Nurse Training Programs, 1943–1948,* Federal Security Agency, USPHS Publication #38. US Government Printing Office, Washington, D.C., 1950, p. 94.

[9] *Ibid.,* p. 53.

accommodations for student nurses. Of that total of over 25 million dollars, the schools (hospitals) expended approximately one-third, and the government, two-thirds.

The Cadet Corps kept intact the American system of nursing education. It contributed a volume of nursing service of better quality than could have been secured by any other method that was suggested. The weaknesses of the program, especially in relation to the selection of students and the assistance given to schools of less than average standards, were widely criticized. But when the work of the corps is appraised in the impersonal light of history, it may be found that the corps provided a fulcrum for the powerful lever of public opinion which expedited the further development of nursing education to meet nursing needs. No comparable body of information about the schools of nursing had ever been built up and made available to those best qualified to use it.[10] The corps demonstrated the value of teamwork between professional associations and federal agencies. It successfully pioneered in "a new relationship between the government and private institutions."

BIBLIOGRAPHY

Anderson, Bernice E.: *The Facilitation of Interstate Movement of Registered Nurses.* J. B. Lippincott Co., Philadelphia, 1950.
"The Bolton-Bailey Bill," *Am. J. Nursing,* **43**:592, 1943.
Henderson, Jean: "One Blueprint for Recruitment," *Am. J. Nursing,* **45**:1002, 1945.
"National Induction as Seen by a Cadet Nurse" (Cadet Nurse's Pledge), *Am. J. Nursing,* **44**:592, 1944.
Newell, Hope: *The History of the National Nursing Council.* National Organization for Public Health Nursing, distributor, New York, 1951.
Petry, Lucile: "The U.S. Cadet Nurse Corps—Established under the Bolton Act," *Am. J. Nursing,* **43**:794, 1943.
———: "Planning the Senior Cadet Period," *Am. J. Nursing,* **44**:57, 1944.
———: "Duties of Nurse Education Consultants," *Am. J. Nursing,* **45**:807, 1945.

[10] Vreeland, Ellwynne M.: "Some Qualitative and Quantitative Factors in Nurse Education," *Pub. Health Rep.,* **63**:1166–1191, (Dec. 24) 1948.

————: "The U.S. Cadet Nurse Corps—A Summing Up," *Am. J. Nursing,* **45:**1027, 1945.

Schaffter, Dorothy: *What Comes of Training Women for War.* American Council on Education, Washington, D.C., 1948.

"Special Report on Nurse Recruitment," *Proceedings of the House of Delegates of the American Hospital Association,* 1944, pp. 43–45.

Stimson, Julia C., and associates: "The Army School of Nursing," *History and Manual of the Army Nurse Corps.* Medical Field Service School, Carlisle Barracks, Pennsylvania, 1937, pp. 72–78.

Switzer, Mary E.: "The Subcommittee on Nursing Goes On," *Am. J. Nursing,* **43:**888, 1943.

The United States Cadet Nurse Corps and Other Federal Nurse Training Programs, 1943–1948, Federal Security Agency, US Public Health Service Publication #38. US Government Printing Office, Washington, D.C., 1950.

"U.S. Cadet Nurse Corps—Regulations Governing Eligibility of Schools," *Am. J. Nursing,* **43:**707, 1943.

Vreeland, Ellwynne M.: "Some Qualitative and Quantitative Factors in Nurse Education," *Pub. Health Rep.,* **63:**1166–91, 1948.

SECTION IX. THE NATIONAL NURSING ORGAN-
IZATIONS DURING WORLD WAR II

Chapter 37

TRENDS IN NURSING AND IN THE PROGRAMS OF
THE NATIONAL NURSING ORGANIZATIONS
DURING WORLD WAR II

A professional association is an association with one object above all others. The members do not come together merely for the pleasure of meeting others of the same occupation; nor do they meet primarily to increase their pecuniary gain; although this may be one of the objects. They have joined in order better to perform their function. They meet:
  To establish standards
  To maintain standards
  To improve standards
  To keep members up to standards
  To educate the public to appreciate standards
  To protect the public from those individuals who have not attained standards or wilfully do not follow them
  To protect individual members of the profession from each other.
These objects of a professional association may be summed up by saying that a profession provides a corporate responsibility.[1]

"ALL PROFESSIONS," says Miss Follett, in discussing the criteria which head this chapter, "have been developed by the work of their own members. . . . There is no one else in the world . . . to create the science, the art, the profession." This book has been based on that premise.

Throughout the war, while the national nursing organizations were participating in the over-all plans and programs of the Na-

[1] *Dynamic Administration*, The Collected Papers of Mary Follett; edited by Henry C. Metcalf and L. Urwick. Harper & Brothers, New York, 1942, p. 136.

tional Nursing Council, they were also pressing forward with some of their own long-range programs. As they strove to adapt nursing to a rapidly changing social order it became apparent that the time had arrived for emphasis on what Miss Goodrich calls *creative nursing*. Some years had elapsed since she had called the attention of the nursing world to three periods of modern nursing, which she termed the emotional, the technical, and the creative. The creative period, according to Miss Goodrich, had begun when a few nursing schools began tapping the resources of institutions of higher education and started weaving the social and health aspects of nursing into the basic curriculum.

The dawn of the creative period was far less rosy than participants in the Winslow-Goldmark study,[2] which pressed for the development of more university schools, had anticipated. Progress was slow. But before World War II various forces had begun to converge on nursing in a way that stimulated more rapid emergence from the "long arid stretches of unremitting toil that boldly and persistently attacked at their base the sores of humanity and laid the foundation for the present dynamic program. . . ."[3] Interest in preventive medicine and public health nursing had been vastly increased by the Social Security Act. The concept of psychosomatic medicine—the interrelationship of the emotional, the mental, and spiritual life of patients with the physical manifestations of disease—was beginning to influence the practice of both medicine and nursing. A study of the social aspects of illness helped to bring the-patient-as-a-person to the attention of doctors, nurses, and social workers. The influence of the psychosomatic theory is clearly revealed by frequent references in the nursing literature of the period to care of "the whole patient" or to "the patient as a person" often without reference to the book in which Dr. G. Canby Robinson popularized that concept.[4]

[2] *Nursing and Nursing Education in the United States.* The Macmillan Company, New York, 1923.

[3] Goodrich, Annie W.: *The Social and Ethical Significance of Nursing.* The Macmillan Company, New York, 1932, p. 314.

[4] Robinson, G. Canby: *The Patient as a Person, A Study of the Social Aspects of Illness.* The Commonwealth Fund, New York, 1939.

As the life span lengthened, due chiefly to the conquest of one communicable disease after another, the degenerative diseases with their psychosomatic connotations called for fundamental adaptations of nursing education and nursing practice. Spectacular advances in medical science were helping to revolutionize the practice of nursing. Chemotherapy and the use of antibiotics call not only for technical proficiency but also for powers of observation sharpened by knowledge of the principles underlying treatment, and the anticipated reactions to therapy. But the Wangensteen drainage apparatus and the positive pressure mark, as well as the trayful of syringes with potent medications, are concrete objects which require mastery; failure to cope with them is measurable. The nurse cannot escape her responsibility. But recognition of the basis of the patient's behavior and the ability to cope with it, in addition to all the other things which make up the art of nursing, are more difficult to teach and much more difficult to practice. Furthermore, although there is an increasing amount of lip service to the psychosomatic concept, physicians and nurse administrators are inclined to minimize the importance of it when time is not available for both. Early ambulation may greatly reduce the amount of time required for some technical nursing procedures while adding others. It emphasizes the importance of an understanding of the physiological principles underlying therapy and of the patient's psychological reaction to the method. "With this method of treatment," said one of the first exponents of early ambulation, "nurses assume a role more appropriate to their intelligence and scientific training. They become supervisors and helpful aides in teaching the patient how to recover, rather than mere servants catering to the patient's physical wants."[5]

"Nursing," said Dr. William Dock, "will become less a matter of caring for bed-fast patients, more a problem of supervising physiological rest, restoring courage and strength, and training patients

[5] Leithauser, Daniel J.: *Early Ambulation and Related Procedures in Surgical Management.* Charles C. Thomas, Publisher, Springfield, Ill., 1946, p. 171.

how to live most comfortably with the chronic disabilities which are sure to recur eventually in many whose lives are saved by modern surgery, endocrine and antibiotic therapy. Rest is the most universally used therapeutic agent for patients who require nursing care; its use, hazards and possible abuse must be thoughtfully considered in every case."[6]

There was an increasing appreciation of the need for helping many patients adjust to the fact that they must live for all their remaining years with certain limitations imposed upon them by conditions that can be controlled but not cured. The population was steadily growing older, and nurses were finding increased numbers of aged patients to be cared for in the hospitals and in their homes. Observant nurses were beginning to realize that lack of emotional satisfactions were at least as often an explanation of the difficult older person's problems as were his physical ailments. Perhaps most important of all, some nurse instructors in hospitals had become aware that the true integration of social and health aspects was, in large part, dependent upon their approach in teaching the care of the patient and that this was, basically, their responsibility rather than that of practicing public health nurses. As a result, the one-time "care study," which had superceded the case study, was beginning to give way to an emphasis upon making a written plan for future living, with the nurse helping the patient and his family work out the details of the restrictions and directions prescribed by the physician. Attempts were being made to show the patient and his family how the handicapped person can live up to the limit of his capacities. Clinics, which formerly emphasized the disease that afflicted the patient, were in many places being replaced by group conferences in which a plan of care for an individual patient was discussed, as well as suggested methods of working out the details of this plan with the patient and appropriate members of his family. In some hospitals it was no longer worthy of special comment when a physi-

---

[6] Dock, William: "Psychological Rest Versus Complete Bed Rest," *Am. J. Nursing*, 45:469, 1945.

cian, a head nurse, a student nurse, and a nutritionist, together with a patient and a member of his family, were observed in conference. At institutes and workshops public health nurses, nurse educators in the basic sciences and in clinical nursing, and other professionals met on the common ground of "patient-centered" teaching.

Changing concepts of care for the handicapped were accelerated by the rehabilitation program developed by Dr. Howard A. Rusk and others for disabled veterans, which he describes as the third phase of medicine (preventive medicine being the second). It has great possibilities, not only for ex-servicemen, but for the many thousands of handicapped persons. No longer, for example, is the victim of a cerebral vascular accident given elementary physical care only. The nurse is a participant in the execution of cooperative and constructive plans for the restoration of the patient to maximum usefulness.

The establishment of the Joint Orthopedic Nursing Advisory Service (JONAS) by the NOPHN and the NLNE in 1941 was an epochal event. For the first time, national nursing organizations developed a program in which individual patients, as persons requiring both preventive and therapeutic care, became the focal point of planning. As Jessie L. Stevenson,[7] the modest but highly expert nurse and physiotherapist, who was responsible for initiating the service, put it: "Every nurse—institutional, private duty, or public health—who gives bedside care or teaches the art of nursing to student nurses or families is responsible for making or preventing crippling."[8] Implicit in that statement lies the distinction between technical and creative nursing. It was supported by evidence that technical nursing, while following physician's orders for treatment and the giving of comfort to bedridden patients without knowledge of body mechanics, could produce disastrously crippling results.

[7] Now Mrs. Harry W. West.
[8] Stevenson, Jessie L.: "What Is Orthopedic Nursing?" *Am. J. Nursing,* **39:** 11, 1939.

Up to this time nurses had been classified in relation to the environment in which they practiced—nursing education, public health, institutional, private duty, or industrial nursing. Emphasis had been placed on advanced preparation for nurse educators and public health nurses. It now became apparent that more attention should be given to clinical nursing, with primary emphasis on individual patient care influencing the development and administration of curriculums and the nursing services. The Maternity Center Association of New York had pioneered in patient-centered teaching, of obstetrical nursing and preparation of the nurse for midwifery, as an advanced phase of nursing. But the national nursing organizations had not previously been directly concerned with the development of such programs. The necessity for preparation, beyond the basic course, for teachers and administrators had long been recognized. "All too often, however," as a committee of the NLNE under the chairmanship of Mrs. Elizabeth K. Porter (later president of the ANA) pointed out, "this has been an advanced superstructure composed of courses in methods of teaching, supervision and the like and imposed upon inadequate preparation and experience in clinical nursing itself."[9]

Following the publication of the *Curriculum Guide* in 1937, a joint committee of the League and NOPHN worked persistently over a period of years on one phase of the problem of converting traditionally technical curriculums into professional ones through the integration of the social and health aspects of nursing. This called for fundamental changes in attitudes, subject matter, and teaching methods. The principles evolved by the committee were presented in a series of articles of such importance to all nurses that they were published simultaneously in the two professional journals. They were supplemented by luminous and practical articles prepared by teachers who had already grasped the concept of creative nursing.

An accelerated trend toward the development of creative or patient-centered nursing, nursing on a professional level, with its

[9] "Advanced Courses in Clinical Nursing," *Am. J. Nursing*, **44:**579, 1944.

connotation of broad social usefulness, may be traced in the following chapters on the major activities of the national nursing organizations during World War II.

BIBLIOGRAPHY

Bixler, Genevieve Knight, and Bixler, Roy White: "The Professional Status of Nursing," *Am. J. Nursing*, **45:**730, 1945.

Courses in Clinical Nursing for Graduate Nurses, Basic Assumptions and Guiding Principles. Pamphlet #1, National League of Nursing Education, New York, 1945.

Dunbar, Flanders: *Mind and Body: Psychosomatic Medicine.* Random House, New York, 1947.

Jones, Florence Terry: "The Nurse's Responsibility in Rehabilitation," *Am. J. Nursing*, **48:**76, 1948.

Rusk, Howard A.: "Implications for Nursing in Rehabilitation, *Am. J. Nursing*, **48:**74, 1948.

Weiss, Edward: "Psychosomatic Medicine," *Am. J. Nursing*, **45:**189, 1945.

Weiss, Edward, and English, O. Spurgeon: *Psychosomatic Medicine*, 2nd ed. W. B. Saunders Co., Philadelphia, 1949.

Chapter 38

THE AMERICAN NURSES' ASSOCIATION

. . . in our endeavor to fulfill obligations for war service, we must not lose sight of responsibilities for the future. The ideals which have motivated the achievements in our profession must be guarded and cherished with zeal and determination. Professional values have significance only in so far as they inspire the finest type of performance. Values relating to nursing education, nursing legislation, personnel practices and distribution of nursing service must be preserved.

JULIA C. STIMSON[1]

WHILE the American Nurses' Association was cooperating with military recruitment and other wartime programs, it did not lose sight of its own long-range objectives or the problems which might be expected to arise in the postwar period of readjustment. It worked continuously to promote improvement in the conditions of employment of nurses. And it endeavored to carry forward its program for the distribution of nursing service through professionally sponsored registries. It expanded its service by the organization of two new units. The Bureau of State Boards of Nurse Examiners was organized in 1943. It functioned under that title until 1949. The title was then dropped, but the program was continued under the guidance of the ANA Special Committee of State Boards of Nursing Education and Nurse Registration.

As the culmination of plans, which had been in the making for almost a decade, the Professional Counseling & Placement Service, Inc. (PC&PS), was established as a wholly owned subsidiary of the ANA in 1945 for the following purposes:

[1] The President's Address, *Proceedings, Thirty-third Convention,* ANA, 1942, p. 41.

To conduct the business of a professional placement and employment agency and employment information office for graduate registered nurses in any state, territory or possession of the United States or in the District of Columbia; to collect and disseminate data concerning the needs for nurses and affiliated workers in the care of the sick in specialized types of service, to be used as the basis of geographic distribution; to collect and refer credentials of nurses and auxiliary workers in the care of the sick, who are qualified.[2]

Membership in the ANA rose rapidly in the strenuous war years. At war's end, 178,000 registered nurses, for whom membership in their alumnae associations was no longer a requirement[3] were looking to the association for assistance in adjusting to postwar conditions.

The component units of the ANA, the state nurses' associations, had provided the foundation for the National Nursing Council's nationwide chain of state and local councils. The council necessarily operated at high speed. As a result, the areas of its responsibility as an emergency organization, in relation to the programs of the established organizations, were not always clearly defined. The resultant misunderstandings in no way impaired the basic structure of the ANA. It is noteworthy that the trend toward the development of joint or collaborative programs, which had begun before the war, rapidly gained momentum and had an important bearing on postwar planning. Discussion in this chapter, however, is restricted to consideration of primary ANA functions during the war.

The collective influence of the state nurses' associations, under the leadership of the ANA, was repeatedly and constructively used in relation to federal legislation pertaining to nurses and nursing. The association supported the successive bills which improved the status of nurses in the Army and Navy Nurse Corps and which

[2] Certificate of incorporation, ANA Professional Counseling & Placement Service, Inc., May, 1945.

[3] Membership in an alumnae association as a requirement for membership in the ANA had been a moot question since 1911 when the name of the Nurses Associated Alumnae of the United States was changed to American Nurses' Association. The House of Delegates voted in 1944 that the requirement be discontinued.

culminated, after the war, in permanently commissioned corps. It worked effectively for the legislation which provided federal aid for nursing education in 1941 (Training for Nurses—National Defense) and in 1943 for the Bolton Act which brought the US Cadet Nurse Corps into existence. When Congress was in session, the ANA was continuously represented in Washington by seasoned observers.

Less obvious, but of fundamental importance, was the association's continuing effort to secure reasonable hours for nurses and improvement in the conditions under which civilian nurses were employed by institutions. The restlessness of nurses, as indicated by frequent change of position by graduate staff nurses, had created a serious administrative problem for institutions before war was declared. This was symptomatic of an unhealthy condition. It had been created by the failure of nurse administrators and of employing agencies to recognize graduate staff service as a basic element in the structure of institutional nursing services which required definition of status and function with personnel policies adapted to its special characteristics.

Changes in medical practice were, quite unintentionally, having a subtly stultifying influence on the development of nursing. As medicine became more and more scientific, it also tended to become impersonal. Technical diagnostic procedures were making almost as heavy demands on nursing time as the treatments which were subsequently ordered for the patients. More and more persons participated in diagnostic and therapeutic procedures under medical direction. Many nurses felt like cogs in an impersonal machine rather than partners with physicians in the care of patients in whom both were vitally interested. As the numbers of patients to be cared for increased, and nursing and other personnel decreased in response to war needs, time for giving nursing care became more and more limited. When hospitals were under pressure to do more and more with fewer nurses it was the nursing care of patients, not the technical procedures and nonprofessional services required of nurses, that suffered most.

Time did not permit that integration of procedures into a plan of nursing care in which the personality of a patient and his emotional needs have as important a place as his physical needs. Distinctions between technical and professional nursing service were to have an important place in postwar planning. But consideration of some of the causes of the unrest of institutional nurses could not be deferred. Efforts to promote the development of personnel policies which would help to stabilize nursing services became one of the most important elements in the ANA's wartime program.

A small study of salaries and personnel policies in relation to institutional nursing services had been made by the AHA and NLNE in 1935. But an ANA study, published three years later, as previously noted, was the first major contribution to the subject.[4] This was followed in 1940 by the AHA's *Job Specifications,* which included important sections on nursing personnel in both nursing education and nursing service. An important study of institutional staff nursing, made under the joint auspices of hospital and nursing organizations, pointed out that:

The patient likes the general staff nurse. Even with the chaotic conditions resulting from the attempt to assimilate a new group for which no preparation has been made, hospitals find that patients like the assurance which comes from the graduate professional worker. . . .[5]

Restless and unsatisfied as she might be, the graduate staff or general duty nurse had become an essential factor in institutional nursing services. It remained for the profession and the employing agencies to create conditions in which nurses could find a reasonable degree of satisfaction and opportunity for professional growth if the services were to be stabilized. The NLNE and ANA collaborated in a study of salaries in 1943. The two organizations, with the AHA, followed through with the report of a study, *Personnel Practices for General Duty Nurses,* the following year.

If the emphasis on salaries and other conditions of employment in the crucial war period seems out of keeping with traditional

[4] *Study of Incomes, Salaries and Employment Conditions.* ANA, New York, 1938.

[5] *The General Staff Nurse,* Report of the Joint Committee of the ANA and the NLNE. ANA, New York, 1941, p. 10.

concepts of nursing and nurses, it must be remembered that the cost of living had soared and that most civilians were enjoying unprecedentedly high incomes. Reports of salary studies and other aspects of personnel administration, in which the ANA and the NLNE cooperated, were published without recommendations or interpretation. The facts spoke for themselves. One by one the state nurses' associations began working on the problems within their own jurisdictions. The California association took aggressive leadership in this movement. Unable to secure the cooperation of the state hospital association in establishing the minimum salary schedule it proposed, the association turned to the War Labor Board (WLB) for assistance.[6]

The following year 21 state nurses' associations reported that they were trying to solve some of the problems created by the outmoded personnel practices of institutions. They developed criteria including time and salary schedules for nurses in the several brackets, general duty and others, and endeavored to secure their acceptance by hospital associations and institutions. The constructive influence of the courses in hospital administration was beginning to be felt in some areas, and nurse administrators were becoming aware of the importance of distinguishing between the administration of nursing schools and hospital nursing services. It was believed that improved personnel policies would stabilize institutional nursing services and, in so doing, improve the care of patients.

The movement was beginning to stimulate the interest of nurse educators in the principles and practice of administration in relation to nursing services, but practicing nurses wanted action. Indeed, a few rebellious nurses had joined trade unions. By 1944, when the House of Delegates of the ANA met in Buffalo, the question "Could the basic economic problems of professional workers be solved through collective bargaining"[7] was of more than academic interest to many delegates.

[6] "W. L. B. Approves Salary Standards of California State Nurses' Association," *Am. J. Nursing,* 43:951, 1943.
[7] Scott, William C.: "Shall Professional Nurses' Associations Become Collective Bargaining Agents for Their Members?" *Am. J. Nursing,* 44:231, 1944.

The attitude of nurses toward the hospitals at this time was colored by the fact that the three national hospital associations had been successful in their efforts to have hospital personnel excluded from the old age provisions of the Social Security Act. Considerable damage had been done to interprofessional relationships by the time that decision had been reversed. The profession as a whole had yet to learn that reasonable hours and adequate salaries, important though they are, would not provide a complete answer to the unrest of institutional nurses. There was imperfect realization that the rapidly growing tendency to sacrifice the art of nursing to the technical requirements of medicine was a more fundamental source of dissatisfaction than either excessive hours or inadequate incomes.

The urgent wartime need for an enormously augmented volume of nursing service brought into focus a problem which antedated the organization of professional nursing, and with which the profession had temporized for almost half a century. This was the question of the preparation and status of nonprofessional workers in the field of nursing. When it was discussed at the historic meeting in Chicago in 1893, courses for trained attendants had already been initiated by the Young Women's Christian Association (YWCA) and established in Brooklyn, Boston, and New York. In 1936, the joint boards of the three national nursing organizations agreed that "responsibility for outlining principles and policies for the control of subsidiary workers in the care of the sick rested with the nursing profession." That pronouncement had been followed, as previously noted, by an ANA board decision that "no formal courses for the preparation of subsidiary workers should be approved until such time as a method for the control of the practice of subsidiary workers is devised."[8] Ten years later only 20 states had provided for the licensure of a second group of workers in the field of nursing, and there was no consensus as to whether the legal designation should be *practical nurse* or some other title.

It will be recalled that both the Winslow-Goldmark committee

[8] Best, Ella: *Brief Historical Review and Information About Current Activities of the A.N.A.* ANA, New York, 1940, p. 64.

and the Committee on the Costs of Medical Care had advocated the preparation of workers to supplement the service of professional nurses, but that the Grading Committee had not approved "the short-course nurse." None of these pronouncements had been followed by positive action. By 1940 about 190,000 persons were employed, under a variety of titles, as practical nurses and hospital attendants.

Mississippi, the first state to do so, had included provision for the licensure of a secondary group of nurses in its nurse practice act in 1914. Following World War I, a few other state associations secured permissive legislation for the licensure of subprofessional workers. The first mandatory act—requiring all who nurse for hire to be licensed—was secured by the New York State Nurses' Association after a five-year "crusade for safer nursing." A succession of waivers, however, deferred the effective date of that legislation to April, 1950. Early in that more than 10-year interval, the ANA and the NLNE had collaborated in the preparation of an invaluable collection of data on the nurse practice acts and the board rules which implement them. A joint committee of the three older national nursing organizations had published several editions of a pamphlet on auxiliary workers and their functions, which were superceded in 1951 by *Practical Nurses in Nursing Services.* This publication was prepared by a joint committee of the five national nursing organizations in cooperation with the National Organization for Practical Nurse Education and Practical Nurses of New York, Inc. (See Chap. 44.)

The development of professionally sponsored registries, as a means of distributing nursing service and of assisting nurses, especially those engaged in private duty, was the major topic of discussion at the second annual meeting of the Associated Alumnae in 1899, and has remained a major interest of the association ever since.[9] For a 10-year period beginning in 1934, materials from the association's carefully compiled studies and reports of registry ac-

---

[9] Best, Ella: "How Are the Goals of Tomorrow's Community Service To Be Realized? Through Registries and Nursing Bureaus," *Proceedings of the American Nurses' Association,* 1936, pp. 561–72.

tivities occupied many pages of the AJN. These statistical reports represented a tremendous volume of bedside nursing by individual nurses. It is the special privilege of private duty nurses to be closely associated with patients and their families. They hear the welcome cry of the newborn. They share the enormous satisfaction of hard-won recoveries from illness, surgical and otherwise. They witness the agony of those left behind when, despite all efforts, life has been cut off too soon. They work with human beings to help them both when they are at their best, as they make a courageous fight against accident or disease, and also when they are at their supine or rebellious worst. But the *Journal* pages of the period, when private duty nursing was being featured as it had not been for many years, carried relatively few articles which interpreted the human interest that is implicit in private duty nursing and that holds many good nurses in that field of nursing although it offers no pecuniary or other evidences of advancement. A comprehensive study of registries, published in 1942, indicated an increasing sense of responsibility to their communities on the part of the nurse registrants and the governing boards of the registries. A growing number of registries had governing boards composed of doctors, nurses, and representatives of community interests. But progress has been slow. Educators and other observers have quite generally considered nurses an inarticulate group, a condition which militated against collaborative planning. But not until mid-century did curriculum planners give serious consideration to the technics of problem solving and the development of communication skills in connection with the basic education of nurses.

The ANA's useful Bureau of State Boards of Nurse Examiners was one of the positive outcomes of the war. It was organized as a clearing bureau on the basis of suggestions made at a conference of state board representatives late in 1942. Among the matters to which it gave immediate attention were: (1) delays in providing for examination and licensure of recent graduates urgently needed for military service, (2) the difficulties experienced by many nurses in securing registration in other states at a time when freedom to move from state to state was extremely important, and (3) acceleration of the basic course and surveys of institutions offering experience for senior cadet nurses. The bureau was established in the ANA office, with a full-time nurse secretary for the first few months. Its work was guided by a large advisory committee and a small working committee; experienced and well-informed Bernice E. Anderson was chairman of both. The bureau's first project was the development of a minimum curriculum which could be used as a basis in evaluating applications for registration by reciprocity. The new agency was successful in securing the interest of state boards in providing more frequent examinations. (As a war measure, at least one of the state boards held an examination every month!) It also helped the state boards to solve some of the problems that arose in connection with the Cadet Corps' requirement for acceleration of the basic programs of nursing schools. Lists of federal institutions, which had been visited and approved by some state boards, in preparation for the assignment of senior cadets, proved to be a time- and travel-saver for other boards. The bureau became a central source of information about the policies, procedures, and results of state board activities. It worked quietly behind the scenes but it made an important contribution to the war effort by facilitating the examination and licensure of the recent graduates, most of whom were destined to be classified 1-A (available for military service) by the Procurement and Assignment Service.

One of the important results of wartime stimuli was the production of the *Guide for Supervision of State Approved Schools of Nursing*. The state boards, within the frame of reference imposed upon them by the nurse practice acts, were in a strategic position to accelerate progressive action. It was, however, a committee of the NLNE, and not of the bureau, which made a study of qualifications for appointment to state boards of nurse examiners. The bureau laid a substantial foundation for a continuing program. As previously noted, the name was dropped in 1949, but the important state board program has been furthered under the guidance of the ANA's Special Committee of State Boards of Nursing and Nurse Education.

Need for counseling and placement services seems to be implicit in professional organizations. In the early period of American nursing, the better known schools rather informally provided the only available placement services. Early registries seem to have made no effort to extend their services to other than private duty nurses. The NOPHN provided somewhat informal counseling and placement service for public health nurses from its earliest days. As we have seen, the three national nursing organizations (Chap. 21) had been confronted with a practical problem, when the ARC discontinued the Bureau of Information it established to meet the needs of ex-service nurses following World War I. That war stimulated the development of counseling services. Counselors had not yet, however, achieved professional status, and little had been published on the subject. The NOPHN established a Vocational Bureau for Public Health Nurses which later cooperated with the American Association of Social Workers to form the Joint Vocational Service, Inc., which, for lack of subsidy, was discontinued in 1939.

The efforts of the ANA and the NLNE to carry on the service for institutional and other non-public health nurses, which had been set up by the ARC, were discontinued. But the midwest division of the ANA became increasingly aware of the need of both employers and nurses for such a service. In 1931 the division established a placement service in Chicago with borrowed funds, a part-time staff, and boundless faith in the project. It was underwritten by the five state nurses' associations that constituted the division. Within four years, Evelyn Wood, the enthusiastic pioneer director of the service, had died. She was succeeded by Adda Eldredge. By this time the debt had been repaid, and already the service was struggling to keep up with requests for assistance from practically every state in the Union. The majority of placements, however, were made in the Midwest. The Ohio State Nurses' Association, which was not a member of the division, had established a placement service in 1927. That association was convinced that the service helped to stabilize nursing within the state. In 1936, against the background of these experiences, an ANA committee began studying the possibility of developing a national counseling and placement service which could be coordinated with the services of professional registries and state placement services. A member of the headquarters staff was assigned from 1938 to 1941 to assist with the development of this program. Wartime shortages put a new emphasis on the whole question of counseling and placement. Tentative plans were discussed with registrars of professional registries meeting in conference late in 1944. They recommended consideration of a long-range plan for placement without fees from members of the association. In that year, also, the ANA conducted a functional experiment at the Midwest Placement Service which provided data for use in formulating a national plan for professional counseling and placement. A majority of state nurses' associations approved the plan. The ANA's Professional Counseling & Placement Service, Inc., was organized and incorporated on May 25, 1945, as a wholly owned, nonprofit subsidiary of the association. Its main office was established in the headquarters office of the association, and a branch office was set up in Chicago following reorganization of the Nurse Placement Service.[10] A majority of the state nurses' associations adopted the program. One of the first acts of the new agency was to enter into an agreement with the Veterans Bureau for the counseling of men and women nurses who had served with the armed forces. It is noteworthy that the VA has annually requested renewal of that agreement.

The ARC nursing service had quite inadvertently severed its long-standing liaison with the ANA when, under extreme pressure to increase enrollments, it replaced the traditional state and local committees with chapter recruitment committees. Efforts to establish some other type of organizational relationship were fruitless. However, this did not then or later interfere with what may be described as a friendly habit of cooperative planning between the two organizations. While plans for the PC&PS were maturing, an extensive two-part study of the postwar plans and aspirations of nurses was made by the ANA and the ARC. More than 40,000 Army

[10] Triggs, Frances Oralind: "A Nationwide Counseling and Placement Service," *Am. J. Nursing,* **45:**467, 1945.

and Navy nurses replied to questionnaires. The returns indicated that although 75 per cent of the nurses expected to remain in nursing, only 16 per cent of them planned to return to their postwar positions, thus blighting the hopes of those who had been counting on returning nurses to relieve the almost intolerably heavy burdens they had been carrying. Almost 50 per cent of these service nurses indicated that they were interested in the educational opportunities which would be made available to them under the liberal provisions of the "GI Bill."[11] A keen observer in the European theater found that public health and psychiatric nurses were the only groups with definite plans for the future. Since these were fields which called for special preparation, the nurses looked forward to study under the terms of the GI Bill. The NLNE and the NOPHN prepared lists of available graduate programs, and the ANA's gay little *W Is for Welcome* pamphlet informed returning veterans of the sources of information about the educational and employment opportunities awaiting them. To balance this study, through the cooperation of the state nurses' associations, questionnaires were sent to all nurses in the US. A sampling of the first 50,000 returned indicated that 54 per cent of those who replied planned to remain in their positions; 21 per cent expected to retire from nursing.[12] In the latter group, it may be assumed, were a considerable number of those who had deferred retirement in addition to those who had come out of retirement to help in the emergency.

There were 17,000 nurses in the European Theater of Operations on V-E Day (May 8, 1945). Patients were transferred to the states with amazing speed, and nurses were sent to redeployment areas for transfer to the states, to the Pacific, or to occupied Germany. The War Department made it possible for the AJN to send an editor, Nell V. Beeby, to visit some of these centers to ascertain how the magazine might help nurses during the period of readjustment. Understandably, the nurses were restless and impatient for "orders." Because they had been unable to keep up to date on developments

[11] Public Law 346, 78*th* Congress, June 22, 1944.
[12] "5,000 Civilian Nurses," from the Research Department of the ANA, *Am. J. Nursing*, 45:1019, 1945.

at home, many of them were apprehensive. They feared competition from the thousands of cadet nurses. They seemed to have little knowledge of the privileges they might enjoy under the "GI Bill." Many of them expressed unwillingness to return to their former positions unless personnel policies had been improved. The military services had treated them as professional women. They would not willingly return to institutions which treated graduate nurses as they had traditionally treated students. Miss Beeby's observations in the ETO corroborated the findings of the ARC-ANA study. But, through the clouds of uncertainty, there shone one glorious fact. Those nurses were almost universally proud, and could always be proud, of the accomplishments of the "outfits" of which they had been a part,[13] for never in any war had the wounded received such prompt and efficient care. It was clear that they would need wise counsel in making readjustments to civilian life. Counseling is helping the other person to help himself. Through the new PC&PS, the ANA hoped to give both ex-service and civilian nurses assistance in adjusting to changing social needs, and in utilizing the educational privileges accorded by "the GI Bill of Rights." Nurses who had anticipated overproduction of nurses by the Cadet Corps quickly discovered that their fears were baseless. There was an abundance of opportunities for placement but there were far too few nurses to meet postwar needs.

BIBLIOGRAPHY

The ANA and You. American Nurses' Association, New York, 1941.
Anderson, Bernice E.: *The Facilitation of Interstate Movement of Registered Nurses.* J. B. Lippincott Co., Philadelphia, 1950.
Annual Salaries and Salary Increases and Allowances Paid to General Staff Nurses. American Nurses' Association, New York, 1943.
"The Bureau of State Boards of Nurse Examiners," *Am. J. Nursing,* 45:458, 1945.
Burgess, May Ayres: "The Short-Course Nurse," *Nurses, Patients and*

[13] Beeby, Nell V.: "My Visit to the Family in the E.T.O.," *Am. J. Nursing,* 45:880, 1945.

Pocketbooks. Committee on the Grading of Nursing Schools, New York, 1928, Chap. 22.

Cook, Lloyd Allen: *Intergroup Relations in Teacher Education.* American Council on Education, Washington, D.C., 1951.

Counseling and Postwar Educational Opportunities. Student Personnel Work Series VI, #5, Vol. VIII, American Council on Education, Washington, D.C., May, 1944.

Deming, Dorothy: *The Practical Nurse.* The Commonwealth Fund, New York, 1947.

Eldredge, Adda: "The American Nurses' Association, a Review of Its Work Since 1922," *Am. J. Nursing,* **26**:533, 1926.

———: "Nursing Bureaus and Professional Counseling," *Am. J. Nursing,* **36**:807, 1936.

Given, Leila I., and Favreau, Claire: *A Guide for Supervision of State Approved Schools of Nursing.* American Nurses' Association, New York, 1948.

Hall, Ruth: "Counseling and Placement Call for Statesmanship," *Am. J. Nursing,* **45**:1039, 1945.

Hampton, Isabel A., and others: *Nursing of the Sick—1893,* chapter by D. J. Kinney on "Association for the Training of Attendants." McGraw-Hill Book Co., New York, 1949, p. 204.

Hicks, Emily J.: "A Crusade for Safer Nursing," *Am. J. Nursing,* **38**:563, 1938.

History of the A.N.A. Professional Counseling & Placement Service, Inc. (mimeographed). American Nurses' Association, New York, 1951.

"Home-Coming Nurses—Your Profession Welcomes You" (editorial), *Am. J. Nursing,* **45**:877, 1945.

Job Specifications for a Hospital Organization. Bulletin #202, American Hospital Association, Chicago, 1940.

Jose, Mary: "Some Army Nurses' Postwar Plans," *Am. J. Nursing,* **45**:596, 1945.

Lewis, Edward McE.: "Educational Benefits for Veterans," *Am. J. Nursing,* **45**:889, 1945.

McGuire, S. H., and Conrad, Dorothy W.: "Postwar Plans of Army and Navy Nurses," *Am. J. Nursing,* **46**:305, 1946.

Manual of Counseling and Placement, A.N.A. Professional Counseling & Placement Service, Inc. (mimeographed). American Nurses' Association, New York, 1950.

"New Salary Scale and Recommended Personnel Practices Adopted in California," *Am. J. Nursing,* **43**:603, 1943.

Nurse Practice Acts and Board Rules, A Digest, prepared by the American Nurses' Association and the National League of Nursing Education. American Nurses' Association, New York, 1940; revised, 1948.

"Nursing Legislation, State Boards, and the War," *Am. J. Nursing,* 43:682, 1943.

Personnel Practices for General Staff Nurses. American Nurses' Association, New York, 1944.

Practical Nurses and Hospital Attendants. Bulletin 203, #5, "The Outlook for Women in Occupations in the Medical Services." US Government Printing Office, Washington, D.C., 1945.

"Report of a Subcommittee to Study Placement Service and Vocational Counseling as an Activity of the A.N.A." (Elizabeth S. Soule, chairman), *Am. J. Nursing,* 44:911, 1944.

Scott, William C.: "The Social Security Act and the Nurse," *Am. J. Nursing,* 44:627, 1944.

"Some Interpretations of Educational Benefits," *Pub. Health Nursing,* 37:628, 1945.

Study of Organization, Control, Policies and Financing of Nurses' Professional Registries. American Nurses' Association, New York, 1942.

Subsidiary Workers in the Care of the Sick. American Nurses' Association, New York, 1940.

Triggs, Frances Oralind: "A Nationwide Counseling and Placement Service," *Am. J. Nursing,* 45:467, 1945.

"'Who Serves the State Boards of Nurse Examiners? Report of Sub-Committee to Set up Recommendations for Minimum Qualifications of Nurse Members of State Boards of Nurse Examiners and for State Educational Directors," *Am. J. Nursing,* 45:141–46, 1945.

"WLB Approves Salary Standards of California State Nurses' Association," *Am. J. Nursing,* 43:951, 1943.

Wood, Evelyn: "Nurse Placement Service," *Am. J. Nursing,* 32:50, 1932.

Chapter 39

THE NATIONAL LEAGUE OF NURSING EDUCATION

We need to cooperate in the interests of the profession, to promote what is good and eliminate what is bad. Much has been accomplished, but much remains to be accomplished; and we must bear in mind that any successful development in the future will lie in unitedly establishing and unitedly keeping the standard of our work at its highest possible point.

LOUISE DARCHE, 1893[1]

MISS DARCHE made the statement quoted above at the historic meeting in Chicago which set the stage for the organization of the National League of Nursing Education. Fifty years later the association was still working unitedly and with determination to safeguard the future of nursing by keeping the standard of nursing education at the highest possible point during the national emergency. At war's end the League, with a membership equivalent to less than 5 per cent of all active nurses, had safeguarded the foundations of the American system of nursing by formulating policies for the adaptation of nursing education to wartime needs. More than 40 state leagues and many local ones were participating in its programs. The League was slowly increasing its lay membership. It had affiliations with about 25 national organizations.

The League was a constituent member of the American Council on Education which, it will be recalled, had been very helpful to nursing in World War I. The council was aware that, in the interval between wars, nursing had made progress in its transition from "a conception of public service in the interests of the institution operat-

[1] Hampton, Isabel A., and others: *Nursing of the Sick, 1893;* Darche, Louise: "Proper Organization of Training Schools in America." McGraw-Hill Book Company, New York, 1949, p. 103.

416

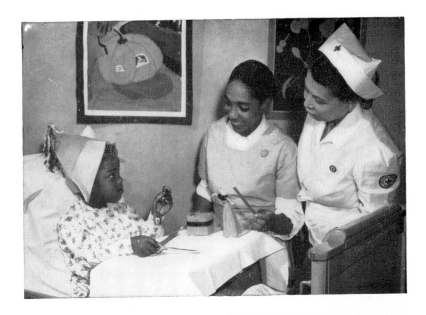

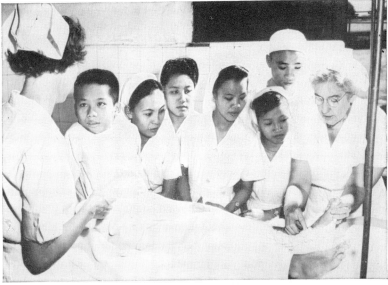

Plate XVII. (*Above*) Recreation therapy is taught in American Red Cross home nursing, mother and baby care, and family health courses (*ARC photo*). (*Below*) American nurses, participating in the health program of the Mutual Security Agency (1952), demonstrate nursing care of a compound fracture to Vietnamese nurses.

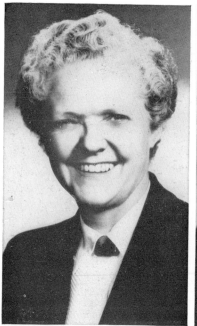

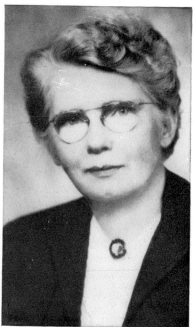

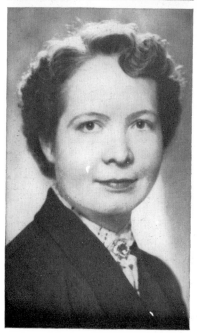

Plate XVIII. Officers of the new National League for Nursing organized in 1952. Ruth Sleeper (*upper left*), president; Marion W. Sheahan (*upper right*), director, Division of Nursing Services; Anna M. Fillmore (*lower left*), secretary and general director.

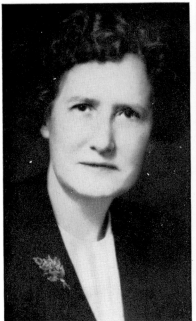
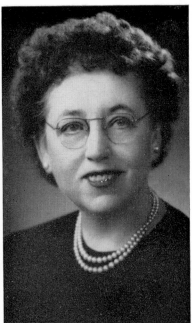
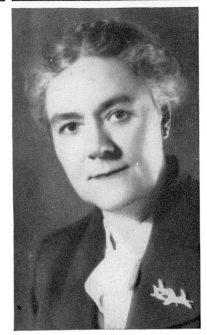

Plate XIX. Elizabeth K. Porter (*upper left*), president, ANA, 1950–   ; Pearl McIver (*upper right*), chairman of the Coordinating Committee which effected the restructuring of the national nursing organizations (*Harris & Ewing*); Ella Best (*lower right*), executive secretary, ANA, 1946–

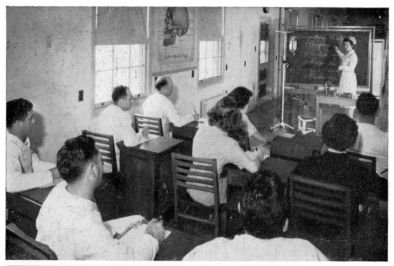

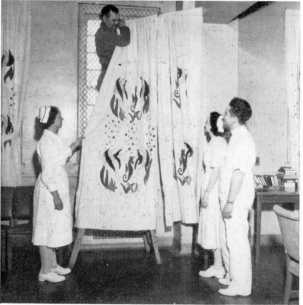

Plate XX. (*Above*) Principles of Wangensteen suction demonstrated by Navy nurse to WAVES and hospital corpsmen (*official Navy photo*). (*Below*) Group activity is important in rehabilitation programs of the Veterans Administration. Patients participated in designing and stenciling drapes.

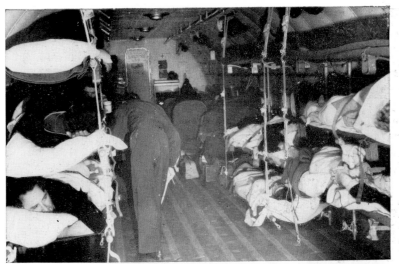

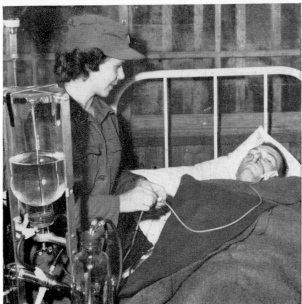

Plate XXI. (*Above*) An Air Force nurse, a captain, caring for patients in an air-evacuation C-54 (*official US Air Force photo*). (*Below*) Army nurse in field uniform with an evacuation hospital in Korea giving a nasal feeding (*US Army photo*).

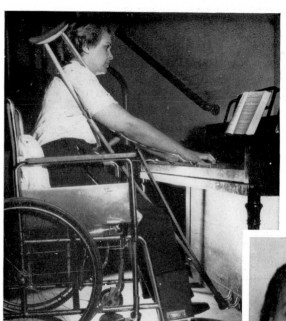

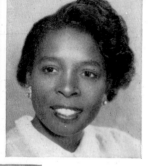

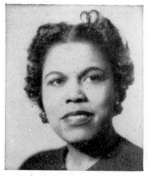

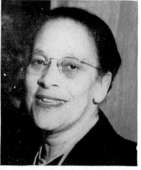

Plate XXII. (*Above*) Paraplegic patient using crutch for piano foot pedal (*courtesy of the Department of Physical Medicine and Rehabilitation, New York University College of Medicine*). (*Below*) Some distinguished Negro nurses: Mary Mills (*center*) (*Department of State photo*); Estelle Massey Osborne (*left*) (*Blackstone Studios, Inc.*); Mabel Keaton Staupers (*right*).

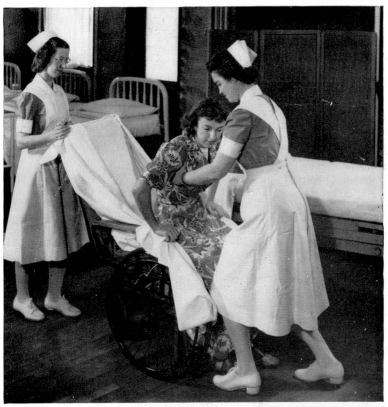

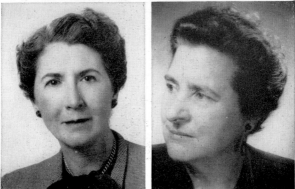

Plate XXIII. (*Top*) Showing correct body mechanics of nurse assisting (self-help) patient (*courtesy of the Nursing Advisory Service for Orthopedics and Poliomyelitis, NLN*). (*Lower left*) Ruth G. Taylor. (*Lower right*) Hazel A. Corbin (*Erich Kastan, 39 West 56 St., New York*).

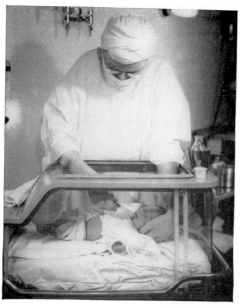

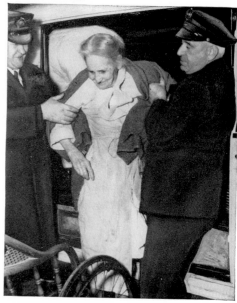

Plate XXIV. (*Above*) Care of premature babies has become an important function of departments of health (*courtesy of the Virginia State Department of Health*). (*Below*) This patient will receive home care under supervision of New York City Department of Hospitals (*World-Telegram, photo by Al. Ravenna*).

ing the school to one of primary concern for the interests of the public as a whole."[2] A conference, requested by the NLNE and the Association of Collegiate Schools of Nursing, was sponsored by the council early in 1942. The report effectively supported the principles and policies for the guidance of nursing schools which had previously been developed by a committee of the Nursing Council on National Defense on which sat representatives of the NLNE and the ACSN. The dissemination of the report among educators encouraged the utilization of the facilities of institutions of higher education for the teaching of the physical, biological, and social sciences. The League expanded the Department of Studies and set up the Department of Measurement and Guidance. The importance of instructional materials was recognized by a revision of *Books Suggested for Libraries in Schools of Nursing,* an invaluable guide to nursing school libraries. A special committee actively cooperated with an agency equipped to produce educational films. *The Guide for the Use of the League Records,* first published in 1938, was revised and reprinted (1942). A desired service to the schools was provided by means of a bulletin, *Nursing Education in War Time,* which proved to be a wartime *tour de force.* It was published under the direction of a special committee of which Nellie X. Hawkinson, director of nursing programs at the University of Chicago, was chairman. The bulletins dealt very practically with every aspect of the administration of an accelerated curriculum beginning with "Curriculum Adjustments" and ending with "Administrative Budget in the School of Nursing." The program of the committee was based on the recommendation of the board of directors, addressed to all schools, that organized instruction in the basic professional program be accelerated. Many factors required consideration in planning an accelerated progam, including "recognition of the importance of student service to civilian institutions whose graduate staffs are becoming more and more depleted." The recommendation that the thirty-six-month period be continued (for high school graduates) but that all organized instruction be completed within thirty months,

---

[2] *Nursing Education for National Service.* American Council on Education Studies, Vol. VI, May, 1942, p. 8.

freeing the last six months for supervised experience, was made with this need in mind.[3] The importance of special efforts to secure affiliations in psychiatric nursing was stressed by the committee, as it had been by the National Nursing Council's Committee on Educational Policies and Resources. The shortage of nurses with psychiatric experience had been conspicuous in World War I. It was more pronounced in World War II. Many of the adjustments approved by the League board had already been tested in a few schools. But schools generally were suffering from depleted faculties and loss of graduate staff nurses. They were resistant to the idea of acceleration until the well-financed and well-publicized US Cadet Nurse Corps (Chap. 36) made it a basic requirement for participation in that program, a stipulation which was accepted by 1125 of the nation's 1300 nursing schools. The ground was somewhat prepared for the cadet program as four of the bulletins had been published before the corps was authorized by Congress in the summer of 1943.

An early bulletin on "Faculty and Facilities" stressed the importance of providing leaves of absence or adjusted hours for faculty members and promising young nurses in order that they might secure the special preparation they needed in order to give maximum wartime service. It had become apparent, at an early date, that faculty replacements had often to be made with less well-prepared people. Beginning in 1941, federal funds were available throughout the war for this purpose, but it was often difficult to persuade administrative nurses that leaves should be granted, to ensure the continuation of good standards of teaching, at a time when vacancies were extremely difficult to fill. Many schools, however, adjusted hours for faculty members who, with federal aid, could secure additional preparation at nearby universities.

The fourth bulletin, "Cooperative Planning by Schools of Nursing," pointed out that when schools got together for joint planning even the least progressive school usually had something to contribute. This bulletin discussed the nine major steps in cooperative planning and the successive steps required in the development of a central

---

[3] "Quality and Quantity Needed," *Nursing Education in Wartime*, Bulletin #1, NLNE, New York, November, 1942, p. 2.

preclinical program or of a central school of nursing. A considerable amount of material had previously been published on both these subjects, but methods of procedure had never been so compactly stated or made so readily available. The collated bulletins, made available as a unit after the war, are an important addition to the literature on the administration of curriculums and of nursing schools.[4]

The bulletins were designed to assist the hospital schools of nursing. In 1944, when the committee had a full-time secretary, a series of nine regional conferences were held to assist the collegiate schools. They were sponsored by the League and the Association of Collegiate Schools of Nursing with the cooperation of the American Council on Education. The reports of the conferences were synthesized and published by the League.[5] The problems of individual institutions could not be considered at such conferences, but the participation of educators from general and nursing education was enlightening to both. The conferences revealed need for clear thinking in the area of aims and philosophy as well as in the more tangible areas of relationships.

The Department of Studies of the League made a valuable contribution to nursing and to the war effort by an almost continuous flow of statistical and other information on such important subjects as enrollment in nursing schools, attrition rates, faculty shortages, weekly time schedules, the educational qualifications of student nurses, and related subjects. Both federal and professional planning agencies depended on the League for this type of basic information about nursing schools. The list of schools approved by state boards of nurse examiners, revised in 1943 by the department, was an extensively used source of information.

There were arguments pro and con for discontinuing the League's accreditation program during the war. The program was not permitted to lag, although some schools were, quite naturally, hesitant about requesting surveys while they were operating under abnor-

[4] *Nursing Education in Wartime.* Complete Series of Fourteen Bulletins, 1942–1945, NLNE, New York, 1945.
[5] *Problems of Collegiate Schools of Nursing Offering Basic Professional Programs.* NLNE, New York, 1945.

mal conditions. Between 1938, when the first surveys were made, and 1945, well over 100 schools had been placed on a list of accredited schools, but a considerable number were provisionally accredited and were due for resurvey. The list was too small to be of significant value to recruitment committees which were in urgent need of materials that would help prospective students to make wise choices. However, interest in the principle of accreditation was much greater than the size of that list would seem to indicate. A special committee on accreditation with representation from the AMA, AHA, and ACS had been formed, at the request of those agencies, to work with the League committee which was responsible for the administration of the program. Early in 1945 the board of directors of the League went on record as approving a first step toward coordinating the accreditation programs of the League, the NOPHN, and the Association of Collegiate Schools of Nursing.[6] Thus was foreshadowed one of the most important of all the activities undertaken in the postwar period, the development of the National Nursing Accrediting Service (NNAS).

The interest of educators and of nurse educators in psychometric tests had grown apace between the wars. Probably the Army school students who took the Army Alpha test in 1919 as a courtesy to a research worker (and whose IQ's were found to be gratifyingly high) were the first student nurses to be so tested. A chapter of the *Curriculum Guide* (1937) was devoted to consideration of the significance and use of objective tests. The following year a joint committee, with Isabel M. Stewart as chairman, representing the League, the ACSN, and Teachers College was appointed "to consider the possibility of developing objective techniques of measuring nursing on a cooperative basis, to take steps to initiate such a cooperative project and to seek funds for its support."[7] The committee received definite evidence that such a service would be welcomed by schools and by many of the state boards of nurse examiners. But efforts to secure foundation support for a service to be set up as a

[6] *Fifty-first Annual Report,* NLNE, 1945, p. 36.
[7] *Forty-fifth Annual Report,* NLNE, 1939, p. 209.

nursing unit of the Test Service of the American Council on Education were unsuccessful.

Miss Stewart, who was working on plans for nursing education in connection with the national preparedness program, resigned in 1940. R. Louise McManus, who had been secretary of the committee, was appointed to succeed her as chairman. Mrs. McManus proceeded, against serious odds reminiscent of those encountered by the founders of the AJN almost a half century earlier, to lay sound foundations for one of the profession's most fundamental and useful services. The committee had been empowered by the board of directors to raise funds. When efforts to interest foundations failed, money was borrowed, at the personal risk of the chairman, to launch the enterprise. Again the cautious challenged the judgment of those who took bold action. But, as in the case of the *Journal,* the enterprise was so soundly conceived it quickly became self-sustaining without initial outlay by the parent organization. The loan was repaid. Work was begun modestly by establishing the NLNE Pre-Nursing and Guidance Test Service in cooperation with committees of the New Jersey League and the Education Section of the Connecticut State Nurses' Association.[8] This particular service was selected as the one most needed by schools under pressure to increase student enrollment.

Teachers College provided space, rent free, during the first year of the committee's work. By 1945 the service had outgrown all available space and was moved to national nursing headquarters. Four different "test batteries" were then in operation:

1. The Pre-Nursing and Guidance Test Service to be used by schools in selecting applicants.
2. The State Board Test Pool in which the member state boards cooperate in producing the tests to be used in the licensing examination.
3. The Achievement Examinations which are intended to be used by students at various points in their course.
4. The Test of Basic Information and Judgment—for graduate nurses.[9]

[8] *Forty-seventh Annual Report, NLNE,* 1941, p. 73.
[9] "National Licensing Examinations?" *Am. J. Nursing,* 45:1035, 1945.

In 1945, 25 boards of nurse examiners had joined the State Board Test Pool;[10] by 1950, when all were members, a long step had been taken toward the solution of the knotty problem of reciprocity. At that time it could be said that no other profession had developed a comparable service. The following year, Elizabeth L. Kemble (University of Cincinnati), who had taught both student and graduate nurses, had been a member of the Psychological Corporation's Nurse Testing Division, and was in the process of acquiring a doctorate in education when she joined the staff. Under her direction the service rapidly reached new heights of usefulness.

From the time the Division of Nursing Education at Teachers College had become independent of the NLNE for financial support until Pearl Harbor, the basic or undergraduate preparation of nurses had been the focal point of all the League's endeavors. No effort had been made to provide standards for collegiate programs for graduate nurses or for the "postgraduate" or added experience courses offered by many hospitals. For many years graduates of substandard schools who wished to become enrolled Red Cross nurses had been advised to take postgraduate courses in the areas of their most serious deficiencies. Nurses who had been required to secure added experience, such as pediatrics, in order to qualify for stipends under the Social Security Act had been perplexed by the lack of criteria or standards for supplementary courses. The question arose again when the Training of Nurses Act of 1941 made provision for various types of programs for graduate nurses. By this time there was also some evidence of a growing interest in clinical specialization.

Institutions desirous of securing graduate nurse service by offering "postgraduate" courses depended on the use of advertising space in the AJN and other nursing publications to carry their message. But there were no professionally authorized criteria by which to judge the merits of their offerings. Acting on the principle that standards should be set by the educational body, the *Journal* appealed to the

---

[10] McManus, R. Louise, chairman, and Sommer, Ida B., secretary: "Report of the Committee on Measurement and Educational Guidance," *Fifty-first Annual Report, NLNE*, 1945, pp. 83–88.

NLNE for assistance. It did not go empty-handed. Throughout the war the drab appearance of the magazine was in sharp contrast to its crackling contents. Enforced limitations on the use of paper made it necessary to utilize narrow margins and the thinnest possible paper in order to pack in its pages the thrilling story of nursing in wartime. But the paper restrictions saved money for the *Journal*. What better investment than in standards for the evaluation of advertisements of postgraduate courses? Could the NLNE provide the *Journal* with the needed criteria? That request resulted in a project which was to have far-reaching significance.

A special committee with Mrs. Elizabeth K. Porter as chairman, then of the University of Pennsylvania faculty, with the aid of subcommittees and many interested nurses scattered throughout the country, produced a series of six pamphlets which have been extensively used.

In its basic assumptions, the committee noted that:

At this particular juncture it is extremely important that advanced preparation should be provided for nurses who wish to qualify themselves for teaching and supervision in a given clinical area. In the past, for want of something better, such preparation has usually taken the form of a superstructure composed of courses in teaching and supervision, imposed on an inadequate knowledge of and experience in clinical nursing itself. As a result head nurses, teachers, and supervisors have often found themselves in the difficult situation of knowing something about *how* to teach without sufficient knowledge of *what* to teach.

The general situation with respect to bedside nursing is equally unsatisfactory. Very little has been done to encourage nurses who excel in this branch of nursing to stay with it, and there has been a tendency to believe that progress for a staff nurse is synonymous with leaving the clinical field.[11]

The reports of that committee, which were published in the *Journal* and in pamphlet form, and the work of the Joint Orthopedic Nursing Advisory Service mark a turning point in nursing education. They placed competence in *nursing* in its proper relation to

[11] *Courses in Clinical Nursing for Graduate Nurses, Basic Assumptions and Guiding Principles—Basic Courses—Advanced Courses.* Pamphlet #1, NLNE, New York, 1945.

teaching. Two distinct categories of courses were considered by the committee: (1) the supplementary and added-experience courses such as had been of special concern to the *Journal* staff, because they seemed to be mere devices to secure hospital personnel, and (2) advanced courses conducted by colleges or universities for the benefit of nurses interested in becoming teachers, supervisors, head nurses, nursing consultants, or expert practitioners in specific clinical areas. In the postwar period a number of universities received grants from the W. K. Kellogg Foundation to develop advanced programs in clinical nursing. It is noteworthy that some universities now make clinical courses a prerequisite for specialization in teaching and ward administration. Most important, however, is the fact that an increasing number of nurses register for these courses with an expressed appreciation of their availability. They pursue their study and nursing practice with an enthusiasm that is heart-warming to instructors who believe that these nurses will inevitably have a potent influence on the evolution of the art of professional nursing.

The work of the important committee on the integration of the social and health aspects of nursing, on which the NLNE and the NOPHN were represented, is discussed in the next chapter. The League was also represented on a variety of joint committees, i.e., committees dealing with matters of concern to it and to other national nursing, medical, and health organizations. Only matters in which the whole profession looked to the League for direct leadership and which posed the way for postwar action have been discussed in this chapter.

BIBLIOGRAPHY

Books Suggested for Libraries in Schools of Nursing, 4th ed. National League of Nursing Education, New York, 1948.
Courses in Clinical Nursing for Graduate Nurses. National League of Nursing Education, New York:
  1. *Basic Assumptions and Guiding Principles—Basic Courses—Advanced Courses.* Pamphlet #1, 1945.
  2. *An Advanced Course in Psychiatric Nursing.* Pamphlet #2, 1945.

3. *Guide for an Advanced Clinical Course in Pediatric Nursing.* Pamphlet #3, 1946.
4. *Guide for an Advanced Clinical Course in Tuberculosis Nursing.* Pamphlet #4, 1947.
5. *Guide for an Advanced Clinical Course in Maternity Nursing.* Pamphlet #5, 1948.
6. *Guide for an Advanced Clinical Course in Orthopedic Nursing.* Pamphlet #6, 1948.

"Curriculum Adjustment—League Board Makes Recommendations for War Emergency," *Am. J. Nursing,* **42**:1182, 1942.

A Curriculum Guide for Schools of Nursing. National League of Nursing Education, New York, 1937.

Essentials of a Good School of Nursing, rev. ed. National League of Nursing Education, New York, 1942.

Faculty Positions in Schools of Nursing and How to Prepare for Them, rev. ed. National League of Nursing Education, New York, 1946.

"Federal Aid for Those Who Teach," *Am. J. Nursing,* **42**:1409, 1942.

Fundamentals of Administration for Schools of Nursing. National League of Nursing Education, New York, 1940.

Guide for the Development of Libraries in Schools of Nursing (mimeographed). National League of Nursing Education, New York, 1952.

A Guide for the Use of League Records. National League of Nursing Education, New York, 1943; supplements, 1943 and 1945.

A List of Schools of Nursing Meeting Minimum Requirements Set by Law and Board Rules as of January 1, 1943, rev. ed. National League of Nursing Education, New York, 1950.

Lorentz, Mildred Irene: "Planning Conferences for Collegiate Schools of Nursing," *Am. J. Nursing,* **44**:877, 1944.

McManus, R. Louise: "How Can We Develop Objective Techniques for Measuring the Professional Achievement of Student and Graduate Nurses?" *Forty-fifth Annual Report of the National League of Nursing Education,* New York, 1939, p. 204; also, discussion, p. 232.

———: *Study Guide on Evaluation.* National League of Nursing Education, New York, 1944.

"Measuring the Outcomes of the Educational Program," *The Curriculum Guide for Schools of Nursing.* National League of Nursing Education, New York, 1937, p. 616.

"Nursing Schools and National Defense" (some principles and policies of guidance in the basic preparation of nurses, Committee on Educational Policies and Resources, National Nursing Council for War Service, Isabel M. Stewart, chairman), *Am. J. Nursing,* **42**:182, 1942.

Pfefferkorn, Blanche, and Rovetta, Charles A.: *Administrative Cost Anal-*

ysis for Nursing Service and Nursing Schools. Sponsored by the American Hospital Association and the National League of Nursing Education, 1940.

Robb, Isabel Hampton: "The Affiliation of Training Schools for Nurses for Educational Purposes," *Am. J. Nursing*, **5**:666, 1905.

Sleeper, Ruth: "The Curriculum in the Emergency," *Am. J. Nursing*, **42**:805, 1942.

Zook, George F.: "Standards and Nursing Education," *Am. J. Nursing*, **42**:928, 1942.

Chapter 40

THE NATIONAL ORGANIZATION FOR
PUBLIC HEALTH NURSING

The primary function of the National Organization for Public Health Nursing is "to stimulate responsibility for the health of the community by fostering the establishment and extension of public health nursing and the education of nurses in public health."

ALMA C. HAUPT[1]

DURING THE WAR, many factors were accelerating the change in emphasis in public health nursing from therapeutic to preventive service. As hospital facilities became more generally available, fewer maternity or acutely ill patients required care in their homes. New antigens, insecticides, and other weapons were reducing the incidence of communicable disease. The function of the public health nurse in assisting the chronically ill to adjust to their handicaps was steadily gaining in importance. By the end of 1944, the National Organization for Public Health Nursing had 349 agencies and approximately 11,000 individual members. Slightly more than 6 per cent of the membership were lay and professional persons who were actively interested in public health nursing. About one-half of all practicing public health nurses were included in its membership. In addition, 188 "contributors" were giving substantial support to the organization.

Because the development of public health nursing as an effective public service has always depended on a working partnership of physicians, nurses, and citizens, the three groups were represented

[1] Haupt, Alma C.: "National Unity in Public Health Nursing," *Pub. Health Nursing,* 37:3, 1945.

on the board of directors of the NOPHN. The organization functioned through the board of directors, an advisory council of which Dr. C.-E. A. Winslow was chairman at the time of which we are writing, and a large number of councils and committees including the council of branches (the state organizations of public health nursing). It also had four sections which were concerned with special interests: (1) board and committee members (of local public health nursing services), (2) school nursing, (3) industrial nursing, and (4) a new nurse-midwife section.

When the nation was preparing for war, less than 24,000 nurses were engaged in public health nursing.[2] The NOPHN strongly advocated support of the principle that the contribution of public health nurses to the health of the nation could be much more important than any aid they might give in military service. Even so, at the height of the war effort, the organization reported that almost 5 per cent of its nurse members and almost an equal number of nurses who had dropped their membership were with the armed forces. Undoubtedly they did good work, but there were few opportunities with the military (and such opportunities were chiefly postwar with the armies of occupation) for the development of services calling for their special skills. The NOPHN policy, based on experiences in World War I, was fully justified by the findings of a study of resources for the care of the sick in their own homes in 16 war communities.

This study was made with the cooperation of all the major agencies requiring the services of public health nurses: the US Public Health Service, the Children's Bureau, and the American Red Cross, in addition to the Metropolitan Life Insurance Company which financed it. The study was urgently needed. The population of one of the communities studied, for example, had been quadrupled by the influx of soldiers, sailors, and industrial workers. In some of these communities it was found that, due to limited hospital facilities, maternity patients were discharged in less than three days after delivery although an eight- or ten-day hospital stay was then stand-

---

[2] "How Many Public Health Nurses?" *Pub. Health Nursing*, 33:21, 1941. (US Public Health Service Annual Census.)

ard obstetrical practice. Such conditions stimulated the development of the Children's Bureau Emergency Maternity and Infant Care Program, which, in turn, increased the demand for public health nursing.

The findings of the 16-community study provided a substantial base for the NOPHN's most distinctive and lasting war service. The organization was one of six national health and welfare agencies which cooperated, as the American War Community Services, in providing service financed by community chests and councils, for wartime communities. Nurse members of the staff went to the assistance of 64 communities. They remained long enough to give practical guidance in the exploration and utilization of community facilities. Successive visits were often necessary. When the war-communities agency was discontinued, six new public health nursing services had been organized, and many inadequate services had been reorganized and developed. Also, as a result of this work, some new services were established at a later date. The immediate results were so impressive that the then new National Foundation for Infantile Paralysis financed the service for a year after the original sponsors had discontinued their support.

Could some of the services performed by public health nurses be delegated to other workers? To answer that problem, in part, a study was made of public health nursing practices in clinics and health conferences. Two hundred and twelve of the five most prevalent types of clinics were selected for the study. These were child health, crippled children, maternity, tuberculosis, and venereal disease clinics. Some voluntary and paid auxiliary workers were employed. But the job analysis showed that public health nurses were doing many things that could have been delegated to non-public health nurses or to auxiliary workers in order to provide more time for teaching and enriching the clinic experience of the patients. The time study showed that two-thirds of the time spent by public health nurses, before and after the clinics, could be saved by delegating activities to auxiliary workers. Examples of jobs which could be efficiently performed by nonprofessional workers were: preparation of examining tables, distribution and care of linen, taking and recording temperatures and weight, cleaning up examining trays. In this connection, it may be noted that a survey of industrial nursing, under other auspices, also found that nurses were performing non-nursing functions in 14 per cent of the plants surveyed.

Industrial nursing was rapidly growing in importance. A study of 42 industrial nursing services in a Pennsylvania county, made for the public health nursing section of the American Public Health Association (1939), indicated a marked lack of standardization. Further work led to a national study which was made for the industrial hygiene section of the USPHS[3] (Chap. 43).

At about the same time, the NOPHN, with financial assistance from several interested organizations, employed an experienced industrial nurse as secretary of its industrial nursing section and assigned to her the preparation of a book for the use of nurses practicing in the varied and complex industrial environments. Mrs. McGrath's practical and comprehensive volume, *Nursing in Commerce and Industry,*[4] was the third book on industrial nursing produced under the sponsorship of the organization.[5] Although the number of industrial nurses was enormously increased during the war, almost one-half of all industrial workers were believed to be in need of occupational health service. They were the workers in the small plants which employed 250 or fewer workers. Authorities were not agreed on the best method for providing health services for them. In 1945 a committee of the industrial nursing section undertook a study of part-time service for small plants with the cooperation of 25 visiting nurse associations which were providing such service. This type of service by VNA's was far from new but had been greatly increased in the prewar and war periods. On the basis of its study, the committee recommended that, "as rapidly as experienced nurses are available, service should be extended to as

[3] Whitlock, Oliver M.; Trasko, Victoria M.; and Kahl, F. Ruth: *Nursing Practices in Industry*, Public Health Bulletin #283, USPHS. US Government Printing Office, Washington, D.C., 1944.

[4] McGrath, Bethel J.: *Nursing in Commerce and Industry.* The Commonwealth Fund, New York, 1946.

[5] The others are: Wright, Florence Swift: *Industrial Nursing.* The Macmillan Company, New York, 1919. Hodgson, Violet H.: *Public Health Nursing in Industry.* The Macmillan Company, New York, 1933.

many small plants . . . as can be convinced of the value of the service."[6] With this report the NOPHN rounded out some 30 years of persistent effort to promote the development of industrial nursing. Many industrial nurses resisted the assumption that their specialized field of nursing was a type of public health nursing rather than a distinct and separate field of nursing; therefore, the American Association of Industrial Nurses (discussed in Chapter 43) was organized in 1942.

During the war approximately one-half of all public health nurses were engaged in school nursing; one-fourth of them devoted full time to it. The other quarter gave service in schools as part of a more general program. Despite the shortages in other fields, the number of nurses employed by departments of education had increased slightly by 1944. This was a field in which developments were being brought about by changing emphasis on the importance of the classroom teacher in the teaching of health. "As health talks are abandoned in favor of integrating health information with the total educational program," said Ruth Freeman, "the nurse must become familiar not only with the subject matter of health, but with the problems and mechanics of classroom teaching that she may effectively assist the teacher with this integration. . . . Changes in the preparation of nurses for school health work have been directed toward the increasing of technical proficiency and leadership ability."[7] A committee of the NOPHN[8] conducted a two-year study of supervision in school nursing which was published in 1945. The participation of state committees, secured with some difficulty under wartime conditions, gave it special value. Trends in the development of school nursing, the council of branches was told, indicated need for closer cooperation between health and education groups at national, state, and local levels.

Two forces are constantly at work in relation to the education of

[6] "Part-time Nursing in Industry. . . as Provided by Visiting Nurse Associations in the United States," NOPHN, New York, 1946, p. 68.

[7] Freeman, Ruth: "Developments in Education of Public Health Nurses for School Health Work," *Pub. Health Nursing*, 37:454, 1945.

[8] Chayer, Mary Ella: "Improving the School Health Program Through Supervision of School Nursing," *Pub. Health Nursing*, 37:75, 1945.

nurses. The first is the response of nurse educators to the stimuli of changing educational philosophy, medical progress, and the constantly changing milieu in which nursing is practiced. The second arises from the dissatisfaction of graduate nurses with basic courses which failed to provide them with a dependable foundation for nursing practice, especially in the broad field of public health nursing or as a basis for positions in teaching and administration. As early as 1915, when NOPHN appointed its first education committee, the organization had recognized these forces. It accepted responsibility for leadership in relation to the preparation of graduate nurses for practice as public health nurses. It was critical of the undergraduate preparation of most nurses and looked to the NLNE for leadership in securing improvement. The NOPHN began approving (accrediting) courses in public health nursing for graduate nurses in 1920. By the following year 15 courses were on the approved list. Twenty years went by, however, before a *Curriculum Guide* in public health nursing was provided. Then, in 1941, the NOPHN sought the cooperation of the USPHS in the preparation of such a publication. Mary J. Dunn was assigned to the project and the *Guide* was published the following year.[9] The list of programs approved by the NOPHN numbered 28 at that time. Meanwhile, a few of the collegiate schools had so thoroughly integrated the social and health aspects of nursing in their basic programs that they considered their graduates qualified for beginning positions in public health nursing services. An application, for approval by the NOPHN, of the Skidmore College basic program presented the organization with a wholly new problem. But by 1952, 14 basic collegiate programs had been approved. The NOPHN had a list of 39 approved programs when it became apparent that the overlapping of accreditation programs was embarrassing some of the schools. The unification of this with other accrediting services, which was an outstanding postwar achievement, is discussed in a later chapter.

[9] *The Public Health Nursing Curriculum Guide*, prepared by a joint committee of the NOPHN and the USPHS. The NOPHN, New York, 1942. (The *Guide* is now [1952] in its fifth printing.)

The NOPHN was constantly stimulated by the opportunities opened to nurses by the public health movement, whereas the NLNE was handicapped in its persistent efforts to improve the basic education of nurses by the traditional demands of both medicine and hospitals for service. But the broader needs of society and the interpretative influence of public health nurses became increasingly apparent in the successive editions of the *Curriculum Guide* prepared by the NLNE.

The committee responsible for the preparation of the *Curriculum Guide* had secured widespread participation in the work of revision by qualified nurses in all fields of nursing education and nursing practice. The book was hardly off the press when the NOPHN was overwhelmed with requests from schools for help in securing affiliations for student experience in public health nursing agencies. But the number of well-organized agencies which had the resources for giving supervised field experience was relatively small, and most of the available experience was needed to provide the field work required as an integral part of the collegiate programs which were preparing nurses for public health nursing. What to do? Steadfastly throughout the period of the war and on into the postwar period a joint committee of the NLNE and NOPHN worked on the fundamental problem of integrating the social and health aspects of nursing throughout the basic curriculum. By 1945 the committee had agreed that "teaching of the health, preventive, and rehabilitative elements of nursing, as well as the curative elements, must be started early in the basic curriculum and in relation to every function and every appropriate learning situation."[10] Guides for instructors were prepared by the committee and published simultaneously in the *American Journal of Nursing* and *Public Health Nursing*.

In the long struggle to establish the concept of undergraduate nurses as students to be taught rather than apprentices to be trained, nurse educators had persistently stressed the educational needs of student nurses rather than the direct care of patients. The committees noted that the time had come for a change of perspective which

[10] "Faculty Preparation in the Health and Social Components of Nursing," *Am. J. Nursing*, 45:564, 1945.

would place the emphasis, in teaching, on the care of the patient. This was, however, but one of the committees which began planning for patient-centered programs while the war was still going on.

The Children's Bureau program for the care of crippled children had already been launched, under the provisions of the Social Security Act, when the National Foundation for Infantile Paralysis was organized in 1938. Few nurses were equipped to work with the social workers, physical therapists, and other specialists in the development of effective programs. A grant from the foundation to the NOPHN in 1939 made possible the appointment of a nurse consultant. Jessie L. Stevenson, a public health nurse equipped with knowledge and experience in both orthopedic nursing and physical therapy, accepted the position. The service, modestly begun by one nurse, became a stimulating force in the improvement of many nursing services. "Every nurse," said Miss Stevenson,—"institutional, private duty or public health—who gives bedside care or teaches the art of nursing to student nurses or families is responsible for making or preventing crippling. . . ." In caring for those already crippled, she pointed out, the nurse "must see beyond the orthopedic defect to the patient as a person."[11] The Joint Orthopedic Nursing Advisory Service, financed by the National Foundation for Infantile Paralysis and administered by the NOPHN, was organized in 1941, and a consultant, Carmelita Calderwood, was engaged by the NLNE to work in cooperation with Miss Stevenson. JONAS provided consultant service to individuals, hospitals, schools of nursing, universities, and nursing service agencies. For several years, it administered scholarship funds provided by the foundation. The service was so successful that, fortunately, it was continued in the postwar period with its mounting incidence of polio. It became the prototype for the Joint Tuberculosis Nursing Advisory Service (JTNAS) which was established shortly after the war. The preparation of handbooks and other publications, of annotated lists of publications, and of visual aids is an important feature of the JONAS service which, after the reorganization of 1952, became the Nursing Advisory

[11] Stevenson, Jessie L.: "What Is Orthopedic Nursing?" *Am. J. Nursing,* **39**:11, 1939.

Service for Orthopedics and Poliomyelitis of the National League for Nursing (NLN).

By this time the NOPHN's experience in planning for nursing in relation to community needs had covered considerably more than a quarter of a century. At war's end, in addition to working with the NLNE on the basic curriculum, it was working in close cooperation with the ACSN on collegiate programs. With the ANA it was working for the inclusion of nursing in prepayment plans for medical care. With the ANA and the NLNE it had representatives on a joint committee on community nursing service. It was also represented on the very active joint committee on practical nurses and auxiliary workers in nursing services, and on other joint committees. It was continuing to add to the long list of health and social agencies with which it enjoyed cooperative relationships. The stage was set for the development of a broader base for further cooperative planning in relation to nursing and health, which is discussed in connection with the restructuring of the nursing organizations.

BIBLIOGRAPHY

Boas, Ernst P.: "The Chronically Sick—the Social and Medical Aspects of Their Nursing Care," *Am. J. Nursing*, **37**:137, 1937.

Bryan, Leah Blaisdell: "Report of the Committee on the Integration of the Social and Health Aspects of Nursing in the Basic Curriculum," *Fifty-first Report of the National League of Nursing Education*, 1945, p. 103.

"Building for the Future in Industrial Nursing," *Pub. Health Nursing*, **37**:117, 1945.

Butzerin, Eula B.: "The Collegiate Council on Public Health Nursing Education," *Pub. Health Nursing*, **36**:31, 1944.

Carn, Irene: "Intergrating Public Health Nursing with Hospital Nursing," *Am. J. Nursing*, **42**:669, 1942.

Curtis, Dorothy E.: "What They Are Doing in Germany," *Pub. Health Nursing*, **37**:503, 1945.

"Faculty Preparation in the Health and Social Components of Nursing, Joint Committee of the N.L.N.E. and the N.O.P.H.N.," *Am. J. Nursing*, **45**:564, 1945; also, *Pub. Health Nursing*, **37**:348, 1945.

Fillmore, Anna M.: "I. Part-Time Nursing Service to the Small Plant," *Pub. Health Nursing,* **37**:130, 1945.

——: "II. Part-Time Nursing Services to Small Industrial Plants," *Pub. Health Nursing,* **38**:453, 1946.

Henricksen, Heide, and Foker, L. W.: "The Small Industrial Health Plant," *Pub. Health Nursing,* **37**:302, 1945.

Hilbert, Hortense: "Public Health Nursing Services in Clinics," *Pub. Health Nursing,* **36**:209, 287, 1944.

Hodgson, Violet H.: *Public Health Nursing in Industry.* The Macmillan Company, New York, 1933.

Jensen, Frode; Weiskotten, J. B.; Thomas, Margaret A.: *Medical Care of the Discharged Hospital Patient.* The Commonwealth Fund, New York, 1944.

Klem, Margaret C.: *Prepayment Medical Care Organizations,* 3rd ed. Bureau Memo #55, Social Security Board. US Government Printing Office, Washington, D.C., 1945.

McGrath, Bethel J.: *Nursing in Commerce and Industry.* The Commonwealth Fund, New York, 1946.

Nyswander, Dorothy B.: *Solving School Health Problems: The Astoria Demonstration Study.* The Commonwealth Fund, New York, 1942.

Report of American War-Community Services, Inc., May 7, 1943, to May 1, 1947. In the files of the National Organization for Public Health Nursing, New York.

Schedule for a Survey of Community Nursing Service, prepared by Joint Committee on Community Nursing Service of the National Organization for Public Health Nursing, the American Nurses' Association, and the National League of Nursing Education, New York, 1939; revised, 1944.

"School Nurse and Community," *Pub. Health Nursing,* **36**:422, 1944.

"Social and Health Aspects of Nursing in the Basic Curriculum":
1. Blaisdell, Leah M.: "We Offer Nursing Service to Industry," *Pub. Health Nursing,* **34**:550, 1942.
2. "The Joint Committee of the N.L.N.E. and N.O.P.H.N.," *Am. J. Nursing,* **44**:62, 1944.
3. Frost, Harriet: "Affiliation and Integration Defined," *Am. J. Nursing,* **44**:168, 1944.
4. Dunn, Mary J.: "Underlying Philosophy and Revised Recommendations," *Am. J. Nursing,* **44**:265, 1944; *Pub. Health Nursing,* **36**:124, 1944.
5. Carn, Irene: "Objectives for the Integration of the Social and Health Aspects of Nursing in the School of Nursing Curriculum," *Am. J. Nursing,* **45**:223, 1945.

Stern, Bernhard J.: *Medicine in Industry*. The Commonwealth Fund, New York, 1946, pp. 102–8.

————: *Medical Services by Government—Local, State, and Federal*. The Commonwealth Fund, New York, 1946.

Stevenson, Jessie L.: "An Orthopedic Service for the Community," *Pub. Health Nursing*, **37**:607, 1945.

Strong, Anne H.: "The Education of Public Health Nurses," *Pub. Health Nursing*, **13**:226, 1921.

"Study of Industrial Nursing Services," *Pub. Health Nursing*, **32**:631, 1940.

Wilson, Alberta B.: "School Nursing Trends," *Pub. Health Nursing*, **37**:160, 1945.

Wright, Florence Swift: *Industrial Nursing*. The Macmillan Company, New York, 1919.

Chapter 41

THE ASSOCIATION OF COLLEGIATE
SCHOOLS OF NURSING

Social necessity certainly created nursing and is now forcing the changes which we are seeking to effect through the university relationship. Upon the nursing profession must and should fall the duty of safe-guarding and perpetuating the best traditions of the profession, while formulating a program through which its achievement may keep step with the progress in medical and other sciences.

ANNIE W. GOODRICH[1]

THE ASSOCIATION of Collegiate Schools of Nursing had been unable to secure the financial support its originators had anticipated. Its programs would have languished during the war had it not been for its close ties with the NLNE and the National Nursing Council. It had, however, achieved an influential position. At the beginning of the war about 80 nursing schools were offering degree programs. The number had practically doubled by 1945.[2] Many of them, however, were not collegiate schools as defined by the ACSN. That organization entered the war period with an active and associate membership of 33 schools. It ended it with 37. These member schools were constituent units of colleges or universities. They offered one or more of three types of programs—basic, combined academic and basic, and advanced. Membership, based on visitation and evaluation of the programs of the schools, carried a connotation similar to accreditation, a complication which had not been foreseen by those who were guiding the League's accreditation program.

The NOPHN's concern with collegiate programs for the prepara-

[1] Goodrich, Annie W.: *The Social and Ethical Significance of Nursing.* The Macmillan Company, New York, 1932, p. 318.
[2] There were 138. *Facts about Nursing.* NIB, New York, 1946, p. 39.

tion of public health nurses, it will be recalled, antedated by more than a decade the organization of the ACSN. It was now found that the programs of the NLNE and the ACSN tended to overlap and thus to confuse issues. Some nurse educators felt that a special department of the NLNE could have dealt as effectively with the development of collegiate schools as a separate organization. To clarify the situation, the ACSN in 1943 reaffirmed the standards or purposes it had adopted in 1935:

1. To develop nursing education on a professional and collegiate level;
2. To promote and strengthen relationships between schools of nursing and institutions of higher learning;
3. To promote study and experimentation in nursing service and nursing education.[3]

The effectiveness of the leadership of the association bore no relationship to either its small size or its limited economic resources. All of its wartime activities were executed in cooperation with one or more organizations. In cooperation with the League, the ACSN asked the American Council on Education for assistance in promoting more effective understanding of nursing and its educational needs. It was a logical request as both organizations were members of the council. The conference, as previously noted, was held early in 1942. Generally speaking, nurse educators did not use the terminology of education. The conference, therefore, got off to a rather slow start. But, "The conference was significant," said the president, Dr. George F. Zook, "not only because it promised needed assistance for nursing schools but also because it helped to build a common understanding between two groups of educators whose interests should draw them more closely together in the future."[4] A brochure based on the proceedings of the conference was published by the council, thus ensuring it an entree to collegiate circles. Nursing, it was pointed out, was in a period of transition "from the older apprenticeship training to professional education; from the control

---

[3] *Proceedings of the Tenth Annual Meeting*, Association of Collegiate Schools of Nursing, 1943, p. 30.

[4] *Nursing Education for National Service*, Series I, Committees of the Council, #17, Vol. VI, p. 8. American Council on Education, Washington, D.C., May, 1942.

of service agencies to professional control; and from a conception of public service in the interests of the institution operating the school to one of primary concern for the interests of the public as a whole." Practical suggestions as to ways by which universities and colleges could help to educate nurses comprise a considerable portion of the text. The recommendations agreed upon by the members of the conference were grouped under general headings—counseling students, preclinical courses, and complete basic and advanced programs.

Educational institutions and nursing schools promptly began to ask for specific assistance. No one organizational pattern had been followed by the pioneer collegiate schools. They were necessarily developed in accordance with the general structure of the universities with which they were connected. Finding an open door to a university had been the primary desideratum; the school or division which gave entrance to it was secondary to it. The stimulating conference report was therefore quickly followed by the publication of *A Guide for the Organization of Collegiate Schools of Nursing.* This was sponsored jointly by the ACSN and the National Nursing Council. It was prepared under the auspices of a committee of the council, of which Isabel M. Stewart was chairman. This *Guide* defined a collegiate school as "a complete structural and functional unit for the conduct of a program of nursing education as an integral part of a college or university. . . . To be an integral part of a college or university, the school of nursing must be financially supported and fully controlled by it, the control operating through the regular lines of authority."[5] The section on curriculum is prefaced by the following statement of basic philosophy:

Nursing is based on an organized body of scientific and practical knowledge and is motivated by a social philosophy which has its roots in the traditions of the charitable and religious orders, as well as in the secular traditions of the family of medicine to which it now belongs. Some traditional concepts of authority and discipline have hampered its progress toward a full democratic philosophy, but the profession is moving in

[5] *A Guide for the Organization of Collegiate Schools of Nursing,* National Nursing Council for War Service and ACSN, New York, 1942. Revised and published by NLNE, New York, 1946.

that direction. Nursing education is rapidly evolving out of a system of modified apprenticeship into a system of direct professional education. To accelerate this development, it needs to strengthen its scientific content, deepen its social understandings, and emphasize more the general cultural aspects of the nurse's preparation. Colleges and universities are in a position to give substantial help in this process.[6]

As in other major wartime programs, it seemed necessary to follow distribution of the printed word with opportunities for discussion. A subcommittee of the NLNE's Committee on Educational Problems in Wartime, as previously noted, took the initiative in arranging a series of regional conferences (1944). The ACSN shared this responsibility, and the conferences were planned with the active cooperation of the American Council on Education. Programs were arranged in accordance with the needs of the regions in which they were held. They were well attended by representatives of hospitals, schools of nursing, and representatives of general education. Since there is a place for experimentation and wide diversity in collegiate schools, educators repeatedly warned against efforts to establish restricted programs for them. The reports of these informal discussions of many phases of collegiate school development were synthesized and published in the form of questions and answers.[7] The report ends with some criteria for evaluating the collegiate school of nursing.

As previously stated, the ACSN accepted responsibility for promoting research in nursing education and nursing practice as a normal function of collegiate schools. In this it was following an established principle of professional education. The application of the principle to collegiate schools of nursing has been well stated by a president of the University of Minnesota:

It is the responsibility of the university to carry on research in the technics of nursing to the end that a steady improvement in nursing practice will result. The 80 college and university schools of nursing may train only a small portion of the nurses, and their hospitals may provide care for a small minority of the patients, but the discoveries they make and the

[6] *Ibid.*, p. 18.
[7] *Problems of Collegiate Schools of Nursing Offering Basic Professional Programs*, Committee on Educational Problems in Wartime, NLNE. The NLNE, New York, 1945.

demonstrations they give of what the best practice can do will probably affect the nursing practice of the entire nation both inside and outside the hospitals. Good hospitals that maintain nursing schools give training in accord with the best tested practice. University schools must go beyond this. They must set up and test new standards.[8]

The conferences stimulated widespread interest in collegiate programs. Need for consultation services became acute. Requests for information and assistance poured in on the deans of the better known schools. The association attempted to make provision for such service by arranging for representatives of member schools to respond to requests for consultation. It was in this small but potent organization that astute observers began to see the face of the future, and the ACSN became an active participant in the program for restructuring the profession.

BIBLIOGRAPHY

"Accrediting Programs of the Nursing Organizations," *Am. J. Nursing,* **47**:698, 1947.
Admission and Matriculation Requirements of Colleges and Universities Offering Advanced Curricula for Graduate Nurses. Association of Collegiate Schools of Nursing, New York, 1941.
Goodrich, Annie W.: "University Schools of Nursing," *The Social and Ethical Significance of Nursing.* The Macmillan Company, New York, 1932, p. 314.
Lorentz, Mildred: "Five Regional Conferences on Problems of Collegiate Schools of Nursing," *Fiftieth Annual Report of the National League of Nursing Education,* 1944, pp. 145–53.
Newell, Hope: *History of the National Nursing Council.* National Organization for Public Health Nursing, distributor, New York, 1951.
Soule, Elizabeth S.: "Building the University School," *Am. J. Nursing,* **38**:580, 1938.
Stewart, Isabel M.: *The Education of Nurses.* The Macmillan Company, New York, 1943, p. 231.
———: "Some Reflections Supplementing the Report on Collegiate School Conferences," *Fiftieth Annual Report of the National League of Nursing Education,* 1944, pp. 154–60.

[8] Coffey, Walter C.: "Education Plans for the Future of Nursing," *Mod. Hosp.,* **61**:62, 1943.

Chapter 42

THE NATIONAL ASSOCIATION OF
COLORED GRADUATE NURSES

N.A.C.G.N. wages the battle for better health on two fronts—against discrimination, and for improved standards of nursing training and hospital care.[1]

WORLD WAR I started the migration of Negroes to industrial centers which reached flood stage during the exciting forties. Race relations rapidly became a matter for national as well as regional consideration. When the nation became involved in World War II, the NACGN was well equipped to grasp the opportunity it brought to Negro nurses. To substantiate that statement, it is necessary to summarize some of the occurrences of the decades between the wars.

Following World War I, as Edwin R. Embree pointed out, there was "a shift from the myth of inferiority to the idea that Negroes had potentialities for growth and development."[2] The program of the Rosenwald Fund, of which Mr. Embree was president, effectively fostered those potentialities by a broad-scale program to improve the education and the health of Negroes. A few Negro nurses had proved their worth in the ANC in World War I. Following that war the ANA and the NLNE began considering the possibility of developing an affiliation between the NACGN, which had only 375 members, and the ANA. But membership in alumnae associations was then a prerequisite for ANA membership, and no data were available to provide a workable basis for affiliation. Of 37 schools then providing training for Negro nurses, 24 were accredited by state boards of nurse examiners. Some of them were accredited by

[1] *N.A.C.G.N.–Four Decades of Service.* The National Association of Colored Graduate Nurses, Inc., New York, 1945, p. 1.
[2] Embree, Edwin R., and Waxman, Julia: *Investment in People*, The Story of the Julius Rosenwald Fund. Harper & Brothers, New York, 1949, p. 162.

very liberal interpretations of the minimum requirements. Fortunately, other agencies were also becoming interested in the preparation and opportunities for Negro doctors and nurses. A short-lived organization called the Hospital Library and Service Bureau made a study in 1925 of educational facilities and opportunities for employment of Negro nurses. This study, although there were a few good schools, showed that facilities for the preparation of Negro nurses were generally lamentably inadequate and that there was little evidence of interest in improving them. The AMA made a study of Negro hospitals in 1928 which revealed serious lack of facilities for the education and practice of Negro physicians. As for nursing, this report states that: "The conditions under which Negro nurses are trained in Negro hospitals are deplorable."[3]

A few years later the Rosenwald Fund compiled data on Negro hospitals from these and other sources. It also arranged with the NOPHN for a comprehensive study of the employment of Negro nurses by public health nursing agencies. More than one-half of the Negro nurses, in the study of 157 agencies, were employed by official agencies. Few of them would have any opportunity to attain supervisory positions. This was only partly due to racial discrimination. Negro nurses in general were in urgent need of better basic preparation and opportunities for postgraduate work. Graduates of Southern schools, it was pointed out, were especially in need of preparation for medical and pediatric nursing. This problem was not, at that time, limited to schools for Negroes since surgery was still the dominant interest in many of the Southern hospitals which were operating schools. Few Negro graduates of Northern schools were interested in practicing nursing in the South where employment conditions were less stable and less desirable. By 1930, it must be remembered, there was a national plethora of poorly prepared nurses, but this report provides interesting data on tenure. Some of the Negro nurses had been in their positions for very considerable periods.

[3] "Investigation of Negro Hospitals; Made under the Direction of the Council on Medical Education and Hospitals of the American Medical Association," *J.A.M.A.*, **92**:1375, 1929.

Two years later, the Rosenwald Fund sent two highly qualified nurses to the Southern states to find answers to the questions: (1) Has the Negro public health nurse in the South proved herself? (2) If so, how can Southern communities be provided with a sufficient number of nurses with good qualifications for the work?[4] The fund was then helping to finance the work of 35 Negro nurses. The report bears eloquent testimony to the high quality of the work of some of the nurses who were observed in action. Health officers reported need for many more of them for both urban and rural positions. The theory that Negroes were especially susceptible to certain diseases was giving way to evidence that the high incidence among them of tuberculosis and venereal disease was due to ignorance, substandard housing, and other social conditions. There were two obstacles to securing adequate numbers of nurses: inadequate financing of public health agencies and lack of facilities in the South for preparation of Negro public health nurses. However, between 1931 and 1940, the decade in which the Social Security Act gave tremendous impetus to the development of public health nursing by official agencies, the number of Negro public health nurses in the US increased by 38 per cent.

The report of a study, subsidized by the Rosenwald Fund, of the employment of Negro nurses by visiting nurse services reveals a constructive picture. Although the associations had improved their services to Negroes, there was no marked increase in the employment of Negro nurses. But six of the organizations that were studied offered a total of 20 fellowships to Negro nurses for postgraduate work. Thirteen fellowships were awarded by the Chicago Visiting Nurse Association, which had been the first organization of its type to employ a Negro nurse (1905).[5] The report stresses the importance of staff education for Negro nurses "since all too often they have had the handicap of poor undergraduate education." In doing health work among Negroes, it was pointed out, there was

[4] Gage, Nina D., and Haupt, Alma C.: "Some Observations on Negro Nursing in the South," *Pub. Health Nursing*, 24:674, 1932.

[5] Jessie C. Sleet Scales was employed in 1900 by the Charity Organization Society of New York to work among her own people. *Am. J. Nursing*, 1:729, 1901.

need for more attention to housing and nutrition and a real under-standing of Negro mores and motivations. "Negro personnel are best able to manage Negro patients," provided they have been ade-quately prepared for the work.[6]

It is not surprising that the investigations of the Rosenwald Fund revealed a lack of leadership among Negro nurses. Provision for nurses was therefore included in the fund's fellowship program. The first of nine fellowships awarded nurses for advanced study was granted in 1929 to one who was destined to become a standard bearer for good nursing and for social equality. This was G. Estelle Massey, then superintendent of nurses at the Homer G. Phillips Hospital, St. Louis, Missouri, who secured a master's degree at Teachers College in 1931. Soon thereafter the struggling little NACGN began to take on national importance. With limited fi-nancial support from the Rosenwald Fund, and office space pro-vided by the National Health Circle for Colored People, the NACGN established headquarters in New York (1934). Estelle Massey (then Mrs. Riddle), was president with the equally zealous Mrs. Mabel Keaton Staupers, a graduate of the Freedmen's Hos-pital School of Nursing, in the key position of executive secretary. The circle worked with the NACGN to secure scholarships for nurses who would prepare for work in the South. Located in the building which housed the three national nursing organizations, there followed years of steadily mounting rapport fostered by the ANA through a committee composed of representatives of all three. The ANA had never excluded qualified nurses from membership on a race basis. When, after the reorganization of 1916, membership was based on membership in a state nurses' association, special provision was made for the continued membership of the alumnae of the Freedmen's Hospital School for Nurses. By 1936 the NACGN had increased its membership 500 per cent and was firmly estab-lished. Then began "ten years of expansion, of collecting facts, of advising the Negro nurse and translating her to the community; ten years of holding conferences and organizing local branches, thus

[6] Cornely, Paul B.: "A Study of Negro Nursing," *Pub. Health Nursing*, **34:** 449, 1942.

merging individual minds into the basic concept of unity, a decade of following up policies and practices thwarting the professional growth of the Negro nurse."[7]

During the life of the National Youth Administration, one of the federal depression agencies, brilliantly dynamic Mary McLeod Bethune, who directed the Division of Negro Education, gave practical assistance and effectively promoted the aspirations of the NACGN. Nor were white advocates of racial equality in this country lacking in other branches of the federal government. Under the pressures of World War II, many doors were opened which had previously been closed to Negroes. The departmentalization of "Negro problems" was recognized by increasing numbers of liberty-loving Americans as an anachronism in a democratic society. Up to that time, the Rosenwald Fund had been the most important single influence in the evolution of Negroes as nurses.

Some of the hopes and dreams of an earlier period became realities when the NACGN became a member of the National Nursing Council for War Service. The activities of the Negro unit of the council, which worked in closest cooperation with the NACGN, have been discussed in connection with the council program. Together with the ANA the council secured the integration of Negro nurses in the two military nursing services. Working with the US Cadet Nurse Corps the council secured the enrollment of approximately 2000 Negro students in schools of nursing. The democratic philosophy of the Cadet Corps and of the national nursing organizations as expressed through the National Nursing Council has had a lasting influence. Whereas only 76 schools admitted Negro students in 1946 (about one-third of them admitted Negroes only) by 1951 the total number had risen to over 300, and the number of enrolled Negro students was higher than it had been at the height of the Cadet program.

In the postwar period, the ANA continued its financial assistance to the NACGN and took successive steps toward its complete integration. Following a unanimous vote at the convention of 1946, the ANA recommended to all state and district associations that

[7] *Four Decades of Service.* NACGN, New York, 1945.

they eliminate racial bars to membership as soon as possible. The Tennessee State Nurses' Association was the first to take the recommended action. By the end of 1948 six other states had done likewise, and the ANA had made provision for the individual membership of professionally qualified nurses barred from state and local organizations. The following year the ANA suggested that the functions and responsibilities of the NACGN be absorbed in the ANA. At its Thirty-fifth Annual Convention, the NACGN voted unanimously to act on that suggestion. The ANA's platform (1950) emphasized "full participation of minority groups in association activities," and the association set up an Intergroup Relations Unit which works in cooperation with the other ANA administrative units, such as public relations, on matters of concern to minority groups. Early in 1951 the NACGN took final action. It celebrated its dissolution with a banquet in New York at which Judge Hastie said, "I can think of no incident which symbolizes the dynamics of constructive social evolution at its best more effectively or more dramatically than this gathering and its occasion."[8] The selfless courage of those who willingly relinquished positions of importance and the social significance of the ANA's leadership were quite generally recognized by the public press. By 1952 only 4 states (Georgia South Carolina, Texas, and Virginia) had not yet followed the lead of their Southern neighbors.

BIBLIOGRAPHY

An American Challenge. American Nurses' Association, New York, 1950.
Barck, Oscar Theodore, Jr., and Blake, Nelson Manfred: *Since 1900. A History of the United States in Our Times,* rev. ed. The Macmillan Company, New York, 1952, p. 832 (Rise of the Negro).
Embree, Edwin R.: *Brown Americans—The Story of a Tenth of the Nation.* Viking Press, New York, 1943.
Facts about Nursing. American Nurses' Association, New York, 1950, p. 47.

[8] Hastie, William W.: "A Farewell to N.A.C.G.N.," *Am. J. Nursing,* **51**:154, 1951.

Hamlin, Donelda R.: *Educational Facilities for Colored Nurses* (mimeographed). The Hospital Library and Service Bureau, Chicago, 1925.

Haupt, Alma C.: "A Pioneer in Negro Nursing" (Estelle Massey Riddle), *Am. J. Nursing*, 35:857, 1935.

"January Board of Directors Meeting, Joint Relations with N.A.C.G.N.," *Am. J. Nursing*, 34:499, 1934.

Landau, Henrietta: "Registered Negro Nurses in the U.S.A.," *Am. J. Nursing*, 43:730, 1943.

McIver, Pearl: "How Many Public Health Nurses?" *Pub. Health Nursing*, 33:21, 1941.

Massey, G. Estelle: "The National Association of Colored Graduate Nurses," *Am. J. Nursing*, 33:534, 1933.

————: "The Negro Nurse Student," *Fortieth Annual Report of the National League of Nursing Education*, 1934, p. 83.

Myrdal, Gunnar: *An American Dilemma, the Negro Problem and Modern Democracy.* Harper & Brothers, New York, 1944.

N.A.C.G.N.—Four Decades of Service. The National Association of Colored Graduate Nurses, Inc., New York, 1945.

Negro Hospitals. Julius Rosenwald Fund, Chicago, 1931.

"The Negro Public Health Nurse" (report of National Organization for Public Health Nursing conference), *Pub. Health Nursing*, 34:452, 1942.

Newell, Hope: "The Council's Negro Unit," *History of the National Nursing Council.* National Organization for Public Health Nursing, distributor, New York, 1951, p. 49.

Osborne, Estelle Massey: "Status and Contribution of the Negro Nurse," *J. Negro Education*, 18:364, 1949.

Rayfield, Stanley: "A Study of Negro Public Health Nursing," *Pub. Health Nursing*, 22:525, 1930.

"Report of Board of Directors of the A.N.A. to the N.A.C.G.N.," *American Nurses' Association Proceedings, Advisory Council*, 1947 and 1948, p. 44.

"Report of the Committee on Training Schools for Negro Nurses," *Thirtieth Annual Report of the National League of Nursing Education*, 1924, p. 214.

Riddle, Estelle Massey: "Negro Nurses: The Supply and Demand," *Opportunity, Journal of Negro Life*, XV:327, 1937.

Salute to Democracy at Mid-Century. National Association of Colored Graduate Nurses, Inc., New York, 1951.

Staupers, Mabel K.: "Story of the National Association of Colored Graduate Nurses," *Am. J. Nursing*, 51:222, 1951.

Thoms, Adah B.: *Pathfinders.* Kay Printing House, New York, 1929.

Chapter 43

THE AMERICAN ASSOCIATION OF
INDUSTRIAL NURSES

Industrial nursing is the practice of the art and science of nursing in industry, to meet the needs of the worker; for the purpose of developing and maintaining the highest potential level of health and efficiency through:
   1. Prompt remedial care of the ill and injured.
   2. Health and safety education.
   3. Cooperation with all health and welfare agencies.[1]

COMMERCIAL and industrial organizations operate for profit. Anything that interferes with the flow of work lessens profit. The success of industrial nursing is therefore measured by the extent to which it contributes to the reduction of loss of time due to injuries and illness and by promoting the physical and emotional well-being of the workers. This, of course, is not to say that industrialists are never influenced by humanitarian motives. It may be said, however, that through well-organized industrial medical and nursing services it has been shown that what is generally considered humanitarian care helps to pay dividends. Essentially, industrial medicine and nursing are preventive medicine and preventive nursing. The growing eminence of industrial nursing can be traced in part to the pioneers in the field and, in part, as is the case with all nursing progress, to extraneous forces.

"The industrial nurse," says the author of *Nursing in Commerce and Industry,* "has enjoyed opportunity and liberty unknown to her sisters in other branches of the profession."[2] This was due largely

[1] *AAIN Newsletter,* American Association of Industrial Nurses, Inc., New York, 1:2, 1949.
[2] McGrath, Bethel J.: *Nursing in Commerce and Industry.* The Commonwealth Fund, New York, 1946, p. xi.

to the competitive nature of commerce and industry which stresses such things as secret formulas and individual differences, and to the fact that, until relatively recently, most industrial nurses began the work without knowledge of the field or preconceived ideas about the opportunities for constructive service. Until World War II, few schools of nursing thought of it as a field for the students they were preparing for practice as graduate nurses. Under the circumstances, it is not surprising that there was a marked tendency to individualism among industrial nurses which caused many of them to resist the concept of standardization which was generally accepted in other types of nursing. When the AAIN was organized in 1942, industrial nursing in the United States was almost fifty years old. The stated purpose of the new organization was "to meet an urgent need for a vehicle through which industrial nurses could work with each other and speak authoritatively on a national scale."[3]

This appears to have been a declaration of independence from the NOPHN which, for purposes of discussion, may be considered one of the extraneous forces which has had an important influence on the development of industrial nursing. As has been shown, the NOPHN at an early date assumed that, since industrial nursing was basically a preventive service, it was a type of public health nursing. This concept, however, was so far in advance of general medical and nursing thought that it was accepted by only a relatively small percentage of industrial nurses. The very substantial contributions of the NOPHN to industrial nursing may be summed up by reference to the three thoroughly practical books which were produced under its sponsorship in 1919, 1933, and 1946. (See Chap. 40.) Experienced industrial nurses concede that the principles discussed in the second volume in this series, if such it may be called, are still valid, while the third one deals with the problems of industrial nursing in more detail.

From 1941, when the expanding war industries had begun to require far more nurses than ever before, until the close of the war, the NOPHN had an experienced industrial nurse on its staff. The

[3] *American Association of Industrial Nurses—A Thumb Nail Sketch.* AAIN, New York, 1950.

services of the consultant nurses who successively held that position were much in demand. The Social Security Act had already created an upswing of interest in the health of industrial workers by providing assistance to state and local health departments for the development of industrial hygiene programs. The USPHS employed its first industrial nurse consultant in 1941. The Indiana and Michigan state departments of health were the first to employ industrial nurse consultants. As the industrial tempo increased and more and more nurses without special preparation were employed in the field of industrial nursing, there were these several sources of much needed nurse consultant service in addition to that provided by some of the large insurance companies in which the industrial companies were insured.

A number of voluntary agencies, whose programs influence nursing, were also interested in industrial health. Through its interest in traumatic surgery the American College of Surgeons (ACS) had set up a committee on industrial medicine and traumatic surgery in 1926. After the passage of the Social Security Act it published minimum standards for the accreditation of medical services in industry comparable to the standards used in accrediting hospitals. The ACS's interpretation of the functions of industrial nurses was, however, extremely limited. It failed to specify that the departments it accredited should employ professionally qualified, i.e., graduate registered nurses. It sharply called attention to a dangerous tendency which was especially noticeable in plants making inadequate provision for medical service, viz., "Nurse and lay first-aid attendants frequently engage in medical and surgical procedures for which they are neither qualified nor licensed."[4] That error may be charged to inexperience and poor basic preparation for nursing. On this point Mrs. McGrath makes the unequivocal statement: "A nurse who fails to get medical orders makes her company legally liable, besides failing to maintain her own professional integrity."[5]

The report of a three-year consideration of standing orders may

[4] Newquist, M. N.: *Medical Service in Industry and Workmen's Compensation Laws.* American College of Surgeons, Chicago, 1938, p. 10.
[5] McGrath, B. J.: *op. cit.,* p. 52.

have some significance in the further development of medical-nursing relationships. It was based on the following principles: (1) Personal medical services involving the establishment of a diagnosis and the definition of treatment, or the performance of specific preventive measures, are functions of the physician. (2) Standing orders serve as authorization for approved routine procedures for common minor conditions, and as a directive for emergency care of more serious or complicated conditions until the physician arrives.

Several years earlier the Council on Industrial Health of the American Medical Association, organized in 1937, had published recommended standing orders for nurses in industry which have been widely used. The Wisconsin State Medical Association, it may be noted, had published such recommendations almost ten years earlier. It may be assumed that nurses with experience in public health nursing, who would naturally be accustomed to the safeguard of standing medical orders, were influential in bringing about that constructive action. However, not all physicians who care for industrial patients have subscribed to the principle of standing orders.

The public health nursing section of the American Public Health Association perceived the need for a body of information about the practice of industrial nursing. The findings of a study of the nursing services in 42 industries in a Pennsylvania county pointed the way to further study. This was followed by the report of a committee to study the duties of nurses in industry, which had representation from every part of the country. These studies led to a comprehensive investigation of nursing practices in industry by the USPHS. The resultant report is a landmark in the evolution of industrial nursing.[6]

The organization of the AAIN in 1942 followed a series of annual conferences that had begun in 1938, when the New England Association of Industrial Nurses, in which Catherine R. Dempsey was the acknowledged leader, instituted a conference with organized

[6] Whitlock, Olive M.; Trasko, Victoria M.; and Kahl, F. Ruth: *Nursing Practices in Industry*, Public Health Bulletin #283. US Government Printing Office, Washington, D.C., 1944.

groups of industrial nurses in New York, New Jersey, and Pennsylvania. There had been an earlier American Association of Industrial Nurses which had its beginnings in Boston in 1916, one year later than the New England association. It is significant that the American Association of Industrial Physicians was also organized at that time although there appears to have been no established relationship between the organizations. By this time (1942), large industries, and therefore industrial nurses, were more widely dispersed throughout the country than ever before.

The value and importance of nursing service in industry had been demonstrated by the gradual but fluctuating increase in the number of nurses employed in this field from 1895 onward. With the increased demands on industrial production and manpower, as a result of the enormous requirements of the military forces during World War II, it became imperatively necessary to consider the nation's human resources and to utilize them to the fullest extent. Early in 1942 the Surgeon General of the US Public Health Service told a convention audience of nurses that health conservation for our industrial army was the most urgent civilian need for the duration of the war. At the peak of wartime production as many as 18 million women were employed, many of them doing work which had previously been considered suitable only for men. Women lose more time than men due to sickness (not, however, due in any marked degree to "feminine ailments") and to nonindustrial accidents. Fortunately, according to experienced industrial nurses, women are, generally speaking, more responsive than men to health teaching. Recognition of the health needs of women broadened the concept of industrial medicine and nursing. It emphasized the relationship between family and community welfare, and the health situation within the plants. Many industrialists who had previously not done so found it necessary to provide health and welfare services for their employees and to utilize community facilities to the fullest extent. By 1945 the number of nurses employed in commerce and industry had reached a previously unimagined total of almost 14,000.

For more than twenty years the NOPHN had valiantly and persistently endeavored to promote the development of industrial nursing through its section on industrial nursing, which functioned also as the nursing section of the National Safety Council between 1930 and 1943. A cooperative relationship persisted after the National Safety Council organized its own nursing section. The NOPHN's efforts were based on the assumption that industrial nursing is a phase of public health nursing. But industrial nursing practice calls for the knowledge and skills derived in varying combinations, depending on the nature of the industry and the type of program it provides for its employees, from both institutional and public health nursing. The milieu in which it is practiced calls for adaptations and relationships quite unlike those in which public health nursing and institutional nursing are practiced. All industrial nurses require practical knowledge of the hazards peculiar to their respective industries, of legislation affecting the worker in his employment, and the relationships of that legislation to their responsibilities. The AAIN is rooted in the soil of the individual experience of industrial nurses. It was nurtured by their aspiration for recognition of their field as a specific component in the over-all field of health and medical care.

When the new association became a member of the National Nursing Council, it promptly informed that body of the need of facilities for the preparation of industrial nurses. The question was referred to the education committees of the NLNE and the NOPHN. Following conferences, it was agreed that the basic curriculum cannot provide for specialization in any field. Nursing schools, however, were urged to emphasize the industrial implications of nursing throughout the course, and some practical suggestions for doing so were provided. By 1945 several universities responsive to the importunities of the industrial groups were offering courses in this special field of nursing, which, in that year, celebrated the fiftieth anniversary of the inauguration of the first industrial nursing service in the US at Proctor, Vermont. Some of these offerings, however, were soon discontinued because interest in them was not sustained. The program at the University of Pittsburgh, located in the area where the first study was made of industrial nursing practices, became pre-eminent in this field.

For the first few years the new organization was largely concerned with the mechanisms of organization and the building up of its membership. It established cooperative relationships with the National Association of Manufacturers and secured a strategic endorsement by that organization of its publication, *Qualifications of an Industrial Nurse.* This was the first of a series of six standard-setting guides published by the AAIN between 1945 and 1950. In 1950 about 11,000 industrial nurses were employed in the US. A few of them were working in personnel departments and a few as visiting nurses, but the great majority were "plant" nurses. Less than a thousand of those reporting had secured experience in public health nursing before entering industry.

Despite all the activities in behalf of industrial nursing of the NOPHN and the AAIN, industrial nurse members of the ANA requested that organization to set up an industrial nurse section. It was so voted, and the section was organized in 1946.[7] By 1950, 30 state nurses' associations had organized industrial nurse sections. The AAIN was one of "the six national nursing organizations," which, under their joint boards, sponsored a number of broad-scale programs after the dissolution of the National Nursing Council. It also participated in the studies of the structure of the national organizations which led to the organization of the National League for Nursing and the expansion of ANA functions in June, 1952. The AAIN, however, withdrew from the group in the spring of 1952. At that time the industrial nurse section of the ANA had the larger membership and could draw upon the resources of other units of the ANA for assistance in the development of its program.

BIBLIOGRAPHY

Baetjer, Anna M.: *Women in Industry, Their Health and Efficiency.* W. B. Saunders Co., Philadelphia, 1946. Issued under the auspices of the

[7] *Proceedings of the American Nurses' Association,* Vol. I, House of Delegates. 1946.

Division of Medical Sciences and the Division of Engineering and Industrial Research of the National Research Council.

Dempsey, Catherine: "Introducing the A.A.I.N.," *Trained Nurse and Hospital Review,* **108**:440–42, 1942.

"Duties of Nurses in Industry," *Am. J. Nursing,* **43**:635, 1943.

"Duties of Nurses in Industry," *Am. J. Pub. Health,* **33**:865, 1943.

"Essentials of Medical-Nursing Services in Industry" (a statement prepared jointly by the American Association of Industrial Nurses, the Industrial Medical Association, and the Council on Industrial Health of the American Medical Association), *J.A.M.A.,* **149**:597, 1952.

Hodgson, Violet H.: *Public Health Nursing in Industry.* The Macmillan Company, New York, 1933.

Hogan, Margaret: "Social Forces and Industrial Nursing," *Nursing World,* **125**:26, 1951.

"Including Industrial Nursing in the Basic Curriculum," *Pub. Health Nursing,* **37**:129, 1945.

"The Industrial Nurse and the War," *Am. J. Nursing,* **43**:57, 1943.

"Industrial Nursing," *Facts about Nursing.* NIB, New York, 1945, p. 67.

"Industrial Nursing Personnel Essential to Maximum War Effort" (Executive Committee, Industrial Nursing Section, National Organization for Public Health Nursing), *Pub. Health Nursing,* **35**:3, 1943.

Klem, Margaret C.; McKiever, Margaret F.; and Lear, Walter J.: *Industrial Health and Medical Programs* (a source book). US Public Health Service Publication #15, Federal Security Agency, Washington, D.C., September, 1950.

Lanza, A. J., and Goldberg, Jacob A. (eds.): *Industrial Hygiene.* Oxford University Press, New York, 1939.

McGrath, Bethel J.: "Fifty Years of Industrial Nursing in the United States," *Pub. Health Nursing,* **37**:119, 1945.

———: *Nursing in Commerce and Industry.* The Commonwealth Fund, New York, 1946.

Markolf, Ada Stewart: "Industrial Nursing Begins in Vermont," *Pub. Health Nursing,* **37**:125, 1945.

Parran, Thomas: "Health Needs of the Nation," *Forty-eighth Annual Report of the National League of Nursing Education,* 1942, p. 60.

Petrinic, Alice J.: "Guidance for the Nurse in Industry—the Industrial Nursing Supervisor," *Pub. Health Nursing,* **36**:533, 1944.

Rood, Dorothy: "The University and the Industrial Nurse," *Am. J. Nursing,* **41**:201, 1941.

Scott, Ruth M.: "State Consultants Serve Industrial Nurses," *Pub. Health Nursing,* **34**:271, 1942.

"Standing Orders for Nurses in Industry," *J.A.M.A.,* **122**:1247, 1943.

Stern, Bernhard J.: *Medicine in Industry.* The Commonwealth Fund, New York, 1946.

"Study of Industrial Nursing Services," *Pub. Health Nursing,* **32:**631, 1940.

Wampler, Fred J. (ed.): *The Principles and Practice of Industrial Medicine.* Williams & Wilkins Co., Baltimore, 1943.

Whitlock, Olive M.: "Nursing Services," *Manual of Industrial Hygiene and Medical Service in War Industries* (William M. Gafafer, ed.). W. B. Saunders Co., Philadelphia, 1943, Chap. 5, pp. 66–87.

Wright, Florence Swift: *Industrial Nursing.* The Macmillan Company, New York, 1919.

Ziano, Joan Y.: "Guidance for the Nurse in Industry—the State Industrial Nurse Consultant," *Pub. Health Nursing,* **36:**528, 1944.

Chapter 44

THE NATIONAL ASSOCIATION FOR
PRACTICAL NURSE EDUCATION

A trained practical nurse is a person trained to care for semi-acute, convalescent and chronic patients requiring service under public health nursing agencies, or in institutions, or in homes; she works under the direction of a licensed physician or the supervision of a registered, professional nurse and is prepared to give household assistance when necessary.

NAPNE, 1947

The practical nurse is a person trained to care for selected convalescent, subacutely and chronically ill patients, and to assist the professional nurse in a team relationship, especially in the care of those more acutely ill. She provides nursing service in institutions, and in private homes where she is prepared to give household assistance when necessary. She may be employed by a private individual, a hospital, or a health agency. A practical nurse works only under the direct orders of a licensed physician or the supervision of a registered professional nurse.[1]

THE NATIONAL ASSOCIATION for Practical Nurse Education (NAPNE) and the National Federation of Licensed Practical Nurses (NFLPN) were not members of the group of six organizations, discussed in the preceding chapters, which organized a joint board of directors in 1949 "to facilitate joint action on matters of common concern." They did, however, have a functional relationship to the joint committees which operated under the aegis of the six organizations, one of which prepared the policy-setting publication quoted at the beginning of this chapter.[2]

[1] *Practical Nurses in Nursing Services*, Joint Committee on Practical Nurses and Auxiliary Workers in Nursing Services (ANA, NLNE, NOPHN, NACGN, ACSN, AAIN, in cooperation with NAPNE, NFLPN) ANA, New York, 1951, p. 11.

[2] "Our Elected Representatives and How They Work," *Am. J. Nursing*, **49**: 129, 1949.

The word nurse was already firmly embedded in the English language when Miss Nightingale began her reforms. For this reason all efforts to restrict its use without some qualifying adjective have failed. The "practical" nurse has existed from time immemorial. The compassionate deaconesses and sisterhoods of the early Christian church had only the knowledge gained by experience. Dickens' Sairey Gamp, a caricature of the practical nurses of his time, called attention to the need for more careful selection of those who were to tend the sick. In our own country, Dr. Alfred Worcester and others wrote with deep appreciation of the "night watcher," the practical, generous-hearted, friendly neighbor of our Colonial and later periods. Volumes have been written about the courageous work of "Mother Bickerdyke" and other practical nurses during the War Between the States. In our own times the group has grown so large and heterogeneous that those whose service has been a blessing to patients and their families have tended to be overshadowed by the less dependable; a condition which is now being combated by organized effort.

Practical nurses and a variety of other nonprofessional workers in the field of nursing have represented an indigenous rather than a planned response to human need. In 1940 there were almost 190,-000 of these workers in the United States.[3] Most of them had not taken organized courses of any kind. Among the exceptions to this generalization were the graduates of a few schools for household or practical nurses. Among the better known schools were those operated by the YWCA in New York which antedated the oldest professional nursing organizations, the widely and favorably known Household Nursing Association in Boston, a school organized by the Thomas Thompson Trust in Brattleboro, Vermont, and the successors to earlier efforts in Detroit and Cleveland. The aim of such schools was preparation of workers for the care of the sick in their own homes, but there was growing evidence that they might usefully be employed by institutions and visiting nurse services. Feeling the

[3] "Practical Nurses and Hospital Attendants," *The Outlook for Women in Occupations in the Medical Services*, Bulletin #203, No. 5, p. 2. Women's Bureau, US Department of Labor, Washington, D.C., 1945.

need for mutual aid, the registered nurse directors of some of these schools met in informal conference in 1938. Out of that and succeeding conferences came the organization in 1941 of the National Association for Practical Nurse Education.[4] This association, with a small membership of professional and practical nurses and non-nurses, has made up in crusading zeal what it lacked in numbers. Financial support has been provided by a number of foundations and other sources interested in meeting a need for less skilled and less costly service than that of graduate professional nurses.

The NAPNE became a member of the National Nursing Council, and for a time Hilda Torrop, the forceful promoter of the new organization, served as consultant to the council. When the council secured the active interest of the General Federation of Women's Clubs in the recruitment of student nurses during the war, the federation promoted enrollment in both professional and practical nursing schools. It will be recalled that the ANA had for some time been encouraging state associations to work for legislation which would help to standardize the preparation and practice of these workers.

In 1944 the NAPNE secured the active interest of the Vocational Education Division of the US Office of Education. The division appointed a working committee made up of qualified representatives from the national nursing, hospital, and educational organizations, from the US Public Health Service, and the US Office of Education. The committee did some hard work under the direction of an expert in vocational education. A job analysis of the practical nurse occupation was undertaken as the essential first step in a constructive program. Nurse educators admitted that working on this committee was a salutary experience. The analysis,[5] published in 1947, was followed in 1950 by the carefully prepared *Practical Nursing Curriculum*. The committee ignored the involved definition in the *Dic-*

[4] "Auxiliary Workers' Instructors Organized," *Am. J. Nursing*, **42**:1211, 1942.

[5] *Practical Nursing, An Analysis of the Practical Nurse Occupation with Suggestions for the Organization of Training Programs*, Misc. #8, Federal Security Agency, Office of Education. Government Printing Office, Washington, D.C., 1947.

tionary of Occupational Titles and used that of the NAPNE which heads this chapter.

There was no uniformity in the legal requirements for the approval of practical nurse schools in the few states which had secured legislation. Some of the best-known schools were in states without such protection. The NAPNE therefore set up an accreditation program. Its requirements were not always in accord with those of the state boards. The National Nursing Council, for its recruitment program, published an inclusive list of the schools approved by the NAPNE, and those approved by state boards of nurse examiners. That list revealed a dichotomy of interests between the NAPNE and the professional organizations. Legal status, based on licenses to practice, provided a bond between practical nurses such as had not previously existed. Organization was the next logical step.

The pioneer association of practical nurses, Practical Nurses of New York, Inc., was organized in 1940. The infant organization had less than 200 charter members but it had constructive ideas. It promptly began working cooperatively with the New York State Nurses' Association through a joint conference committee which functions as a clearing bureau on matters of mutual interest. The Milbank Memorial Fund financed an important study of the counseling and placement of practical nurses for the association in 1945. The report called attention to the highly significant fact that progress for the group had been the result of lay and medical leadership rather than that of either practical or professional nurses. Investigation of the service provided for practical nurses by professionally sponsored registries revealed limited facilities and only mild interest in the provision of counseling and placement service for practical nurses. This observation could have been substantiated by reference to the ANA's study of registries in 1942. Little more than one-half of all the professionally sponsored registries were then providing service for nonprofessional nurses. The recommendation that the minimum salary of practical nurses be 75 per cent of that of professional nurses was subsequently adopted by the association. This pioneer state association of practical nurses spearheaded the movement which resulted in the affiliation of 13 state associations of practical nurses to form the National Federation of Licensed Practical Nurses in 1949. The following year the ANA encouraged all state nurses' associations to work with practical nurses in relation to improvement in preparation and conditions of employment.

As Dorothy Deming, in the Preface to her admirably comprehensive study, *The Practical Nurse,* has said: "Patients have always wanted and will always want practical nurses for certain types and stages of illness."[6] Why then has the profession so reluctantly accepted responsibility for the preparation and supervision of a second group of workers in the field of nursing? The causes are deep-seated. They stem from the stultifying poverty and restricted aims of nursing schools which were organized to serve the needs of particular institutions rather than to prepare nurses to meet community needs. The professional and periodic economic insecurity of the very considerable numbers of nurses prepared in schools which met only the minimum standards set by law understandably has been a serious deterrent to liberal thought and courageous action. But, as we shall see in our discussion of postwar nursing needs and resources, practical nurses seem destined, in team relationships, to provide an increasingly important part of the nursing service required to maintain the health and welfare of the American people. If they are to avoid making some of the mistakes that have hampered the development of professional nursing, there must be, and there are abundant evidences that there will continue to be, constructive and friendly collaboration between the two groups of practitioners.

The NAPNE was not a participant in the study of structure of the national nursing organizations which culminated in the organization of the NLN. Because its interest, as its name implies, is in the *education* of practical nurses, it is hoped that its functions may be fused with those of the NLN in the near future.

BIBLIOGRAPHY

Accreditation of Schools of Practical Nursing. National Association for Practical Nurse Education, New York, 1949.

[6] Deming, Dorothy: *The Practical Nurse.* The Commonwealth Fund, New York, 1947.

"A.N.A. Cooperates with N.F.L.P.N." (National Federation of Licensed Practical Nurses), *Am. J. Nursing,* **51:**259, 1951.

"Annual Report of the President," *Practical Nurse News,* **7:**1–2, 1950.

Bradley, Richard M.: "Household Nursing in Relation to Other Similar Work," *Am. J. Nursing,* **15:**968, 1915.

Given, Leila I.: "Licenses for Nursing—Professional and Practical," *Nursing World,* **75:**186, 1951.

Goulding, Fern A.: *A Selected Bibliography to Accompany the Practical Nurse Curriculum.* Office of Education, US Government Printing Office, Washington, D.C., 1950.

Jarrett, Mary C.: *A Brief Study of Counseling and Placement of Practical Nurses in New York State.* Published under a grant from the Milbank Memorial Fund by the Committee for Recruitment and Education of Practical Nurses of New York, Inc., New York, 1945.

Kuster, Lillian E.: "National Federation of Licensed Practical Nurses," *Nursing World,* **75:**189, 1951.

Phillips, Elisabeth C.: "Developments in the Field of Practical Nursing—Professional Organization Activities," *Am. J. Nursing,* **52:**73, 1952.

Practical Nurse Education: Manual for State and Local Leagues (mimeographed). National League of Nursing Education, New York, 1949.

Practical Nurses in Nursing Services. Prepared by the Joint Committee on Practical Nurses and Auxiliary Workers in Nursing Services in cooperation with the National Association for Practical Nurse Education and the National Federation of Licensed Practical Nurses. American Nurses' Association, New York, 1951.

Practical Nursing Curriculum, Suggestions for Developing a Program of Instruction Based upon the Analysis of the Practical Nurse Occupation. Miscellaneous Publication #11, Federal Security Agency, Office of Education. US Government Printing Office, Washington, D.C., 1947.

Study of the Employment of Graduates of the Michigan Practical Nurse Training Program. Wayne University College of Nursing, Detroit, 1951.

Study of Organization, Control, Policies and Financing of Nurses' Professional Registries. American Nurses' Association, New York, 1942.

Torrop, Hilda M.: "The First Ten Years of NAPNE," *Nursing World,* **75:**188, 1951.

———: "NAPNE Reports," *Am. J. Nursing,* **52:**72, 1952.

Worcester, Alfred: *Nurses for Our Neighbors.* Houghton Mifflin Co., Boston, 1914.

SECTION X. THE ATOMIC AGE   1945 – 1952

Chapter 45

NURSING IN TRANSITION

War is a catalyst, not a creator. It rarely, if ever, initiates new forces. It accentuates and accelerates processes already in operation.

C.-E. A. WINSLOW[1]

Nursing is one of the services for the care of the sick, the prevention of illness and for the promotion of health which is carried on under medical authority. Nursing is designed to provide physical and emotional care for the patient; to care for his immediate environment; to carry out treatment prescribed by the physician; to teach the patient and his family the nursing care which they may have to perform; to give general health instruction; to supervise auxiliary aides and co-ordinate the services of other workers contributing to patient and family care. This service may be given in hospitals or other institutions for the care of the sick, in homes, in community health agencies, in industries or in schools.[2]

WORLD WAR II was indeed a catalyst as described by Professor Winslow. International and national forces already in operation in the field of health were greatly accelerated by it. The program of the World Health Organization (WHO), for example, which inherited the functions of the Health Organization of the League of Nations and of the Health Division of the United Nations Relief and Rehabilitation Adminstration (UNRRA), is far more extensive than the sum of the earlier programs. Discussion of nursing in connection with it and other international agencies may be found in Chapter 51. In the US, wartime health programs—military and civilian—had

---

[1] Winslow, C.-E. A.: "Postwar Trends in Public Health and Nursing," *Am. J. Nursing*, **45**:989, 1945.

[2] Report on the program of "Temporary Accreditation of the National Accrediting Service," Part II, p. 19. National League for Nursing (Division of Nursing Education), New York, 1952.

made citizens more health conscious than ever before. They were enjoying the highest standard of living the world has ever known, and increasing numbers of people were beginning to regard health protection and medical care as a basic human need comparable to food, shelter, and clothing. Powerful labor organizations were demanding health benefits and in so doing were accelerating the development of prepayment health and medical care programs. At mid-century a few of them had established highly organized health centers. One was reported to have the erection of a chain of hospitals under consideration. The acceleration of processes already in operation was clearly revealed by data on hospital admissions. Whereas the population increased by 14.5 per cent in the wartime decade, the number of patients annually admitted to hospitals more than doubled between 1935 and 1950.[3]

Almost twenty years had been added to the life expectancy of persons born at mid-century as compared with those born in 1900. The Surgeon General of the USPHS declared that the health of adults, in sharp contrast with the emphasis on child care in the early part of the century, had become the nation's primary health problem. The infant death rate for 1950 was the lowest ever recorded, and community programs for the care of premature infants were calling for nurses with special preparation. But there was still much to be done for children. As the mid-century White House Conference pointed out, physical health is not enough. That important conference was devoted to consideration of the development of healthy personalities. Rehabilitation of the handicapped and medical care programs adapted to the needs of an aging population were broadening the scope of nursing. Heart disease and cancer had displaced pneumonia and tuberculosis as the principal causes of death. Venereal diseases were yielding to penicillin and sulfa drugs. The fluorination of water supplies was beginning to reduce dental decay, one of the most common ailments. Arthritis and other disabling conditions were demanding more and more attention. The hormones—ACTH and cortisone—had been added to the list of amaz-

[3] "Hospital Service in the United States, The 1951 Census of Hospitals," *J.A.M.A.*, **149**:11, (May 10) 1952 (reprint).

ing mid-century therapeutic agents. Success in treating a few tuberculosis patients with antibiotics and isoniazid made exciting news. Years of usefulness could be added to the lives of cancer patients by early diagnosis and treatment, and the later stages relieved by miraculous advances in surgery. Although the average hospital stay was steadily being reduced, surgical advances, such as those in cardiovascular and neurological surgery, required longer periods of hospitalization and the highest degree of nursing skill. The increasing number of poliomyelitis patients, adults as well as children, was also challenging the skills of nurses. There had been a time when the inclusion of the elements of physics in the curriculum was questioned. The problem had ceased to be debatable, not only in relation to the use of the Respir-aid rocking bed but also the "iron lung" for polio patients. Many surgical procedures required the postoperative use of transfusions, infusions, and the use of suction. Parenteral medication was demanding more and more time.

The average hospital stay of patients had been shortened by early ambulation and the newer therapies, but the number and complexity of the diagnostic tests and the surgical and other treatments they received had been greatly increased. While the volume of medical care was being enormously expanded by advances in medical science, in psychosomatic and in physical medicine, the medical profession, as represented by its national organization, had not encouraged any marked increase in the number of doctors. As a result, by mid-century there were almost a score of health professions. Doctors necessarily became the leaders of health teams (not always recognized as such) composed of nurses, nutritionists, social workers, occupational therapists, physical therapists, and other professionally and technically prepared workers in varying combinations. Nursing, faced with the necessity for devising new technics and new patterns of nursing service, found it essential to re-emphasize the importance of preparing professional nurses for competence in nursing practice and for leadership in nursing education, nursing service, and in community relationships.

Nurses shared the pervasive sense of postwar disillusion and lack of direction, but not for long. The catalytic force of the enormously increased demand for nursing service accelerated action in relation to curriculum revision and patterns of nursing service. Consideration of the reconstruction of the national nursing organizations, held in abeyance during the war, was actively resumed at the earliest possible date. The superb work of the Structure Committee, which was carried forward concurrently with the basic programs of the organizations, especially that of the National Committee for the Improvement of Nursing Services, is discussed in Chapter 49. The ANA, in the first formally stated platform ever adopted by its House of Delegates (1946), balanced consideration of ways and means for meeting the demand for nursing services with concern for the welfare of nurses. The congress of the International Council of Nurses, for which the ANA was hostess in 1947, had an inspirationally tonic effect on the whole profession.

By the middle of 1946 almost 45,000 nurses had been released from military service.[4] Enrollment in nursing schools early that year stood at the all-time high of 129,000 students, most of whom were members of the US Cadet Nurse Corps. But the National Nursing Council estimated that 41,700 more nurses were required than appeared to be available.[5] The Veterans Administration was rapidly adding to its roster of patients and needed many more nurses; but the clamor for nurses, for clamor it was, was created by physicians and by the civilian hospitals which continued to operate at capacity. Both groups had anticipated a swift restoration of prewar staffing and were not easily persuaded that the "shortage" of nurses was due to the increased demands for nurses in all fields, including the offices of physicians.

Nursing was credited by Surg. Gen. Scheele with being the first professional group to make a critical analysis of its problems and to formulate a constructive program. This was recognition of the postwar program of the National Nursing Council which had been released to the state associations and other agencies coincidentally with the bombing of Hiroshima.[6] Well-established nursing councils,

[4] *Facts about Nursing,* 1945, NIB, p. 22.
[5] *Facts about Nursing,* 1946, NIB, p. 32.
[6] "A Comprehensive Program for Nationwide Action in the Field of Nursing," *Am. J. Nursing,* **45**:707, 1945.

such as those in existence in Boston, Detroit, and some other metro-politan areas, were especially well prepared to carry forward com-prehensive programs. But the overwhelming magnitude of the post-war demand for nursing service had not been anticipated by either the council or the employing agencies. A well-attended National Health Assembly (1948) whetted citizen as well as professional in-terest in health and medical care programs. The assembly and the ten-year health program, subsequently prepared for President Tru-man by the Federal Social Security Administration,[7] aroused parti-sanship on the highly controversional question of compulsory versus voluntary insurance as a method for paying for medical care which was steadily becoming both more scientific and more costly. At that time more than 30,000,000 persons were enrolled in Blue Cross (hospital) plans. This and other prepayment plans, in which some 90,000,000 people were enrolled by 1952, constituted an important factor in the mounting demand for nursing service.

Shortage of nurses! In that irritatingly recurrent phrase, which was to be replaced by the more accurate "increased demand for nursing service," may be found the motivation for sharp acceleration of processes in both nursing education and nursing services which were already in existence. The special characteristics of the evolving postwar program were summarized as: (1) recognition of nursing as a service to be planned in relation to community needs, (2) the preparation and licensure of practical nurses, (3) critical evaluation and reconstruction of educational programs—basic and advanced—for professional nurses, (4) removal of nursing schools from the con-trol of service agencies to an appropriate place in the educational system of the nation, (5) reorganization of the professional organi-zations to ensure unity of action within the profession and in inter-professional and community relationships in the development of nursing education and nursing service, and in promoting the welfare of the members of the profession.

The social significance of nursing is indicated by the variety of agencies which made estimates of the nation's need for nurses in this

[7] Ewing, Oscar R.: *The Nation's Health—A Ten-Year Program.* US Govern-ment Printing Office, Washington, D.C., 1948, p. 38.

period. The President's Commission on Higher Education used data prepared by the US Women's Bureau. Those prepared for the Conference on the Nation's Health were based on the current ratio of nurses, both professional and practical, to population (one for every 280 persons) in the 12 states "at the top of the ladder." Following the passage of the National Defense Act in 1947, nursing was again declared an essential service; military nursing services were expanded and nurses were called upon to participate in the civil defense program. The NLNE responded to this new emphasis on preparation for disaster by preparing a guide for instructors. It was, however, the state nurses' associations that accepted responsibility for implementing the program by means of which thousands of nurses received special instruction. Nurses in the National Capital learned that civil defense planning was really effective when a train plunged through the concourse of the Union Station shortly before President Eisenhower's inauguration. With the invasion of South Korea in 1950, the nurses of the armed forces—Army, Navy, and the new Air Corps—were again called upon to care for wounded men. The harsh realities of war were in no wise assuaged by the fact that the military action in which US troops participated was not officially designated "war," nor by the symbolism of the flag of the United Nations under which they served. A pervasive sense of crisis accelerated the trend toward the reconstruction of nursing during the period of "the cold war" between the ideologies of the freedom-loving Western world and Communism in which the US was forced to play a principal role. The Committee on Nursing in National Security,[8] using the ANA's 1949 inventory of nurses as a basis, found a deficit of 65,000 nurses without making provision for increases in the military services in case of total mobilization. The National Security Resources Board, on the basis of a more comprehensive study, arrived at approximately the same conclusion and indicated that the situation would become increasingly critical.

But the profession had no firm base on which to estimate the nation's need for nurses. The ANA therefore launched a five-year study

[8] Composed of representatives of the six national nursing organizations: ANA, AAIN, ACSN, NACGN, NLNE, and NOPHN.

of nursing functions at mid-century. The NCINS (discussed later) was encouraging realistic regional planning, and (1952) the USPHS began a two-year study which is expected to provide a new formula for estimating needs for public health nurses.[9] Since it was increasingly apparent that the number of students and therefore of graduate nurses could not be greatly increased, it was necessary to find effective methods for utilizing and supplementing their services. The nursing team, of professional nurses and nonprofessional workers, which may be the answer to that problem is discussed in the chapter on nursing education. In the meantime (1952) President Truman appointed a commission of fifteen persons (Marion W. Sheahan the only nurse) to investigate the health 'requirements of the US and report within the year. The report is not available at this writing. While these long-range programs were being developed, methods of meeting the immediate situation were being accelerated. Before discussing them, some of the causes of the enormously increased demand for nursing service in the postwar period must be summarized.

The Hospital Survey and Construction (Hill-Burton) Act of 1946 made millions of dollars available for the construction of hospitals and health centers under prescribed conditions with emphasis on the needs of rural areas. The states lost no time in securing legislation which would permit the use of such funds within their jurisdictions. Unlike the Mental Hygiene Act, effective the same year, the act made no provision for the preparation of personnel. The new installations, with those of the Veterans Administration, promptly began adding to the nursing deficit. By 1951 the nation had over 1,000,000 acceptable hospital beds, exclusive of 190,000 in federal government hospitals. But Hill-Burton estimates indicated need of an additional 874,000 beds, and this at a time when the low birth rate of the depression years was seriously affecting the potential supply of student nurses. Then, too, as the need for nurses increased, competing opportunities for young women were also increasing. It was obvious that, if nursing was to attract and hold its

---

[9] For more than a quarter of a century the generally accepted ratio of public health nurses to population has been 1 to 5000 unless nursing care is included in the program when it is 1 to 2500.

fair share of each year's high school and college graduates, it would
be necessary to do several things: (1) accelerate changes in nursing
education such as had been recommended by the Winslow-Goldmark and later studies, (2) improve the administration of nursing
services, and (3) improve the economic status of nursing. The
second point was brought into sharp focus by advances in the theory
and practice of hospital administration. What the profession proposed to do about them will be discussed in subsequent chapters.

Among the highlights of this fertile period in the hospital and
health field were the publication of *Hospital Care in the United
States*, the *College Curriculum in Hospital Administration*, and the
Administrative Internships in the Hospital. Hospital Care is the report of an independent commission which received its initial impetus from the AHA. Its studies were carried forward in cooperation
with the USPHS. The basic recommendations were in line with
those in a report prepared for the APHA and a series of reports
published by the USPHS.[10] The recommendations relating to nursing education were in general accord with principles advocated
by the nursing organizations.

The recommendations of the "pilot" study of hospitals, made in
Michigan for the Hospital Commission, were based on the principle
that all necessary services could be made available within a designated area or region by associating smaller institutions with larger
ones in some type of integrated pattern. This was in keeping with
the concept of health service areas advocated by the USPHS. In the
postwar period the APHA and the AHA, for the first time, formally
recognized the need for coordinated planning for hospitals and health
centers. The professionalization of hospital administration (at mid-
century a dozen universities were offering programs in this field)
and the trend toward interprofessional planning were a stimulating
challenge to the nursing profession.

It was, however, the report of the study which had been initiated in connection with the postwar planning of the National

<hr/>

[10] Emerson, Haven, and Luginbuhl, Martha: *Local Health Units for the
Nation.* The Commonwealth Fund, New York, 1945.

Nursing Council which gave the nursing profession a dynamic sense of direction and an exciting action program. This, "the Brown report,"[11] was made possible by the Carnegie Corporation and the Russell Sage Foundation. The potency of its recommendations was augmented by "the Ginzberg report"[12] on the function of nursing and the report of the Committee on Nursing of the American Medical Association.[13] Esther Lucile Brown, the brilliant social anthropologist who prepared the report, was already well known to many nurses through her studies of nursing and other professions. Having pointed out that nursing is both a complex and an "emotionally explosive" subject, Dr. Brown was unconditionally authorized to make an objective study to determine *the needs of society* for nursing. Following the publication of *Nursing for the Future*, which climaxed the work of the National Nursing Council, that organization was promptly dissolved (1948). Responsibility for over-all leadership in nursing reverted to the national nursing organizations. Having learned the value of a united front as, for example, in interesting the Kellogg Foundation in the work of the council and of the Carnegie Corporation and the Russell Sage Foundation in the study of nursing, the joint board of "the three national nursing organizations" voted itself out of existence and was succeeded by a joint board of six national nursing organizations,[14] which, in turn, went out of existence in 1952, when the national nursing organizations were restructured. Four major activities believed to have implications for all nursing were placed under the aegis of the joint boards. They were the programs of: (1) the Committee on the Unification of Accrediting Services, (2) the Committee on Careers in Nursing, (3) the Joint Committee on Practical Nurses and Auxiliary Workers

[11] Brown, Esther Lucile: *Nursing for the Future*. The Russell Sage Foundation, New York, 1948.

[12] *A Program For the Nursing Profession*, Committee on the Function of Nursing. The Macmillan Company, New York, 1948.

[13] "Committee on Nursing Problems," *J.A.M.A.*, 137:877, 1948.

[14] To the original three (American Nurses' Association, National League of Nursing Education, and National Organization of Public Health Nursing) were added the boards of the American Association of Industrial Nurses, the Association of Collegiate Schools of Nursing, and the National Association of Colored Graduate Nurses.

in Nursing Services,[15] and (4) the National Committee on the Improvement of Nursing Services, originally named the Committee on the Implementation of the Brown report.

There were other important indications that nursing was moving rapidly from one era toward another. The remarkable changes in the international scene are discussed in Chapters 50 and 51. Among those in the American scene were the commissioned status of the Army, Navy, and Air Force nurses which gave added prestige to the whole profession; the reconstruction of the program of the ARC nursing service, and the announcement (1950) that the Metropolitan Life Insurance Company (followed by a similar statement of the John Hancock Life Insurance Company) would discontinue its annual expenditure of $4,000,000 for nursing service at the end of a two-year period during which it would assist the many nursing agencies with which it had contracts to readjust their programs.

In 1947, by Congressional action, members of Army and Navy Nurse Corps were placed in commissioned grade, and the services became responsible for their own recruitment and established their own Reserves. The Air Force Nurse Corps, established two years later, was granted the same privileges and assumed similar responsibilities. Contrary to popular belief, not all members of this corps become flight nurses. Those who do are given a rigorous course in aeromedical nursing. All three corps responded, in the highest military and nursing traditions, to the Korean crisis of 1950.

Under the administration of community-minded Ruth B. Freeman the ARC nursing service, which had recruited nurses for military service since 1909, established a new enrollment to meet ARC requirements only. The expanded instructional program calls for nurses prepared to teach in the home nursing and nurses' aide programs; public health nurses and nurses with special preparation for the care of polio patients are needed for disaster service; and very considerable numbers of nurses are required for the blood donor service. Nurses now earn the privilege of becoming enrolled ARC

[15] The National Association for Practical Nurse Education and the National Federation for Licensed Practical Nurses were also represented on this committee.

nurses by giving some type of service. In accordance with a long-standing policy all ARC public health nursing services were discontinued in 1951.

The nature of the social ferment of the period was revealed in the variations in the 35 state-wide surveys of nursing which are discussed in the following chapter. The first one, made for the Michigan Nursing Center Association, paralleled the pilot study of hospitals made in that state for the Commission on Hospital Care. The utilization of surveys as a basis for regional planning was vigorously endorsed by the Brown report.

Although agencies of the federal government had increased their employment of registered professional nurses from less than 8000 in 1940 to over 23,000 in 1950, they had 4000 less than their authorized quotas. The USPHS continued its interest in nursing education and became a powerful influence in that field following the termination of the Cadet Nurse Corps. When (1949) Lucile Petry was appointed Chief Nurse Officer and assistant to the Surgeon General she was the first nurse in the world to bear the title General.

Despite the universal apprehensiveness due to the international political situation, the professional climate of the period acquired an electric quality which was stimulating to all types of nurses. Planning groups sought counsel from other professions. No longer were major decisions based on the reports of relatively small committees. Conferences, institutes, and workshops at which the technics of group dynamics and socio-drama were used became the order of the day. The importance of these and other technics of communication were stressed by educators. The interested participation, on invitation, of "resource people" from many other fields such as education, the social sciences, hospital administration, and management, was one of the most significant evidences of the dawn of a new era. Nursing had learned that it could not lift itself by its own bootstraps! *A Thousand Think Together* was the meaningful title of the report of conferences held in connection with Dr. Brown's study of nursing education. Opinionnaires were extensively used to obtain a cross section of participation in the "Structure Study." A series of articles in the *Journal* by the well-known publicist Edward

L. Bernays revealed conflicting concepts of nursing. These materials stimulated interest in the development of public relations programs and gave the profession an increasing sense of partnership, in relation to the nation's health, with the other health professions and with the public. The NIB, as previously noted, was dissolved during this period, and the preparation and publication of the handbook, *Facts about Nursing,* became a function of the ANA's statistical department. The ANA developed a broad-scale public relations service which included provision for instruction in public relations technics for constituent organizations requesting assistance. The NOPHN capped years of fruitful public relations work with the publication of Mrs. Wensley's manual.[16]

There were many evidences that nursing had become a recognized social force when the nation faced the crisis of 1950. In both world wars, nurses had found it necessary to take the initiative in securing federal recognition of nursing as a service requiring comprehensive planning during a national emergency. But when the National Security Resources Board set to work to meet the mid-century crisis, the board secured the services, "on leave" for a brief period from the ARC, of Ruth Freeman, as director of a nursing unit. Dean Ruth P. Kuehn, of the University of Pittsburgh, was appointed to represent nursing on the advisory committee to the board. Federal plans for the participation of nurses in the civil defense program and for the utilization of nurses in case of national emergency were made in accord with established policies of the national nursing organizations. Within the profession, acceptance of the philosophic principle that in union there is strength overcame the strong potentialities for self-perpetuation of three national organizations,[17] and brought into existence the National League for Nursing which is discussed in Chapter 49. The new organization, it was believed, could work more effectively than any one of its elements in promoting the education of nurses, the extension and administration of nursing services,

[16] Wensley, Edith: *Building Sound Public Relations.* NOPHN, New York, 1949.

[17] The National League of Nursing Education (established in 1894), the National Organization for Public Health Nursing (1912), and the Association of Collegiate Schools of Nursing (1932).

and the development of interprofessional and community relationships. The administration of institutional nursing services, for the first time in nursing history, began to receive as much attention as the administration of nursing schools. Furthermore, the program of one organization instead of three could be more effectively coordinated with the expanding program of the ANA.

A number of important anniversaries fell within the six-year period which ended with the convention of 1952. All were celebrated as challenges, not as memorials. This had been true too of the fiftieth anniversary of the NLNE (1943). That had been signalized by the inauguration of the Mary Adelaide Nutting award which is conferred for "leadership in nursing education." The ANA quietly celebrated its half century of constructive work for nurses and nursing in the first postwar year. It was in that year that Ella Best (St. Luke's, Chicago, and Teachers College), who had capably served the association in various positions for 16 years, succeeded Alma H. Scott as executive secretary. Mrs. Scott had served the organization with passionate devotion since 1933.[18] But in 1948 the association went "all out" to celebrate the Diamond Jubilee of Nursing, the seventy-fifth anniversary of the founding of the three pioneer Nightingale schools, and the graduation of "America's first trained nurse." In connection with the Jubilee a "nursing progress" week was celebrated by many state associations. The evolutionary process at work in nursing education is clearly revealed by the status and program, at mid-century, of the pioneer schools. The last class of the Connecticut Training School for Nurses had been graduated (1926) with the first class of the Yale School of Nursing which superceded it and has now graduated more than a thousand nurses. The Bellevue School of Nursing and the Mills School for Men Nurses (1888) have jointly been identified since 1942 as the Division of Nursing of the College of Medicine of New York University. The Massachusetts General Hospital School of Nursing, where able Sally Johnson was succeeded by modest but richly endowed Ruth Sleeper (1947), has always been one of the most influential hospital schools of nursing in this country. It is now (1952) conducting an outstanding experi-

[18] "Tribute to Alma H. Scott," *Am. J. Nursing*, **50**:789, 1950.

ment in basic nursing education and has an affiliation, with a limited enrollment, with Radcliffe College. Two other schools in existence in 1873, although not organized in accordance with the Nightingale principles, also merit attention. The school from which Linda Richards was graduated (1873) at the New England Hospital for Women and Children had an honorable history when it was discontinued at mid-century. The primary interest of those who organized the school had been in providing an institution in which women could practice medicine, rather than the education of nurses. The school of the Women's Hospital, Philadelphia, is on the list of schools approved for temporary accreditation.

The Division of Nursing Education of Teachers College, Columbia University, which had led educational thought in nursing for half a century, very appropriately devoted its three-day semicentennial anniversary program to "The Future of Nursing Education." On the retirement of Isabel M. Stewart (1947), whose professional life "has been incredibly full of service to nurses and nursing education,"[19] brilliant R. Louise McManus became the third director of that internationally famous "school." Realizing that the times called for changes in the curriculum Mrs. McManus asked the administration of the college, as a first step, for a committee to study the functions of nursing. The immediate result of that request was the Ginzberg report to which reference has been made.

In its golden anniversary issue (October, 1950) the *American Journal of Nursing* gave the profession a comprehensive overview of fifty years of nursing. Mrs. Eleanor Roosevelt and Gerda Höjer of Sweden, president of the ICN, were honor guests at the anniversary dinner. The board of directors had already taken steps to ensure a broad base for the magazine's service to the profession in its second half century. Nell V. Beeby, after 14 constructive years on the editorial staff, had succeeded the retiring editor Mary M. Roberts (1949), who was designated Editor Emeritus. The magazine, in recognition of her long service, established the Mary M. Roberts

[19] "The Future of Nursing Education." *Proceedings*, Fiftieth Anniversary Celebration of Nursing Education in Teachers College, Columbia University. New York, 1950.

Fellowship to encourage interpretative writing on professional subjects by nurses in active practice. It was, however, the thorough reorganization of the internal mechanisms of the *Journal* and the appointment of Sims Gaynor as business manager that established a historic administrative precedent at national nursing headquarters. The business of the magazine, the largest and most widely read nursing publication in the world, was so adeptly reorganized by Mr. Gaynor that an early ambition of M. E. P. Davis, to whom the *Journal* owes its sound foundation, was realized. The American Journal of Nursing Company, of which the ANA is the sole stockholder, by accepting responsibility for the production of two new magazines, became to all intents the "publishing house for the profession" of which she had dreamed. Miss Beeby, continuing as editor of the AJN, became also the first executive editor of the American Journal of Nursing Company. *Nursing Research* was launched under the aegis of the Association of Collegiate Schools of Nursing (1952) and became a responsibility of the NLN when the ACSN was absorbed in the new organization.

Plans were made for an official publication of the National League for Nursing which would be called *Nursing Outlook* which would absorb *Public Health Nursing* magazine (January, 1953) and carry on its fine traditions and service. These developments had been greatly facilitated by the establishment (1950) of national nursing headquarters at 2 Park Avenue, New York. The *Journal* and the nursing organizations occupy adjoining offices in space, which then seemed spacious and is now crowded, which is the equivalent of one-third of a city block.

In this period of transition, in which the major external forces were the establishment of the World Health Organization, the passage of the Hill-Burton Act, the National Defense Act, and the invasion of South Korea, matters under the direct control of the profession moved forward quickly but with due caution. The integration of the NACGN with the ANA (1951) and plans for the fusion of the NLNE, NOPHN, and ACSN to form the National League for Nursing (1952) were carried forward with vision, zeal, courage, and the adventurous spirit of pioneers. Having consolidated their forces, nurses were prepared to move forward on a united front to strengthen the American system of nursing education and to coordinate new patterns of nursing service with the services of other members of the health team.

BIBLIOGRAPHY

Abdellah, Fay G.: "State Nursing Surveys and Community Action," *Pub. Health Rep.*, **67**:554, 1952.

The Administrative Internship in the Hospital. Joint Commission on Education (American College of Hospital Administration and American Hospital Association), Chicago, 1947.

America's Health (National Health Assembly—A Report to the Nation). Harper & Brothers, New York, 1948.

"A.N.A. Platform," *Am. J. Nursing*, **46**:729, 1946.

A.N.A. Public Relations Planning Kit. American Nurses' Association, New York, 1951.

The American Nurses' Association 1896–1946—Tomorrows and Yesterdays, as told on the fiftieth anniversary of the association's founding. American Nurses' Association, New York, 1946.

Armstrong, Donald B., and Haupt, Alma C.: "A Forty-Year Demonstration of Public Health Nursing by the Metropolitan Life Insurance Company," *Pub. Health Nursing*, **43**:41, 1951.

Becker, Harry: "Organized Labor and the Problem of Medical Care," *Ann. Am. Acad. Polit. & Soc. Sc.*, **273**:122, 1951.

Bernays, Edward L.: Fourteen articles dealing with the nursing profession and public relations, beginning May, 1945, and terminating November, 1947, *American Journal of Nursing*.

——: *Public Relations.* University of Oklahoma Press, Norman, Okla., 1952.

Bixler, Genevieve Knight: *Nursing Resources and Needs in Michigan—A Survey.* Prepared for the Michigan Council on Community Nursing, 1946.

The Book of States, 1950–1951, Vol. VIII. Council of State Governments, Chicago, 1950.

Chayer, Mary Ella: *Nursing in Modern Society.* G. P. Putnam's Sons, New York, 1947, Chap. 2.

Children and Youth at the Midcentury, Fact Finding Report, a Digest. Mid-Century Conference on Children and Youth, Washington, D.C., 1950.

The College Curriculum in Hospital Administration. Joint Commission for the American Hospital Association and the American College of Hospital Administrators. The Physicians Record Co., Chicago, 1948.

"Coordination of Hospitals and Health Departments, American Hospital Association and American Public Health Association," *Am. J. Pub. Health,* **38**:702, 1948.

Dewhurst, J. Frederic, and associates: *America's Needs and Resources.* The Twentieth Century Fund, New York, 1947.

Dublin, Louis I., and Speigelman, Mortimer: *The Facts of Life from Birth to Death.* The Macmillan Company, New York, 1951.

Dunham, Ethel C.: *Premature Infants.* Children's Bureau Pub. #325, US Government Printing Office, Washington, D.C., 1948.

The Effects of Atomic Weapons. US Government Printing Office, Washington, D.C., 1950.

Emerson, Haven: *Local Health Units for the Nation.* The Commonwealth Fund, New York, 1945.

Fagin, I. D.; Miller, Myrtle; and Fisk, Bernice: "The Health Institute of the UAW-CIO," *Pub. Health Nursing,* **38**:466, 1946.

Flagg, Maurice: "They Showed the Way," *Red Cross Magazine,* **1**:27, 1951.

Freeman, Ruth B.: "Civil Defense Planning and Nursing," *Am. J. Nursing,* **50**:531, 1950.

Ginzberg, Eli: "Perspectives on Nursing," *Am. J. Nursing,* **47**:474, 1947.

Hawley, Paul R.: *Non-Profit Health Service Plans.* Blue Cross Commission, Blue Shield Commission, Chicago, 1949.

Herrold, Kenneth F.: "Conference Planning and Action Through Use of the Group Process," *Pub. Health Nursing,* **42**:199, 1950.

Higher Education for American Democracy, Report of the President's Commission on Higher Education, 6 vols. US Government Printing Office, Washington, D.C., 1947, Vol. 1, p. 78.

"Hospital Beds in the United States," *Pub. Health Rep.,* **67**:312, 1952.

Hospital Care in the United States. The Commission on Hospital Care. The Commonwealth Fund, New York, 1947.

Hospital Nursing Service Manual. American Hospital Association and the National League of Nursing Education, 1950.

"Hospital Survey and Construction Act," *Am. J. Nursing,* **48**:361, 1948.

Illness and Health Services in an Aging Population. U.S. Public Health Service Pub. #170, US Government Printing Office, Washington, D.C., 1952.

Kernodle, Portia B.: *The Red Cross Nurse in Action, 1882–1948,* "Blueprint for Change." Harper & Brothers, New York, 1949, Chap. XXX.

Kuehn, Ruth P.: "Nurse Power in Mobilization—An Analysis of the Over-all National Nursing Needs as Revealed by the Health Resources Advisory Committee," *Am. J. Nursing,* **51**:395, 1951.

"Linda Richards, 1949 Version," *Am. J. Nursing,* **49**:457, 687, 1949.

Man and His Years, An Account of the First National Conference on Aging. Sponsored by the Federal Security Agency, Health Publications Institute, Inc., Raleigh, N.C., 1951.

"The Mary Adelaide Nutting Award," *Am. J. Nursing,* **43**:762, 1943; **44**:587, 1944.

Medical Aspects of Civil Defense. Council on National Emergency Medical Service, American Medical Association, Chicago, 1952.

"Mobilization of Nurses for National Security," *Am. J. Nursing,* **51**:78, 1951.

Mountin, Joseph W., and Greve, Clifford H.: *Public Health Areas and Hospital Facilities, A Plan for Coordination.* US Public Health Service Pub. #42, US Government Printing Office, Washington, D.C., 1950.

Mountin, Joseph W., and Hoge, Van M.: *Health Service Areas, Requisitions for General Hospitals and Health Centers.* Public Health Bull. #292, US Government Printing Office, Washington, D.C., 1945.

Muller, Theresa Grace: *Dynamics of Human Behavior.* Boston University School of Nursing, Boston, 1950.

Munson, Helen W.: "Linda Richards," *Am. J. Nursing,* **48**:551, 1948.

The Nurse in Civil Defense. Federal Civil Defense Administration (Technical Manual), US Government Printing Office, Washington, D.C., 1952.

Nursing During Disaster, A Guide for Instructors in Basic Professional Programs and Practical Nurse Programs. National League of Nursing Education, New York, 1951.

"Plans of General Hospitals for the Coordinated Hospital System," *Hospitals,* **22**:49, 1948.

Platform Recommendations and Pledge to Children. Midcentury White House Conference on Children and Youth, Washington, D.C., 1950.

Porter, Elizabeth K.: "Salute to the Future," *Am. J. Nursing,* **52**:978, 1952.

Requisitions for General Hospitals and Health Centers. Public Health Bull. #292, US Government Printing Office, Washington, D.C., 1945.

Russell, E. Kathleen: "Fifty Years of Medical Progress, Medicine as a Social Instrument: Nursing," *New England J. Med.,* **224**:439–45, 1951.

Russell, James Earl: *Federal Activities in Higher Education after the Second World War.* King's Crown Press (Columbia University), New York, 1951.

Senn, Milton J. E. (ed.): *Symposium on the Healthy Personality.* Josiah Macy, Jr. Foundation, New York, 1950.

Shalit, Pearl R.: "The Nurse and the National Mental Health Act," *Am. J. Nursing*, **47**:709, 1947; **50**:94, 1950.

Shryock, Richard Harrison: *The Development of Modern Medicine—An Interpretation of the Social and Scientific Factors Involved*, 2nd ed. Alfred A. Knopf. New York, 1947.

Stieglitz, Edward J.: *The Second Forty Years*. J. B. Lippincott Co., Philadelphia, 1946.

"Temporary Accreditation" (NNAS releases list of 627 programs approved for temporary accreditation), *Am. J. Nursing*, **52**:997, 1952.

United States Government Organization Manual, 1951–1952. US Government Printing Office, Washington, D.C.

Wallace, Helen M.; Losty, Margaret A.; and Wishile, N.: "Prematurity as a Public Health Problem," *Am. J. Pub. Health*, **40**:41, 1950.

Watkins, Arthur L.: "Current Trends in Physical Medicine and Rehabilitation," *New England J. Med.*, **247**:91, 1952.

Wensley, Edith: *Building Sound Public Relations*. National Organization for Public Health Nursing, New York, 1949.

Wright, Jessie, "Respir-aid Rocking Bed in Poliomyelitis," *Am. J. Nursing*, **47**:454, 1947.

"Yale University School of Nursing," *Pub. Health Nursing*, **43**:666, 1951.

Chapter 46

EVOLUTIONARY ADJUSTMENTS
IN NURSING SERVICES

The single, unaided physician is no longer the principal source of medical care in the United States. Modern medicine is furnished by a team of nurses and technical assistants headed by the physician, who in turn is aided by the research worker.[1]

To be part of a team means that one must be extemely well prepared in his own field, that he must see himself in relation to the contribution of others, that he must sense constantly the changing needs of the individuals whom he and the group are serving, that he must accept the corresponding changes in his contribution and the contributions of the other team members to those needs, that he must have the courage to say what he can do and why he feels that he can do that thing better than another, that he must have the grace to give up what he likes to do if another can do it better. It means further, that he must learn to do things which do not come too easily if they can best be done by him for the good of all. It means the will to pull with others and the integrity to withdraw from those parts of an undertaking which are not his. It means the enduring belief that together we can do things which no one of us individually could do alone, and that the together-ness makes possible a concept of the job which is greater than the sum of the individual parts.[2]

WE ARE HERE concerned with postwar nursing service and the forces which accelerated its growth and its adaptation to the nation's need. In the interval between the wars, when successive studies which emphasized the need for educational reforms were being made, admin-

[1] Dickinson, Frank G.: "The Medical Care Team." *Ann. Am. Acad. Polit. & Soc., Sci.*, 273:25, 1951.
[2] Hubbard, Ruth W.: "The Nurse on the Healing Arts Team," *Am. J. Nursing*, 49:27, 1949.

istration had become a science with a body of principles which are applicable in an extraordinary variety of situations. Conditions which led to the profession's recognition of its need for assistance in solving problems, from administration and other social sciences, provide much of the subject matter of this chapter.

Generally speaking, nurses in administrative positions, especially those in hospitals, were not equipped with requisite administrative skills for effecting the smooth integration of large numbers of volunteers and other nonprofessional workers into existing patterns of nursing service. Competent observers have noted, however, that they were not given adequate credit for the courage and tenacity of purpose with which they kept civilian nursing services operating throughout the war. Institutions which were forced to close departments lacked personnel of all types. The end of the war brought no respite because hospital admissions increased rapidly. At mid-century, although there were more registered professional nurses actively engaged in nursing than ever before, there were serious deficits in all fields of nursing. The most urgent needs were those of the hospitals although, collectively, they had added 50,000 registered nurses to their rosters in the postwar period. By 1950, according to the AMA, hospitals were augmenting the services of well over 200,000 professional nurses and approximately 100,000 student nurses with those of about 225,000 practical nurses, attendants, and nurses' aides.[3] The distressingly low ratio of professional to nonprofessional workers in mental—approximately one-half of all patients were in mental hospitals—and tuberculosis hospitals was a matter of increasing anxiety to the American Psychiatric Association and to the National Tuberculosis Association. The influence of these and other agencies concerned with clinical specialties is discussed in the chapter on nursing education. A condition described by Katherine De Witt many years earlier, in 1909 to be exact, prevailed in many institutions. It was as unsatisfactory to patients as it was unrewarding to nurses. "Probably the hospital atmosphere with which most of us are familiar is one of strain and stress—so many

[3] "Hospital Service in the United States, The 1951 Census of Hospitals," *J.A.M.A.*; **149**:13, 16 (May 10) 1952.

things to be attended to, so many duties, so many demands, so many interruptions, so much left undone we had hoped to accomplish. . . . There are always too many patients, too few nurses, and too little time for the amenities of life."

Symptomatic of that condition was the oft-repeated statement that patients preferred volunteer aides or other nonprofessional workers because they seemed less hurried and more interested than nurses. Many nurses were aware of the need for study and clarification of the functions of nursing and of the basic philosophy of the profes-

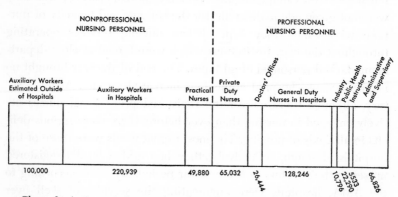

Chart 2. Active nursing personnel in the United States and territories by fields of nursing, 1950. Professional, total 325,167; nonprofessional, total 370,819. (National Committee for the Improvement of Nursing Services, *News Letter*, April-May, 1952.)

sion. Both were complicated by the economic status of the profession. Of the latter the Ginzberg report states bluntly that a major reason for the shortage of nurses was "the traditional tendency to minimize economic incentives in rewarding nurses."[4]

A factual basis for that opinion could be found in the comprehensive study of the economics of nursing made under the aegis of the National Nursing Council. The handicap to augmenting professional resources by the recruitment and education of more students was succinctly stated as follows: ". . . there are occupations requiring much less training that provide earnings equal to or above those of

[4] *A Program for the Nursing Profession*, Committee on the Function of Nursing. The Macmillan Company, New York, 1948, p. 98.

nurses."[5] Under these circumstances, in a period of keen economic competition for workers and one in which the number of high school and college graduates was relatively low (due to the low birth rate of the depression) it was impossible to recruit greatly increased numbers of students. The financial insecurity of precedent-setting voluntary hospitals (a subject of special study in 1952) helped to obscure this issue. The general reluctance of institutions to face the problem of the economic insecurity of nurses in the excessively competitive wartime situation had caused the ANA to launch an economic security program (Chap. 38) immediately following the war. As demands for nursing service increased, methods for integrating the services of nonprofessional workers in comprehensive programs of nursing service became of paramount interest to all planning agencies. This inevitably put a new emphasis on administrative practice in relation to nursing service and on the education of nurses in relation to their changing functions. We shall return to that point after consideration of other elements in the total fabric of mid-century nursing service in the United States.

The number of public health nurses rose steadily after the war, but, in 1951, children and adults in the rural areas of more than 1100 counties and a few small cities were without the protection and service of a single full-time public health nurse. Fortunately existing patterns of public health nursing could readily be adapted to changing conditions. An important evidence of mid-century adaptation is indicated by changes in structure of state health departments. Many of them consolidated their nursing activities in divisions of nursing. Their programs were no longer restricted to public health nursing since, in most states, the health departments had been made responsible for the hospital survey and planning programs made possible by the Hill-Burton Act. As a result, nurse consultants in "hospital planning, construction, and licensure" had been appointed in approximately half the states by the middle of 1952. Never before

[5] *The Economic Status of Registered Professional Nurses, 1946–1947.* US Labor Bureau Statistics. Articles based on the study: "Economic Status of the Nursing Profession," *Am. J. Nursing,* **47**:456, 1947; "Economic Status of Public Health Nurses," *Am. J. Nursing,* **47**:585, 1947; "Economic Status of Private Duty and General Staff Nurses," *Am. J. Nursing,* **47**:669, 1947.

had American nurses had such an opportunity to facilitate the administration of nursing services through participation in architectural and personnel planning.

The number of nurses employed in safeguarding the health of industrial workers remained at a high level, but many of the small industries, which in the aggregate employed a high percentage of the nation's workers, provided no such service. The number of office nurses employed by doctors, according to the ANA's 1951 inventory, had risen with astonishing rapidity until it practically equaled the total number of public health nurses! Many nurses left the practice of nursing to become nurse anesthetists or some other type of medical technician. The American Association of Nurse Anesthetists reported a demand far exceeding the supply in 1950.

The ANA recorded (1951) that the number of active nurses engaged in private duty nursing had dropped to approximately 20 per cent of the total number. Many of these independent practitioners were restricting their work to special duty service in hospitals although they sometimes served as staff nurses for brief periods. The private duty picture is incomplete because no data are available from registries which are operated in connection with hospitals or alumnae associations or from the very considerable number which are operated for profit. Approximately one-half of the 164 registries sponsored by state nurses' associations, which report to the ANA, were providing consultation and placement service for practical nurses. At mid-century less than two-thirds of the calls to professionally sponsored registries were for professional nurses.

In the spring of 1952 the ANA, which sets minimum standards for professionally sponsored registries, approved a new "Statement of Principles for Nurses Professional Registries" which is designed to stimulate constructive action in relation to their organization and use. It emphasizes a principle which is in accord with that of the ANA Professional Counseling & Placement Service, Inc., viz., that service shall be rendered "on a non-profit basis to qualified professional and practical nurses without regard to race, creed, color, school of nursing, or length of residence in the area." It is assumed that well-planned action based on the new statement will, among other things, improve the quality of nursing care in the communities by promoting educational programs such as institutes and workshops for the registrants; will result in cooperation with all programs of the state and national associations for the welfare of the registrants and in the interest of promoting better nursing service; and that the registries will make every effort to integrate their services with those of state and national counseling and placement services so as to provide better distribution of nursing personnel.

Since many private duty nurses restrict their practice to special duty in hospitals, the relationship of the registries to the hospitals is important. It appears, however, to be dependent on local conditions. Some hospitals pay, on a per capita basis, for the service they receive from them—many do not. The hospitals may, or may not, have representation on the governing boards of the registries. The special duty nurse often has an equally anomalous relationship to the hospital which employs her. She may, for example, be almost continuously on duty in one institution without participating in any way in staff or other conferences in the departments to which she may be called. Few hospitals have as yet attempted to develop special conference programs for these nurses.

To return to consideration of institutional nursing. The potential for important developments in the second half century may be predicated on the evolution of "the medical care team"; increasing specialization in clinical nursing; rapid developments in the theory and practice of hospital administration; the development of nursing teams as part of an aroused interest in the administration of nursing services as distinct from, although often cooperating with, the administration of schools of nursing.

At mid-century the long-established tradition that the hospital is "the workshop of the doctor" was giving way to the concept of patient-centered institutions. "Consider the patient as a person," says a report on medical education, "was merely a platitude in medical schools until relatively recently."[6] Today that concept is an increas-

---

[6] Curran, Jean A., and Cockerell, Eleanor (cochairman): *Widening Horizons in Medical Education,* a Study of the Social and Environmental Factors in Medicine, 1945–1946. The Commonwealth Fund, New York, 1948.

ingly dynamic force in all programs for comprehensive patient care. Participation in planning is implicit in the team concept. Effective planning is possible only when the members of the team are equally well prepared in their respective fields. Fortunately the trend toward clinical specialization in nursing paralleled the trend toward medical teamwork to which the Children's Bureau has given notable impetus. Increasing numbers of nurses qualified to do what Miss Goodrich calls *creative nursing* were available to initiate experiments in comprehensive programs for patient care.

By mid-century excellent examples of medical teamwork (not to be confused with the nursing team) could be found in pediatric departments such as the one in which the order for "TLC" (tender, loving care) first appeared on a patient's chart and in many departments caring for polio patients. The results of teamwork were apparent in obstetrical departments where "rooming-in" and natural childbirth were making the care of obstetrical patients and their babies a warmly human experience for all concerned. It could be observed in a few institutions where psychiatric teams, composed of psychiatrist, psychiatric social worker, clinical psychologist, and psychiatric nurse, were democratically sharing professional knowledge and information about their patients as a basis for the development of therapeutic plans of action.

"The modern concept of adequate patient care," says the *Hospital Nursing Service Manual*, "interprets that care in terms of total patient needs, whether these needs be diagnostic, preventive, or therapeutic, physical, psychological, spiritual, or social. It recognizes the patient as a person, with an individual personality and with individual needs, who has come from a recognized place within the family and the community and must be helped to make his adjustment to his condition and to his new environment. The ultimate objective of adequate patient care is to return the individual to his family and community restored to health and productive capacity. The broad, social concept of total patient needs has many implications for the nursing department, as to both its activities and the competence and attitude of its staff."[7]

[7] *Hospital Nursing Service Manual*, AHA and NLNE, 1950, p. 1.

Through teamwork in giving patient-centered care, the encapsulation of the several professions in their immediate interests is being broken down. A psychiatrist offers an illuminating explanation of the condition which had been a barrier to wholesome interprofessional relationships and also, in the case of nursing, between professional and practical nurses. He says: "Our education, our training, our professional status have become psychological aspects of ourselves. In order to enter fully into an exchange of ideas, it was as though we had to relinquish something of our personalities."[8]

At war's end hospital administrators were increasingly adapting the principles and technics of administration to their extremely complex organizations. But, as the Ginzberg report pointed out, the nursing services were less affected by them than other departments of the hospital. This was attributed, in part, to the failure of administrative consultants to perceive the need for reform and, in part, to the resistance of nurses to change. However, institutions which had not already done so found that central supply rooms could effect important economies in nursing time as well as in equipment and supplies. Postoperative recovery rooms were an innovation which assured patients of superior care after major surgery and also helped to keep nursing service in the nursing units on an even keel. So, too, did the postdelivery rooms which were provided in connection with some maternity departments.

A study of hospital staffing, still unpublished at this writing, has already had wide influence on nursing services because some of the very practical results have been shared generously at workshops and through the pages of hospital and nursing publications. Marion J. Wright, who directed that study at Harper Hospital, Detroit, had capped faculty experience in the school of nursing by securing a degree in hospital administration. She had the assistance and guidance of management engineers in planning and conducting the study. One of the immediate results—there are many others—was the establishment of a central messenger service which released many hours per day of nursing time for service in the nursing units. Be-

[8] Bartemeier, Leo H.: "Working Programs in Mental Hospitals." Third Mental Hospital Institute, American Psychiatric Association, 1951, p. 3.

cause other departments participated in the study, it was possible to assign to historically younger departments, such as housekeeping and dietary, functions properly belonging to them but traditionally performed by nurses. Released from non-nursing responsibilities, all nursing personnel spend full time in giving nursing service. Furthermore, the principles and technics of work-simplification are being applied continuously in all services.

The nursing deficit was generally attributed to increased use of hospital facilities. But alert nurse administrators could not operate their services on the basis of a generalization. As reports of researches directed toward the identification of more specific causes began to appear in the professional publications it became quite generally apparent, as research workers at the University of California Hospital demonstrated, that patients were needing *more,* but different, care.[9]

Patients needed more care because of the steadily broadening scope of medical practice, as, for example, in rehabilitation programs and rapid changes in therapy. Early ambulation, the use of isotopes, blood derivatives, antibiotics, and other new therapeutic agents made greater demands on the nursing services than older methods. The use of parenteral medication and transfusions was enormously increased. Postoperative routines, standardized for a relatively long period of bed care, were replaced by frequent changes in medical orders. Time and sympathetic understanding are required to allay the fears and resistances of patients for whom early ambulation and the newer therapies are ordered by physicians. In the strenuous days of the war many institutions had begun streamlining their nursing procedures. As ward manuals were revised, it was found that once standard procedures were no longer in use. Those that superceded them, including some formerly performed by doctors, required a broader base of information, greater skill in performance, and keener observation of results. The tendency to transfer relatively routine medical procedures to nurses was not without the danger of transgressing legal restrictions on nursing. It was, however, in connection

[9] Binhammer, Hannah M., et al.: "Our Patients Require More Care," *Am. J. Nursing,* 48:366, 1948.

with the civil defense program that the *Journal* focused attention
on the subject by inviting discussion of the question, "Should the
nurse do venipuncture?"[10]

Little had been written on the general subject of the administration of nursing services before the war. As noted in an earlier chapter, until well into the forties the subject was almost invariably
taught in relation to the administration of nursing schools and therefore of services staffed in varying degrees by students. The functions of head nurses, however, had been a matter of concern since
the late twenties when a committee of the NLNE, of which Mary M.
Marvin was chairman, considered the question and decided that
universities offering programs for graduate nurses should be encouraged to make provision for the preparation of head nurses. The
teaching function of the head nurse which was considered, by the
committee, to be at least as important as her administrative function was given major emphasis until the advent of the teaching
supervisor and special provision was made for ward teaching. Expertness in the clinical field in which she functioned was placed
high on the list of requirements for head nurse positions. Miss Marvin (later Mrs. Wayland), had won distinction as a teacher of nursing. Her book, the *Hospital Head Nurse,* published in 1938, was an
important addition to the then meager literature of the profession.
It is of interest that the second edition, revised with the aid of collaborators and published in 1944, refers to the nursing team but
without elaboration.

The university schools were, naturally, the first to stress the importance of making a clear distinction between the functions of a
nursing school and a nursing service. As Erma A. Holtzhausen, then
director of nursing service at Vanderbilt, pointed out in a clarifying
discussion of the administration of a nursing service, *a nursing service is patient-centered whereas the student is the center of a school
program.* Therein lies the dichotomy that still plagues the directors
of hospital schools of nursing because of the extreme difficulty of
dealing justly with both when they are directed by one person.
The University Hospitals in Cleveland were among the first in the

[10] "Should Nurses Do Venipunctures?" *Am. J. Nursing,* **51**:603, 1951.

postwar period to turn to management engineers for assistance with their staffing problems. They learned, and shared their discovery that nursing can learn from industry, with *Journal* readers. Frances Reiter (Kreuter) of the Teachers College faculty effectively focused widespread attention on the most obvious trouble spot in the administration of nursing services in general hospitals. After intensive study of the almost fantastic aggregation of functions which many head nurses were expected to perform, she persuaded an artist to portray her conception of current practice. That set of cartoons[11] aroused more interest and stimulated more action than thousands of words could have done. Shortly thereafter the USPHS responded to a request from a well-known institution for "an analysis of the head nurse function to see what can be done to relieve the head nurse either by reallocation of duties or by adding personnel to the ward staff to reduce the demands made upon her."[12] Head nurses participating in the collection and analysis of data found that they were better able to see (1) how they could organize their plans more effectively, (2) why and how they could delegate more work, and (3) the need for studying and reorganizing the ward secretary's work. The latter point became self-evident when it was discovered that work occupying 18 per cent of head nurses' available time could be reassigned. The technics and the findings of this study were promptly shared with the profession through the *Journal*. A division of the USPHS, under the brilliant direction of Margaret G. Arnstein, provides both statistical information and assistance, when requested by appropriate agencies, with research in nursing. The division's impressive contribution to current knowledge of nursing resources, through consultation or participation in state surveys, is discussed in connection with regional planning and nursing education.

While these "administrative tools" were in preparation, the basic problem of providing nursing service which would be satisfactory to the patient and satisfying to those who gave the care was being

[11] Reiter, Frances: "Where Is The Head Nurse?" Artist's Conception. *Am. J. Nursing*, 48:156–157, 1948.

[12] *Head Nurse Activities in a General Hospital, 1950*, Public Health Monograph #3, Pam. 336. USPHS, Washington, D.C.

studied in many institutions and by many groups. One committee
stated this problem as follows:

The functions of nursing may be conceived of as being of a spectrum
range. Many functions involve the performance of skills and techniques
varying in difficulty and complexity and extending on a continuum, from
the simplest performed by the mother and others, and easily picked up
without training, to the most complex function demanding a very high
degree of skill and expertness that can be developed only with considerable training. Many functions also demand judgment ranging from that
based upon common knowledge to judgment that can be arrived at only
by bringing to bear upon the professional problems pertinent knowledge
from the extensive reservoir of scientific information derived from many
fields of study. . . .[13]

The nursing team is an administrative device for providing service of spectrum range, as needed, by the individual patients in a
group assigned to a team by the head nurse. Nursing teams are
composed of at least one professional nurse, who is the team leader,
and other workers, such as student nurses, practical nurses, and attendants in varying combinations. Team leaders function as truly
professional people since success depends on diagnosing each patient's *nursing* needs and making, with the team, a comprehensive
plan to meet them. Nursing teams cannot be created overnight!
Plans for change inevitably meet with resistance from those who
are expected to participate in a new setup if they have not shared in
the planning. As an expert in the field of administration puts it:
"To expect loyalty and confidence and willingness to contribute
their services from people whose feelings of personal integrity have
been damaged—no matter how unwittingly—is to ask for the
moon."[14] Nurse educators are well aware of their responsibility for
the preparation of team leaders who can secure and maintain the
confidence of the workers, practical nurses, nurses' aides, or others,
who become members of nursing teams. Is the nursing team the

[13] *Regional Planning for Nursing and Nursing Education*, p. 54. (Work
Conference, Teachers College, Columbia University, June 1950.) Bureau of
Publications, Teachers College, New York, 1950.
[14] Roethlisberger, F. J.: *Management and Morale*. Harvard University Press,
Cambridge, Mass., 1952.

answer to unsatisfactory conditions in institutional nursing? At this time it may be said that there is a growing body of evidence in its favor.

The nation has never had enough public health nurses to meet its potential needs. Highly qualified nurses were accepting WHO and other assignments for pioneer work in other countries. It was difficult to replace them. However, although the USPHS reported that salaries in public health nursing were too low to be attractive the number, and preparation, of public health nurses was steadily rising. Some notable developments marked the mid-century as the beginning of a new era in public health nursing.

Approximately 90 per cent of public health nurses were employed by official (tax-supported) agencies, a remarkable reversal in trends within the quarter century which had seen the nursing services of the USPHS and the Children's Bureau developed. Through their national and regional offices they had established networks of consultative services to state agencies and to educational institutions. The level of preparation for nurses holding supervisory positions in state health departments and related agencies had risen appreciably. The census of public health nurses (1952) indicated that the most significant increase shown at each census period was in the employment of nurses by local departments of education. Approximately 30 per cent of school nurses had completed an educational program approved for public health nursing. Among them were the "nurse-teachers" and the "teacher-nurses" of New York and New Jersey, respectively, who, although not usually classroom teachers, had secured the preparation and status of faculty members.

Prior to 1942, public health nursing in health departments and in voluntary agencies (usually called visiting nurse services), with a few exceptions, had developed separately but side by side. The care of the sick in their homes on a part-time basis was the essential service of the voluntary agencies although they had added to it, at an early date, the teaching of preventive measures and health principles. The primary function of health departments is the prevention of disease, and their nurses gave no bedside care. They were occupied with giving instruction in the homes and, depending on the programs of the departments, in many types of clinics. School nursing was an important function where such service was not an established responsibility of the department of education. But in 1942 the North American Conference of State and Territorial Health Officers and the APHA both sponsored the principle that bedside nursing is an essential community service. During the depression, it will be recalled, federal emergency agencies had broken with the tradition that official public health nursing agencies might not give bedside care. In the first postwar year a committee, representing all the federal and national agencies interested in public health nursing, prepared a statement which placed emphasis squarely on family needs. Two decades had gone by since studies had shown that it was desirable, and more economical, to have one qualified nurse (instead of two or more specialists) visit a home. But health departments had feared that if bedside nursing were accepted as a function, it might deflect interest from the preventive services. The recommendations of the committee, set forth against a historical background, in "Desirable Organization of Public Health Nursing for Family Service,"[15] have already had a profound influence on the evolution of public health nursing and the development of combination services. The recommendations are prefaced by the statement: "In the future development of public health nursing, it is important to carry out those principles which will help assure an adequate and sound public health nursing service, and which will make it possible for one public health nurse to give health guidance and bedside care to the entire family." The NOPHN followed the publication of that report with a series of valuable studies[16] which most effectively rounded out its service before it was fused with other organizations to form the NLN.

[15] "Desirable Organization of Public Health Nursing for Family Service," reprinted from *Public Health Nursing*, Aug., 1946; with Revision, Part II, Principle 7, October, 1947.

[16] (1) Rusby, Dorothy A.: *Study of Combination Services in Public Health Nursing*, NOPHN, 1950. (2) *Cost Analysis for Public Health Nursing Services*, NOPHN, 1950. (3) *Public Health Nursing for Your Community—A Guide to Establishing a Public Health Nursing Service*, NOPHN, 1950. (4) Wensley, Edith: *The Community and Public Health Nursing*, Handbook for Boards and Committees. The Macmillan Company, New York, 1950.

In his Foreword to Miss Rusby's study of combination services, Eduard C. Lindeman said: "We have here an example of democratic adaptability. Qualitatively, strong private institutions and agencies are essential for democratic survival. But, in order to be strong, private institutions need not practice isolationism. Indeed, their real strength is revealed in their capacity to collaborate, to blend their services in the interest of efficiency."

These "tools," prepared for use in facilitating the evolutionary process which was at work throughout the public health nursing field, were therefore available when the Metropolitan Life Insurance Company made the startling announcement in 1950 that its 40-year nursing service would be discontinued January 1, 1953. (The John Hancock Company made a similar announcement six months later.) These services, it will be recalled, were developed in most places on the basis of contractural arrangements with established visiting nurse services. Home care of maternity patients had ceased to be important since a very high percentage of such patients was being hospitalized. The acute communicable diseases which had taken a terrible toll of children's lives when the service was established had virtually been eliminated. The number of policyholders who asked for the service was steadily decreasing. The MLI, which had maintained a pleasantly collaborative relationship with the NOPHN, arranged to transfer some of its experienced field supervisors to that organization's staff in order to ensure the additional consultation services which would surely be requested of the NOPHN. Two and one-half years were allowed for the conferences with community chests and councils, which helped to support many nursing services, and for conferences on the readjustment of the budgets and services of the affiliated nursing services. It was assumed, and the assumption was fully justified, that consultant services would be especially valuable in communities which had depended almost entirely on MLI nurses and therefore might be interested in establishing permanent services. With highly competent guidance from the NOPHN's augmented expert staff, the withdrawal of MLI support has stimulated citizen, medical, and nursing interests to new efforts with the resultant organization of 11 new visiting nurse services. The interest of physicians in part-time nursing service was aroused by an article prepared by MLI physicians for the *Journal of the American Medical Association.* As MLI and John Hancock services were being withdrawn, other programs for the utilization of part-time service were being developed. The Home Care Program of the Veterans Administration, for example, makes contracts for nursing service with existing agencies.

Over a period of years the ANA and the NOPHN have studied and promoted the inclusion of nursing in prepayment plans for medical care. Blue Cross is now conducting experiments in the utilization of visiting nurse services, and a number of large insurance companies are including it in certain types of policies. Also, since a very high percentage of industrial workers are employed in small plants, it is believed that visiting nurse agencies may find opportunities for increasing their services in that area.

Experiments with new programs seemed to offer other expanding opportunities for visiting nurse services. The Montefiore Hospital of New York, which had pioneered years before in giving scientific institutional care to "chronic" patients, undertook an experiment (1947) in home care for selected long-term patients which has aroused widespread interest. When the director of the program and the social worker have found that a patient is medically and socially suitable for home care, and the visiting nurse has investigated the home and found that the family is receptive to the idea, the patient is returned to the home but remains under the jurisdiction of the hospital. Such patients may receive any or all of the following services: medical and nursing care, social service, housekeeping service, occupational therapy, dietotherapy, physical therapy, x-ray service, and laboratory examinations. The nursing service is provided, on contract, by the Visiting Nurse Service of New York. "The hospital," as the director of the program puts it, "has integrated its facilities with those of the community for the benefit of the patient."[17]

The Montefiore experiment was so successful that the method

[17] Cherkasky, Martin, and Randall, Marian G.: "A Community Home Care Program," *Am. J. Nursing*, 49:650, 1949.

was adopted by the municipal hospital system of New York. The visiting nurse services of Brooklyn and New York provide nursing care. These and similar experiments in a number of other cities are not only providing superior care for the patients but they accomplish it at a much lower cost than hospital care while releasing beds for patients who require hospitalization. (About thirty years had elapsed since an AHA committee suggested that a study of home care might reveal the possibility of reducing hospital costs!) The concept of comprehensive patient care, so effectively exemplified in these programs, was providing a focal point for nursing education as the profession swept onward to the second half of the twentieth century.

The federal government is the world's largest employer of professional registered nurses. It also provides consultant services which are progressively helping to improve the quality and distribution of nursing services throughout the nation. Its principal service agencies[18] are the three military services, the Nurse Corps of the Army, Navy, and Air Force; the hospital (marine hospitals) service of the USPHS; and the Veterans Administration. Although some 5000 nurses had been added to these services between 1950 and 1952, all were then operating at less than their authorized strength. The organization of the new Air Force Nurse Corps (1948) and the reorganization of the VA nursing service were outstanding events in the postwar period.

Immediately following World War II, Army nurses in occupied areas in Europe and Asia became deeply interested in helping local nurses to re-establish their educational and service programs. Some of them, especially in Japan, laid the foundations for lasting international friendships. Following the invasion of Korea, articles in the public press about the superb work of nurses with the armed forces in Korea and Japan made other nurses proud of them but did not stimulate recruitment appreciably. The long-continued "emergency" was not conducive to recruitment for military service. The ANA, it will be recalled, is on record as favoring a draft of nurses should such legislation again be put forward. The basic problem

[18] For complete list see *Facts about Nursing*, 1952, ANA, pp. 36–37.

goes back, as it always does in emergencies, to who or what agency is responsible for assuring the nation a reasonable supply of nursing service. In an effort to find an answer, the military services are working cooperatively with both the ANA and the NLN.

Dorothy V. Wheeler, under whose direction the reorganization of the VA service which is now (1952) authorized to employ over 15,000 nurses was carried forward, credits Gen. Paul R. Hawley with the foresight which made the reorganization possible. The VA was given its own Professional Standards Board which functions in much the same fashion as the Civil Service Commission. The revitalized service has attracted some of the nation's ablest nurse educators and administrators. It provides affiliations, especially in tuberculosis and psychiatric nursing, for approximately 100 schools of nursing. Its liberal salary schedules and other personnel policies have tended to improve conditions for nurses in civilian institutions in the neighborhood of veteran facilities. The service endeavors to stress excellence in bedside nursing by making it possible for nurses —who like to give direct care to patients but have won the privilege of promotion—to progress in grade and income while continuing to do bedside nursing. Historically, such recognition of good nursing is long overdue. Unfortunately, the VA finds that the profession's tradition of honoring position, rather than competency in the practice of nursing, is resistant to change.

Since World War II all government nursing services have operated on the basic principle that the service of professional nurses must be utilized at the highest level of efficiency. This general policy was made official in 1952 by a directive from the Department of Defense which interdicted the performance of non-nursing functions by nurses and instructed the military departments to train sufficient practical nurses and auxiliary personnel to perform the functions from which nurses were relieved.

Through research, grants-in-aid, and consultant services federal agencies, respecting "states rights," promote national upgrading of nursing and its adaptation to changing needs. The USPHS and the Children's Bureau are the sources of such assistance. The Division of Nursing Service of the USPHS was created in 1946. The Cadet

Nurse Corps had entered the terminal stage of its program which had been so brilliantly and modestly directed by Lucile Petry (Leone). Miss Petry had participated in the revision of the NLNE's *Curriculum Guide,* and held a succession of university positions, including that of assistant to the dean of the school at the University of Minnesota, and was a member of the board of directors of the NLNE. Possessing an extraordinarily comprehensive knowledge of nursing education, organization, and relationships, she was the logical person to be made responsible, as director of the new division, for coordinating the nursing activities which had been established under the jurisdiction of various units of the USPHS. These covered the gamut of nursing: nursing education, hospital nursing, and public health nursing. Margaret Arnstein, who had participated in planning both the wartime programs in nursing education, was appointed director of the new Bureau of Nursing Resources. Pearl McIver, who had organized the Division of Public Health Nursing (1934) and directed the first wartime nursing education program, continued as director of that division. Numerous references have already been made to the participation of the USPHS in the development of nursing services. Some of its practical demonstrations of teamwork will be amplified in the discussion of nursing education.

The medical care team idea is well illustrated by the compact program of the Children's Bureau in which four professions participate—medicine, nursing, nutrition, and social work. The primary interests of the bureau are maternal and child welfare and the care of crippled children. Although commonly thought of as a public health service, Ruth G. Taylor, director of the nursing unit since the early forties, has insisted that consideration be given to all phases of nursing service related to the health of mothers and children regardless of locale, whether in homes, hospitals, clinics, or convalescent homes. Because of the inclusiveness of this concept, Dr. Edwin F. Dailey, director of the Division of Health Services of the bureau for many years, credited Miss Taylor with effecting "one of the most significant changes in attitude toward public health programs during the past decade."[19] Like the USPHS, the bureau provides consultative services, through its regional offices. It has had a significant influence on the education of nurses and the quality of nursing service through grants for advanced programs in obstetric and pediatric nursing.

In the midst of many efforts to adapt nursing resources to the rising demands for nursing service, the National Committee for the Improvement of Nursing Services (NCINS) (1948) became, to use Professor Winslow's term, a powerful catalytic agent. By 1952, as shown in the next chapter, it had effectively promoted "the acceleration of forces already at work" in nursing education. It had also lived up to its promise that "every activity of the committee will be used as an opportunity to bring about a better understanding of the problems of nursing as they affect interprofessional groups and of the avenues open for cooperation."[20] Good nursing is dependent upon well-prepared personnel. This was the basic premise on which the committe built its program.

The first phase of its work, when the committee was still called the Committee on Implementing the Brown Report, was financed by the nursing organizations. Enthusiastic Helen W. Goodale (Florentine), who became executive secretary of the committee late in 1948, prepared two study guides to encourage careful analysis and use of the book.[21] The work of a Subcommittee on School Data Analysis which produced the Interim Classification of Schools of Nursing is discussed in the chapter on nursing education.

In 1949 Marion W. Sheahan, then recently retired from the Division of Nursing of the New York State Department of Health where she had achieved distinction as an administrator and was widely known for her statesmanship, accepted appointment as director of programs of the NCINS. She and Miss Goodale spent four

[19] Dailey, Edwin F.: Address before Children's Bureau Advisory Committee on Maternal and Child Health and Applied Children's Services, Washington, D.C., Sept. 14, 1948. (Mimeographed.)

[20] Sheahan, Marion W.: "A Program for the Improvement of Nursing Services," *Am. J. Nursing,* **50:**794, 1950.

[21] Brown, Esther Lucile: *Nursing for the Future.* Russell Sage Foundation, New York, 1948.

months in the field to interpret and guide the reactions to the Interim Classification of Schools. Miss Goodale resigned from the committee in 1951 to direct a new nursing service education program at the University of Minnesota. Following the field experience, Miss Sheahan began programs which could secure the united backing of the boards of directors of the six national organizations. The planning was so sound that the W. K. Kellogg Foundation granted $200,000 for a three-year program. The committee was enlarged to include 40 representatives of medicine, dentistry, hospital administration, public health, general education, social science, and various citizen interests.

The committee began at once to promote state or regional planning through the development of similar committees in the states. Data on nursing resources were graphically presented in a sparkling newsletter which aroused interest and stimulated use of the materials in relation to local situations. The Joint Commission for the Improvement of the Care of the Patient, which had been organized on the initiative of the medical and hospital organizations with nursing representation, served as an interprofessional advisory committee to the NCINS. The commission has no executive power. Action is dependent on the acceptance of commission recommendations by the boards of directors of the medical, hospital, and nursing organizations represented on it. The word "nursing" does not appear in the name of the commission. Its primary purpose, however, is the consideration of problems related to nursing service. By the summer of 1952, through the work of subcommittees, there was general agreement between the commission and the NCINS that improvement of nursing service depends on:

1. Well prepared nurses for faculty of schools and for administrative and supervisory services.
2. Effective in-service education to improve workers on the job.
3. More practical nurses properly prepared.
4. Experimentation in nursing curriculums. [Two-year program was specified.][22]

[22] *NCINS News Letter*, Vol. 2, No. 2, April–May, 1952.

As this is written, although the several boards of directors had not yet taken official action, it was thought that the nurse members were not overoptimistic in believing that the four points would be accepted by all the participating organizations as the basis for an ongoing program for the improvement of nursing service.

The Inter-Association Committee on Health, which represents six national organizations,[23] had already adopted a statement of principles for the improvement in quantity, quality, and distribution of nursing personnel to meet civil and military needs.

Through the appointment of experienced Marian G. Fox as nursing specialist on the staff of the AHA, an effective liason was established between that organization and the NCINS. A historic precedent was established when the NCINS and the AHA jointly began sponsoring week-long regional institutes (three) on nursing service administration. The faculties included experts from many fields in addition to hospital administration and nursing. Planned for the participation of hospital administrators and directors of nursing service, they provided a forum for consideration of the practical application in local situations of the results of national and other studies. Regional workshops on the functions of head nurses in which the USPHS also participated were provided for groups restricted to nurses who were to direct head nurse studies, state nurse consultants, and faculty members of universities which were conducting programs in education for administration of nursing service.

Following the restructuring of the national organizations in June, 1952, the NCINS became the Advisory Committee to the Nursing Service Division of the National League for Nursing. The programs of the committee had successfully stimulated an objective approach to problems which previously had been emotionally charged; they had opened up new vistas of usefulness through interprofessional relationships; they made it possible for nursing service to attain the overt place of honor in the national nursing organizations to which it has always implicitly been entitled.

[23] Members represent the American Dental, Hospital, Medical, Nurses', Public Health, and Welfare Associations. *Am. J. Nursing,* **52:**763, 1952.

By the middle of 1952, the closing date for this volume, some encouraging trends in the evolution of nursing service had emerged from the vortex of postwar nursing.

1. The results of research were beginning to replace traditions in the philosophy and administrative practice in nursing services.

2. There were encouraging evidences of growing accord among the professions with which nursing is most closely associated in medical care teams.

3. There was a marked trend toward liberalizing institutional personnel policies with resultant, although uneven, improvement in time and salary schedules.

4. There was general acceptance by registered professional nurses of the need for the preparation and licensure of practical nurses.

5. The usefulness of the nursing team, composed of professional and nonprofessional workers, as an administrative device for providing comprehensive patient-centered care, had been effectively demonstrated.

6. There was increasing utilization of nursing service in prepayment and other part-time home care programs.

7. Effective utilization of nursing resources was shown in the trend toward a development of public health nursing services "which will make it possible for one public health nurse to give health guidance and bedside care to the entire family" and in the utilization of nursing teams, especially in institutional nursing.

8. The supportive interest of the federal government, through consultation services and grants-in-aid of nursing education, as a means for improving nursing service, had "accelerated forces already in operation," especially in the fields of maternity, pediatric, orthopedic, and psychiatric nursing.

The most specific action taken by any national body to improve the administration of nursing services was that of the W. K. Kellogg Foundation which, in 1950, invited 14 universities to participate in a two- to five-year program for the improvement of the preparation of administrators of nursing services. The foundation, it will be recalled, had practically maintained the National Nursing Council; it had financed a five-year program in clinical nursing at

10 universities; and it had supported the NCINS. It seems probable that future historians may consider the Kellogg program in the administration of nursing service a milestone in the evolution of nursing comparable to the Winslow-Goldmark report of 1922. Its stimulating influence on nursing education is discussed in the next chapter.

BIBLIOGRAPHY

Abramson, Judith: "Orientation to the Home Care Program," *Am. J. Nursing*, **52:**739, 1952.

"Administration of Home Nursing Care of the Sick by Health Departments," *Pub. Health Nursing*, **37:**339, 1945.

Aims of Nursing Administration. Catholic University of America Press, Washington, D.C., 1947.

Barron, Mabel: "Twenty-Eight Years of Team Work," *Am. J. Nursing*, **49:**225, 1949.

Barton, Walter E.: "The Nurse as an Active Member of the Psychiatric Team," *Am. J. Nursing*, **50:**714, 1950.

Benderoff, Olga C.: "A Look at Nursing Service," *Ohio Nurses' Review*, July–Aug., 1952.

Berger, Harriett, and Johnson, Marjorie: "Developing the Nursing Team at St. Luke's, Chicago," *Am. J. Nursing*, **49:**442, 1949.

Brackett, Mary E.: "The Nursing Team Satisfies," *Hosp. Management*, **72:**80, 1951.

Bredenberg, Viola C.: *A Functional Analysis of the Nursing Service Team.* Catholic University of America Press, Washington, D.C., 1949.

———: "Experimental Research in Nursing Service," *Am. J. Nursing*, **50:**661, 1950.

Carnevali, Doris, and Sheldon, Nola Smith: "How Early Ambulation Affects Nursing Service," *Am. J. Nursing*, **52:**954, 1952.

Casper, Thelma A., and Cawley, Marie: "Early Ambulation and Postpartum Care," *Am. J. Nursing*, **52:**1210, 1952.

Deming, Dorothy: "The Professional Examination Service," *Am. J. Pub. Health*, **42:**299, 1952.

De Witt, Katharine: "Hospital Atmosphere as It Impresses an Outsider," *Pacific Coast J. Nursing*, **5:**151, 1909.

"The Economic Status of the Nursing Profession," *Am. J. Nursing*, **47:**456, 1947.

Finer, Herman: *Administration and the Nursing Services.* The Macmillan Company, New York, 1952.

Flagg, Maurice: "They Showed the Way," *Red Cross Magazine,* 1:27, 1951.

Fluent, Marion A., and Cadmus, Robert R.: "Nursing Learns from Industry," *Am. J. Nursing,* 49:350, 1949; also in *Hospitals,* 23:35, 1949.

Foley, Margaret (ed.): *Nursing Service in Catholic Hospitals.* The Catholic Hospital Association, St. Louis, 1952.

Fraser, Mary A.: "A Report on Functional Analysis in a Naval Hospital," *Nursing World,* 126:115, 1952.

Frasher, Charles B.: "The A.B.C.'s of the Nursing Service Merit System," *Pub. Health Nursing,* 42:273, 1950.

Freeman, Ruth B.: "Nursing Plus—American Red Cross Nursing Service," *Am. J. Nursing,* 48:12, 1948.

Frost, Harriet, and Overholser, Margery: "Referral of Patients for Home Nursing," *Am. J. Nursing,* 49:329, 1949.

Gillian, Ruth I.: "Effective Organization of the Nursing Service Leads to Improved Patient Care," *Mod. Hosp.,* 76:49, 1951.

Gillian, Ruth I., and Tibbitts, Helen G.: "Whose Job Is the Head Nurse Doing?" *Am. J. Nursing,* 52:298, 1952.

Ginsburg, Ethel L.: *Public Health Is People.* The Commonwealth Fund, New York, 1950.

Griffin, Margaret J., and Sobotka, Irene A.: "Care for Patients at Home," *Am. J. Nursing,* 52:717, 1952.

Guide for Inclusion of Nursing in Medical Care Plans. American Nurses' Association and National Organization for Public Health Nursing, New York, 1950.

Guide Outlines for Courses of Instruction in Training Hospital Aides in Veterans Administration Nursing Service. Veterans Administration, Washington, D.C., 1950.

Hamilton, James A.: "Success or Failure in Nursing Administration?" *Am. J. Nursing,* 49:496, 1949.

Hampton, Peter J.: "An Introduction to Job Description," *Am. J. Nursing,* 47:411, 1947.

"The Harper Hospital Study," *Am. J. Nursing,* 52:984, 1952.

Haupt, Alma C., and Connors, Helen: "Nursing in Medical Care Plans," *Am. J. Nursing,* 51:357, 1951.

The Head Nurse Looks at Her Job. US Public Health Service Pub. #227. US Government Printing Office, Washington, D.C., 1952.

Health Service Areas—Requirements for General Hospitals and Health Centers. Public Health Bull. #292. US Government Printing Office, Washington, D.C., 1945.

Holtzhausen, Erma A.: "Nursing Service in a Teaching Hospital," *Am. J. Nursing*, **46**:550, 1946.

Hospital Nursing Service Manual. American Hospital Association and the National League of Nursing Education, 1950.

"Hospital Survey and Construction Act," *Am. J. Nursing*, **48**:361, 1948.

Job Descriptions and Organizational Analysis for Hospitals and Related Health Services. US Department of Labor in cooperation with the American Hospital Association. US Government Printing Office, Washington, D.C., 1952.

Kemble, Elizabeth S.: "Shorter and Sharper Testing Tools for the Prenursing and Guidance Test Services," *Am. J. Nursing*, **47**:327, 1947.

Kempf, Florence C.: "Evaluating the Performance of Nursing Personnel," *Am. J. Nursing*, **49**:707, 1949.

———: *Manual on Performance Evaluation of Nursing Service Personnel.* University Hospitals of Cleveland, 1950.

Kennedy, Johanna E.: "A Health Department Develops a Generalized Service," *Pub. Health Nursing*, **44**:513, 1952.

Kroeger, Louis J., and associates: *The Nursing Function in California Hospitals.* Part I of a report on a study for the California State Nurses' Association (mimeographed), May, 1952.

Kuntz, Mary N., and Rogers, Mary: "Planning Assignments for Nursing Teams," *Am. J. Nursing*, **50**:526, 1950.

Leavell, Hugh R.: "Contributions of the Social Sciences to the Solution of Health Problems," *New England J. Med.*, **247**:885, 1952.

Leino, Amelia: "Organizing the Nursing Team," *Am. J. Nursing*, **51**:665, 1951.

———: "Team Functioning of Hospital Nursing Personnel," in *Problems of Graduate Nurse Education*, Work Conference Report #2. Bureau of Publications, Teachers College, Columbia University, New York, 1952.

Magoun, F. Alexander: "New Ways in Personnel Administration," *Am. J. Nursing*, **46**:751, 1946.

Marvin, Mary M.: "The Position and Preparation of the Head Nurse," *Am. J. Nursing*, **28**:818, 1928.

Measuring Nursing Resources. Division of Nursing Resources, US Public Health Service, Federal Security Agency, Washington, D.C., 1949.

"The Military Nursing Services" (requirements for reserve commissions), *Am. J. Nursing*, **51**:449, 1951.

Mountin, Joseph W.: "Changing Patterns of State Health Services," *Am. J. Pub. Health*, **41**:516, 1951.

The Nation's Health—A Ten-Year Program. A report to the President by Oscar R. Ewing, US Government Printing Office, Washington, D.C., 1948.

O'Malley, Martha, and Orem, Dorothea: "Diagnosis of Hospital Nursing Problems," *Hospitals*, **26**:63, 1952.

Part-Time Nursing in Industry as Provided by Visiting Nurses Associations in the United States. National Organization for Public Health Nursing, New York, 1946.

Perkins, Dorothy, and Heslin, Phyllis: "Nursing Service and Nursing Education Advance Together with the Team Plan," *Am. J. Nursing*, **52**:185, 1952.

Petry, Lucile: "The Nursing Survey, an Essential for Sound Planning," *Am. J. Nursing*, **51**:380, 1951.

Pigors, Paul, and Myers, C. A.: *Personnel Administration, a Point of View and a Method*, 2nd ed. McGraw-Hill Book Co., New York, 1951.

Practical Nurses in Nursing Services. Prepared by the Joint Committee on Practical Nurses and Auxiliary Workers in Nursing Services, New York, 1951.

A Program for the Nursing Profession, Committee on the Function of Nursing. The Macmillan Company, New York, 1948.

Psychiatric Nursing Personnel, Facts and Figures for 1950. American Psychiatric Association, New York, 1951.

The Public Health Service Today. Federal Security Agency, US Public Health Service, Washington, D.C., 1952.

Randall, Marian G.: "Nursing in Health Service Plans," *Pub. Health Nursing*, **36**:311, 1944.

"Recommended Adjustments for Public Health Nursing Services in the National Security Program," *Pub. Health Nursing*, **43**:259, 1951.

Registry Manual. American Nurses' Association, New York, 1949.

Roethlisberger, F. J.: *Morale and Management*. Harvard University Press, Cambridge, 1952.

Schafer, Margaret K., and Galbraith, T. P.: "Recovery Room Services— A Guide for Planning," *Hospitals*, **26**:65, 1952.

Seyffer, Charlotte (ed.): *The Organization of Hospital Nursing Services*. Catholic University of America Press, Washington, D.C., 1952.

Shepard, William P., and Wheatley, George M.: "Visiting Nurse Service —Community Asset for Every Physician," *J.A.M.A.*, **149**:554, 1952.

"Should Nurses Do Venipunctures?" *Am. J. Nursing*, **51**:603, 1951.

Smillie, Wilson G.: *Preventive Medicine and Public Health*, 2nd ed.; Sec. VI, "Public Health Administration." The Macmillan Company, New York, 1952.

Smith, Harriet H.: "The Nurse Consultant in Hospital Planning," *Am. J. Nursing*, **51**:441, 1951.

Staffing the General Hospital—25 to 100 Beds. Division of Medical and

Hospital Resources, US Public Health Service, Federal Security Agency, Washington, D.C., 1949.

Standard Nursing Administrative Procedures for VA Hospitals. Veterans Administration Manual M. 10–9, Washington, D.C., 1950.

Standards for Psychiatric Hospitals and Clinics. American Psychiatric Association, New York, 1951.

Stokes, John H.: "The Question of Venipuncture," *Am. J. Nursing,* **52:** 307, 1952.

Struve, Mildred, and Lindblad, Anne Hahn: "The Nursing Team in the Hospital," *Am. J. Nursing,* **49:**5, 1949.

Tead, Ordway: *The Art of Administration.* McGraw-Hill Book Co., New York, 1951.

"Training for Nursing Service Administration," *Am. J. Nursing,* **51:**11, 1951.

Tuckey, Ruth: "The Practical Nurse in a Public Health Agency," *Am. J. Nursing,* **48:**647, 1948.

Urwick, Lyndall: *The Elements of Administration.* Harper & Brothers, New York, 1944, Chap. 46.

Vreeland, Ellwynne M.: "Fifty Years of Nursing in the Federal Government Nursing Services," *Am. J. Nursing,* **50:**626, 1950.

Waagen, Louise, "Basic Nursing Service Policies," *Hospitals,* **26:**74, 1952.

Wayland, Mary Marvin; McManus, R. Louise; and Faddis, Margene O.: *The Hospital Head Nurse,* 2nd ed. The Macmillan Company, New York, 1944.

Wensley, Edith: *The Community and Public Health Nursing.* The Macmillan Company, New York, 1950.

"What Is Posdcorb?" *Am. J. Nursing,* **38:**444, 1938.

Williams, Ralph Chester: *The United States Public Health Service, 1798–1950.* Published by the Commissioned Officers Association, US Public Health Service, Bethesda, Md., 1951.

Wright, Marion J.: "Messenger Service at Harper Hospital, *Am. J. Nursing,* **52:**172, 1952.

Chapter 47

NURSING EDUCATION AT MID-CENTURY

Schools of nursing should be maintained—not for the sake of hospitals, or any other institutions, not for the sake of the nursing profession, or students of nursing, nor any other limited group—but for the present and future welfare of society as a whole.[1]

Within a democratic society there is no person, group of persons, or organized voluntary body that has power to order sudden and drastic change. Such changes as are effected will result from long and careful planning at the conference table of national, state, and local nursing associations and other bodies, and of state boards of nurse examiners. More importantly, they will issue from the persistent and courageous efforts of hundreds of nurse educators working within their own schools and communities.

ESTHER LUCILE BROWN[2]

THE POVERTY of nursing schools (in 1949 the typical school still had no separate budget) and the inadequacy of the technical prewar pattern of nursing education, with its major dependence on approximately one-fifth of the nation's hospitals, were thrown into sharp relief by the enormously increased demands for nursing service which have been discussed in the preceding chapter. The public, through donations or tax funds, bears approximately half the expense of all other forms of higher education but contributes only 7 per cent of the costs of nursing education. The revolutionary changes in social philosophy and in medical care previously noted called for an enrichment of programs for the preparation of professional nurses with special emphasis on the psychosomatic aspects of medicine, on interpersonal and interprofessional relationships,

[1] *Fundamentals of Administration for Schools of Nursing*, NLNE, 1940 (reprinted, 1947), p. 204.

[2] Brown, Esther Lucile: *Nursing for the Future*. Russell Sage Foundation, New York, 1948, p. 14.

and on the technics of communication. The enormously increased demand for service, necessitating the integration of large numbers of nonprofessional workers in nursing services, put a new emphasis on the importance of the administrative and teaching functions of professional nurses. The profession had not wholeheartedly supported its own policies in relation to the preparation of practical nurses nor, at mid-century, was it fully prepared to develop the continuous staff education programs and the in-service programs required in connection with the evolving patterns of nursing service. It is not probable that nursing schools can be released from the obligation to provide excessive amounts of hospital nursing service until such programs have been well developed.

With the turn of the mid-century, a wealth of stimulating material became available to nurse educators and others concerned with the reforms in nursing education advocated by the Brown report. In addition to the studies already enumerated, and the almost photographically descriptive *Nursing Schools at the Mid-Century,* there were the report of the President's Commission on Higher Education and, in 1951, the reports of the Committees on Nursing Services Administration which are a distillate of the thinking of the participants in the five-month Nursing Service Administration Seminar made possible at the University of Chicago by the Kellogg Foundation. There were also the reports of two nationally sponsored curriculum conferences and two work conferences sponsored by Teachers College, Columbia University.[3,4]

It is not possible to appraise the potential influence on nursing of the report of the President's Commission. It proposed that the number of community (junior) colleges be increased and their activities multiplied. It recommended that such community colleges offer terminal programs on a semiprofessional (technician) level for the preparation of personnel to meet the increased demand for

[3] *Nursing Organization Curriculum Conference,* Curriculum Bulletin #1, and *Joint Nursing Curriculum Conference,* Curriculum Bulletin #2. NLNE, New York, 1950 and 1951, respectively.
[4] Work Conferences: (a) *Regional Planning for Nursing and Nursing Education,* (b) *Problems of Graduate Nurse Education,* Work Conference #2. Teachers College, Columbia University, New York, 1950 and 1951, respectively.

personnel in medicine, dentistry, and nursing. Teachers College, Columbia University, received an anonymous grant for a five-year experimental program based on these recommendations. The first two-year program leading to an associate degree was undertaken in New York (1952) where the nurse practice act requires only a two-year preparation for licensure. Proponents of this type of program believe that it is a logical step toward securing a recognized place for nursing in the nation's educational system. The Ginzberg report, for example, advocates this type of program anticipating that *in time* there would be professional nurses (with at least a baccalaureate degree) and semiprofessional nurses, presumably with associate degrees, but no licensed practical nurses. Mildred L. Montag, author of *The Education of Nursing Technicians,*[5] is director of the pilot program. The announcement of the Teachers College program promptly raised such questions as: If semiprofessional nurses, eligible for licensure, can be prepared by tax-supported community colleges, what will be the influence of that movement on the preparation of practical nurses? Prophecy is not a function of a historian. At this writing (1952) further development of practical nursing is an important element in the programs of the professional organizations and of the NAPNE. The ANA has reported that 39 states and territories are providing for the licensing of practical nurses (or other workers of similar preparation). The laws, in six of the seven states which have separate laws for nonprofessional nurses, are mandatory. In 18 states the body legally responsible for the accreditation of nursing schools is responsible for both types.

In 1951, between 8000 and 10,000 student nurses were enrolled in junior colleges.[6] The greater number were in cooperative programs in which academic education was given in the college and the clinical experience in a local hospital. The number of junior colleges offering programs in nursing was then increasing throughout the nation. Out of approximately 400, about one-fourth were offering terminal or semiprofessional courses; the others, preparatory or

[5] Montag, Mildred L.: *The Education of Nursing Technicians.* G. P. Putnam's Sons, New York, 1951.

[6] Bogue, Jesse P. (ed.): *American Junior Colleges,* 3rd ed. American Council on Education, Washington, D.C., 1952.

preprofessional programs. In California, where the junior college movement has had its greatest growth, schools of nursing (with the notable exception of the two schools of the University of California) are hospital schools, and affiliations of both types have been arranged with junior colleges. The increase in the number offering nursing courses was found to be due to the development of hospital facilities in cities which previously had none. It may be noted that the number of state colleges offering four-year programs is also increasing, as pointed out some time ago by Lenore Bradley, then of the New York board of examiners. Although some nurse educators believe that these and other small liberal arts colleges can offer desirable opportunities for the preparation of nurses, the question is still a subject for debate.

The Brown report, which spearheaded the movement for mid-century educational reform, was published in the autumn of 1948. Many pages of the AJN for the following year bear testimony to the speed and earnestness with which the nursing organizations responded to its provocative challenge. The initial response of the six national nursing organizations was the organization of the four major committees noted in Chapter 45, one of which, the National Committee for the Improvement of Nursing Services, was originally called the Committee on Implementing the Brown Report. The key question to which Dr. Brown's advisory committee had agreed she should find an answer was: "Who should organize, administer, and finance professional schools of nursing?" She reported that persons conversant with the trend in professional education in the US were practically unanimous in the opinion that the preparation of professional nurses belongs in institutions of higher learning. Students of nursing history were well aware that this was not the radical suggestion that many persons, who had accepted nursing's traditional use of "professional" and "registered" as synonymous terms, believed it to be.

The Winslow-Goldmark report, *Nursing and Nursing Education in the United States,* had advocated collegiate schools for the preparation of leaders in nursing. Miss Goodrich had told a nursing audience in 1934 that, within a decade, every nursing school should be definitely associated with a college or university or be discontinued! In the early forties, Isabel M. Stewart had pointed out in her admirable history of nursing education that "the time seemed not far distant when the bachelor's degree must be a basic requirement for the professional nurse as it is for librarians and other young professions, and also that a decision must be reached about the preparation of more than one grade of nurse."[7] The Bixlers, too, in their incisive analysis of nursing, indicated that the professional status and social usefulness of nursing should be increased by determined effort to secure a place for nursing education in institutions of higher learning.

The introduction of many thousands of practical nurses and unprepared personnel into nursing services put new emphasis on the importance of preparing professional nurses for leadership in all nursing situations and relationships, beginning with the team relationship at the bedside of hospitalized patients.

Due to its incandescent quality, intrinsic merit, and the enthusiasm with which its sale was promoted by the profession, the distribution of the Brown report exceeded that of any other social study known to Dr. Brown. The first reaction of many readers, who overlooked the statement which heads this chapter, was fear—fear of immediate demotion of the social and professional status of many nurses and schools of nursing. Through the NLNE and the NCINS, which were to have a dynamic influence on the evolution of nursing as a community service, the profession took quick action. The National Nursing Accrediting Service had been established in 1948 with Hazel A. Goff and Julia M. Miller successively carrying the program on a temporary basis until July, 1950. Miss Miller then succeeded Adelaide W. Mayo, who was retiring, as executive secretary of the NLNE. Helen Nahm, director of the Division of Nursing Education of Duke University, who had been appointed some months earlier, became director of the service. Miss Nahm, a Ph.D., with experience in both large and small schools, was temperamentally, as well as academically and professionally, unusually well

[7] Stewart, Isabel M.: *The Education of Nurses.* The Macmillan Company, New York, 1943.

qualified for this exacting and influential position. In the summer of 1951 the NLNE and the NNAS put a "flying squadron"[8] in the field to explain three major programs. These were Accreditation, Evaluation and Guidance (Tests and Measurements) and the NLNE's new Department of Services to Schools of Nursing. Workshops were held in various parts of the country, and the *Manual on Accrediting Educational Programs* was published. The NCINS acted promptly to provide a sound foundation for an action program based on Dr. Brown's recommendation that ". . . nursing make one of its first matters of important business the long overdue official examination of every school; that the lists of accredited schools be published and distributed as far as possible to every town and city of the United States. . . ."[9] A subcommittee—Louise Knapp, (chairman), director of the Washington University School of Nursing—was appointed to make a study of basic nursing education which was known as the "School Data Analysis." The NCINS, at this stage, was neither staffed nor financed for a comprehensive study. Staff assistance was requested of the USPHS which promptly and generously responded by providing a highly competent staff to work under the direction of the subcommittee in preparing a classification of schools of nursing (1) to furnish a basis for the planning of nursing services, (2) to provide a list of schools for which the profession would be willing to recruit students, (3) to distinguish degree and diploma programs. The NCINS accepted responsibility for securing information for its own use and that of other committees. The collaboration of the USPHS made possible the *Interim Classification of Schools of Nursing Offering Basic Programs* (1949) and, the publication the following year of *Nursing Schools at the Mid-Century,* an impressive milestone marker.

Thanks to the wholehearted support of local and state nursing groups and of hospital administrators, 97 per cent of all schools (1156) voluntarily participated in the questionnaire study. Schools were classified in two groups. Group I included approximately 25 per cent of all schools; Group II included 50 per cent of them. About

[8] Helen Nahm, Ruth Bishop, and Kathryn W. Cafferty.
[9] Brown, Esther Lucile: *op. cit.,* p. 116.

300 schools, including those with the lowest national standings, were not classified.[10] By previous arrangement, the National Nursing Accrediting Services (Lucile Petry was chairman of the Joint Committee on the Unification of Accrediting Activities) published its first list of accredited schools[11] just one month in advance of the *Interim Classification*. This was merely a compilation of the programs, both basic and advanced, which had been approved for the purpose by the four agencies which had been fused to form the NNAS. Comparative lists, such as the *Interim Classification* had long been needed by the Committee on Careers in Nursing, by counselors and by institutions offering advanced programs for graduate nurses. But the *Interim Classification* was received with shocked surprise, rebellious disbelief, and considerable misunderstanding by persons unaccustomed to thinking in comparative terms. Then, too, some confusion was created by the publication of the two lists at approximately the same time.

By this time Mary Ellen Manley had succeeded Mary Connor as chairman of the NCINS, and Marion W. Sheahan had become director of programs. High aspirations and a shortage of funds! This was the situation, by no means unique in nursing history, which confronted her. Experienced in interprofessional and intergroup relationships, Miss Sheahan spent some weeks in the formulation of programs which would at once have the unified support of the joint boards of the national nursing organizations and be of sufficient scope to justify foundations in providing financial aid. Substantial grants were obtained for the development of a program under the NCINS and for the accreditation program.[12] These grants may be considered the impressive first fruits of the growing unity of purpose which was being fostered by the Structure Committee. The National Nursing Accrediting Service was set up with four boards of review: basic noncollegiate professional nursing education, basic collegiate

[10] "Interim Classification of Schools of Nursing Offering Basic Programs, 1949," *Am. J. Nursing,* 49: adv. 34–36, 1949.

[11] Petry, Lucile: "We Hail an Important First," *Am. J. Nursing,* 49:630, 1949.

[12] Contributed by the Kellogg Foundation, the Rockefeller Foundation, the Commonwealth Fund, and the National Foundation for Infantile Paralysis.

professional nursing education, public health nursing education, postgraduate professional nursing education. It is hoped that the time may be not far distant when a board will also be required for nonprofessional (practical) nursing education. The hardworking and conscientious personnel of these boards represent a cross section, both professional and geographic, of current thinking and practice in their respective categories.

A growing list of fully accredited schools was published in the *AJN* each year from 1949 until 1953 when such publication became a privilege of *Nursing Outlook*. During the furor over the *Interim Classification*, hospital administrators and directors of schools of nursing recommended that all schools be visited and that the list of schools be made a part of the accreditation program. With foundation support the NNAS developed a five-year plan for temporary accreditation on the assumption that, with assistance, many basic schools of nursing, if desirous of improving their facilities and programs, could do so. A concerted effort was being made to give such assistance. The many regional conferences arranged by the NNAS for faculty and other representatives of nursing schools were a stimulating source of information and guidance. State boards of nurse examiners were encouraged to develop more flexible criteria and were becoming actively interested in the "upgrading" rather than mere standardization of the schools within their jurisdictions. The NLNE's Department of Services to Schools of Nursing, under the direction of Kathryn W. Cafferty, has become an important source of practical assistance, especially in relation to curriculum. The first list of basic schools granted temporary accreditation for a five-year period was published in 1952.[13] Although 25 per cent of the 1103 programs evaluated by NNAS were not approved for temporary accreditation, 85 per cent of all students were enrolled in fully or temporarily accredited programs. Schools which appeared to be the sole source of supply of nurses for a considerable area were given special consideration by NNAS. In general, two types of reaction to the omission of a school from the list of those temporarily accredited have been noted. Omission is a boon to

[13] "Temporary Accreditation," *Am. J. Nursing*, **52**:997, 1952.

schools which accept the challenge and secure assistance from the NNAS and other sources in formulating plans for securing community interest and support of efforts toward improvement as, for example, by some type of centralized program. Omission from the list is a bane to the complacent and to those who disregard the fundamental obligation of schools to educate students for a broader range of service than that required to meet the service needs of any one institution. Fortunately those that accept the challenge seem to be in the majority. Mid-century national policy, in other words, was to assist schools, both hospital and collegiate, to attain their highest level of educational achievement in relation to the nation's needs for nursing. In this effort the profession has the support, in principle, of the AHA.[14] This policy is not a negation of the principle that nursing education should be the obligation and prerogative of institutions of higher education. It is recognition of the fact that time will be required for that change to be effected by democratic processes.

To revert to consideration of the place of nursing in institutions of higher learning as envisioned in the Brown report! The educational needs of nursing, Dr. Brown discovered, were not very well understood in academic circles. Dean Margaret Bridgman of Skidmore College, who had been closely associated with the school of nursing, was engaged by the Russell Sage Foundation to serve as interpreter and advisor on nursing education to institutions of higher education. She subsequently became a consultant on the staff of the new National League for Nursing. Miss Bridgman was shocked to find that some colleges and universities had made "concessions to nursing" instead of insisting on work of a quality equivalent to that required in other disciplines. Her book, *Collegiate Education for Nursing*, addressed primarily to educators, was planned for publication by the Russell Sage Foundation early in 1953. The fallacies in the type of amiable generosity disclosed by Miss Bridgman have been painfully revealed by the NNAS; of 117

[14] "Report of the American Hospital Association Convention," *Am. J. Nursing*, 52:1351, 1952.

degree programs (1952) only 45 were fully accredited; 22 were not acceptable for temporary accreditation.

It may be asked: What effect will the national accreditation program have on the function of state boards of nurse examiners? Will nursing adopt the pattern of other professions which restrict the functions of the legally constituted bodies to the procedures of licensure and punishment of infractions of the law while depending on professional organizations for the advancement of educational standards? At mid-century, there is little evidence of a trend in that direction. The fluid state of nursing education has created both problems and opportunities for state boards of nurse examiners. State nurses' associations are constantly alert to the importance of securing legislative action when social change indicates the desirability of changing the minimum standards set by law. State boards are in a strategic position to advise on such matters as the utilization of clinical and educational community resources in the development of central schools or other centralized programs. The rigidities of their time requirements have been considered, by nurse educators, a stumbling block to progress. Some boards have, however, approved the philosophy of experimentation by collegiate and hospital schools with each proposal requiring special consideration. The reports of the annual state board conferences, sponsored jointly for many years by the ANA and the NLNE and since 1947 by the ANA with representation from the League, indicate marked improvement in the preparation of state board personnel and an increasingly cooperative relationship between the boards and the professional organizations. The State Board Conference of 1948, for example, was preceded by a carefully planned work conference on the implications, for the boards, of the Brown report. More recently the subject of collegiate schools has received special attention. As previously noted, all state boards had become members of the State Board Test Pool by 1950, one of the several services of the NLNE's Department of Measurement and Guidance which had been superbly organized by Elizabeth L. Kemble,[15] and is now, under Dr.

[15] Now dean, school of nursing, University of North Carolina.

Ruth Bishop, providing a service not equaled by that of any other profession. This relieves the boards of an enormous load of technical work. All students take the same state board examinations but the respective boards set their own "passing marks." This practice is helping to solve the problem of reciprocity, so important to a migratory profession, for the nurses of the future. Out of long and studious experience in state board work, Bernice Anderson suggests that state boards should "spend less time looking backwards and trying to patch up the inadequacies of the past."[16] Representatives of the Department of Measurement and Guidance and of the NNAS regularly attend the annual state board conferences.

The length of time required to prepare a student for the practice of professional nursing has long been a controversial subject. The Brown report re-emphasizes one of the principal recommendations of the Winslow-Goldmark report by recommending that: "Experiments in simultaneously shortening the period of training but improving the course of study are particularly needed. Scientifically controlled tests of the educational value of nursing practice in selected areas of concentration and in diverse environmental situations merit initiation. Especially recommended as transitional steps toward the future are the creation of central schools of nursing, and utilization of the teaching resources of junior colleges."[17]

Considerable interest in educational experimentation with a shortened course had already been aroused by the Metropolitan School experiment conducted under the auspices of the Canadian Nurses' Association at Windsor, Ontario. This school, financed by the Canadian Red Cross, graduated nurses at the end of 25 months who were eligible for registration in all the provinces of Canada. The sponsors concluded that nurses could be prepared in less than the traditional three years provided the school were operated and financed as a school and not as a service agency. Because experiments might be inhibited by the requirements of the nurse practice acts or state board rules, schools desirous of undertaking experi-

---

[16] Anderson, Bernice: "The Problem of Interstate Licensure," *Am. J. Nursing*, 52:587, 1952.

[17] Brown, Esther Lucile: *op. cit.*, p. 127.

mental programs find it advantageous to arrange for early conferences with their respective state boards. For example, in Massachusetts, where the school of the Massachusetts General Hospital
is under the democratic and farsighted leadership of Ruth Sleeper,
there is being conducted a new program in which the three-year
requirement of the state board is one of the decisive factors.[18] The
new basic program is concentrated in a 28-month period and is followed by an eight-months' internship in which the students (interns) perfect their skills and secure practical experience in such
services as the operating rooms and eye, ear, nose, and throat services. They also have the privilege of electing a service in which they
wish additional experience. There is no formal classwork but the
nurse-interns help to plan a ward teaching program which accords
with their needs. Stipends are provided during this period. Is this
program a success? The school is attracting far more well-qualified
candidates than the national average. The students, the school, and
the hospital like the program!

Planning for the development of nursing education to meet the
nation's need for nursing service was by no means restricted to the
national nursing organizations and the federal government. The
state surveys of hospital resources required in connection with the
Hospital Survey and Construction (Hill-Burton) Act inevitably
stimulated interest in nursing resources. When the pilot hospital
survey was being made in Michigan (1946), the Detroit Council
on Community Nursing (later the Michigan Nursing Center Association) swung into parallel action and had a survey of nursing resources made by a well-known educator.[19] But the report roused
little interest outside nursing circles until the Brown report was
published. When that report recommended that "appropriate nursing bodies initiate planning on a state-wide basis for the distribution of the kinds of schools that are designed to meet state needs"[20]
Michigan nurses found themselves in the vanguard of progressive

[18] Sleeper, Ruth: "We Study Our Basic Program," *Am. J. Nursing,* **51:**681, 1951.

[19] Bixler, Genevieve Knight: *Nursing Resources and Needs in Michigan,* 1946.

[20] Brown, Esther Lucile: *op. cit.,* p. 186.

planning. The report stimulated interest in "centralization of instruction in basic programs," as a substitute for small schools, with a pooling of nursing students for assignment to hospitals needing nursing services and properly staffed with clinical supervisors, coordinators, and counselors.[21] Among the important results which may be attributed to that survey are: (1) the state-wide chain of programs for practical nurse education which was established in connection with the state Department of Vocational Education, (2) the program of the College of Nursing at Wayne University which was reorganized (1947) to better meet the needs of the state for nurses with advanced preparation. This was accomplished with assistance from the Children's Bureau, the USPHS, and the Kellogg Foundation. At the University of Michigan the three-year and five-year programs have been replaced by a basic four-year program combining general and professional education and leading to the B.S. degree.

Schools with university relationships appear to be increasingly interested in the four-year type of program. Since no two states are alike, each requires a program adapted to its special needs. In Mississippi, where nurses were already aware of need for reform, they worked with the State Hospital Commission which took the initiative in securing a broad base of citizen interest in a survey of nursing resources. In a five-year period the number of schools was reduced by one-third and the enrollment of students increased by 170 per cent. The state legislature voted funds for the establishment of a degree program in the state university. It also provided a very substantial sum for scholarships for nurses who would return to the state after securing advanced preparation.

By the end of 1949, the USPHS had prepared a manual for use in making studies of nursing resources and, on invitation, had provided consultant or field service for most of the 35 states and Hawaii which had made surveys. Nineteen of the reports were made available for analysis. The general purposes of the surveys were to (1) determine if the number of nurses in each major field of nursing

[21] *Ibid.*, p. 67.

practice was adequate to meet the state's needs, (2) ascertain if the facilities for nursing education could produce enough well-prepared nurses, (3) determine if graduate nurses in hospitals, schools of nursing, public health, and industry are trained for the jobs which they are performing.[22]

The surveys revealed acute shortages of professional nurses of all types. The highest need per patient was found in mental and tuberculosis hospitals. The highest numerical need was in the general hospitals which habitually employ the largest numbers of professional nurses. Data on the distribution of public health nurses confirmed the generally known fact that many rural communities had no public health nursing services. *Lack of prepared teaching personnel* was the most serious of all the problems revealed in these surveys. Among the more immediate results of some of them were refresher courses for graduates and new affiliations for student nurses in mental and tuberculosis nursing. Following the surveys several states (with assistance from the Kellogg Foundation) set up new programs for practical nurse training in public vocational schools. Several states increased the number of public health nurses who had completed a year or more of work in approved programs. The report of a study made for the University of Washington, following the state survey, by Dr. Jean A. Curran and Helen Bunge is especially notable for its emphasis on methods for improving interprofessional relationships.

It is highly significant that the greatest progress toward achieving survey goals has been made in the 13 states where "citizens and citizen leaders, in addition to nurses, planned the early stages of the survey and followed through on the post-survey recommendations." Legislative response to the findings of some of the surveys has been impressive. The legislatures of Mississippi, Alabama, and Wyoming led the way in providing appropriations for new nursing programs in their respective state universities. Due chiefly to the initiative of the nursing organizations, those of Connecticut, Mississippi, Minne-

[22] Abdellah, Faye G.: "State Nursing Surveys and Community Action," *Pub. Health Rep.*, 67:554, 1952.

sota, and Wisconsin provided for generous scholarship aid, an example not lost on the other state associations. South Dakota restricted state aid to psychiatric nursing.

A number of state surveys had been completed when a work conference on regional planning was held in the summer of 1950.[23] The conference was planned by the Division of Education of Teachers College and directed by a well-known social scientist. In addition to nursing, the fields of medicine, hospital administration, sociology, economics, research analysis, and college administration were represented by persons from about one-half of the states. The principles evolved at that conference were adopted by the National Committee for the Improvement of Nursing Services which actively encouraged further regional planning by its affiliated committees. The report has been an important guide and stimulant to mid-century planning.

Thus far we have discussed regional planning on a state-wide basis, but regional or areal planning arises out of a common interest and may disregard political boundaries. A regional plan sponsored by the Commonwealth Fund and the Council of Rochester Regional Hospitals (1946) has successfully demonstrated the value of collaborative planning. In New England, the extremely interesting Boston University School of Nursing–Bingham Associates–Kellogg Foundation regional nursing program is being developed in Maine and Massachusetts on the basis of the well-established Bingham Associates regional program for the improvement of medical knowledge and medical care.

The conference on regional planning pointed out that the scope of areal planning may be based upon governmental, national, or societal factors and agreed that "the borderline of state boundaries might be crossed in order to realize the fullest benefits necessary for sound planning." It recommended that "regional planning for nursing education by the nursing profession utilize the same regional areal units as are used in the planning of higher education." Prosperity has come to the Southern states. Alert nurse educators in the

[23] *Regional Planning for Nursing and Nursing Education,* Report of Work Conference, Division of Nursing Education, Teachers College, held at Plymouth, N.H., June, 1950. Bureau of Publications, Teachers College, New York, 1950.

South, where the state universities, along with Vanderbilt, Duke, Emory, Meharry, and other institutions of higher education, were increasingly interested in nursing education, were already acting on that principle. When the Southern Regional Education Board[24] was organized (1948) as a central planning agency in graduate and professional education, they had been quick to take action. They organized a Southern Conference of State Leagues and sought the cooperation of the Regional Education Board. Recognizing nursing as an important social force, that agency set up a Committee on Nursing representative of the 14 Southern states. In its recommendations the committee has included consideration of the region's need for programs leading to the master's degree and for a nursing research center. It is hoped that plans under way for regional cooperation in higher education among the Western states may provide similar opportunity for cooperative planning in the field of nursing.

The seven-point fundamental philosophy of the NCINS[25] was based on the principle that good nursing service depends upon nursing personnel who have received sound preparatory training for their functions. Following the Conference on Regional Planning the committee decided to explore further the possibilities of such planning. By 1952 practically all states had committees of varying composition and titles working in cooperation with the NCINS.

A new edition of the *Curriculum Guide,* according to tradition, was due in this period. But thinking in relation to nursing education, along with philosophies and methods in both general and professional education, was changing rapidly. A national guide, concerned with curriculum content, tends to set a uniform pattern and thus to hinder experimental curriculum development. The NLNE (1950) adopted the educational philosophy that the development of a curriculum is the responsibility of the faculty of each school, not of the profession as a whole. Each would be planned on the basis of the aims and resources of the individual institution. All, it was assumed, would be concerned with the preventive and rehabilitative as well

[24] *Book of the States 1950–1951,* Vol. VIII, The Council of State Governments.

[25] Sheahan, Marion W.: "A Program for the Improvement of Nursing Services," *Am. J. Nursing,* **50**:794, 1950.

as with the curative aspects of medicine and with nurses as members of the health team.

Collegiate schools were considering the relative merits of curriculums in which elements of general and professional education are integrated and those in which blocks of time, in varying arrangements, are devoted to each. The NLNE, instead of revising the *Guide for the Organization of Collegiate Schools of Nursing* (1946), published descriptions of eight successful schools. These were designed, primarily, to assist administrators of institutions of higher education who, in increasing numbers, were becoming interested in nursing education.[26] The *American Journal of Nursing* in the same year published descriptions of four new patterns in nursing education, including the four-year basic program developed at Loretto Heights College (Colorado) through the cooperation of three religious orders and the discontinuance of two hospital schools of nursing. The others describe types of utilization of the facilities of hospitals, junior colleges, and universities which were being developed in Mississippi, Wyoming, and in connection with the University of Southern California. But the NLNE was keenly aware of its responsibility for leadership in the midst of a constantly changing social structure. It published a useful set of guiding principles, later revised, which took cognizance of the need for standards in both basic and advanced education of professional nurses and for the preparation of practical nurses.[27] It also, as previously noted, established a Department of Services to schools which quickly found that their greatest problems lay in the area of curriculum development.

Beneath the growing emphasis on specialization in the clinical areas in both medicine and nursing, there was increasing evidence of concern about the social, psychological, and spiritual needs of patients. The sick body, to quote Miss Nightingale, is something more than "a reservoir for storing medicines. . . ." It is also some-

[26] *Descriptions of Eight Basic Collegiate Schools of Nursing.* National League of Nursing Education, New York, 1952.

[27] "Platform of the National League for Nursing Education," *Am. J. Nursing,* **47**:247, 1947.

"N.L.N.E. Principles on Organization, Control and Administration of Nursing Education," *Am. J. Nursing,* **50**:396, 1950.

thing more than an aggregation of "systems." *Journal* articles reveal the growing influence on nursing of psychosomatic medicine. Articles on curriculum stressed the importance of correlation of subject matter. After years of effort the social and health aspects of nursing had been integrated throughout the curriculums of the better schools. Authorities on nutrition pointed out that nutrition is too vitally related to everyday living to be taught as an isolated subject. The point could be made with equal cogency about mental hygiene. A few specially qualified public health nurses were joining the faculties of nursing schools to promote the integration of social and health aspects, to familiarize students with community health and social resources, to encourage the development of referral systems and that ongoingness of thought that places a patient's hospital experience in its right relationship to his total health needs and experiences.

Important changes were occurring in the teaching and practice of clinical nursing. They were due, in part, to the NLNE's Committee on Postgraduate Clinical Nursing Courses and in part to "specialist" agencies. The Maternity Center's teaching about "natural childbirth" and the careful preparation of both parents for shared experiences in relation to childbirth were beginning to exert a profound influence on the evolution of maternity nursing. JONAS was not only giving expert assistance when needed during epidemics of polio. Through its field program and its extensive list of publications and visual aids it stimulated improvement in the care of polio and orthopedic patients. It won approval from the League's board of directors for the inclusion of the care of patients with poliomyelitis in the basic curriculum. By 1952 the disease was so prevalent that, although the experimental use of gamma globulin was offering hope of control, it was felt that efforts to prepare nurses to care for stricken patients should be increased. The Joint Tuberculosis Nursing Advisory Service had followed *Safer Ways in Nursing to Protect Against Tuberculosis* with an instructional plan for nursing schools.[28] The encouraging results of experiments with the use of streptomycin and isonicotinic acid (isoniazed) in the treatment of

[28] *Instructional Plan for Basic Tuberculosis Nursing.* NLNE, New York, 1949.

tuberculosis in no way lessened the need for nurses who could see beyond the patient with diseased lungs to the person emotionally disturbed by separation from his family and the prospect of being out of circulation for a considerable period. The Psychiatric Nursing Project, financed by the National Institute of Mental Health and sponsored by the NLNE and NOPHN, had made a study of the qualifications of psychiatric nurses as a preliminary to constructive planning.[29] It is especially noteworthy that, although the preparation of specialists was essential to the development of the preventive, therapeutic, and rehabilitation aspects of the care of patients in these categories, these programs also enriched the main stream of nursing service.

When the NLNE adopted the philosophy that nurse educators should be encouraged to help themselves, it disbanded the Curriculum Committee which had been working with many subcommittees on a unit basis. Special committees were appointed to compile bibliographies. Although they are not annotated, they provide a spacious background for every aspect of basic and advanced curriculum study. They constitute significant evidence of the increasing scope and quality of the literature of the profession.

The reports of two curriculum conferences sponsored by the League and attended by representatives of all the national nursing organizations and the NAPNE were widely used. The earlier one reveals an extraordinary diversity of interests and the dangers implicit in the fragmentation of a curriculum. A definition of nursing was needed to provide a focal point for the discussion. Out of the confusion, an analyst of the conference noted that there was "some semblance of one of the first steps in problem solving—recognition of problems."[30] A definition of nursing was formulated at the second more productive conference which has been used, with modifications, by other conference groups. (It may be found at the head of Chap. 45.) "Nursing," it was pointed out, "is facing a major development in its educational program. Whether the development will be

[29] *Inventory and Qualifications of Psychiatric Nurses.* NLNE, New York, 1950.

[30] *Curriculum Bulletin No. 1.* Nursing Organization Curriculum Conference. NLNE, New York, 1950.

merely an organizational shift or a basic improvement depends upon what is done toward developing and improving curricula in nursing."[31] The following philosophy of nursing education was adopted by the second conference group. "Nursing education should be reviewed as a whole in its setting in current society. It should be designed to meet present needs and develop attitudes and skills to meet future demands made upon the graduate nurse. This involves deciding what nursing students should know, do and be in relation to the world in which they live and in the special nursing fields for which they may prepare. It is important to help students gain an attitude for solving day-to-day problems and to provide opportunities to help students learn how to solve problems of the nursing profession as a whole."[32] The new emphasis on teaching students to recognize problems and to devise methods for solving them was in sharp contrast to the didactic methods of an earlier day. Issues were clarified by agreement on definitions of curriculum terms, basic assumptions, and the formulation of principles. There was repeated emphasis on the need for reducing the lag in curriculum development through research. The conference recommendations, which included statements of specific areas in which research was most urgently needed, have stimulated experimentation. Following the conference, the ACSN worked energetically to bring to fruition its plans for the periodical, *Nursing Research* (1952). Awareness of need for research pointed up the need for more nurses endowed with intellectual curiosity and equipped by training to undertake or to participate in exploratory programs. This need will be met, at least in part, by a grant of $100,000 from the Rockefeller Foundation to the Division of Nursing Education of Teachers College (1952). A center has been planned for the administration of a program of research, experimentation and field service in nursing education, and for studies of ways and means to improve nursing services. The center is expected to provide the nursing profession with a service similar to that of research agencies which serve edu-

[31] Caswell, Hollis: *Problems in Curriculum Development*, Curriculum Bulletin No. 2. NLNE, New York, 1951, p. 11.
[32] *Op. cit.*, p. 29.

cation in the medical, engineering, and other well-established professions.

The growing maturity of the profession was well illustrated by its interest in and support of studies and research. A statement of guiding principles for research in nursing, prepared by a joint committee of the national nursing organizations, was published in the AJN.[33] The ANA, for example, had published its first inventory of nurses in 1949. It launched its nationwide five-year program for the study of nursing functions by allocating funds for clearly defined research projects in six widely separated states.[34] The ANA's statistical department also set up a clearing house for studies.

A study of the abilities needed by nurses, it was agreed, was a necessary first step toward curriculum construction. Such a study would be supplemented, it was thought, by the ANA study of functions. The NCINS financed this project which was conducted under the direction of the NLNE. Several thousand nurses, most of them members of nursing school faculties, although nurses in all fields were invited to participate, took part in this study which was implemented by a carefully prepared check list.[35] The completed study was planned for publication in the autumn (1952) issue of *Nursing Research*. Some of the outcomes of the study were immediate and important. There was better and more widespread understanding of the educational philosophy which had been evolved by the relatively small groups who participated in the two curriculum conferences. There had been marked stimulation of interest in the evaluation of curriculums in individual schools and among local groups of nurses. These groups are interested in proficiency in nursing skills and have had an opportunity to indicate the skill-areas which are of greater, and of lesser, importance to them.[36] The next steps in curriculum study, whatever they are to be, will be developed under the aegis of the new NLN. In the meantime, it must be remembered

[33] "Research in Nursing—Philosophy and Plan of Action," *Am. J. Nursing*, **52**:601, 1952.

[34] *Facts about Nursing*, 1951, ANA, p. 108.

[35] *A Check List on the Abilities Needed by Nurses with Suggestions for Continued Curriculum Study*. NLNE, New York, 1951.

[36] Shields, Mary: "What's Next in Curriculum Study?" *Am. J. Nursing*, **52**: 1085, 1952.

that the adaptation of the curriculum of a school to changing needs and resources is a primary function of the faculty. The faculties of the better schools offering a three-year program were mindful that the Brown report (p. 127) had recommended that "experiments in simultaneously shortening the period of training but improving the course of study are particularly needed." Changes in progressive educational philosophy, in addition to the ferment of change in all phases of nursing, stimulated a lively interest in methods of teaching. This was indicated by an increased volume of material, periodical and other, on the subject. In the title of a book by Maude B. Muse we find the key to new thinking about method, viz., *Guiding Learning Experience*.[37]

Thus far we have been concerned with basic nursing education. A review by the National Nursing Accrediting Service of the programs offered to graduate nurses by departments or divisions of nursing in colleges and universities also revealed a confused and confusing situation. There are no legal requirements to stimulate the development of standards for the postdiploma education of nurses. The number of institutions offering such courses had almost doubled in the postwar period, but, except in public health nursing, the profession had not developed criteria for their guidance, although the NLNE had made a beginning in relation to programs in clinical nursing.[38] The influence of the Association of Collegiate Schools had extended only to those nursing education divisions or departments which sought membership. Among the problems identified by the NNAS was the disconcerting fact that frequently there was little differentiation between the programs leading to a baccalaurate degree and those leading to the master's degree! In such instances the master's was found to be little more than a symbol indicating that the nurse had previously earned a bachelor's degree. The findings resulted in a cogent set of recommendations[39] from which the following is quoted:

[37] The Macmillan Company, New York, 1950.

[38] *Courses in Clinical Nursing for Graduate Nurses, Basic Assumptions and Guiding Principles*. NLNE, New York, 1945.

[39] "Some Problems Identified" (a report on programs for graduate nurses by a board of review of the NNAS), *Am. J. Nursing*, **51**:338, 1951.

. . . programs leading to a master's or higher degree should be in accord with those for higher degrees in other professional fields . . . should begin where the well-developed basic collegiate programs leave off. . . . Programs leading to higher degrees should be established as a result of regional studies and planning. . . . The baccalaureate degree should be in harmony with programs for other types of professional and general education. To that end they should be primarily supplemental in nature. . . .

The directors of some of the well-established departments and divisions had already begun evaluating and adjusting their programs to meet changing needs. The programs in nursing at the University of Chicago were organized on the divisional level leading to a master's degree. Most of the others were offering programs leading to both the bachelor's and the master's degrees. Nurses working for doctorates usually found it necessary to work in the school of education or some other department of the university. The Ginzberg study, as has been noted, had been made to provide the Division of Nursing Education at Teachers College with the basis for a reconstruction of its curriculum. Following a three-year study by the faculty and consultants that curriculum was realigned. Ten major programs were synthesized into three main areas of study on the graduate (master's) level with one "prespecialization" program on the bachelor's level.[40] Prespecialization is interpreted to mean the general preparation required for practice as a professional nurse and is comparable to that of the better basic collegiate schools. The voluminous report of a two-weeks' work conference on Problems of Graduate Nurse Education which was held at Teachers College in the summer of 1952 suggests that "regional planning and research may help in some areas to break the present bottleneck of costs for initiating, for maintaining and for expanding graduate education."[41]

The NCINS included provision for a conference on graduate education for public health nursing in its long-range planning for the improvement of nursing service. The report of the conference, sponsored by the education committee of the NOPHN, includes an

[40] Nursing Education Division, Teachers College, Columbia University, *News Notes of Alumni #4*, May, 1951.
[41] "Problems of Graduate Nurse Education," *Work Conference Report No. 2.* Bureau of Publications, Teachers College, Columbia University, 1952.

excellent historical sketch of the consistently progressive educational program which the NOPHN had conducted almost from its inception. Emphasis throughout had been on preparation for practice as public health nurses rather than on preparation for administrative, consultative, and other leadership positions. [42] On the basis of earlier statements of policy and criteria this conference formulated a set of guiding principles for developing graduate programs (leading to the master's degree), pointing out that large numbers of such programs in public health nursing might not be needed to prepare the desired leadership but that variation in patterns, diversity, and experimentation are desirable.

The most serious problem in the whole field of nursing education was the scarcity of well-prepared faculty. *Nursing Schools at the Mid-Century* reveals that, in 1949, only 55 per cent of all nurse instructors had academic degrees! Deplorable though this is in relation to present-day standards in both general and professional education it represents considerable progress in a 20-year period. In 1929 the Grading Committee had found that less than 4 per cent of all nurse instructors had a background of four or more years of college education. But nursing had been caught in the swiftly moving stream of social change. How can the preparation of nurses for positions of leadership be accelerated? This became a burning question. Data compiled by the NLNE showed that for the five-year period beginning in 1947 (the first year for which such data were made available) the total number of graduate nurses annually enrolled in programs leading to degrees had reached approximately 12,000 with approximately 2300 graduated each year. Of this number approximately 300 received master's degrees. By 1951, the number securing their education under the GI Bill (18 per cent of the whole) was beginning to decrease. In that year 31 nurses were working for doctorates and over 1200 for master's degrees.

Two-thirds of all graduate nurses who were working toward degrees in 1951 were studying on a part-time basis. The courage and persistence of such nurses reveal one of the glories of the profes-

[42] *Report of Conference on Graduate Education in Public Health Nursing.* NOPHN, New York, 1951.

sion, but it is a socially wasteful process. Too often the degrees represent little more than an aggregation of credits instead of a balanced program leading toward a planned professional objective. If scholarship aid and professional counseling were more generally available nurses could more quickly achieve the higher competency which is so greatly needed. The number who completed programs that prepared for advanced nursing practice, teaching, supervision, and administrative posts in 1951 was 1449, a figure described by the League as "microscopic" when compared with the nation's need.

As this is written, the National Committee for the Improvement of Nursing Services, most influential and far-reaching of the postwar agencies, has in preparation a handbook which will serve as a guide to regional planning for the improvement of nursing service and of basic and advanced nursing education. One of the first projects planned for the new NLN was a work conference on graduate nurse education. Sources of scholarships and fellowships for graduate nurses are extremely limited. No federal agency is now providing any considerable amount for stipends for advanced work. An Office of Education publication indicated that some 300 scholarships and 50 fellowships were available in institutions of higher education. Even these small numbers were unevenly distributed with more than one-third of the scholarships restricted to one institution and more than one-half of the fellowships to another.[43] The number of scholarships was augmented by the state-aid programs previously discussed, but, in most states, the provision of scholarships and fellowships was dependent on the initiative of individual institutions. A consideration of the cost of nursing education and of responsibility for it may be introduced at this point.

The cost of nursing education, in relation to the relative values of a student's service to a hospital and the education she received for it, had been a contentious subject until the professions of hospital administration and of nursing developed pertinent evaluation tech-

[43] Wilkus, Theresa Birch: "Scholarships and Fellowships Available in Institutions of Higher Education," Office of Education, Federal Security Agency, Bulletin #16, 1951, p. 29.

nics. By mid-century, when rising demands for nursing service were paralleled by the increasing cost of medical care, a principle which had been formulated by the Grading Committee a quarter of a century earlier was beginning to gain credence. "No hospital should be expected to bear the cost of nursing education out of funds collected for the care of the sick. The education of nurses is as much a public responsibility as is the education of physicians, public school teachers, librarians, ministers, lawyers and other students planning to engage in professional public service, and the cost of such education should come, not out of the hospital budget but from private or public funds."[44]

The AHA and NLNE had collaborated on an important study of cost analysis in 1940. But the Cadet Corps found that cost accounting had not been widely adopted among hospitals. It therefore provided a manual for use in connection with the allocation of federal funds for the education of cadet nurses. Since that time a few cost studies have appeared in hospital publications.

On the basis of predictions for increased demands for nursing service in the postwar period, the National Nursing Council had been convinced that federal aid for nursing education should be continued, when the Cadet Corps was discontinued, in order to ensure the quality and quantity of nursing care needed by the nation. The nursing organizations took over responsibility for the formulation of basic principles and the development of a program for securing federal aid for nursing education. The NLNE prepared a statement of objectives in relation to federal aid in which emphasis was placed on improvement of nursing education programs, both basic and advanced. The AHA formally recognized the need for federal aid "in the national emergency" and reaffirmed its position in 1950. It is, however, opposed to any type of federal control of nursing education.

A forceful statement on nursing education was included in the 1950 platform of the ANA, and, in that year, the NLNE adopted a revised statement of principles which includes the following:

[44] Burgess, May Ayres: *Nurses, Patients, and Pocketbooks.* The Committee on Grading of Nursing Schools, New York, 1926, p. 447.

It is recognized that a majority of the schools of nursing in the country are now controlled by hospitals. It is anticipated that this situation will change as those schools with adequate faculty and clinical facilities take steps to enrich their programs, to reorganize them, and to seek university or college support for their administration and control. . . . Programs for practical nursing education should be administered and controlled by an educational institution with appropriate contractual arrangements with service agencies for nursing practice. . . . As the education of citizens is a public responsibility, money from public and private sources should support nursing education. Funds should be made available for the development of instructional facilities, scholarships, research.[45]

Nursing Schools at the Mid-Century[46] showed that 65 per cent of the cost of nursing education was being borne by hospitals, 24 per cent by tuition and fees, 3 per cent by gifts and endowments, 4 per cent from state and local funds, and 4 per cent from university and college funds. These data and the several statements of policy provided the ANA with the basic materials for an approach to Congress. The ANA had not completed the formulation of its proposal when bills, emanating from other sources, were introduced shortly after Congress convened. When it became clear that an omnibus bill, designed to provide aid for medical, nursing, and other schools in the health group, which was vigorously opposed by the AMA, would fail of passage, the ANA swung into action and sought the assistance of the Honorable Frances Payne Bolton. After conferences with representatives of all interested groups, a bill to be known as the Nursing Education Act of 1951 (H.R. 910) was hopefully introduced. It was sponsored by the nursing organizations but did not have the unqualified support of the AHA.

Once again the nursing profession was commended for the excellence of the material presented at congressional committee hearings. But the political climate of the eighty-second Congress was unfavorable to aid for professional education and the bill was tabled. As written, the bill would have provided assistance for the four types

[45] "Organization, Control and Administration of Nursing Education," *Am. J. Nursing*, 50:241, 1950.

[46] West, Margaret, and Hawkins, Christy: *Nursing Schools at the Mid-Century*. National Committee for the Improvement of Nursing Services, New York, 1950.

of educational programs: advanced, basic-collegiate, basic-hospital, and practical nursing. Before the eighty-third Congress was convened, the national organizations began laying the groundwork for further effort. Quite undaunted, the ANA, which had exceeded its own best efforts in alerting the state nurses' associations and in providing them with factual information on the progress of the effort and suggestions for action in relation to H.R. 910, was preparing a new approach to the nation's lawmakers.

It is apropos to note here that the federal government engages in two types of educational activity.[47] It operates its own programs, as at Annapolis and West Point, but principally it aids states and territories in financing education. It may be noted that two nursing schools, those at St. Elizabeth's (psychiatric) and the Freedman's Hospital, in Washington, are operated under federal auspices. Two other schools offering basic programs have been closed: the Army School of Nursing (1918–1931) and the one inaugurated by the USPHS after World War I which, after a few months, was discontinued and its students transferred to the Army school. The US Cadet Nurse Corps pioneered in a new relationship between the government and private institutions.

Frequent reference has been made to the substantial support of nursing projects by the W. K. Kellogg Foundation. Nursing, however, is but one of its several interests. Hospital administration is another. Following up on the studies of the Commission on Hospital Care, the foundation financed a curriculum study in hospital administration and assisted universities offering programs in that field to increase their enrollments following the release of desirable candidates from service in the hospital corps of the armed forces. It was no secret that tensions often existed between hospital administrators and nursing service administrators, who were also responsible for the administration of nursing schools, and that such tensions had been exacerbated by the increasing use of hospital facilities.

Keenly aware of the situation, Mildred L. Tuttle, the farseeing

---

[47] *Federal Educational Activities and Educational Issues Before Congress*, Vol. I, Parts 1 and 2. US Government Printing Office, Washington, D.C., 1951.

director of the Division of Nursing of the foundation, invited a small group of consultants from the field of nursing service administration to meet with her for the purpose of identifying pertinent problems in nursing service administration and content areas which should be included in educational programs to prepare nursing service administrators. It is noteworthy that, in this instance, representatives of the profession had not taken the initiative. The successive steps taken by the foundation are therefore of special interest. The results of the conference were discussed with the general director of the foundation and members of the foundation staff, especially those in the Divisions of General Education and Hospitals. The subject was then presented to the Nursing Advisory Committee of the foundation and invited guests, including Dr. Ralph Tyler, dean, Division of Social Sciences, University of Chicago, and Professor Herman Finer, Division of Political Sciences, also of the University of Chicago. Selected representatives of 14 universities were then invited to attend a two-day institute at the University of Chicago which was directed by Professors Tyler and Finer. The plan for a seminar on the administration of nursing services, which was presented to this group for suggestions and approval, provided the basis for a five-month seminar directed by Professor Finer at the University of Chicago beginning in January, 1951. Out of this careful planning a program of such potentialities evolved that history may appraise it as the foremost event in the postdiploma education of nurses since the NOPHN began evaluating programs in public health nursing. The group of seminarists included, in addition to two representatives from each of the 14 universities, a representative from each of the federal nursing services. Work began with a preliminary survey of current university offerings. Their limitations and the paucity of literature on administration in relation to nursing services quickly confirmed the convictions of seminarists and faculty about the importance of the work which they had undertaken.

The reports of five seminar committees (published for the use of the participating universities) are a stimulating distillate of the thinking of the carefully selected participants. The subjects considered by the committees were: Content of Nursing Service Education; Component Fields That Constitute the Study of Administration; In-Service Education; Administration of the Basic Nursing Program, and, in accordance with good practice in connection with all types of instructional programs, there was a Committee on Education. The first recommendation of the last-named committee directed attention to the need for research in nursing service administration. A book by the director of the seminar, based on research in connection with the seminar, has now been published.[48]

The seminar laid the foundation for a two- to five-year program in the participating universities. In financing the programs the foundation made provision for additional faculty in these schools. Members of the seminar anticipated drawing upon education (as a matter of course!) and such other fields as business, economics, industrial relations, and statistics and research in setting up new programs. No two universities are alike, but representatives of a variety of disciplines are participating with keen interest in the new programs.

The comprehensive objective formulated by the foundation was the development of programs in:

  I. In-service education (credit and noncredit)
    a. Consultant service to hospitals
    b. Workshops, institutes, conferences on campuses and in regional areas
 II. Programs leading to the bachelor's degree (for head nurses and supervisors)
    a. Expansion and extension of existing programs
    b. Development of new programs
III. Programs leading to the master's degree (for administration of nursing services)
    a. Expansion and strengthening existing programs
    b. Development of new programs

In general terms, the programs would be both on campus and off campus with each enriching the other. The principle of areal

[48] Finer, Herman: *Administration and the Nursing Services.* The Macmillan Company, New York, 1952.

or regional planning, which had been useful in teacher training programs, was adopted.

The 14 universities defined their potential areas of influence, in cooperation with other agencies such as nearby universities and professional organizations. One of them, for example, was happy to find that its area coincided with that of a hospital council which promptly provided a channel for the development of community relationships.

In order that they might share experiences, a conference of representatives of the participating institutions was held about a year after the conclusion of the seminar. All had made significant contributions to the improvement of nursing services in their areas. The programs, of course, were not identical since they were based on areal needs and resources. Refresher courses for general duty nurses, actual or potential, had been followed by a request for similar assistance for private duty nurses in one area. Requests for in-service programs not only provided assistance for the institutions making the requests, they also provided stimulating material for those who were teaching the new courses in administration. Fifty nurses, in addition to the required 20, enrolled for a requested extension program in one area. In another, the director of the program has described the extramural program in her area as "similar to bits of yeast" which stimulate interest in improving nursing service in institutions which had not previously known how to analyze their problems or to secure assistance in meeting them. Work conferences at which problems of immediate concern, such as interpersonal relationships, are said to have been especially rewarding. It is of related interest, in this connection, that the University of Minnesota, one of the participating universities, had previously made a significant study of the potentialities for nursing education in rural hospital affiliations with a university school.

Two further aspects of nursing education remain to be discussed —the selection and recruitment of students. By 1950, prenursing and guidance tests made available by the League's Department of Measurement and Guidance, or similar psychometric tests, were being used extensively. The cumulative record form on which the results of League tests are returned to the schools was being used as a guidance tool throughout the student's stay in the school since space is provided for records of the results of achievement tests, and also for the graduate nurse test battery, and for the results of state board examinations. The attrition rate, for the country as a whole, was distressingly high. However, among the schools there appeared to be a growing number of impressive exceptions to that generalization. They are schools which are truly "student-centered"; students participate in planning the programs in which counseling is an important factor.

A recent study reveals the startling fact that, on the basis of current practice (1952), only 38 out of 100 girls who enter nursing schools will be active in the profession two years after graduation and only 29 will be so engaged five years thereafter.[49] A comparison with data compiled by the Grading Committee shows that, although more nurses drop out of active practice early, those who stay in remain longer. The average professional life expectancy is approximately 1.5 per cent lower than in 1927. The high matrimonial rate among young nurses might be used as an argument for interesting more men in nursing as a career. But, although nursing provides a superb preparation for matrimony, that is not the function of a nursing school. That function is to prepare students for careers in nursing which may, or may not, be interrupted by matrimony. No study has been made of the number of nurses who have returned to practice when their children no longer need them. Present interest in refresher courses seems to indicate that if they were made more generally and continuously available within defined areas, they might attract "inactive" nurses and be both an important source of needed "nurse power" and of fulfillment and satisfaction to individual nurses.

When the joint boards of the six national nursing organizations set up the National Committee on Careers in Nursing, the profession accepted responsibility for leadership in the recruitment of student nurses, but, collectively, they lacked the resources for the extensive

[49] West, Margaret, and Crosby, Edwin L.: "An Action Program . . . Answer to the Nursing Shortage," *Hospitals*, **26**:66 (May) 1952.

program for which there was obvious need. Theresa I. Lynch (dean of the University of Pennsylvania School of Nursing) accepted the chairmanship of the committee, and Mrs. Muriel C. Henry, an enthusiastic expert in public relations, became the director of the program (1948). It is a large committee. On it sit representatives of the nursing, hospital, and medical organizations, also individuals or representatives of organizations especially interested in the activities of women. There are, too, experts in public relations, and high school and college counselors. Fortunately, the committee inherited the interest in nursing of the Advertising Council (which assists service programs such as, currently, the ARC Blood Donor Program) and of Anson Lowitz. Mr. Lowitz has directed the council's nursing program, in cooperation with successive recruitment committees, since the early days of World War II. Through the freely contributed imaginative and technical "know-how" of the council, American business has contributed radio and television time and advertising space valued at many millions of dollars.

There is no more striking recognition of the social usefulness of nursing than the continuing interest of the Advertising Council and the sources of financial support of the recruitment program. United Community Defense Services, a "Red Feather" Agency,[50] has become the principal contributor to the budget of the committee. This agency was established in 1951 to put the experience and skill of national health and welfare agencies at the disposal of communities affected by the national mobilization. "Trailertowns," for example, were again presenting a whole series of social and health problems. The National Foundation for Infantile Paralysis, however, has been a generous contributor over a longer period. Blue Cross and the American Cancer Society have been contributors, but not continuously. The budgets of the nursing, hospital, and medical associations permit only nominal contributions to the committee's budget.

The five-year program developed in 1950 has two phases: (1) the use of mass appeal technics which is directed by the Advertising Council in cooperation with the Careers Committee and (2) stim-

[50] Member of Community Chests and Councils of America.

ulation of state and local interest in the development of coordinated programs adapted to local conditions. There has been great diversity of interest and of effort in these areas. With an increased budget (1951) a field program was initiated through which, by means of regional institutes and consultant services, local efforts are being strengthened and coordinated. It was anticipated, for example, that the interested groups or agencies might establish a single post office address in each state for inquiries about nursing schools.

The preparation of materials for the use of state and local groups has been an important segment of the committee's work. Chief among them is the pamphlet (now in its second edition), *Schools of Nursing in the United States, 1952*. This is a list of state-accredited schools carefully coded to provide maximum information about them in little space. It is noteworthy that no such list was possible before the interim classification of schools was made in 1949. Major emphasis has necessarily been placed on interesting high school graduates. The committee has not, however, overlooked the importance of programs directed to college counselors and students. Enrollment in collegiate schools has practically doubled since the war. Many of the strong hospital schools which attract college women, as well as the collegiate schools, could admit larger classes. The National Nursing Council, it will be recalled, had found that only persistent and well-directed effort could be expected to secure any really significant response from this group. Appeals to the interest of Negroes have been incorporated in all basic materials as well as in "copy" prepared especially for them. Special materials on opportunities in nursing for men have been made available.

The committee has been urged to develop a program to recruit, viz., to interest graduate nurses in securing supplementary or advanced preparation. The need for many more well-prepared nurses is self-evident. If, for example, the schools had a higher percentage of well-qualified faculty members, it is probable that the serious loss of students (approximately one-third), so wasteful of both human and educational resources, could be reduced. The usefulness of such a program would be contingent upon the availability of data about programs for graduate nurses, comparable to that included in the list of undergraduate schools in the United States. The NNAS is now in possession of such data. Such a program would, however, inevitably fall short of its objective if scholarships and fellowships are not made more generally available.

Eighty years of amazing technical and social changes have passed into history since the famous trio of "Nightingale schools" was established. Has nursing education, burdened as no other profession has ever been by demands for student service, kept pace? By what yardstick shall it be measured? The evolution of nursing education[51] is discussed in 20-year periods, in the *Curriculum Guide*. The first, or pioneer period, ended in 1893 with the beginning of organized effort to set goals for its improvement. The years of unrestrained and unstandardized expansion, called the "boom period," terminated in 1913. By that time a majority of states had secured nurse practice acts. However, as the Grading Committee found, the number of schools continued to increase rapidly until well into the twenties. The third period, ending in 1933, was one of "standard setting and stock taking." It was indeed a period of stock taking, as shown in earlier chapters, in the whole field of health and medical care. The League's curriculums of 1917 and 1927 provide abundant evidence of the profession's effort to set educational standards. It is pertinent to conjecture about the term future appraisers may apply to nursing education in the twenty years now ending. Adjustment was the key word to the reconstruction of the *Curriculum Guide* (1937). Does *adjustment* best describe nursing education in the period in which the profession met the successive challenges of the Great Depression, World War II, and the technical and social phenomena of the Atomic Age? Only time can give the necessary perspective for evaluation. At close range the phrase "adjustment with an eye to the future" seems applicable.

In a period of conflicting pressures, marked progress has been made in the uphill struggle to secure for nurses the type of education required to fit them for the myriad needs of society rather than

[51] Elaborated in Isabel M. Stewart's *Education of Nurses*. The Macmillan Company, New York, 1943.

for the immediate service of institutions. Standards established by the profession provided a foundation for the spectacular work of the US Cadet Nurse Corps. The "American system" of nursing education has been immeasurably strengthened by the work of the League's Department of Measurement and Guidance and by the National Nursing Accrediting Service. The profession has gained the assistance and respect of philanthropic foundations through its unity of purpose and collaborative efforts to improve nursing education as a means for improving nursing service. It has aroused the active interest of an increasing number of institutions of higher education in nursing education. Finally, on the eightieth anniversary of the introduction of modern nursing in the United States, it may be said that nursing had begun to make significant progress toward professional partnerships, in the care of those in need of health and medical care, with the other members of the medical team.

BIBLIOGRAPHY

Abdellah, Faye, G.: "State Nursing Surveys and Community Action," *Pub. Health Rep.*, **67:**554, 1952.

"Advanced Preparation in Psychiatric Nursing and Mental Hygiene" (grants by the US Public Health Service to ten universities), *Am. J. Nursing*, **47:**497, 1947.

Bernard, Harold W.: "Recent Emphases in Educational Practices," *Am. J. Nursing*, **47:**243, 1947.

Biehusen, Irma: "Alumnae Associations in Action," *Am. J. Nursing*, **46:**662, 1946.

Bishop, Ruth: "Bird's-Eye View of the First Ten Years of the League's Testing Services," *Fifty-eighth Annual Report of the National League of Nursing Education*, 1952, p. 110.

Bixler, Genevieve K.; Austin, A. L.; and Bunge, H. L.: "Research and Nursing Education," *Am. J. Nursing*, **48:**45, 1948.

Bixler, Genevieve K., and Bixler, Roy W.: "The Professional Status of Nursing," *Am. J. Nursing*, **45:**730, 1945.

Bogue, Jesse Parker: *The Community College.* McGraw-Hill Book Co., New York, 1950.

Bradley, H. Lenore: "Central Schools for Rural Areas," *Am. J. Nursing*, **43:**447, 1943.

Bridgman, Margaret: "Achievements and Potentials in Nursing Education," *Am. J. Nursing,* **52**:980, 1952.

Burgess, May Ayres: *Nurses, Patients, and Pocketbooks.* Committee on the Grading of Schools of Nursing, New York, 1928, p. 55.

Cafferty, Kathryn W. (ed.): *Workshop on the Coordination of Education and Nursing in Centralized Programs.* Catholic University of America Press, Washington, D.C., 1950.

————: *A Dynamic Basic Nursing Curriculum.* Catholic University of America Press, Washington, D.C., 1951.

Cancer Nursing in the Basic Professional Nursing Curriculum. US Public Health Service Pub. #147. US Government Printing Office, Washington, D.C., 1951.

Carn, Irene, and Mole, Eleanor W.: "Continuity of Nursing Care," *Am. J. Nursing,* **49**:388, 1949.

Coffey, Hubert S.: "Role Playing in Exploring Relationships," *Pub. Health Nursing,* **42**:267, 1950.

"Completion of an Education Program in Nursing Approved for Public Health Nursing," *Pub. Health Nursing,* **43**:97, 1951.

Corey, Stephen M.: "Fundamental Research, Action Research, and Educational Practices," *Teachers College Record,* **50**:509, 1949.

Cost Analysis of Schools of Nursing, A Manual of Methods and Procedures. US Public Health Service, Federal Security Agency, US Government Printing Office, Washington, D.C., 1947.

Crenshaw, Virginia P.: "Teaching Patients," *Am. J. Nursing,* **50**:666, 1950.

Curran, Jean A., and Bunge, Helen: *Better Nursing.* University of Washington Press, Seattle, 1951.

Dade, Lucy, and Wolf, Lulu K.: "A New Approach to the Teaching of Nursing Arts," *Am. J. Nursing,* **46**:404, 1946.

Deming, Dorothy: *The Practical Nurse.* The Commonwealth Fund, New York, 1947.

"Doctoral Degrees," *Am. J. Nursing,* **50**:377, 1950.

Faculty Positions in Schools of Nursing and How to Prepare for Them. National League of Nursing Education, New York, 1946.

Feider, Ruth E.: "Nursing in Junior and State Colleges," *Am. J. Nursing,* **50**:236, 1950.

Ferguson, Marion: "Research in Nursing," *Am. J. Pub. Health,* **41**:716, 1951.

Fidler, Nettie D.: "The Metropolitan School of Nursing," *Am. J. Nursing,* **51**:51, 1951.

"Field Instruction," *Pub. Health Nursing,* **43**:206, 1951.

The Field Practice Period in the University Public Health Program of

Study. Division of Nursing Education, Teachers College, Columbia University, New York, 1949.

Fundamentals of Administration for Schools of Nursing. National League of Nursing Education, New York, 1940 (second printing, 1947).

Gelinas, Agnes: *Nursing and Nursing Education*. The Commonwealth Fund, New York, 1946.

Goodman, Lois: "Preparing Public Health Nurses to Teach Home Nursing," *Am. J. Nursing*, 49:498, 1949.

Goodrich, Annie W.: "The Changing Order and Nursing," *Proceedings of the Twenty-ninth Convention of the American Nurses' Association*, 1934, p. 88.

"Graduate Nurses in Colleges and Universities," *Am. J. Nursing*, 52:1096, 1952.

Guide for the Development of Libraries in Schools of Nursing. National League of Nursing Education, New York, 1952.

Hereford, Julia J., and Wolf, Lulu K.: "A Laboratory in Clinical Experience," *Am. J. Nursing*, 49:799, 1949.

Higher Education for American Democracy, A Report of the President's Commission on Higher Education. Vol. I, "Establishing the Goals"; Vol. III, "Organizing Higher Education." US Government Printing Office, Washington, D.C., 1947.

Hollister, William G., and Husband, Grant W.: "Sociodrama: A Way of Teaching Mental Health Skills," *Pub. Health Nursing*, 43:490, 1951.

Holtzhausen, Erma A.: "Nursing Service in a Teaching Hospital," *Am. J. Nursing*, 46:550, 1946.

Hopkins, L. Thomas: "Dynamics in Research," *Teachers College Record*, 50:339, 1950.

Hughes, Everett C.: "Studying the Nurse's Work," *Am. J. Nursing*, 51:294, 1951.

"The Inventory of Psychiatric Nurses," *Am. J. Nursing*, 51:309, 1951.

Kelley, Earl C.: *The Workshop Way of Learning*. Harper & Brothers, New York, 1951.

Kraus, Bernadine: "Patient Referral System," *Am. J. Nursing*, 44:387, 1944.

Leino, Amelia: "A New Basic Nursing Program," *Am. J. Nursing*, 52:834, 1952.

Lentz, Edith M.: "Patterns of Supervision in Hospitals," *Hospitals*, 26:74, 1952.

McManus, R. Louise: "Action Research," *Am. J. Nursing*, 51:739, 1951.

Mann, Estella P.: "The Head Nurse as a Leader," *Am. J. Nursing*, 49:626, 1949.

Manual of Accrediting Educational Programs in Nursing. National Nursing Accrediting Service, New York, 1949.

Marvin, Mary M.: "Research in Nursing," *Am. J. Nursing,* 27:331, 1927.

————: "The Position and Preparation of the Head Nurse," *Am. J. Nursing,* 28:818, 1928.

Mereness, Dorothy: "Preparation of the Nurse for the Psychiatric Team," *Am. J. Nursing,* 51:320, 1951.

Minnesota Rural Programs for Students in Nursing. University of Minnesota, Minneapolis, 1952.

Morrissey, Alice B.: "Psychosocial and Spiritual Factors in Rehabilitation," *Am. J. Nursing,* 50:763, 1950.

Mullane, Mary Kelly: "From Blueprint to Bedside," *Am. J. Nursing,* 52:875, 1952.

Murchison, Irene: "A Four-Year Basic Collegiate Program," *Am. J. Nursing,* 52:481, 1952.

————: "State Boards and Collegiate Programs," *Am. J. Nursing,* 52:1217, 1952.

Nahm, Helen: "Accreditation Now," *Am. J. Nursing,* 51:523, 1951.

Neilson, Marie E.: "Case Method of Assignment," *Am. J. Nursing,* 49:576, 1949.

Nutting, M. Adelaide: *A Sound Economic Basis for Schools of Nursing.* G. P. Putnam's Sons, New York, 1926.

Oglevee, Christine L.: "A Coordinated Nursing School," *Am. J. Nursing,* 52:213, 1952.

Parran, Thomas: "Professional Nursing Needed," *Am. J. Nursing,* 45:133, 1945.

Patterson, Lillian B.: "University of Washington Starts an Experimental Program," *Washington State J. Nursing,* 25:8, 1952.

Peplau, Hildegard E.: "Toward New Concepts in Nursing and Nursing Education," *Am. J. Nursing,* 51:722, 1951.

Perkins, Dorothy: "A Program to Develop Team Leaders," *Am. J. Nursing,* 52:309, 1952.

Perkins, Dorothy, and Heslin, Phyllis: "Nursing Service and Nursing Education Advance Together in the Team Plan," *Am. J. Nursing,* 52:185, 1952.

Peterson, Rosalie, et al.: "Inservice Education in Cancer Nursing," *Pub. Health Nursing,* 43:255, 331, 386, 1951.

Petry, Lucile: "Nursing Education in Higher Institutions of the North Central Association," *North Central A. Quart.,* Vol. XV, April, 1941.

Petry, Lucile; Arnstein, Margaret; and McIver, Pearl: "Research for Improved Nursing Practices," *Pub. Health Rep.,* 67:183, 1952.

Pfefferkorn, Blanche, and Rovetta, Charles A.: *Administrative Cost Analy-*

sis for Nursing Service and Nursing Education. American Hospital Association and the National League of Nursing Education, 1940.

Phillips, Elisabeth C.: "A Practical Plan for Education of Practical Nurses," *Mod. Hosp.*, **74**:58, 1950.

———: "Developments in the Field of Practical Nursing," *Am. J. Nursing*, **52**:74, 1952.

Practical Nurse Education—Manual for State and Local Leagues. National League of Nursing Education, New York, 1949.

"Preparation of the Instructional Staff in Schools of Nursing," *Am. J. Nursing*, **47**:695, 1947.

"Priorities in Public Health Nursing Education—A Statement of Recommendations by the NOPHN Education Committee." *Pub. Health Nursing*, **43**:34, 1951.

Problems of Graduate Nurse Education, Report of Work Conference, Division of Nursing Education, Teachers College, 1952. Bureau of Publications, Teachers College, Columbia University, 1952.

Proceedings of Work Conference, Collegiate Council of Public Health Nursing Education (National Organization for Public Health Nursing), October 10–13, 1951. Milford, Michigan.

"Programs of Nursing Education Approved by the National Nursing Accrediting Service," *Am. J. Nursing*, **49**:631, 1949.

"Psychiatric Nursing and Mental Hygiene, 1900–1948," *Am. J. Nursing*, **49**:739, 1949.

Read, Grantly Dick: *The Birth of a Child.* Vanguard Press, New York, 1950.

"Recommended Qualifications for Public Health Nursing Faculty and Teaching Personnel," *Pub. Health Nursing*, **43**:141, 1951.

Regional Planning for Nursing and Nursing Education, Report of Work Conference held at Plymouth, N.H., June 12–23, 1950. Bureau of Publications, Teachers College, Columbia University, New York, 1950.

"Regional Planning—the N.C.I.N.S. Answers Some Questions," *Am. J. Nursing*, **52**:206, 1952.

Render, Helena Willis: "Creative Aspects of Psychiatric Nursing," *Am. J. Nursing*, **50**:433, 1950.

Report of Conference on Graduate Education in Public Health Nursing, April 30–May 4, 1951, National Organization for Public Health Nursing, New York.

Reports of the Committees on Nursing Services Administration, Nursing Service Administration Seminar, University of Chicago, January 15–June 8, 1951.

"Research in Nursing, Philosophy and Plan of Action," *Am. J. Nursing*, **52**:601, 1952.

Rugg, Harold: *Foundations for American Education.* World Book Co., Yonkers, N.Y., 1947.

Russell, E. Kathleen: "Fifty Years of Medical Progress, Medicine as a Social Instrument: Nursing," *New England J. Med.,* 224:439–45, 1951.

Rynbergen, Henderika: "Nutrition in the Nursing School Curriculum," *Am. J. Nursing,* 50:282, 1950.

Shalit, Pearl: "The Nurse and the Mental Health Act," *Am. J. Nursing,* 50:94, 1950.

Smith, Dorothy M.: "Patient-Centered Teaching in Medical and Surgical Nursing," *Am. J. Nursing,* 50:314, 1950.

Spalding, Eugenia K.: "Appraising Basic Collegiate Programs in Nursing," *Am. J. Nursing,* 50:796, 1950.

"State Aid to Nursing Education" (editorial), *Am. J. Nursing,* 51:691, 1951.

Stewart, Isabel M.: *The Education of Nurses.* The Macmillan Company, New York, 1943.

Swiss, Margaret Tobin: "The Nursing Intern and the Team Plan," *Am. J. Nursing,* 52:221, 1952.

Taylor, Ella A.: *Withdrawal of Students—A Three-Year Study of Withdrawal of Students from Schools of Nursing.* National League of Nursing Education, New York, 1951.

"Teaching Aids for Clinical Instructors in Psychiatric Nursing," *Am. J. Nursing,* 48:664, 1948.

Temporary Accreditation, Report on the Program of the National Nursing Accrediting Service. Part I, "Study of Basic Programs Offered by Schools of Nursing"; Part II, "Summary of Nineteen Conferences, Summer, 1952." National League for Nursing, New York, 1952.

Thompson, Esther M.: "A Regional Nursing Program," *Am. J. Nursing,* 52:58, 1952.

Tschudin, Mary O.: "What Is a Sound Basic Collegiate Program in Nursing Education?" *Am. J. Nursing,* 52:986, 1952.

Tyler, Ralph W.: "Trends in Professional Education," *Am. J. Nursing,* 49:50, 1949.

———: *Basic Principles of Curriculum and Instruction.* University of Chicago Press, Chicago, 1950.

Vosloh, Lillian: "One Pattern in Nursing Education," *Am. J. Nursing,* 52:333, 1952.

West, Margaret D.: "Estimating the Future Supply of Professional Nurses," *Am. J. Nursing,* 50:656, 1950.

Whitehall, Albert V., and Foster, Marion J.: "Nine Strikes Against Federal Aid for Nursing Education," *Hospitals,* 26:55, 1952.

Wilson, Dorothy: "Staff Education; Principles and Purposes," *Pub. Health Nursing*, 41:126, 1949.

Witmer, Helen L. (ed.): *Pediatrics and the Emotional Needs of the Child*. The Commonwealth Fund, New York, 1948.

Wolf, Anna D.: "Making Democratic Principles Effective in Nursing Schools," *Forty-eighth Annual Report of the National League of Nursing Education*, 1942, p. 174.

Chapter 48

NURSING PRACTICE IN THE ATOMIC AGE

We have talked of our rights. We have guarded our freedom. Our highest virtues have been service and sacrifice. Are we not now thinking of these virtues somewhat differently? The spirit of a new age is fast gripping every one of us. The appeal which life makes to us today is to the socially constructive passion in every man. . . . This is a great affirmative. Sacrifice sometimes seems too negative, dwells on what I give up. Service sometimes seems to emphasize the FACT *of service rather than the* VALUE *of the service. Yet service and sacrifice are noble ideals. We cannot do without them. Let them, however, be the handmaids of the great purpose of our life, namely, our contribution to that new world we wish to see rise out of our present chaos, that age which shall bring us individual freedom through collective control.*[1]

NURSING is in a constant state of adaptation to the needs of society. But, as indicated in the chapters on service and education, more changes had been effected since Pearl Harbor than in all the years between the wars. Nursing in this was not unique. To dramatize the swift pace of technological and social change ushered in with the bombing of Hiroshima, a noted editor declared that "modern man is obsolete."[2] Concurrently with the arrival of the Atomic Age many nursing technics and practices were becoming obsolescent.

Individuals fear rapid change because it seems to threaten their security. This chapter, therefore, is concerned with the individual nurse as a practitioner in the rapidly expanding house of health at the mid-century. The number of nurses in active practice in 1941

[1] *Dynamic Administration—The Collected Papers of Mary Parker Follett*, edited by Henry C. Metcalf and L. Urwick. Harper & Brothers, New York, 1940, Chap. XIV, "Individualism in a Planned Society," p. 314.

[2] Cousins, Norman: "Modern Man Is Obsolete," *Saturday Review of Literature*, 28:5–9, (Aug. 18) 1945.

was 173,000. Ten years later there were over 334,000 (not including those with the armed forces). Almost 49 per cent of them were employed by hospitals. Approximately 21 per cent were in private duty practice, which was increasingly tending to become an institutional rather than a general community resource,[3] although private duty nurses retained their status as independent practitioners.

"The fundamental responsibility of the nurse," says the Code for Professional Nurses, "is to conserve life and to promote health," which the World Health Organization defines as "a state of complete physical, mental and social well-being and not merely the absence of disease or infirmity." The promotion of health is the major concern of nurses who are at work in a wide range of health services which, since it begins with prenatal care, is more comprehensive than social work's concept of "cradle to the grave service." Public health nurses, working in homes, hospitals, and clinics, are increasingly concerned with the physical and mental health of the whole family rather than with that of a single member; and the school nurses, while providing preventive services, are constantly on the alert for correctible defects of sight, hearing, teeth, nutrition, and emotional balance. In this group are the industrial nurses with programs adapted to combat the varied health hazards of millions of employed persons while promoting optimum health. Here are many of the profession's specialists—in maternity and child welfare, in tuberculosis, veneral disease, polio and orthopedics, rehabilitation, and, more recently, in cancer and cerebral palsy. Nor can we overlook the pervasive influence of nurses who teach the Red Cross classes and in home care of the sick and mother and baby care.

About 80 per cent of all nurses are employed persons. They are subject to the over-all policies of employing agencies, such as hospitals, nursing homes, and other institutions—both voluntary and tax-supported; departments of health—state, county, and municipal; departments of education; and the whole gamut of commercial and industrial organizations. As professional persons they are under moral obligation to maintain and promote good standards of nursing practice. Progress in nursing has often been due to persistent

[3] *Facts about Nursing*, 1952, ANA, p. 3.

effort to reconcile the conflicting loyalties created by diverse employment conditions. It has been stimulated by the WHO's definition of health. Citizen demand for more and more health service has caused three facts to stand out above all others. (1) The economic status of nursing must be improved; (2) professional registered nurses and student nurses must continue to share the privilege of providing nursing service with nonprofessional workers; (3) professional nurses find it obligatory to take leadership in developing methods for the democratic integration of the several types of workers into effective patterns of nursing service. These call for more effective patterns of nursing education.

This chapter attempts to show: (1) How external forces are influencing the professional and technical development of nursing practice and (2) some of the ANA's more important efforts to assist the individual nurse to make her best contribution to the nation's health services. The analysis may appropriately be prefaced by consideration of the increasing momentum of a fundamental change in the economic status of women. Married women constituted 55 per cent of all women workers in 1951,[4] but "professional nurses," says the edition of *Facts about Nursing* for that year, "may be characterized as both young and married. About 62 per cent of all the nurses are married and over half are under 40 years of age."[5] In the late twenties, the Grading Committee's best guess had been that only one out of five active nurses was married.[6]

Schools of nursing are, necessarily, now adapting their policies to the high incidence of early marriage and encourage students who marry to complete their programs. Directors of nursing services are searching for methods for resolving the conflict between the normal desire of young people for socially acceptable hours off duty and the professional obligation to meet the round-the-clock needs of patients. These administrators are beginning to realize that nurses cannot be expected to feel a personal sense of obligation to share

[4] *Status of Women in the United States, 1952.* Women's Bureau, US Department of Labor, D-55 (mimeographed).

[5] *Facts about Nursing,* 1952, ANA, p. 14.

[6] Burgess, May Ayres: *Nurses, Patients, and Pocketbooks.* Committee on the Grading of Nursing Schools, New York, 1928, p. 245.

the less desirable hours if they are not fully informed of the importance of the situation in terms of human needs, rather than of administrative expediency, and have shared in making plans for meeting them.

In developing its postwar program, the ANA has been keenly aware of the importance of promoting job satisfaction and of improving the career potentialities of nursing. This, for example, was the dual motive that caused the organization to work for professional status for nursing under federal civil service and for Old Age and Survivors coverage under the Social Security Act. Before discussing the ANA program, however, it will be helpful to focus attention on some of the major changes in nursing practice which were evident at mid-century. For illustrative purposes three seemingly disparate subjects have been selected. They are: the bed bath, the nursing team, and the responsibility of professional nurses for their own acts.

The changed status of the bed bath symbolizes a fundamental change, due to several causes, that began at about the time of Pearl Harbor. Prior to that time the bed bath was the focal point of the care of bed patients. In the early days of the war, hospital nurses who omitted the daily bath from sheer lack of time did so with a sense of guilt. At about that time, paralleling the growing emphasis on psychosomatic concepts of treatment, came early ambulation. Both placed emphasis on helping patients to help themselves, psychologically and physically. Maternity patients and some others for whom early ambulation was ordered could take showers if carefully safeguarded. Many of those who could not were expected to manage at least a partial bath. In losing its position of eminence, in plans for patient care, the bed bath seemed to be in danger of becoming a lost art. But in institutions where early ambulation was the general policy, its practice as a distinctive nursing art was, of course, required to maintain hygiene of the skin of polio, neurosurgical, and other critically ill patients requiring complete bed rest.

Just as the routine bed bath was passing from the center of the picture, nurses generally were beginning to appreciate the psychological value (visiting nurses had long known it) of that quiet period of close association with their patients. Good nurses had always used the bath period to develop rapport with their patients. Some of them, in common with Miss Nightingale, recognized the importance of psychological supportive care although they didn't have a name for it. Miss Nightingale described it in *Notes on Nursing* as follows: "Apprehension, uncertainty, waiting, expectation, fear of surprise, do a patient more harm than any exertion. Remember he is face to face with his enemy all the time, internally wrestling with him, having long imaginary conversations with him."[7] Good practice therefore requires that in developing skills and empathy, students shall be taught, and graduates practice, the delicate art of encouraging patients to talk freely of their anxieties and to record significant findings. The seeming disinterest of nurses who have not yet developed this skill is causing considerable criticism of nurses by patients who, taking technical skill for granted, are extremely sensitive to the mental attitudes of those who care for them. As the average hospital stay grew shorter, social workers, with doctors and nurses, began to think of the period of hospitalization as just one phase of a continuum of patient care. Information acquired by nurses during that quiet period could provide an important part of the information needed in the planning for successive stages of care. The referral of patients through social service channels to visiting nurse or other community agencies gave reality to the theory of a continuum of care.

"All professional nurses should possess the essential knowledge and the ability to teach measures to conserve health and to restore health."[8] So said a study made for the Grading Committee, a principle which was elaborated by the *Curriculum Guide*. The bath period was generally accepted as an excellent time for the teaching of health principles, and for interpretation of medical orders, especially those related to the posthospitalization period of patients who were being taught how to live with a handicap. The availability of community resources and the functions of visiting nurses, social

[7] Woodham-Smith, Cecil: *Florence Nightingale, 1820–1910.* McGraw-Hill Book Co., 1951, p. 229.

[8] Johns, Ethel, and Pfefferkorn, Blanche: *An Activity Analysis of Nursing.* Committee on the Grading of Nursing Schools, New York, 1934, p. 38.

workers, physical therapists, and other specialists often require interpretation to patients and their families. Without the bath period, making provision for time for productive conversation and teaching requires considerable skill in planning. Specific attention to the art of communication and the allocation of time for it is now a definite part of the daily program of patient care in well-managed nursing services. Administrators of institutional nursing services find it necessary to devise in-service programs (a well-established practice in public health nursing services) for nurses whose basic preparation had stressed technical skills at the expense of interpersonal relationships.

The *nursing team* (discussed in an earlier chapter) is an administrative device which a growing number of nurses believe can be used to improve both the service and the job satisfaction of nurses and other members of nursing teams. The psychological and social as well as the physical needs of patients are grouped, with the medical orders, to provide the focal point of nursing planning when the team method of assignment is used. The patient, as an individual for whom a complete nursing plan has been made, acquires greater importance and seems more interesting than a person whose needs are assumed to have been met when the instructions on lists—medicine, treatment, diet, etc.—have been fulfilled. The nursing plan is a far more stimulating challenge to a nurse's skills than an aggregation of medical orders can ever be. Patient-centered care can, of course, be provided without formally organized teams. It is believed, however, that the team concept provides greater opportunity for staff nurses, as members of a team or as team leaders, to exercise and develop their skills and capacity for wholesome interrelationships in a truly professional manner. In other words, it fulfills the third and fourth of the fundamental needs of nurses which the Grading Committee pointed out years ago, viz., reasonable hours, adequate income, constructive leadership, opportunity for growth.

The mid-century emphasis on patient-centered care indicates a resurgence of the motivation (helping others) which is one of the most precious heritages of the profession. It places on professional nurses responsibility for developing democratic and mutually helpful relationships with the nonprofessional members of the nursing team, comparable to those which they would like to enjoy with other members of the health team. But planning for nursing teams does not begin with the individual. It begins when top-level administrative groups become convinced that a determined and enlightened effort must be made to improve interpersonal relationships "in the very highly controlled hospital environment."[9]

Professional responsibility. The growing tendency of the public to sue nurses for alleged negligence and for the courts to hold nurses responsible for their own acts indicates a significant trend in the changing status of nurses. The subject was discussed by the House of Delegates of the ANA in 1950.[10] The association completed arrangements in 1951 for liability insurance for nurses desiring it. Five state associations have their own liability insurance plan apart from the ANA plan.

This raises the question, previously discussed in other connections, "What is nursing? How shall it be defined?" For example: Does a procedure become a nursing procedure merely because physicians in specific situations find it convenient to delegate to nurses medical procedures which have become routine? Historically, this has been accomplished without formal recognition by either profession of the transfer of responsibility. For example, the question of venipuncture has been discussed pro and con, without definite conclusions in relation to the civil defense program. The technic is not intricate. Considerable numbers of nurses have become highly expert, notably in the blood donor service of the ARC. The situation appears to be somewhat similar to that of the nurse anesthetist whom many believe should more appropriately be classified as a medical technician than as a nurse. Nurses required by medical orders to give intravenous therapy admit grave concern about the responsibility thrust upon them when powerful drugs, such as heparin and Levophed are prescribed. The question of having nurses

[9] Simmons, Leo W.: "The Manipulation of Human Resources in Nursing Care," *Am. J. Nursing*, **51**:453, 1951.

[10] ANA *Proceedings*, House of Delegates, Vol. 1, 1950, p. 167.

(nurse-midwives) made responsible for normal deliveries in hospitals is another matter which may be rising on the horizon of nursing. There will be more such problems as the ratio of interns to hospitalized patients grows smaller. If nursing is a profession, should it be expected to define its area of competence in order to avoid violations of the medical practice acts? Studies of the functions of nurses, now being made under the aegis of the ANA's remarkably farseeing research program, may confidently be expected to provide answers to this and many related questions.

The ANA's plan for professional liability insurance is only one evidence of the association's concern for nurses as individuals who have won the right to practice as registered professional nurses. Its total program is predicated on the needs of society for nursing service with emphasis on the status and conditions of employment of the individual nurse. The ANA's total program is based on three documents: The Certificate of Incorporation,[11] the Platform[12] (subject to revision every two years), and the Code for Professional Nurses.[13] In relation to the nation's need for nursing, as previously noted, the ANA makes inventories of nurses, is responsible for studies of nursing functions, and has established the PC&PS. It may initiate or sponsor federal legislation. The association maintains an office in Washington where a staff member serves as ANA representative and handles many questions referred to the ANA from the nation's capitol. She also serves as an observer in Washington to ensure prompt action in relation to any legislation which may have a bearing on nursing or which might be influenced by the association. It maintains cooperative relationships with the federal nursing services and that of the American Red Cross. The ANA's public relations program is a "two-way street" since it interprets nursing to the public and the public to nurses. As shown in the following chapter the ANA's program is carefully coordinated with that of the NLN. Frequent reference has been made to ANA activities throughout

[11] Certificate of Incorporation and Bylaws, Amended June, 1952.
[12] "The ANA Platform," *Am. J. Nursing*, **52**:953, 1952.
[13] "Code for Professional Nurses," *Am. J. Nursing*, **52**:1247, 1952.

this book. A brochure, now in preparation, which will replace Miss Best's well-known *Brief Historical Review*,[14] will provide comprehensive information about the ANA in compact form.

But we are here concerned with the ANA programs which have a direct relationship to the practice of nursing by individual nurses. The uncertainties of the mid-century indicated imperative need for a code of ethics. The preparation and publication of a code had been one of the initial purposes of the association, but action had been deferred until the organization should have a body of experience on which to build. Tentative codes had been published, for discussion preliminary to formal action, in 1926 and 1940,[15] but neither was completed. Early teaching of ethics had placed emphasis on specific loyalties, such as to "the doctor," "the hospital," "the training school," rather than on the basic principles of ethical conduct and the fundamental interprofessional and nurse-patient relationships. The inhibiting influence of early teaching, which tended to result in subserviency and conflicting loyalties, is still evident to philosophic observers of nursing practice.

The Code for Professional Nurses, published by the ANA in 1950, was prepared by a committee headed by Sister Berenice Beck of Marquette University after suggestions had been received from some 5000 persons, chiefly nurses representing a cross section of the profession. It is prefaced by a series of declarative statements of which the following is the first:

Professional nurses minister to the sick, assume responsibility for creating a physical, social, and spiritual environment which will be conducive to recovery, and stress the prevention of illness and promotion of health by teaching and example. They render health service to the individual, the family, and the community and co-ordinate their services with members of other health professions involved in specific situations.

There is no taint of subserviency in the code. Note the relationship of the professional nurse to the physician—"The nurse is ob-

[14] Best, Ella: *Brief Historical Review and Information about Current Activities of the American Nurses' Association, Including Certain Facts Relative to the National League of Nursing Education.* ANA, New York, 1940.
[15] "A Suggested Code," *Am. J. Nursing,* **26**:599, 1926. "A Tentative Code," *Am. J. Nursing,* **40**:977, 1940.

ligated to carry out the physician's orders intelligently, to avoid misunderstandings or inaccuracies by verifying orders, and to refuse to participate in unethical procedures. The nurse sustains confidence in the physician and other members of the health team. . . ."

Principles and factual statements, in and of themselves, do not solve problems. Following the convention of 1952, the committee began publication in the *AJN* of a series of interpretative articles based on the 17 principles in the code, which are prefaced by the statement that:

Service to mankind is the primary function of nurses and the reason for the existence of the nursing profession. Need for nursing service is universal. Professional nursing service is therefore unrestricted by consideration of nationality, race, creed, or color.

Several planks of the ANA platform[16] rest solidly on this foundation. The Intergroup Relations Program, instituted after the ANA had taken over the functions and obligations of the NACGN (see Chap. 42) is implemented by plank 14 which recommends:

Promoting the inclusion and full participation of minority groups in association activities, and eliminating discrimination in job opportunities, salaries, and other working conditions.

Interest in this ANA program is widespread; approximately 22,-000 copies of its superb brochure, *An American Challenge,* have been distributed. The ANA is, of course, not working alone in this field. Federal agencies have gone far, in the past few years, toward integrating Negro nurses in their services as have state and municipal institutions and agencies in many parts of the country. Voluntary institutions have variable policies.

The inauguration of the ANA Professional Counseling & Placement Service (1945) is discussed in Chapter 38. By 1952 one-half of the constituent state associations had established such service. Nurses in other areas could secure assistance from the branch office of the ANA PC&PS in Chicago. Counseling and placement service is provided without cost to individuals and employers. Some states

[16] "Platform of the American Nurses' Association," *Am. J. Nursing,* 52:953, 1952.

make a small charge for compiling credentials. The primary purposes, it will be recalled, are to provide educational, vocational, and professional counseling for nurses and to promote a better distribution of qualified nursing service. It is noteworthy that clients of PC&PS may be registered nurses, practical nurses, and prospective candidates for either professional or practical nursing schools. To limit service to members of the ANA would be inconsistent with the broad purposes for which the service was established. PC&PS is increasingly useful to employers of nurses as a source of information on acceptable personnel policies as well as on the availability of personnel.

The development of state PC&PS services is based on the logical assumption that knowledge of and interest in local conditions facilitates guidance in placement and stimulates improvement of employment conditions. This development has been relatively slow, chiefly because of financial considerations and difficulty in finding nurses qualified by interest, temperament, education, and experience for these important positions. From the beginning of the new service the ANA thought of registries sponsored by district associations as potential cooperating units of the state PC&PS. In a few states registries are now participating local units of the state's PC&PS and carry on complete placement services. In others the registries cooperate only to the extent of using the national PC&PS application forms for their registrants. Following the Biennial Convention of 1952, ANA PC&PS undertook a special study to determine specific factors relating to the counseling and placement of the older nurse. These senior citizens, it was believed, might prove to be a valuable source of needed nurse power. The service of PC&PS cannot be fully evaluated, at a time when demand greatly exceeds supply, in terms of the number of placements. Moreover, the counseling aspects of the service cannot be adequately measured by statistics. But its files contain the professional credentials of approximately 40,000 nurses, an ever-ready source of information for would-be employers.

The PC&PS is steadily gaining in usefulness and prestige. It is less well known than it deserves to be. Any important change in the economy of the nation, such as war or depression, would reaffirm the judgment of those who have labored to establish this broad-scale service on a firm foundation.

The dynamic Economic Security Program of the ANA is one of the most important and controversial programs ever undertaken by it. Time will probably show that the methods employed by the association created far more opposition than the principles on which the program was developed. As the Grading Committee had pointed out years before, "The fact that nursing is an idealistic profession does not render it immune to economic law. If nursing is to retain its high idealism, it must make sure that its members are free from undue economic pressure."[17] The ANA had persistently acted on that principle but with small result until the skyrocketing cost of living forced the issue. The conditions which led the association to embark on its economic security program in 1946 are discussed in Chapter 32. The basic principle on which it has been built may be found in the code of ethics: "The nurse has an obligation to give conscientious service and in return is entitled to just remuneration." It is important to keep in mind both facets of the ANA's effort to secure economic justice for nurses. One is concerned with potential nurses, the other with nurses in active practice. The nation wants more nurses! Current efforts to improve the education of nurses are expected to have an important bearing on the future supply by reducing the loss of students after they have been enrolled in nursing schools. In this materialistic age, however, many potential students (or their families) make vocational choices on the basis of the economic rewards that follow the expenditure of time and money for preparation. Improvement in the economic status of nurses and in employment conditions, the ANA believed, were urgently needed to promote the recruitment of students.

The goals of the ANA's economic security program are: (1) wider acceptance of the 40-hour week and the establishment of minimum salaries; (2) increased participation of nurses in the actual planning and administration of nursing service; development of nurses' associations in the role of exclusive spokesmen for nurses in matters

[17] Burgess, May Ayres: *Nurses, Patients, and Pocketbooks.* The Committee on the Grading of Nursing Schools, New York, 1928, p. 433.

affecting their employment; (3) the development of collective bargaining technics by state nurses' associations; (4) the restriction of the membership of a nurse to only one organization which can act as a bargaining agent; (5) the elimination of barriers to the employment of minority racial groups.

The use of the term "collective bargaining" set off an electrical charge of considerable proportions among nurses and between nurses and employing agencies, the hospitals in particular. But the words were used deliberately, after careful thought, since no alternative term would so clearly indicate the determination of the ANA to secure improvement in the conditions under which many nurses were employed. "Most people do not know the meaning of the words 'collective bargaining,'"[18] says a well-known writer on this subject, adding that of those who have some idea of the meaning, many frequently have an incorrect idea. The dreadful potentiality of the strike has made collective bargaining effective in industry. But the ANA program is unique. It relies on collective bargaining or negotiation to secure results *without* the strike. In 1950 the association voted that:

In recognition of the fact that the nursing profession and employers of nurses share responsibility for the provision of adequate nursing service to the public, the American Nurses' Association, in conducting its economic program (1) *reaffirms* professional nurses' voluntary relinquishment of the exercise of the right to strike and of the use of any other measures wherever they may be inconsistent with the professional nurses' responsibilities to patients; and (2) reaffirms its conviction that the voluntary relinquishment of measures ordinarily available to employees in their efforts to improve working conditions imposes on employers an increased obligation to recognize and deal justly with nurses through their authorized representatives in all matters affecting their employment conditions.

"Conflict," said the president of the ANA in discussing the policy, "can be constructive. It is through the clash of ideas that new understandings and new principles for action eventually emerge."[19]

[18] Heron, Alexander R.: *Beyond Collective Bargaining.* Stanford University Press, Stanford, Calif., 1948.

[19] Porter, Elizabeth K.: "A Realistic 'No-Strike' Policy," *Am. J. Nursing,* 51:539, 1951.

What, then, *is* collective bargaining? Students of the subject ad-
.mit that it is difficult to define although the Taft-Hartley Act provides a legal definition. Heron says that ". . . collective bargaining
means, first of all, a process in which there is a delegation of authority to negotiate, on behalf of a larger number of persons than
are actively engaged in the negotiations."[20] It is in this sense that
the term is used in the ANA program. Rev. Joseph D. Munier, who
has eloquently supported the ANA program at two biennial conventions of the association, using quotations from official canon law of
the Catholic Church to support his position, says that "Collective
bargaining . . . means . . . replacing the dispensable individual
with the indispensable group when talking business in regard to
the economic facts of life for nurses."[21]

Income, time schedules, and hours of work provide units of
measurement which are universally understood. "It is fruitless to
talk about capitalizing on the spiritual values of work, adjusting
work conditions to provide psychological satisfactions, or promoting
mutual understanding between management and workers if income
for work does not provide adequately for the physical needs of the
worker and his family, . . ."[22] says Glen U. Cleeton. The ANA had
reached an identical conclusion about nurses and the conditions of
their employment.

Representatives of the association conferred with legal counsel,
economists, sociologists, and industrial and public relations experts
before setting up the program. Its research department provided
factual information. Data provide the backbone of an economic program, as the association pointed out in articles prepared for the
Journal.[23] There was no escaping the fact that inequities existed as,
for example, in a state where the cost of living rose 28 per cent between 1946 and 1948 and there was no change in the income of

[20] Heron, A. R.: *op. cit.*, p. 7.
[21] *Proceedings of ANA*, Vol. II, 1952, p. 263.
[22] Cleeton, Glen U.: "The Human Factor in Industry," *Ann. Am. Acad.
Polit. Soc. Sci.*, 274:17, 1951.
[23] Patterson, Lillian B.: "The Economic Brief," *Am. J. Nursing*, 49:421,
1949; and Titus, Shirley C., and Marrich, Sylvia: "Economic Security for
Nurses in Tax-supported Institutions," *Am. J. Nursing*, 49:425, 1949.

nurses. It is true, too, that today's facts can be tomorrow's delusion as, for example, in relation to a spiraling cost of living. The state associations are recognized, in the initial statement of policy, as "qualified to act and should act as the exclusive agent of their respective memberships in the important fields of economic security and collective bargaining." The ANA set up policies and criteria and provided a staff to serve in a consultative capacity to the state associations. The wartime experience of the California State Nurses' Association (see Chap. 38) provided a dramatic background for the new program which California's zealot, Shirley C. Titus (executive secretary of the California State Nurses' Association), describes as "a social engineering job in the field of economics." Social engineering, as Edward L. Bernays taught the profession in the first postwar years, calls for expert use of public relations technics. The pool of public good will toward nursing, he pointed out, was very large but it was also very shallow because the public was poorly informed about nursing. The public is, however, thoroughly familiar with the economic yardstick of the relation of income to cost of living. The California association found that an informed public could be the nurses' best friend in relation to the economic status of nurses in specific hospital and public health nursing situations.

By 1949 the economic program was also making real headway in Minnesota and Washington. It had aroused interest in all states and stimulated action in many of them. A salary study made that year, by the ANA, indicated that the incomes of nurses throughout the country had been improved considerably since the findings of the Department of Labor study had been made known two years earlier. The extent to which improvement could be attributed directly to the program could not be appraised since other influences, including improvement in the salaries for the large number of nurses employed by the Veterans Administration, were at work. No later national study of incomes has been made. Neither has any study of "turnover" or other measurable data been made to ascertain the relation between time schedules and income, and the stability of the nursing services provided for patients. Slow improvement in time schedules caused the ANA to vote for vigorous promotion of the 40-hour week at the 1952 convention.[24]

A study, completed in preparation for the convention of 1952, shows the result of six years of effort by the ANA. Of 44 reporting state associations, 22 had adopted programs which were in essential agreement with that of the ANA. A few nurses had lost their positions in the struggle for a cause in which they believed. The state programs were in various stages of development. Five of the 22 had signed a total of 84 collective bargaining contracts covering 196 hospitals and other nurse-employing agencies. They were the associations of California, Minnesota, Pennsylvania, Washington, and Wisconsin. Of the other 22 state associations which reported, 8 had programs which depart in principle from that of the ANA; the others then had no program. State associations which recognize the need for an economic program but eschew the collective bargaining technic have set up minimum standards of employment for the major categories of nurses. They seem to depend chiefly on conference technics and public opinion. They are making some headway toward their objectives. With the background of experience indicated by the report, the production of a manual for an economic security program (for the use of state associations) was begun immediately following the convention.

There can be no doubt that it was necessary to improve the economic status of nurses in order to maintain good standards of nursing service. Why then has the method adopted by the ANA for coping with the problem been described as one of the most controversial subjects in the association's history?[25] The reasons and emotions are much too complex for definitive analysis. As indicated elsewhere in this book, hospital traditions had caused many institutions to be laggard in facing the changing status and the economic facts of nursing. In common with many industrial employers, hospital administrators were reluctant to grant their nurse employees

[24] "A Resolution Calling for the 40-Hour Week for Registered Professional Nurses," *Am. J. Nursing,* **52**:963, 1952.
[25] Titus, Shirley: "Economic Facts of Life for Nurses," *Am. J. Nursing,* **52**: 1109, 1952.

the right to participate in planning the conditions under which they could most efficiently care for patients. There was an intense emotional response among hospitals and some nurses to the term collective bargaining, which denoted either fear of strikes or distaste for applying industrial practices to professional workers. Some nurses thought the whole discussion of economics unethical, because they confused ethics with tradition. Also, the forthrightness of the Brown report had caused many graduate nurses to be fearful of loss of professional status. "The immediate objective of professional service is the welfare of the client or patient," says Taeusch, "and any realistic as well as justifiable system of professional ethics should be similarly oriented."[26] The ANA was convinced that the care of patients could not be stabilized and improved without marked improvement in the economic and other conditions of employment of nurses. In the conviction that it was basing its action on a sound ethical principle, it therefore embarked on a program such as few other professional groups have attempted. The ANA, in courageously advocating collective bargaining *without use of the strike*, blazed a new trail in employer-employee relationships.

The tangibles which are the immediate objective of collective bargaining provide a foundation for the psychological job satisfactions that hold nurses in their positions and thereby stabilize and improve nursing service. "Job satisfaction," which is a morale-building and stabilizing force in any nursing service, depends in part on the basic motivation of the individual (there are some misfits in nursing just as there are in other groups) and on the administrative skills in the line organization. This is the point at which "collective planning," which is still a new concept in interpersonal and interprofessional relations, takes over. "Many collective bargaining agreements include honest recognition of the mutual interest of employees and employers in the efficient and economical operation of the business. None of them has ever created the will to work efficiently and cooperatively. They may clear away obstacles to cooperation. They may cure conditions which have generated resist-

[26] Taeusch, C. F.: "Professional Ethics," *Encyclopedia of Social Sciences*. The Macmillan Company, New York, 1934, p. 472.

ance to cooperation and efficiency. But they do not in and of themselves generate efficient work by individual employees."[27] This profound truth has been recognized by the professional organizations.

The ANA, through its Economic Security Program, has worked persistently to "cure conditions which have generated resistance to cooperation and efficiency" and thus to promote stability of nursing services. Many types of collective planning, through regional conferences and the like, are now in operation. Chief among them, in relation to the economic security program of the ANA, is the program of the NCINS which, it will be recalled, had been set up by six national nursing organizations. In collaboration with the Joint Commission for the Improvement of the Care of the Patient, it developed programs which could be integrated in those of the new NLN which place illuminating emphasis on the administration of nursing services. As shown in the next chapter, the programs of the ANA and NLN are geared to mesh as they move forward in a joint effort to secure the development of the amounts and kinds of nursing service the nation needs with a reasonable degree of job satisfaction for those who participate in the services.

BIBLIOGRAPHY

American Nurses' Association:

An American Challenge. American Nurses' Association, New York, 1951.
"The ANA Economic Security Program," *Am. J. Nursing*, 47:70, 1947.
"The ANA Economic Security Program—Criteria for the Evaluation of State Programs in Relation to Official National Policy," *Am. J. Nursing*, 49:656, 1949.
ANA PC&PS Manual. American Nurses' Association, New York, 1953.
"Brotherhood Has to Be Lived," *Am. J. Nursing*, 52:163, 1952.
Certificate of Incorporation and By-Laws, Amended June, 1952. American Nurses' Association, New York.

[27] Reprinted from *Beyond Collective Bargaining* by Alexander R. Heron, with permission of the author and of the publishers, Stanford University Press. Copyright by the Board of Trustees of Leland Stanford Junior University.

"Economic Facts of Life for Nurses," *Am. J. Nursing,* **52:**1109, 1952.
I. Titus, Shirley; II, Munier, Joseph D.; III, Mermelstein, Thelma M.

"The Individual, the Section, and the State Nurses' Association in Collective Bargaining," *Am. J. Nursing,* **51:**540, 1951.

"Meet the ANA," *Am. J. Nursing,* **50:**357, 1950.

"A Nationwide Counseling and Placement Service," *Am. J. Nursing,* **45:**467, 1945.

Northrup, Herbert R.: "The ANA and the Negro Nurse," *Am. J. Nursing,* **50:**207, 1950.

"Platform of the ANA," *Am. J. Nursing,* **52:**953, 1952.

"PC&PS Statement of Principles," *Am. J. Nursing,* **52:**48, 1952.

Ballard, Berton J.: "The Nurses' Staunchest Friend Could Be the Public," *Am. J. Nursing,* **46:**586, 1946.

Bishoff, Mary W., and Connolly, Mary G.: "New Skills Are Needed," *Am. J. Nursing,* **51:**576, 1951.

Carn, Irene: "We Must Nurse People Better," *Am. J. Nursing,* **47:**148, 1947.

Carn, Irene, and Mole, Eleanor W.: "Continuity of Nursing Care. An Analysis of Referral Systems with Recommended Practice," *Am. J. Nursing,* **49:**388, 1949.

Corbin, Hazel: "Changing Maternity Service in a Changing World," *Pub. Health Nursing,* **42:**427, 1950.

Feinsinger, Nathan P.: "Labor Legislation, Economic Security, and Individual Freedom," *Am. J. Nursing,* **52:**426, 1952.

Gilbreth, Lillian: "Management Engineering and Nursing," *Am. J. Nursing,* **50:**780, 1950.

Gillingham, J. B.: "Collective Bargaining and Professional Ethics," *Am. J. Nursing,* **50:**214, 1950.

Hall, Reina F.: "Interviewing as a Nursing Procedure," *Am. J. Nursing,* **52:**707, 1952.

Hart, Joseph L.: "Economic Security for Nurses," *Am. J. Nursing,* **38:**391, 1938.

———: "Drift—Conflict—or Education?" *Am. J. Nursing,* **38:**544, 1938.

Heron, Alexander R.: *Beyond Collective Bargaining.* Stanford University Press, Stanford, Calif., 1948.

———: "Constructive Policies of Labor Relations," *Ann. Am. Acad. Polit. & Soc. Sc.,* **274:**166, 1951.

Heyel, Carl: "Personnel Organization No Substitute for Good Personnel Relationships," *Hospitals,* **20:**80, 1946.

Holfeltz, Katherine M.: "Nurses' Professional Registries and the Professional Counseling and Placement Service," *Am. J. Nursing,* **48:**364, 1948.

Karabasz, Victor S.: "Industrial Management and Nursing," *Am. J. Nursing*, **52**:442, 1952.

Kidneigh, John C.: "The Philosophy of Administrative Process and the Role of the Consultant," *Pub. Health Nursing*, **43**:474, 1951.

Koos, Earl Loman: "What Society Demands of the Nurse," *Am. J. Nursing*, **47**:306, 1947.

Leino, Amelia: "Planning Patient-Centered Care," *Am. J. Nursing*, **52**:324, 1952.

Lippitt, Ronald: *Training in Community Relationships.* Harper & Brothers, New York, 1949, Chap. 5, "Planning the Workshop Curriculum and Procedures."

Loevinger, Ruth Howe: "The Minnesota Story of Economic Security," *Am. J. Nursing*, **51**:228, 1951.

Lotspeich, Ruth L.: "Why Do General Duty Nurses Resign?" *Am. J. Nursing*, **51**:468, 1951.

Lyons, Veronica: "Understanding the Psychological Components of Health Care," *Am. J. Nursing*, **52**:80, 1952.

Magoun, F. Alexander: "New Ways in Personnel Administration," *Am. J. Nursing*, **46**:751, 1946.

Menninger, William C.: "Opportunities in Nursing for a Satisfying Life," *Am. J. Nursing*, **48**:525, 1948.

Muller, Theresa Grace: *Dynamics of Human Behavior* (pamphlet). Boston University School of Nursing, Boston, 1950.

Nelson, Thomas H.: "Changing Concepts of Administration," *Am. J. Nursing*, **49**:70, 1949.

Northrop, Herbert R.: "Collective Bargaining and the Professions," *Am. J. Nursing*, **48**:141, 1948.

Patterson, Lillian B.: "The Economic Brief—An Important Technic in Collective Bargaining," *Am. J. Nursing*, **49**:421, 1949.

Perlstein, M. A.: *The Problem of Cerebral Palsy Today.* National Society for Crippled Children and Adults, Chicago, 1947.

Phillips, Elisabeth C.: "Nursing Service Needs Can Be Met," *Am. J. Nursing*, **49**:504, 1949.

Reider, Norman: "Human Needs and Nursing," *Pub. Health Nursing*, **42**:388, 1950.

Roethlisberger, Fritz J.: *Management and Morale.* Harvard University Press, Cambridge, 1941.

Sheppard, Harold L., and Sheppard, Audrey P.: "Paternalism in Employer-Employee Relationships," *Am. J. Nursing*, **51**:61, 1951.

Titus, Shirley C., and Marrich, Sylvia: "Economic Security for Nurses in Tax-Supported Institutions," *Am. J. Nursing*, **49**:425, 1949.

Weiner, Florence R.: "Professional Consequences of the Nurse's Occupational Status," *Am. J. Nursing*, **51**:614, 1951.

White, Edwin E.: "Collective Bargaining and the Democratic Process," *Ann. Am. Acad. Polit. & Soc. Sc.*, **274**:85, 1951.

Williamson, S. T., and Harris, Herbert: *Trends in Collective Bargaining*. The Twentieth Century Fund, New York, 1945.

Chapter 49

THE RESTRUCTURING OF THE
NATIONAL ORGANIZATIONS

*How can nurses achieve professional unity and at the same time preserve
the diversity within that unity which permits stimulation and growth of
the various phases of nursing, nursing education, and community nursing
service, as well as professional welfare of nurses? How can nurses secure
maximum cooperation from the public they serve in achieving all these
ends—ends as important to the public in need of nursing care as to the
nurses themselves?*[1]

CONCURRENTLY with day-by-day effort to provide an increasing
volume of nursing service amid the swift-moving and sometimes
turbulent currents of postwar activities discussed in the preceding
chapters, the profession carried forward a deeply probing study of
the structure and functions of the six national nursing organizations.
In scope and social motivation the study was believed to be without precedent among professional organizations. As a result, in
1952, the almost 60-year-old NLNE, the 40-year-old NOPHN, and
the 20-year-old ACSN were combined to form the National League
for Nursing; the sturdy structure of the ANA was adapted to provide for a more comprehensive and democratic program which
would be coordinated with that of the NLN.

"Every social agency," says Raymond B. Fosdick, "carries within
itself not only the seeds of possible decay, but a tendency to exalt
the machinery of organization above the purpose for which the organization was created."[2] But no nurse who attended the epocal

[1] *New Horizons in Nursing* (Foreword). The Macmillan Company, New
York, 1950.
[2] Fosdick, Raymond B.: *The Story of the Rockefeller Foundation.* Harper
& Brothers, New York, 1952, p. 293.

convention of 1952 can ever forget the sense of dedication to a
greater service which pervaded the meetings at which well-loved
organizations, to which nurses with special interests had given
years of devoted service, were voted out of existence in order that
the NLN, inheriting the traditions, resources, and ongoing programs of three organizations might be born to fulfill, in cooperation
with a stronger ANA, the challenge of ever-widening horizons.
Those who have traced the evolution of nursing through these pages
will agree that some such confluence of the various streams of interest and activity was inevitable. As the president of the ANA told
a huge convention audience, decisions based on the structure
study were "the logical outcome of historical events."³ Interrelationship with many other professional bodies and agencies, as well as
an ever-increasing number of joint nursing projects, had created the
situation which caused thoughtful nurses to ask the questions which
head this chapter.

Consolidation of the professional organizations was by no means
a new idea. For various reasons it had been considered, as previously
noted, in 1909 and in the mid-twenties. At the earlier date the members of the Superintendents' Society (NLNE), who enjoyed their
small and intimate conventions, decided against a merger with the
Associated Alumnae because they feared loss of identity. When the
offices of "the three national organizations" had been established
under one roof in the mid-twenties (Chap. 21), careful consideration was given to a proposal, based on the assumption that administrative economies could be effected, that the organizations and
their programs be merged. Each of the associations decided that the
time was not then ripe for such a change. Hospitals were operating
more than 2000 schools, and the ANA and NLNE were making a
determined effort to secure a reduction in their number and improvement in their quality. The NOPHN's decision was especially
specific. The public health movement was rapidly gaining momentum, and the organization was keenly aware of it's opportunity to
guide the development of nursing as a community service. NOPHN
members were asked "would a divorcement (as nationally handled)

³ Porter, Elizabeth K.: "Salute to the Future," *Am. J. Nursing*, **52**:978, 1952.

of the professional interests (education, standardization, etc.), from the function of pure service to the community strengthen or weaken public health nursing in the country?"[4] The answer was unequivocal. From that time forward the programs of NOPHN were developed on the basis of clearly defined objectives (1) for improving the preparation and status of public health nurses and (2) for assisting with the development of nursing as a community service. In the early thirties, although the NLNE voted to become the Department of Education of the ANA (without loss of autonomy) neither organization changed its bylaws. Results, therefore, were not impressive although the educational body began for the first time to participate in state board conferences.

By 1939, when a state nurses' association asked the ANA to investigate the possibility of conserving the time, effort, and resources of nurses by a merger of the three organizations (ANA, NLNE, and NOPHN), the functions and potentialities of nursing had been increased enormously. The movement toward collegiate education for nurses was on the march, and a fourth organization, the ACSN, had been established. The question was referred to a special committee of which Mary Beard was chairman. The committee reported[5] that four important developments seemed to indicate need for unity of action. These were: the National Health Program, the growing interest of American universities in nursing education, the interest of organized labor in nursing (small groups of unhappy nurses were joining unions believing they could solve problems created by inept personnel policies such as have been discussed in earlier chapters), and the question of legal recognition of a subsidiary group of workers in the field of nursing. World events prevented immediate action. Early in 1944, when the end of World War II was believed to be in sight, the joint boards of the three older organizations voted "to undertake a joint survey of their organization structure, administration, functions, and facilities to determine whether a more effective means can be found to promote and carry forward the

[4] Gardner, Mary S.: "Report of a Six-Months Study of the NOPHN," *Public Health Nurse*, 18:374, 1926.
[5] ANA—Reports to the House of Delegates, 1940.

strongest possible program for professional nursing and nurses."[6] The NACGN, the ACSN, and the new AAIN accepted invitations to participate in the study. At this time the National Nursing Council, of which the six organizations were members, was preparing to release its comprehensive program[7] for the postwar development of nursing. The council, since it was an emergency organization, was not represented on the committee set up by the national organizations to consider reconstruction, but its activities and its comprehensive program stimulated spacious thinking. Out of a superabundance of source materials, only the highlights of the sequence of events which led to the series of historic decisions of 1952 can be considered here.

Established organizations are notable for their tenacious hold on life and their deeply grooved habit patterns, but only a few nurses remembered that it had required the brilliant leadership of Miss Goodrich, and several years of subsequent effort, to convert the Nurses' Associated Alumnae, which had been renamed the American Nurses' Association, into a federation of state associations. It was agreed that specialists in social studies should be engaged to make the initial survey of the structure, resources, and programs of the six participating organizations.[8] The sociologists who undertook the task were much impressed by the readiness of individual nurses to contribute funds to finance the study. Plans called for a preliminary report at the biennial convention of 1946. But, such was their enthusiasm for the potentialities inherent in a restructured profession, as they envisioned it, that the Raymond Rich Associates rushed their report[9] to completion in order to have it published in the AJN in time for presentation at the convention.

The thousands of nurses who attended the biennial of 1946 were

[6] *Am. J. Nursing*, 44:517, 1944.

[7] "A Comprehensive Program for Nationwide Action in the Field of Nursing," *Am. J. Nursing*, 45:707, 1945.

[8] American Nurses' Association, National League of Nursing Education, National Organization for Public Health Nursing, National Association of Colored Graduate Nurses, Association of Collegiate Schools of Nursing, and American Association of Industrial Nurses.

[9] Raymond Rich Associates: "Report on the Structure of Organized Nursing," *Am. J. Nursing*, 46:648, 1946.

in effervescent spirits. Restrictions on travel had interdicted large meetings throughout the war. They were enjoying the first postwar opportunity to share experiences and were happy in the discovery that, for the profession as a whole, wartime stresses had resulted in far more unity than disharmony. Then, too, the ANA, although without fanfare, because the war was so recently ended, was celebrating its golden anniversary. Prompt action on a number of important matters indicated that nurses were in a receptive and constructive state of mind. The report on structure was presented to several audiences. But it was couched in unfamiliar terminology which fell on minds wholly unprepared to consider the radically different type of organization which was recommended. The report created more bewilderment and resistance than enlightenment and was referred to committees for further study.

A special meeting of the House of Delegates of the ANA, the first in the organization's history, was held the following summer to discuss the subject. Katharine J. Densford, the president, a stickler for parliamentary procedure who had been confronted with many wartime problems, presided. Intensely emotional resistance to change was somewhat offset by the earnestness with which some of the better informed members pleaded for unity of thought and action. In view of its predominant size, provision was subsequently made to treble the representation of the ANA on the Structure Committee.[10] Provision was also made for financial support of the work of the committee on a per capita basis by the participating organizations, the ANA making an immediate contribution to facilitate the work. When the committee made its final report (1949), approximately $100,000 had been expended for meetings, travel, special studies, publications, staff, and office space. Never had so much material, including opinionnaires to secure free expression of ideas as the work progressed, been made available in connection with a single project for use by individuals and at institutes, workshops, conventions, and other gatherings. State associations organized structure committees, and they, in turn, promoted study of the whole question by district committees and other local groups.

[10] Committee on the Structure of National Nursing Organizations.

When it became clear that the trend of opinion was definitely toward the goal of a single national organization, to replace the six which were participating in the study, the committee produced a new and tentative plan for one organization.[11] In accordance with the insistence of many nurses that the democratic district—to state—to national type of organization which had been so successfully developed by the ANA should not be relinquished, the tentative plan provided for that type of structure. The plan was published and distributed well in advance of the convention of 1948. Action taken by the three older organizations seemed to indicate that the profession wanted two things:

1. One organization which would offer membership (a) to all graduate registered nurses, and (b) to non-nurses, schools of nursing and nursing services.

2. Continued membership in the ICN.[12]

There were, however, important obstacles to the development of a single organization. (1) It was found that donors could not deduct, for income tax purposes, gifts or grants to an organization which engaged in legislative programs in the interest of its members. (2) Inquiry revealed that the ICN (which is made up of national organizations of professional nurses only), in the interest of nurses in countries where there was fear of "outside influence" in the affairs of nurses, could not consider admitting an organization which included non-nurses. The organizations were united in their desire to retain membership for American nurses in the ICN which, in a period of serious international uncertainties, had enhanced the status and usefulness of nursing by securing official relationship with the World Health Organization in June, 1948 (Chap. 51). The legislative program of the ANA, as repeatedly indicated in this text, is important to all nurses and to the "consumers" of nursing service. It is equally true that nursing could not have achieved its present position of eminence as an essential social service without the aid of

[11] "A Tentative Plan for One National Nursing Organization," *Am. J. Nursing,* **48**:321, 1948.

[12] *Handbook on the Structure of Organized Nursing,* 2nd ed. Prepared by the Committee on Structure of the National Nursing Organizations, New York, August, 1949, p. 4.

the tax-free philanthropic foundations. From its earliest days some NOPHN projects and more recently projects of the NLNE and those sponsored by the boards of directors of two or more organizations had depended on grants and contributions. Some hospitals and many nursing agencies were dependent, in some degree, on community chests and councils for support. In the postwar period the Brown report, and the important programs set in motion as a result of it, would not have been possible without the stimulating understanding and financing of foundations.

Recognizing the fundamental nature of these problems, the boards of directors of the six organizations, meeting with the Joint Committee on Structure (January, 1949), voted unanimously to present a plan for two organizations to the members of all the organizations. A handbook was made readily available to encourage study of the new plan by individuals as well as by local, state, and national groups. Nurses took their "homework" on structure seriously. It was said, after the convention of 1950, that the House of Delegates of the ANA (representing over 175,000 nurses) had never seemed so well informed or so mature in its judgments. Requests from the General Duty and Private Duty Sections that the House vote against any change were overridden to the ultimate advantage of both sections. The House of Delegates voted to go forward with plans for two organizations with the important proviso that the ANA retain its corporation and that any changes in ANA functions be accomplished through the revision of, or amendments to, its existing bylaws.

Most of the 60 nurses appointed to represent the several organizations on the Structure Committee, who were members of the committee when it disbanded late in 1949, had served throughout four strenuous years of democratic effort to reconcile differences of opinion and to devise a structural pattern which all types of membership in the existing organizations—nurses, non-nurses, nursing schools, and nursing services—could accept. Hortense Hilbert served as chairman throughout, having been re-elected when the committee was revitalized following the first frustrating wave of disagreement and resistance to change. The presidents of the organizations in the later stages of the committee's work were Mary Delehanty (AAIN), Elizabeth S. Bixler (ACSN), Pearl McIver (ANA), Mabel K. Staupers (NACGN), Agnes Gelinas (NLNE), and Ruth Hubbard (NOPHN). The work of the historic committee was hastily summarized for the committee and was published under the title *New Horizons in Nursing.*[13]

This record represents, however, only the first stage of a two-stage effort. By the time the committee was disbanded, Mrs. Elizabeth K. Porter (director of advanced programs, Frances Payne Bolton School of Nursing, Western Reserve University) had succeeded Pearl McIver as president of the ANA, and Emilie Sargent (executive director of the Detroit VNA) had followed Ruth Hubbard of Philadelphia's similar service as president of the NOPHN. Each of the six organizations promptly organized a committee on structure. It was agreed that the six chairmen, with the presidents and executive secretaries of the organizations, should function as a Joint Coordinating Committee. This committee, working steadily on the basis of ever-expanding *areas of agreement*, reviewed and harmonized the proposals from the six organization committees. Miss McIver was a logical choice for chairman of the committee. Few nurses were so well known; also, she had been a member of the original committee to consider restructuring the organizations and of the Committee on Structure. As president of the ANA for a single term (1948–1950) she devoted so much time to the work of the association, at headquarters and in the field, that she could not permit consideration of re-election. Under her leadership many issues were clarified and during her term the membership of the ANA pulled out of its postwar slump and added more than 25,000 nurses. As chairman of the committee, Miss McIver made effective use of her gift for clear exposition to explain the philosophy and technical planning of the committee to many audiences. Concurrently a series of informative articles, prepared for the committee by its executive secretary, Mrs. Edith Wensley, was published in the *AJN* and other appropriate media.

[13] *New Horizons in Nursing.* Compiled by Josephine Nelson. The Macmillan Company, New York, 1950.

In planning for the new NLN, the boards of directors of the three organizations involved agreed that the charter of one of the participating agencies would be used as a foundation because certain legal and financial problems could thus be avoided. Plans for the proposed structure of the NLN were therefore constructed on the foundation of the NLNE. Before taking the final step of submitting material to the regularly constituted committees on constitution and bylaws, a special meeting of representative nurses from all the states was arranged in order that the committee might have assurance that its proposals were in line with the thinking of the various occupational groups in the profession. That Minneapolis conference was a master stroke. Residual doubts of the proposed restructuring were resolved when some of those in attendance realized, for the first time, that all barriers were down and that professional registered nurses would be eligible for membership in either or both organizations. Shortly thereafter about 100 private duty and general duty nurses joined the NOPHN in order that they might become charter members of the proposed NLN! Whether a nurse joined the ANA or the NLN, or both, would be a matter of individual choice and interest. Since the ANA provides the foundation structure for organized professional activities it was anticipated that a very high percentage of all active nurses would continue membership in it. It was hoped that many nurses, in addition to those engaged in nursing education and public health nursing, would also become members of the more specialized organization.

When the report on structure was presented for final decision at the convention of 1952, the 10-year old AAIN had decided to withdraw from the proposed union with the organizations which would be fused to form the NLN. The NACGN had already been absorbed by the ANA (Chap. 42), and the number of state nurses' associations which did not make provision for membership of Negro nurses had been reduced from eleven, in 1948, to four.

The structural changes in the ANA which converted the sections from conference groups into administrative units made it a more democratic organization and ensured "diversity within unity." The bylaws provide that "the voting body shall consist of the regularly accredited delegates *from each section* of the state nurses' association. . . . Each section of a state nurses' association shall be entitled to one delegate for every two hundred active members or fractional part thereof . . . state nurses' associations shall be entitled to three delegates at large. . . ."[14] This means a smaller House of Delegates in which the *nurses who nurse,* as well as the consultants, administrators, instructors, and the like, are assured representation.

Provision was made for seven sections: (1) educational administrators, consultants, and teachers; (2) general duty; (3) industrial; (4) institutional nursing service; (5) private duty; (6) public health; (7) special groups. Three of the seven were new and held organizational meetings during the convention. The men nurses' section, as previously noted, and the government nursing section were discontinued. Although the AAIN had decided to continue its independent existence, the ANA Industrial Nurse Section, which had been organized on request of the association's industrial nurse members following the war, now had the larger membership. Members of the section encourage membership in the NLN in anticipation of the time when a department of industrial nursing can be organized within the division of nursing service of that organization. The USPHS has replaced the designation "industrial nursing" with the more descriptively inclusive term *occupational health nursing,* but a change has not yet been considered by the national organizations. Following the convention, the development of sections on the new basis promptly became a major activity of most of the state nurses' associations. Out of the dozen specified functions of the sections, one of the most important is "to define the functions, standards, and qualifications for practice within the occupational field . . . as, for example, for private duty, general duty nursing, or for public health nursing positions.

Requirements for membership in sections must necessarily be compatible with the general membership requirements of the ANA. Each section is responsible for the preparation of a program of work and a statement of the annual budget required to execute it. All of

[14] ANA Certificate of Incorporation and Bylaws, Rules for Sections. Amended June, 1952, p. 30.

the ANA's well-established services, such as research, public relations, legislation, counseling and placement, and economic security, stand ready to assist the sections, but the initiative must come from the occupational groups which comprise them. The fundamental purposes of the ANA, to improve the quality and promote the distribution of nursing service and to upgrade the status of nurses can be accomplished only on the home front, viz., in the cities, towns, villages, and rural areas in which nurses live and work. To accomplish this broad objective it works in cooperation with the NLN.

The NLN is unique among professional organizations in its scope and provision for "diversity within unity." Its object is:

. . . to foster the development and improvement of hospital, industrial, public health, and other organized nursing services and of nursing education through the coordinated action of nurses, allied professional groups, citizens, agencies, and schools to the end that the nursing needs of the people shall be met.[15]

In order to fufill its purposes democratically, its provisions for membership, although classified in two groups, are equally broad. They are based on NOPHN's 40 years of successful experience in promoting the development of nursing as a community service and on its educational aims as well as those of the NLNE and the ACSN. Members are classified as individual and agency. Individual members may be professional nurses, non-nurses (there are 19 qualifying clauses), and student nurses. The history of the NOPHN provides convincing evidence of the positive values of non-nurse membership in an organization set up to do those things for the welfare of society which a profession can do only in close cooperation with others. Agency membership is available to (1) organizations or other groups that are administratively engaged in providing nursing services and (2) schools, divisions, and departments that provide educational programs in nursing. The exchange of ideas due to the membership of public health nursing agencies in the NOPHN was one of the fundamental sources of its strength. The ACSN was composed solely of collegiate schools. Charter membership was conferred on members in good standing of both groups, agencies

[15] Certificate of Incorporation, NLN.

and schools, and on individual members when the NLN bylaws were adopted. They provide for a board of directors of 21 members which shall include nurses engaged in administration, supervision, teaching, and in giving direct care to patients. The first board of directors includes representatives of general duty, private duty, and public health staff nurses, as well as a hospital administrator, a physician, and specialists in psychiatry and tuberculosis. The lay members, men and women, represent a cross section of the people of the United States including religious and minority groups. Racial discrimination is interdicted. All standing committees have nurse members who are engaged in giving direct care to patients.

The AHA studied the proposed structural organization, functions, and methods of financing the NLN in advance of the convention of the nursing organizations. *Hospitals,* its official organ, announced that the board of trustees of the association was "fully in accord with the over-all aims of the NLN" but that it did not favor "institutional membership for hospitals in organizations that are essentially personal membership associations of professional or technical groups."[16] The NLN continues to believe, however, that hospital schools and hospital nursing services can derive values from membership comparable to those which are known to have accrued to agency members of the NOPHN.

The practitioners of nursing, especially the great groups of general duty and private duty nurses, now have an opportunity to demonstrate their capacity to develop leadership and to promote professional growth in relation to the needs of society in both ANA and NLN. By keeping the larger objective in view both organizations hope to secure correction of conditions which have had a frustrating influence on individual nurses and therefore on the advancement, in usefulness, of the profession.

The ANA and the NLN will go forward together. A coordinating council provides a means for promoting desirable developments and for reconciling differences. Broadly speaking, matters that relate to nurses as individual practitioners are properly the concern of the

[16] "Hospitals and the League for Nursing," *Hospitals,* Vol. 26, No. 6, Part I (June, 1952) p. 74.

professional organization composed exclusively of registered professional nurses, the ANA. The over-all purpose of the NLN has already been stated (Chap. 47). Almost 1000 students attended the historic convention. Those who represented student organizations in their home states voted for a separate organization to be placed under the aegis of the coordinating council. Further action was deferred to the NLN convention of 1953. The poise, judgment, and enthusiasm of the students offered bright promise for the future of nursing.

In anticipation of a favorable decision by the several organizations and in order to ensure smooth transition from the old to the new structure, the Committee on Agreements, on the basis of legal advice, arranged for necessary administrative officers to staff the NLN until the board of directors could be elected and make appointments. Anna Fillmore, the farseeing and objective general director of the NOPHN, who some years earlier had been a member of the ANA staff, was appointed general director of the NLN. Few nurses are so well equipped by education and experience for that demanding office. Her experience includes practice in the fields of private duty, institutional, and industrial nursing, also public health nursing with both official and nonofficial agencies. Miss Fillmore has consistently and progressively added to her professional background by study at the University of California and at Teachers College, New York. She concluded her formal education with work at the Harvard School of Public Health where she earned the degree of master of public health. Marion W. Sheahan, recipient of an honorary degree from Adelphi College and of the Lasker award from the APHA, who had effectively developed the programs of the Committee on the Improvement of Nursing Services, was made assistant to the general director and director of the Division of Nursing Services. Julia M. Miller, experienced in the methods of hospital and collegiate schools (most recently at Emory University), then executive secretary of the NLNE, became director of the Division of Nursing Education.

In the period of transition these officers necessarily had dual functions. They carried their heavy burdens with optimistic fortitude.

The positions, it should be noted, are administrative and not elective, a point about which there was some confusion at the time. A truly Herculean task was performed under heavy pressure but with an extraordinary degree of equanimity. In addition to bringing together in one organization the staffs of the NLNE and NOPHN and combining the programs of these organizations, with that of the ACSN, there were also a number of special projects with their own administrative staffs to be fitted into the new structure. The National Nursing Accrediting Service, with gentle but sagacious Helen Nahm serving under a new title, was made an administrative unit of the new organization. The active program of the NOPHN would continue under the direction of efficient Ruth Fisher, almost without a break, as the Department of Public Health Nursing. The work of the NCINS had been carefully planned to fit into a program for the new Division of Nursing Services. But there was no organized unit of membership or of service to be transferred by any organization to the Hospital Nursing Department. Time would be required to build up its membership. Service would be developed on the basis of the cooperative philosophy of the NCINS, already working like yeast throughout the country. The work of the Joint Committee on Practical Nurses and Auxiliary Workers in Nursing Services was placed within the NLN, but an administrative practical nurse unit was not provided for in the plan accepted in 1952. It should be noted, however, that the pros and cons of practical nurse membership in the NLN were reviewed at the very first business meeting of the new organization. The delegates approved, in principle, the inclusion of practical nurses in the membership. A committee was appointed to consider the steps to be taken in cooperation with the other interested organizations—the NAPNE and the National Federation of Licensed Practical Nurses. It was anticipated that positive action on including practical nurses as members of the NLN might be taken at the 1953 convention. Action relative to a Department of Industrial Nursing in the Division of Nursing Services was discontinued (temporarily, it is hoped) when the AAIN withdrew from the study of structure.

The Careers Committee, energetically carrying forward the five-year program which had been authorized by the joint boards of the six organizations (Chap. 47), was arousing a more general interest in nursing than any previous peacetime program. Without that program the schools of nursing could not, conceivably, have enrolled 7 per cent of the girls graduated each year from the nation's high schools as they did in the early fifties. Because recruitment of students was considered a responsibility of society and of allied professions, as well as of nursing, decision as to the appropriate place of the Careers Committee in the new structure was deferred for consideration and action at the 1953 convention.

In addition to the four joint committee projects, several other administrative units under joint sponsorship were incorporated in the NLN. JONAS, the highly successful result of cooperative planning by NOPHN, NLNE, and the National Foundation for Infantile Paralysis, which finances it, became the NLN's Nursing Advisory Service for Orthopedics and Poliomyelitis (NASOP). The NLN's Tuberculosis Nursing Advisory Service (TNAS), formerly the JTNAS which was sponsored by the same two nursing organizations, is financed by the National Tuberculosis Association. The Mental Health and Psychiatric Nursing Project of the NLNE and NOPHN, operated since 1946 on a grant from the National Institute of Mental Health (USPHS), was also made part of NLN.

The organization chart of the NLN shows nursing services, for the first time in nursing history, equated with nursing education. Professional interest in hospital nursing services can no longer be restricted, as it has tended to be, to institutions which operate or are affiliated with nursing schools. The Division of Nursing Services with its Departments of Hospital Nursing and Public Health Nursing, is balanced by the Division of Nursing Education which has a Department of Diploma and Associate Degree Programs and one of Baccalaureate and Higher Degree Programs.[17] Each department has its own steering committee which is elected by its own membership. The structural organization of the NLN makes quite extraordinary provision for diversity within unity. The membership re-

[17] National League for Nursing, Certificate of Incorporation and By-laws. Adopted June, 1952.

quirements ensure diversity because "an individual or agency applying for membership in the National League for Nursing shall also apply for membership in one division and one department within that division." They may, however, attend appropriate meetings of the other divisions and the other departments of the organization. Ruth Sleeper, an ex-president of the NLNE, who is known for her generosity of spirit, the judicial quality of her mind, and her devotion to the highest ideals of nursing, was elected first president of the NLN.

The ANA, which had emerged from the period of stress and strain stronger than ever before, enthusiastically re-elected its president, Mrs. Elizabeth K. Porter. Staunch and energetic Ella Best continued to serve as the association's efficient executive secretary. The structure and major programs of the association had been recognized as fundamental to the development of nursing in the United States. Its position as the representative of American nursing in international relationships had been reaffirmed. Katharine J. Densford, as president, had been privileged to witness the birth of the United Nations at San Francisco (1945), and saw its great purposes written into the preamble of its constitution:

to save succeeding generations from the scourge of war . . .
to reaffirm faith in fundamental human rights, in the dignity and worth
    of the human person . . .
to promote social progress . . .
to practice tolerance . . .

Subsequently a representative of the association (the executive secretary) was granted observer status at the United Nations (UN). This means that the association is supplied with information which can be shared with its constituent organizations and members. In this way it fulfills the first part of the obligation imposed by the following plank in the ANA platform: "Continuing to support the United Nations and its specialized agencies, particularly the World Health Organization, through the International Council of Nursing." The intrinsic assumption underlying the program based on this direct relationship between the UN and the ANA is that nurses are good citizens.

The program of the ICN is discussed in the following chapter. It seems appropriate, however, to consider at this point some of the more intimate relationships between the ICN and the ANA. Back in the twenties the ICN had discussed, without reaching a decision, the need for what may be called a program of international hospitality. Following the congress of 1947 the Committee on the Exchange of Nurses developed an excellent program which, in the US, is the principal responsibility of the International Unit at ANA headquarters. Service is restricted to nurses who are members of their respective national organizations. Under the ICN program there are several categories of exchange privileges:

(1) Matriculation in a university for advanced study in nursing education or public health nursing

(2) Short periods of observation

(3) Additional clinical experience under supervision

(4) Regular salaried employment for those who enter the country on permanent immigration (not visitor) status.

In relation to the fourth category, the International Unit cooperates with the ANA Professional Counseling & Placement Service. Obviously a comprehensive knowledge of the nurse practice acts is a prerequisite to placement. In 1952, in cooperation with the ICN, the ANA assisted 72 nurses from 13 countries and helped 8 American nurses to secure opportunity for study in 5 other countries. The ICN program was already under way when the Department of State announced (1949) the regulations under which the nation's broad-scale exchange-visitor program would be operated. The ANA has been designated a sponsor of the federal program. No less than six programs, of which "Educational Exchanges under the Fulbright Act" is the best known, are classified as exchange-visitor programs. "They are all designed to insure direct communication between the United States and other nations through the personal contact of carefully selected representatives of the nations concerned."[18] To participate in these programs, educational and other institutions must first be approved for the purpose by the Department of State.

[18] *Two-Way Street*. Report of the US Advisory Commission on Educational Exchange. US Government Printing Office, Washington, D.C., June 30, 1950, p. 21.

The obligations of citizenship demand that the programs offered shall be truly educational and suited to the needs of those who come as strangers and whom we hope will become our friends. There are some evidences that a few nurse-hungry institutions look upon exchange-visitor programs as an opportunity to augment their nursing resources. But most of the institutions and agencies accepting nurse-visitors from other countries give the needs of the visitors priority over their own need for service. They have found that the visitors come with the spirit of ambassadors of good will and that they have a pleasantly stimulating influence.

Through the international unit the ANA participates officially in the US Department of State's exchange-visitor program. Planning programs of study, observation, and work for nurses from other countries constitutes the major part of the activity of this busy unit which works in close cooperation with both the voluntary and federal agencies that have a similar or related programs. Although the international programs provide a "two-way street," the traffic toward the US is heavier than that away from it. A few American nurses have gone to other countries as students or lecturers under the Fulbright Act.

The base of the ANA's international relationships is constantly expanding. Miss Best was a participant in the first postwar meeting of the International Hospital Federation Congress in The Netherlands (1949). The organization has sent representatives to meetings of a number of other international organizations including that of the World Federation for Mental Health, Geneva (1949); the Congress of the Inter-American Commission of Women, Buenos Aires (1949); and the second Gerontological Congress in St. Louis (1951). Further discussion of international relationships will be found in Chapters 50 and 51.

This account of the evolution of American nursing ends with the history-making convention of 1952. The plan for restructuring the professional organizations had been arrived at after many months of arduous effort by the most democratic methods it had been possible to devise. The signals of two coordinated national nursing organizations and their constituent units, now representing more than 177,-

000 registered nurses, public health nursing services, hospital nurs- ing services, collegiate and hospital schools of nursing, and nursing specialties, have been set at "Go" for the advancement of nursing as a multiphase service to society and for improvement in the pro- fessional status of nurses. The new structure has a broad base which will support the increasingly comprehensive programs required by mid-century developments in the field of social welfare. It makes provision for active participation, in the planning and administra- tion of nursing services and nursing education, of practitioners of nursing as well as of teachers and administrators. It provides for the stimulation of nursing thought by that of non-nurses who are con- structively concerned with the provision of adequate nursing service for the American people. There are many encouraging evidences of the readiness of the constituent units of the two national organiza- tions to follow the green light into a future of expanding profes- sional growth and social usefulness. An abundance of hard work will be required of state and local groups in both organizations. In the ANA much of the burden of developing sections will fall on the state and district associations. However, most of the state associa- tions are well equipped for the task. The technically efficient ANA headquarters promptly released copies of the certificate of incorpo- ration and the revised bylaws to its constituent units and offered them consultation services. The NLN faced a much more com- plicated situation. The headquarters staffs of the NLNE and NOPHN (ACSN had no staff) and those of the joint projects and committees were combined in what seemed, to onlookers, like record time. Within a month of the convention the bylaws adopted at the convention and other informative materials were on their way to the state leagues and the state organizations for public health nursing which had already begun working on bylaws for the leagues. Unlike the state nurses' associations and some of their larger districts, neither the state and local leagues nor the state organizations for public health nursing had established head- quarters. Time, therefore, will be required to build up membership and to perfect and then decentralize the structure for which the foundation has been so painstakingly laid. In all program planning,

it would be necessary to keep in mind the importance of community relationships.

One of the most important contributions of NOPHN to the new structure, membership in the National Social Welfare Assembly and the National Health Council, two organizations concerned with the over-all social welfare and health needs of the nation, was transferred to the NLN. In the larger cities it will also be necessary for the new units of the NLN to come to some agreement about functions and programs with the nursing councils, each of which has been relatively independent of the nursing organizations. In the meantime the major elements in the programs of both national organizations are being carried forward with inspiring enthusiasm. "Cooperation" continues to be the key word and, as Professor Ashley Montagu told the first NLN audience on that June day in 1952, "cooperation, love, and security are one, and they motivate human behavior from birth." Shortly after the end of the war the AJN noted that: "The opportunities for nursing in the next decade transcend anything we have ever known. The extent to which they are realized will depend, in large measure, on the nursing profession itself. Is nursing, through its organizations, equipped for effective leadership in the new era?"[19] The answer is an exuberant, "Indeed it is!" In six crowded years of enlightened, forceful "composite leadership" the profession has made impressive progress toward new horizons of social usefulness.

BIBLIOGRAPHY

"AAIN for Two Organizations," *Am. J. Nursing*, **50**:756, 1950.
The American Nurses' Association 1896–1946—Tomorrows and Yesterdays, as told on the fiftieth anniversary of the association's founding. American Nurses' Association, New York, 1946.
"Change in the Structure Voted," *Am. J. Nursing*, **50**:390, 1950.
Educational Exchange Grants. Superintendent of Documents, US Government Printing Office, Washington, D.C., 1953.
Gardner, Mary S.: "Report of a Six-Months Study of the NOPHN," *Public Health Nurse*, **18**:374, 1926.

[19] *Am. J. Nursing*, **45**:985, 1945.

Haupt, Alma C.: "National Unity in Public Health Nursing," *Pub. Health Nursing*, **37**:3, 1945.

——: "The Structure Study; Facts and Fallacies," *Pub. Health Nursing*, **39**:345, 1947.

"History of the Structure Study," *American Nurses' Association Proceedings, Special Sessions, Advisory Council and House of Delegates*, 1947, pp. 108–30.

"Institute of International Education," *Thirty-third Annual Report*, New York, 1952, "Fulbright Program," p. 14.

"Joint Advisory Committee to Give Attention to the Joint Survey of the National Professional Nursing Organizations," *Pub. Health Nursing*, **36**:372, 1944.

"Let's Look at the League," *Am. J. Nursing*, **48**:246, 1948.

McIver, Pearl: "Report of Joint Co-ordinating Committee on Structure," *American Nurses' Association Proceedings*, Vol. I, House of Delegates, 1952, p. 84.

Melby, Elizabeth, et al.: "What Type of Organization Will Best Further Ideals and Standards in Schools of Nursing and Meet the Needs for Nursing Education in the Different States?" *Thirty-ninth Annual Report of the National League of Nursing Education*, 1933, pp. 98–114.

"New ANA Industrial Nurses Section," *Am. J. Nursing*, **46**:733, 1946.

"NOPHN Resolves," *Pub. Health Nursing*, **44**:421, 1952.

"Nurses Unite for Service" (editorial), *Am. J. Pub. Health*, **42**:993, 1952.

"Preface to Co-ordinated Action," *Am. J. Nursing*, **48**:10, 1948.

Proceedings of the Thirty-eighth Convention of the American Nurses' Association, Vol. I, House of Delegates, "International Interests," 1952, p. 69.

"Report of the ANA Special Committee to Consider the Possibility of Consolidation of Three National Nursing Organizations" (Mary Beard, chairman), *American Nurses' Association Proceedings, Special Sessions*, 1940.

"Report of Committee on Closer Union of Nursing Societies" (Mary E. Gladwin, chairman), *Fifteenth Annual Report, American Society of Superintendents of Training Schools for Nursing* (National League of Nursing Education), 1909, p. 26.

"Report of the Industrial Nurses' Section," *American Nurses' Association Proceedings*, Vol. I, House of Delegates, 1946, pp. 147–49.

"Report of the Industrial Nurses' Section," *American Nurses' Association Proceedings*, Vol. II, Advisory Council, 1948, pp. 641–96.

"Report of Joint Committee (ANA, NLNE, and NOPHN) on Self-analysis," *American Nurses' Association Proceedings*, 1926, p. 22.

"Report of Promoting Committee for Study of Structure of National

Professional Nursing Organizations," *American Nurses' Association Proceedings*, Vol. I, 1946, pp. 191–93.

"Report on the Structure of Organized Nursing, Raymond Rich Associates," *Am. J. Nursing*, 46:648, 1946.

Sargent, Emilie: "What It Means to Become a Charter Member in the National League for Nursing Through Your Membership in the NOPHN," *Pub. Health Nursing*, 44:307, 1952.

"The Six Organizations to Be Studied" (editorial), *Am. J. Nursing*, 46:279, 1946.

Sleeper, Ruth: "The Time Is Now," *Fiftieth Annual Report of the National League of Nursing Education*, 1944, p. 50.

Structure:

"Progress in Structure Planning," *Am. J. Nursing*, 51:80, 1951.

"The Two Organizations in the New Structure," *Am. J. Nursing*, 51:288, 1951.

"Your Place in the New Structure," *Am. J. Nursing*, 51:561, 1951.

"The ANA in the Proposed Structure," *Am. J. Nursing*, 51:594, 1951.

"The NLA in the Proposed Structure," *Am. J. Nursing*, 51:647, 1951.

"Special Interest Groups in the ANA and NLA," *Am. J. Nursing*, 51:731, 1951.

"Non-Nurses and Agencies in the NLA," *Am. J. Nursing*, 52:181, 1952.

"Answers to Some Questions about Structure," *Am. J. Nursing*, 52:313, 1952.

"Proposed Amendments to Certificate of Incorporation of the National League of Nursing Education," *Am. J. Nursing*, 52:463, 1952.

"Proposed Bylaws of the National League for Nursing," *Am. J. Nursing*, 52:463, 1952.

"Structure of National Organizations and the ICN," *Am. J. Nursing*, 49:635, 1949.

"Structure Program in 1950," *Am. J. Nursing*, 50:230, 1950.

"The Structure Study—A Look at the Records," *Pub. Health Nursing*, 38:441, 1946.

"A Tentative Plan for One National Nursing Organization," *Am. J. Nursing*, 48:321, 1948.

Thompson, Ella M.: "Should Qualified Practical Nurses be NLN Members?" *Am. J. Nursing*, 52:594, 1952.

Trading Ideas with the World. Report of the US Advisory Commission on Educational Exchange. US Government Printing Office, Washington, D.C., 1949.

"A Two-Organization Structure," *Am. J. Nursing*, 50:741, 1950.

Two-Way Street. Report of the US Advisory Commission on Educational Exchange. US Government Printing Office, Washington, D.C., 1950.

SECTION XI. HEALTH—A UNIFYING
WORLD FORCE

Chapter 50
NONGOVERNMENTAL ORGANIZATIONS—
AND WORLD HEALTH

Health is a state of complete physical, mental and social well-being and not merely the absence of disease or infirmity.

The enjoyment of the highest attainable standard of health is one of the fundamental rights of every human being without distinction of race, religion, political belief, economic or social conditions.

The health of all peoples is fundamental to the attainment of peace and security and is dependent upon the fullest co-operation of individuals and States.[1]

The stage of development of nursing varies greatly from culture to culture. It is limited by the stage of development of medicine and public health. It is interesting to note, however, that in countries where medicine is highly developed and nursing is not, the health status of the people does not reflect the advanced stage of medicine. Nursing is essential to the vitalization of the health program.[2]

THE FOUR MAJOR FORCES—Christianity, war, and the biological and social sciences—which have helped to make professional nursing an essential social service are nowhere more apparent than in the complex network of international governmental and nongovernmental health programs. The early service of missionary nurses, the foundation of many later efforts, has been discussed in earlier chapters. So, too, has the wartime and postwar civilian service of American nurses in Cuba and the Philippines following the Spanish-American

[1] From the constitution of the World Health Organization.
[2] Report on the first session, Expert Committee on Nursing, World Health Organization, Technical Report Series, #24, WHO. Geneva, 1951, p. 5.

War and in Europe and the Near East during and following World War I. Such services were increasingly conditioned by expanding social philosophies and by scientific advances in medicine, nutrition, and in sanitary and other measures for the control of communicable diseases. Although the rapid rise of the public health movement is one of the glories of the twentieth century, the goals established by the World Health Organization are still far distant. We are therefore concerned with the role of nurses in the international health movement and the relationship between nursing organizations and services and international health agencies.

The remarkable prescience of the founders of our national nursing organizations and of the ICN (Chap. 8) is revealed in the 1909 amendment to the preamble to the constitution of the International Council of Nurses.

We nurses, representing various nations of the world, sincerely believing that the profession of nursing will be advanced by greater unity of thought, sympathy and purpose, do hereby unite in a federation of associations to improve our work in the service of the sick, *to promote the health of the nations*, and to advance the best interests of our beloved profession.

The significance of the phrase which was inserted at that time and is here italicized lies in the fact that nursing had no relationship with the one and only international health organization then in existence. This was the Pan American Sanitary Bureau (PASB), established in 1902, which took on the functions of a regional office of the World Health Organization a half century later. Like it the International Office of Public Health, established in Paris in 1909 and ultimately absorbed in the health section of the League of Nations, was also concerned chiefly with quarantine.

The Rockefeller Sanitary Commission, forerunner of the International Health Division of the Rockefeller Foundation, which was to become one of the world's most influential agencies in the field of public health, and therefore in the promotion of nursing, began working toward the eradication of hookworm in the Southern states in 1909. By 1912 a flood tide of interest in public health nursing in the United States, stimulated in part by the foundation's interest in the development of county health units, was moving toward a crest which resulted in the formation of the National Organization for Public Health Nursing in that year.

By mid-century international health programs, according to authorities in that field, had entered the fourth phase of their development. The first had been the period of quarantine and sanitary measures. The organization of the Health Section of the League of Nations (1923) ushered in the second phase. However, between the wars, as the Health Section had no division of nursing, nursing was more directly influenced in the second phase by the Nursing Division of the League of Red Cross Societies (1919) and the Rockefeller Foundation. The US was not a member of the League of Nations nor did it officially recognize its very efficient Health Organization. In the interest of hemispheric development, the US organized the Institute of Inter-American Affairs in 1942. World War II interrupted all other international health programs. Public health services, including nursing, therefore became an important part of the program of the United Nations Relief and Rehabilitation Administration (1943–1947) which was organized to ameliorate the tragic plight of millions of refugees and displaced persons in liberated countries. Some parts of the program developed in this third phase of international health work were merged with the health programs of the fourth phase, namely those of the United Nations— the World Health Organization and the United Nations International Children's Emergency Fund (UNICEF), which were well developed by mid-century.

With this background we can now return to consideration of the ICN and the fundamental relationship of American nursing with it. The early history of the ICN has been summarized in Chapter 8, "Nursing Organizations Build for the Future." Its organization was essentially a part of the movement which had brought the ANA and NLNE into existence following the World's Fair in Chicago in 1893. Miss Nutting, writing of those who attended the last ICN Congress held before World War I darkened the world, said:

The permanent picture before me is of women of striking vigor, power and ability, of women of marked spiritual quality, of high souled courage and over and over again I am impressed by the similarity of our problems. We are really one in all of the things that really matter. . . .[3]

Such was the quality of the pioneers and of their followers who, by mid-century, had made the ICN the largest organization of professional women in the world and had brought it into official relationship with WHO (1948). Their accomplishment gains perspective, in a materialistic world, when it is noted that not until 1939 was the ICN able to ensure the attendance of even two officers at meetings by defraying their expenses.

The simple structure of the ICN was well planned. Its work is complicated by the universal need for improvement in means of communication between peoples of varied cultures and traditions. In nursing, as in all other human relationships, as the world grows smaller—transportation-wise—interrelationships become more complex. The ICN is a federation of national organizations of professional nurses, one to a country. In 1951 the ANA was one of 30 national organizations in active membership, and there were 16 associate members. The board of directors is made up of the usual elected officers plus the presidents of the member organizations. The voting body, the Grand Council, consists of the board of directors and four representatives of each member organization. Representatives of associate members (national organizations which are working toward membership) may attend meetings of the Grand Council but have no vote.

The ICN is maintained by per capita dues, equivalent to 8 pence in British currency, paid by the national organizations. Fluctuations in exchange complicate matters for the treasurers and for those who plan the budget! To date (1952), 12 cents per capita has been the maximum required of the ANA. Since approximately one-half of the world's nurses are in the US[4] and the ANA now has over 177,000 members, it is naturally the major source of support. However the percentage of nurses who contributed to the ICN, through membership in their national nursing organizations, is far higher in

[3] Report of Delegate to the Congress of the ICN, *19th Annual Report of NLNE*, 1913, p. 47.
[4] *Facts about Nursing*, 1951, ANA, p. 91.

some of the smaller countries such as Denmark. But the ICN's income from an aggregate membership of approximately 400,000 is seriously inadequate for the support of a fact-finding, standard-setting, and coordinating organization of world-wide scope and influence. This problem has been met, in part, by making the Florence Nightingale International Foundation (to be discussed later) a legal entity within the ICN. On the basis of its demonstrated competence, the FNIF can receive grants and provide services, based on signed agreements, for agencies concerned with determining the volume and quality of nursing service. It can, and should, receive grants for research.

A continuous program of work is carried forward by the headquarters staff under the direction of the executive secretary and by the committees. But, until recently, the ICN has been more widely known in the US for its quadrennial congresses than for its program. Meetings of the board of directors and the Grand Council are held in connection with the congresses and at such other times as they may be required. The organization has also held interim conferences in times of great nursing activity, as, for example, in Stockholm (1949). Three times the ICN has been invited to hold a congress in the US. Its first one was held in Buffalo (1901) in connection with the Pan-American Exposition. The one scheduled for San Francisco in 1915 in connection with the Pan-Pacific Exposition was canceled by the outbreak of World War 1; World War II blocked out plans for 1941. It was fitting, therefore, that this country, physically undamaged by the war, should be the hostess in 1947 with devoted Effie J. Taylor, former dean of the Yale School of Nursing, who had been elected president in London in 1937 and who had kept alive the flame of interest throughout the war, as the presiding officer.

Five congresses and two interim conferences had been held since World War I. Heroic little Finland, entertaining its first international gathering in 1925 with Baroness Mannerheim, a graduate of the Nightingale School in London, presiding, set a standard of hospitality that is still a challenge to hostess organizations. The facts, previously unknown to many citizens of the US that Finland's standard of literacy was higher than our own and that Finnish nurses had achieved an enviable professional status, were both enlightening and stimulating. The opportunity to savor the culture of other countries enhances enormously the interest of nurses in the congresses.

The Canadian Nurses' Association, of which Mabel F. Hersey of the Royal Victoria Hospital (Montreal) was president, was hostess to the Montreal congress in 1929, but the presiding officer was an American, Nina D. Gage, who had been elected president when the Nurses' Association of China had anticipated that privilege and Miss Gage had been its president. The report of a study of public health nursing in the member countries, presented by Mary S. Gardner, chairman of the Committee on Public Health Nursing, was an important contribution to the program. A communication from Miss Nutting, who had retired from active participation in nursing affairs, set in motion an important train of events. She reminded Miss Gage and other officers that the recommendation that an educational memorial to Miss Nightingale be founded in the country where she had done her greatest work had been acclaimed with enthusiasm at the Cologne congress in 1912 but that nothing had yet been done about it. Mrs. Bedford Fenwick, who, with Miss Nutting as co-sponsor, had made that recommendation, was appointed chairman of a committee to consider the matter with results which will be considered shortly.

The attendance at Montreal had been so overwhelming that the nursing associations of France and Belgium combined forces to entertain the 1933 congress in Paris and Brussels when Mlle. Chaptal of France was president. Mrs. Karin Neuman-Rahn of Finland presented a superb report from the Committee on Mental Hygiene and Mental Nursing of which she was chairman. The first of a series of recommendations, well in advance of developments in this country, emphasized the need for making the inclusion of mental nursing in the basic program a compulsory requirement.[5] At this meeting Hazel A. Goff presented the report of a study of public health nursing in ten nonindustrial European countries. The study had been

[5] *Proceedings,* ANA, 1938, p. 387.

made under the auspices of the League of Nations by means of a special grant made available through the ICN.[6]

Alicia Lloyd-Still (later Dame Alicia), matron of famous St. Thomas's Hospital, was the president of the hostess organization when (1937) the nurses of the world converged by the thousands on London, the cradle of modern nursing. Enthusiastically immersed in the forward march of the profession, and with little awareness of the rising tide of political discord in various parts of the world, that congress adjourned with Dame Alicia's prophetic watchword *"loyalty"* ringing in their ears. Loyal to nursing and its compassionate function they certainly were through years of horror caused by international jealousies and conflicting national loyalties. Ten years were to elapse before they met again, like free spirits united by the durable bonds of a common aspiration, in Atlantic City. The United Nations had come into being only two years earlier. A session on World Organization in the Fields of Health, Education, and Science was the outstanding feature of that congress.[7] It provided an exciting backdrop against which to project plans for the development of nursing in the fourth phase of the international health movement. At this time the Grand Council and the board of directors came to grips with (1) certain problems of administration which were pointed out in a special study expertly made, on request, by Mrs. Alma H. Scott, executive secretary of the ANA, and (2) with problems connected with the postgraduate education of nurses which will be discussed in connection with the nursing section of the League of Red Cross Societies.

One of the early aspirations of the ICN had been brought to fruition between the wars. This was the preparation of an educational program which might be used as a guide by nursing schools,

[6] Goff, Hazel Avis: "Report of a Study of Public Health Nursing in Europe," *The International Nursing Review*, Vol. IX, Nos. 1–4, 1934, p. 31.

[7] *Proceedings*, 9th Congress, ICN, Atlantic City, N.J., 1947, p. 35. Speakers: Harold E. Snyder, United Nations Educational, Scientific and Cultural Organization (UNESCO), director, Commission on International Education Reconstruction; Aake Ording, United Nations director, United Nations One Day's Pay Plan (for the rehabilitation of children); Wilbur A. Sawyer, director of health, United Nations Relief and Rehabilitation Administration.

especially in countries in which modern nursing was still in its infancy. *The Educational Programme of the School of Nursing*, prepared by Isabel M. Stewart, was first published in 1934. Its adoption by the nursing division of the League of Red Cross Societies added to its prestige and greatly extended its usefulness. An amended edition was published four years later and a revised edition under a new title,[8] after World War II, when postgraduate (postdiploma) education and advanced nursing education were sharing the limelight with basic nursing education in many countries. Miss Stewart, who had succeeded Miss Nutting as chairman of the Committee on Education, had performed a monumental service for the ICN almost concurrently with a comparable service which resulted in the *Curriculum Guide* of the NLNE. The members of her committee, which began work during the Helsinki congress, represented a cross section of the varied experiences and educational philosophies of the world's nurse educators. A preliminary draft of a report, discussed at Montreal four years later, was subsequently published in seven languages and distributed for critical analysis by nurses in all countries having nursing schools. By this time nursing surveys were being made in Canada and other countries as well as in the US. A mass of material, therefore, required analysis before a final report could be written. A gratifying demand for the successive editions was considered adequate recompense by those who had contributed almost unbelievable amounts of time and effort to that project.

The vitality of the ICN seemed to be at a low ebb following World War I. The organization of the Nursing Division of the League of Red Cross Societies (1920), to be discussed later, appears to have had a stimulating effect on it. Ten years had elapsed between meetings of the board of directors when the board was convened in Copenhagen (1922) with Mrs. Henny Tscherning of Denmark (who had succeeded Miss Goodrich) as the presiding officer. To their delighted surprise those present found that the unity of purpose of the member organizations had not been impaired by either the war or the gap in time. A Grand Council meeting

[8] *The Basic Education of the Professional Nurse*. The ICN, 19 Queens Gate, London, S.W., 7, England, 1949.

and an interim conference were held in the same city the following year.

Miss Dock, who, as secretary, had been a power behind the throne from the inception of the ICN, resigned in 1922. (Concurrently she resigned the post of editor of the *AJN*'s Foreign Department. An ardent pacifist, she had "boycotted the war" in that department!) Christiane Reimann, a scholarly and financially independent Danish nurse, was appointed to succeed her. Not, however, until after the highly successful Helsinki congress was an office established in Geneva with Miss Reimann in charge. The first major project undertaken was the publication of a magazine in the three official languages of the ICN—English, French, and German. *The ICN*, later renamed *The International Nursing Review*, published from June, 1926, to December, 1939, (with an interregnum of some months) became a valuable compendium of international information. In addition to material from authoritative sources in many countries, it published committee reports and the results of studies. It stimulated interest in nursing education. In countries where nursing was young, it aroused the interest of nurses in the ICN and in the development of national associations as a preliminary to affiliation with it. But the magazine did not secure the circulation that its merits warranted. Financial difficulties resulted in its suspension for a few months in 1935 and the removal of the headquarters from Geneva to London. The move facilitated business transactions as the position of treasurer of the ICN has traditionally been held by a British nurse. Also the London office was thought to be more readily available to international visitors. Miss Reimann resigned in order to live on the continent and was succeeded by Princess Anna Schwarzenberg, an accomplished linguist and a graduate of the Rudolfinerhaus, Austria's pioneer school of nursing. She was also an "Old International" (see p. 609) and, like Miss Reimann, had done postgraduate work in the US. Publication of the magazine, on a quarterly basis, was resumed.

When the board of directors met in London in the summer of 1937, with the president, Effie J. Taylor, presiding, there were many evidences of political discord throughout the world. The Congress of the US, for example, had just passed a Neutrality Act "to keep us out of war." But the secretary of the ICN was authorized to accept invitations to meet with nursing organizations in South Africa and India. The cataclysmic invasion of Poland in September, 1939, set off the train of events which plunged mankind into World War II. The secretary was recalled from South Africa. The leading editorial of the December issue of *The International Nursing Review* tells the story:

The outbreak of war ends abruptly many of the activities of the ICN, among them the publication of *The International Nursing Review* which ceases to appear for an indefinite period—the Council is leaving London for a neutral country.

Miss Schwarzenberg was given an indefinite leave of absence and Calista Banwarth (Salmon), an "Old International" and the American member of the staff, accepted responsibility for transporting the council's most valuable records to the US. Working with Miss Taylor in New Haven, she helped her to keep open all possible channels of communication with nurses of other countries. In 1944 Miss Schwarzenberg was recalled, and a small office was established in New York in anticipation of the termination of the war. Publication of the *International Nursing Bulletin*,[9] to replace the more ambitious magazine of prewar years, was begun as soon as possible after V-J Day, the first issue appearing in October, 1945. Published quarterly, this inexpensive bulletin is limited in scope but it provides the member organizations and their publications with basic information about the increasingly ramified activities of the ICN.

The *Bulletin* effectively stimulated interest in the Atlantic City congress. The proximity of the ICN office to that of the ANA at that time facilitated coordinated planning. Canadian and American donors, including the ARC, the Rockefeller Foundation, and many nurses and nursing organizations, contributed to a travel fund for representatives of national organizations who would otherwise not have been able to attend. Local groups on the Atlantic seaboard made themselves responsible for hospitality. All told, 40 nationalities

[9] *International Nursing Bulletin*. The ICN, 19 Queens Gate, London, S.W., 7, England.

were represented. Many of those nurses had been in military service, some had been imprisoned, a considerable number knew war at its uttermost bestial worst. The congress, fully described elsewhere,[10] revivified the spirits of nurses depressed by their war experiences. It was a truly inspiring experience for the nurses of the hostess country. Regardless of all other loyalties, fidelity to the finest traditions of nursing transcended all other emotions in that great gathering. The joy in reunion of nurses of many tongues was an unforgettable experience.

Energetic and liberal-minded Gerda Höjer, of Sweden, was elected president at Atlantic City. Plans for a meeting of the Grand Council and an interim conference in Stockholm were quickly under way. Nurses everywhere were looking for guidance in the confused state of the postwar world. Ruth Sleeper became chairman of the Education Committee[11] which, at Stockholm, presented educational standards for the use of the Committee on Membership in determining the eligibility of a national organization for membership in the ICN. The first criterion is that the school, or schools, in a country desirous of membership shall be accredited by an official agency or by the educational section of the national nursing organization. The committee also set up minimum standards for use in countries where basic programs are being established. The major issue at Stockholm, however, was consideration of a report on the relationships and functions of the ICN and the Florence Nightingale International Foundation. This takes us back to 1919 and the organization of the League of Red Cross Societies (LORCS).

The extensive activities of the ARC in Europe during and following World War I have been discussed in earlier chapters. They seemed to indicate that Red Cross societies could develop useful peacetime programs. The League of Red Cross Societies was planned at a conference of representatives of national Red Cross societies at Cannes, France (1919). The meeting was attended by Lillian D. Wald and by several American nurses then in postwar ARC administrative positions in Europe, and by nursing representa-

---

[10] "Forty Nations—and One World," *Am. J. Nursing*, **47**:438, 1947.
[11] "The ICN and Nursing Education," *Am. J. Nursing*, **50**:385, 1950.

tives of other national societies. Miss Delano, whose presence had
been anticipated, was then suffering her last illness at Savenay,
France. Dr. William H. Welch, always a staunch advocate of public
health nursing, gave impressive support to a recommendation for a
department of public health nursing under the direction of a professional nurse. The LORCS was established in Geneva the following
year. The new organization carefully avoided infringing on the
status and functions of the International Red Cross Committee
(inspired by Henri Dunant and established in Geneva in 1863)
which is concerned with such matters as the status of the Red Cross
societies in relation to the Geneva conventions and such neutral
activities as the care of prisoners of war. The LORCS was animated
by a driving altruism inspired by the tragic plight of millions of persons in the war-torn countries, and, as Kernodle points out, "circumstances made the association of nursing service with European
countries more lasting than that of other [ARC] services."[12] A
division of nursing was made an integral part of the new LORCS.
Alice L. Fitzgerald, with European background and American
training, who had effectively coordinated the service of ARC nurses
with France's Service de Santé, became director. Some of the Red
Cross societies were strongly in favor of volunteer amateur nursing
for war service whereas the ARC nursing service, to which Miss
Fitzgerald belonged, and the ICN were making determined efforts
to ensure the status of the "trained" or professional nurse. There
was therefore considerable friction between the groups on the subject of nursing education. But, as we have seen, there was urgent
need for a substantial development of public health nursing in
many European countries. Miss Fitzgerald secured authority and
funds for the establishment of a course in public health nursing at
Kings College for Women of the University of London (1920–1921),
which was transferred to Bedford College the following year. A
course for training nurse administrators and teachers in schools of
nursing was added in 1924. Scholarships were provided by the
LORCS, and the National Red Cross societies were encouraged to

[12] Kernodle, Portia B., *The Red Cross Nurse in Action, 1882–1948.* Harper
& Brothers, New York, 1949, p. 180.

do likewise. Enrollment was limited by the capacity (20) of the residence provided at 15 Manchester Square. Miss Fitzgerald was succeeded by her assistant, Katherine Olmstead, at the end of the first year, and she in turn by a British Red Cross nurse, Mrs. Maynard Carter, in 1927.

By 1933, the courses had attracted over 200 nurses from 41 countries. Their professional, social, and cultural backgrounds varied enormously. Courses which required the most concentrated effort on the part of some of the participants seemed elementary to others. But they provided a means of communication between nurses of many nations and fulfilled a major objective of the LORCS, especially in relation to some of the European countries. A considerable number of the "Old Internationals" (as they became known after 1925 when the alumnae organized under that title) became leaders in pioneer nursing situations. Also, the international courses had been the means of encouraging some of the National Red Cross societies to take an active interest in the development of professional nursing. The LORCS was about to discontinue the program at just the time Mrs. Bedford Fenwick and her committee began their efforts to implement the ICN's reactivated interest in a memorial to Miss Nightingale. As an initial step, the committee secured approval of the following statement from the board of directors of the ICN:

That the Foundation should be in London, that it should be of an international character, and a living memorial, not a museum. The suggestion which appeals most to the directors . . . is that the memorial should take the form of an endowed foundation for postgraduate nursing education.[13]

Acceptance of the LORCS courses as the first step toward a more substantial educational program seemed logical to persons not familiar with the trend toward advanced nursing education (as contrasted with postdiploma or postcertificate programs) in a number of countries. It is not surprising that there was not complete unanimity about the proposal to accept the LORCS courses as the nucleus of a program for the memorial foundation.

The fact that the ICN did not take over full responsibility for the development of the foundation later became the source of consider-

[13] Minutes, Board of Directors, ICN, Paris, 1933.

able confusion. The wisdom of a "marriage" or partnership between such unlike organizations as the strictly professional ICN and the broadly humanitarian LORCS with its emphasis on volunteer service had not been very adequately debated by the units of the participating organizations when, on July 5, 1934, in London, the Florence Nightingale International Foundation was brought into being. Of the ten stated objectives of the foundation, the more important are as follows:

(1) To establish and maintain a permanent International Memorial to Florence Nightingale in the form of an endowed trust for post-graduate nursing education either in continuation of the post-graduate courses for nurses hitherto organized by the League of Red Cross Societies and conducted in conjunction with the College of Nursing[14] by Bedford College for Women (University of London) or otherwise. (2) The maintenance and development of facilities for post-graduate education for selected nurses from all countries.[15]

The complex structure of the FNIF established it as a second international organization without a' clear line of demarcation between its functions and those of the sponsoring ICN. The governing body was a grand council composed of five representatives of each of the parent bodies (the ICN and the LORCS) and two representatives of each of the national Florence Nightingale Memorial Committees contributing to the foundation. Executive powers were delegated to the Committee on Management. In addition to the ICN and the LORCS, the British Red Cross and the British Council of Nurses were represented on the Committee on Management. This, in addition to the participation of the College of Nursing in the program, caused some nurses to feel that both structure and program were British rather than international. The LORCS gave a long-term lease and the furnishings of the pleasant residence at 15 Manchester Square to the FNIF. It was generally considered a costly program and credit should be given the British Red Cross for generously making up such deficits as occurred. Olive Baggallay, a grad-

[14] The College of Nursing (since 1939 the Royal College of Nursing) is a membership organization which offers educational programs in a broad range of nursing subjects.

[15] The Florence Nightingale International Foundation Constitution and By-Laws.

uate of the Nightingale school at St. Thomas's (later the first chief of the Nursing Section of WHO), was appointed secretary, i.e., administrator, of the FNIF. Nan L. Dorsey, a former director of the Public Health Nursing Association of Pittsburgh and an early graduate of the LORCS course, continued to serve as warden or house mother at Manchester Square.

National committees were supposed to be made up of representatives of the national nursing organization and of the National Red Cross society, the committees reporting directly to the FNIF. Their primary function was considered to be the procurement of endowment and scholarship funds and selection of applicants. Many national nursing organizations found this a confusing and ineffective arrangement. It was never formally accepted by the ARC although representatives of that body gave generous assistance in the early years of the program. In practice, the American committee functioned as a special committee of the ANA. To secure an endowment, an immediate goal of £50,000 (then approximately $250,000), and an ultimate goal of four times that was established. Quotas were allocated to the national committees on the basis of membership in the representative national nursing organizations. Fund-raising efforts were based on belief in the importance of international cooperation. The House of Delegates of the ANA (1938) voted unanimously to accept the quota of $88,575 allocated to the United States. The amount was reallocated to the state associations on the basis of their respective memberships. A few were unresponsive. Most of them responded as nurses almost invariably do to an accepted and specifically stated professional objective. A considerable number of states had completed their quotas when the war interrupted all such activities. All but five states have now (1952) reached and many have exceeded their quotas. The ANA has received over $76,000 of the national quota and has forwarded $50,000 to the FNIF. It is anticipated that means to complete the quota will be available before the 1953 congress in Brazil.

When the courses were necessarily discontinued in the autumn of 1939, the nurses who had completed one-year courses under the aegis of the FNIF raised the number of "Old Internationals," including some half dozen nurses from the US, to over 300. Some of the "Old Internationals" have made, or are making, important contributions to the development of nursing within the international community of nations. The house on Manchester Square was destroyed by bombs. But the FNIF was kept alive! Between 1944 and 1947, provision was made for 24 nurses to study under FNIF auspices in five countries—Canada, England, New Zealand, Sweden, and the US, scholarships having been provided, through the LORCS, by a few of the Red Cross societies.

The period between the wars had been one of rapid change in many countries. Where nursing was well established there was a growing interest in postcertificate work and in the development of both basic and advanced university programs. In the US, as we have seen, the period was characterized by the rise of collegiate schools and the organization of the Association of Collegiate Schools of Nursing. Notable progress was being made in a number of other countries. Acting on the principle that the FNIF courses provided little more than a focal point for a larger development, a committee was appointed to study the facilities in London for advanced nursing education and to give consideration to the future development of the foundation. The Rockefeller Foundation, then actively promoting the development of nursing in Europe, made it possible for Miss Goodrich (honorary president of the ICN and a vice-president of the FNIF) and Miss Baggallay to visit nursing centers in 10 European countries. Miss Goodrich became enthusiastic about the potentialities of the FNIF. The Rockefeller Foundation provided a fellowship for Daisy C. Bridges (now executive secretary of the ICN), a distinguished graduate of St. Thomas's, who studied at the University of Toronto and visited universities in the United States in preparation for a position as instructor in the FNIF program. War intervened before proposed changes could be effected.

The prompt development, after World War II, of the World Health Organization clearly indicated need for a clarification of international nursing policies and programs. Intellectual and emotional opinions about the FNIF varied widely in that period of rapidly accelerating professional and social change. An objective study was indicated, and the foundation was fortunate in securing the services of experts.[16] Their report is remarkable for its perceptive interpretation of the nuances of nursing thought and for the convincing logic of its recommendations. These are too detailed for inclusion here, but the first and the concluding sentences merit quotation:

(1) The emergence of the World Health Organization as a coordinating agency for all health services makes it imperative that the International Council of Nurses be strengthened, united, and representative of all countries of the world, in order to promote the best interests of professional nursing throughout the world. . . . A memorial created within the framework of the International Council of Nurses could stimulate that organization to give to nurses such leadership as Florence Nightingale gave in her own day. Thus the memorial, by service to the profession, would honor the name and perpetuate the work of the greatest of nursing leaders.

The results of the two studies requested by the ICN were coordinated by a joint planning committee. Some of the administrative changes recommended in Mrs. Scott's report were effected. At Stockholm (1949) the FNIF, firmly established as an endowed trust, became a legal entity within the ICN. It retains its trust deed and its trust funds. The endowment fund, in 1948, was £26,458— far short of the £50,000 anticipated as a first goal in 1934. The board of directors of the ICN functions as the board of the FNIF which also has a council of not less than seven or more than nine members. It is specified that one member of the council shall represent the LORCS and that two shall be chosen for their competence to direct educational activities. Some of the world's most eminent nurses were appointed to the first council. They were Kathleen Russell, formerly director, school of nursing, University of Toronto; Mrs. R. Louise McManus, director, Division of Nursing Education, Teachers College, New York; Mary I. Lambie, formerly director, Division of Nursing, Department of Health, New Zealand; Venny Snellman, director of nursing education, Depart-

---

[16] Hamley, H. R., and Uprichard, Muriel: *A Study of the Florence Nightingale International Foundation.* Welbecson Press, Ltd., London, 1948.

ment of Health, Helsinki, Finland; Marjorie Duvillard, director, Bon Secours School of Nursing, Geneva, Switzerland; Yvonne Hentsch, chief, Nursing and Social Service Bureau, LORCS, Geneva. Ellen J. Broe, formerly educational director, Graduate School, Aarhus University, Aarhus, Denmark, who has had unusually broad experience and opportunity for study in a number of countries, was appointed director of the FNIF. In general, the FNIF is responsible for the long-term educational activities of the ICN. Its principal objectives are "to promote research, to create a center of information on educational activities, to establish and stimulate the award of scholarships and to develop a section of the library of the ICN devoted specifically to Florence Nightingale."[17] The first major project undertaken by the FNIF, functioning within the framework of the ICN, is a study of advanced programs in nursing education which was requested by WHO and based on signed agreements between the two organizations.

A further word about the Red Cross and its influence on professional nursing. Variations have been due to the culture, and the position of the Red Cross itself, in the various countries. The stalwart support of professional nursing standards by the ARC in the teens and twenties has been recorded in earlier chapters. As Miss Hentsch pointed out at the Atlantic City congress of the ICN, the Red Cross in some countries has pioneered in establishing schools for professional nurses. In some it has pioneered in establishing public health nursing service. But Dunant's original purpose, at a time when there were no professional nurses, was to provide volunteers for service in time of war or emergency. Nonprofessional persons who were prepared for such service were often excellent organizers who were accustomed to positions of leadership. It is not unnatural that, in some countries, they reluctantly relinquished leadership to professional nurses. But the trend was everywhere toward the development of leadership by professional nurses with recognition, at mid-century, that the preparation of volunteer nurses' aides and

---

[17] "Reorganization of the Florence Nightingale International Foundation within the International Council of Nurses," *The International Nursing Bulletin*, Vol. VIII, #3, Autumn issue, 1952.

other auxiliary workers and their integration in nursing services are extremely important functions of professional nurses for which they require special preparation.

The ICN has long had representation on the advisory committee of the nursing service of the LORCS. As previously stated, the FNIF, functioning within the ICN, has a representative of the LORCS on its advisory council.

The relationship of foundations to the development of nursing may appropriately be considered in this chapter on nongovernmental agencies. The influence of the Rockefeller Foundation, since its organization in 1913, has been described by some experts in the field of health as comparable to that of the official international health organizations and by others as the pilot which showed them the way. The broad term "international health" came into the American language with the organization of the International Health Commission (now the International Health Division) of the Rockefeller Foundation. Since 1942, the W. K. Kellogg Foundation (organized in 1930) has also had an increasingly important influence on nursing outside the United States. The purpose of the Rockefeller Foundation, "the Welfare of Mankind Throughout the World," appears on its seal. The fundamental relationship of health to welfare accounts for the foundation's pervasive influence on nursing. A number of references have already been made to the foundation's relation to the development of nursing in the US. They are summarized here as a preface to a consideration of its international contribution to the advancement of nursing. The foundation's first contribution to American nursing, it will be recalled, was financial assistance to the infant NOPHN (1914). The foundation, in a determined effort to place responsibility for health and sanitation on government agencies, was then promoting the development of county health units for which public health nurses would be needed. Through this and other agencies the seeds of public health nursing service in official agencies were being sown. The NOPHN was the logical organization to develop standards.

It was to answer the need for better preparation of nurses for participation in public health programs that the foundation initiated the Winslow-Goldmark study.[18] Conclusions based on that study may be found in Appendix II. That history-making volume not only charted a course for nursing in the US; it stimulated analytical study of nursing in other countries. Plans for the experiment at Yale were in the making before the book came off the press! That school's success (Chap. 19) caused the foundation to give endowment aid to two other university schools and developmental assistance to a number of others.[19] Fellowships were provided to enrich the preparation of faculty members. The General Education Board of the foundation, which is interested in the education of Negroes, has given financial assistance to the schools at Meharry Medical College, the Division of Nursing at Dillard University, the School of Nursing Education at the Florida Agricultural and Mechanical College, and St. Philip Hospital School of Nursing in Richmond.

The foundation contributed to the Grading Committee, the National Nursing Council for War Service, and, more recently, to the Committee on the Improvement of Nursing Services. The foundation's interest in nursing in other countries, always incidental to larger social programs, began in China only a little later than in the United States. The nursing school, established (1920) as a division of the Peiping Union Medical College, ranked with the best American collegiate schools. The foundation had previously made it possible for the well-established Nurses' Association of China to have nursing textbooks translated. In the Far East assistance was also given to the St. Luke's Hospital School in Tokyo, the school at the Chulalongkorn University in Siam, and some assistance was given in the Philippines where a college of nursing is now in operation at the Philippine University. In the South Pacific the foundation has given fellowships and travel grants to nurses in the Fiji Islands, New Zealand, and Australia. The Ana Nery School in Rio de Janeiro (1921), Brazil's pioneer school, was established to help meet the

[18] *Nursing and Nursing Education in the United States.* Report of the Committee for the Study of Nursing Education (C.-E. A. Winslow, chairman) and Report of a Survey by Josephine Goldmark, secretary. The Macmillan Company, New York, 1923.

[19] The Vanderbilt and the University of Toronto schools were endowed; and the schools at Skidmore College, Western Reserve University, Peabody College, and the University of Washington were among those that received assistance.

nation's recognized need for public health nursing. This was followed by assistance to the Edith Cavell School and the University School of Nursing at St. Pierre Hospital, Brussels. Later the foundation helped to establish schools in three other South American countries and gave developmental aid to two more. Here, as elsewhere, fellowships have been provided for the preparation of nurses for teaching and administrative positions.

In Europe, F. Elisabeth Crowell's expert work with the Commission on Tuberculosis (1917–1922) was followed by her appointment to the staff of the Paris office of the foundation. From that time until her retirement in 1940, nursing programs were developed in cooperation with national governments in accordance with a basic policy of the foundation. During her tenure modern schools were aided in nine European countries. This included the construction of school and residence buildings. Mary Beard, a member of the committee which was responsible for the Goldmark report, directed the foundation's nursing program from the New York office from 1924 to 1938. She was succeeded by Mary Elizabeth Tennant, the present director of the program, who had joined Miss Crowell in Paris in 1928 and had been transferred to the New York office six years later. The governments, educational institutions, and nurses of many countries have sought council of these nurse-statesmen who have been assisted by a number of other highly qualified nurses.

Since World War II, assistance has been given to six established schools, some of them for work in advanced nursing education. Health centers—rural and urban—were established, and 200 European nurses received scholarships (or fellowships). By 1950 the foundation had helped nursing to acquire better resources and higher standards in 5 countries in Asia, 14 in Europe, and 10 in the Americas (including Canada and the United States). In India, where there is desperate need for teachers as well as for public health nurses, the foundation has had a nurse adviser since 1944. It is of interest that, in this enormous and thickly populated country, there are now two collegiate centers of nursing education. The College of Nursing of Delhi University has been assisted by the Rockefeller

Foundation. Students at a school established at Vellore under American missionary auspices early in the century may now choose between a three- and a four-year program, the latter leading to a B.S. degree, with a major in nursing, from the University of Madras.[20]

Many American nurses have participated in programs in other countries which have had assistance from the foundation but only, as in the case of the PUMC School in China, the first of its international nursing education projects, until indigenous nurses can be prepared to take leadership. But it may be that the foundation's pervasive international influence is chiefly due to the continuing fellowship program which was started in the twenties. By means of it, carefully selected nurses of many nationalities have been sent to universities and nursing centers for study and observation. The exchange of ideas and the interest in research which is stimulated by such experiences have had an exceedingly potent influence on nursing thought and educational practice. This influence has been felt not only in the countries of origin and in the countries visited but in the national and international nursing organizations.

The Kellogg Foundation restricts its programs to three areas—medicine, hospital administration, and nursing in the Americas. It works cooperatively with governmental agencies and foundations having similar interests. It is chiefly concerned with the strengthening of professional schools. Mildred L. Tuttle, director of the division has been alert to opportunities for promoting nursing education. The foundation's contributions to nursing in the US have been mentioned frequently. It may, however, be recalled that immediately after World War II this foundation made three-year grants to 11 universities, two in Canada and the remainder in the US, to help them expedite postwar adjustments and to improve the teaching of clinical nursing. It is currently (1952) giving assistance to 14 American universities for work in the administration of nursing services.

Since 1942 the Kellogg Foundation has provided fellowships for

[20] Culver, Elsie Thomas: "A Nursing School in South India," *Am. J. Nursing,* **50:**172, 1950.

91 Latin American nurses and for 71 Canadians for study in Canada or the United States. The earlier ones were chiefly for preparation for teaching basic sciences, nursing arts, or the clinical specialities. The trend now is toward preparation for the administration of nursing education or of nursing service. Ten schools in South America and one in Haiti are now (1952) receiving assistance. Four are in Brazil, one in Uruguay, one in Colombia, and one in Chile. Both foundations work cooperatively with national governments and with the official international health agencies which are discussed in the following chapter.

BIBLIOGRAPHY

Forman, Douglas N., and Dodd, Edward M.: "The Nurse in Mission Work," *Am. J. Nursing*, **51**:307, 1951.

Fosdick, Raymond B.: *The Rockefeller Foundation—A Review for 1947.* The Rockefeller Foundation, New York, 1947.

———: *The Story of the Rockefeller Foundation.* Harper & Brothers, New York, 1952.

Maxcy, Kenneth F. (ed.): *Rosenau's Preventive Medicine and Hygiene,* Sec. IX, "Public Health Organization and Activities." Appleton-Century-Crofts, Inc., New York, 1951.

Sawyer, Wilbur A.: "Nursing and World Organization in the Fields of Health, Education and Science," *Proceedings of the Ninth Congress of the International Council of Nurses,* 1947, p. 43.

Winslow, C.-E. A.: "International Cooperation in the Service of Health," *Ann. Am. Acad. Polit. & Soc. Sc.,* **273**:191, 1951.

Florence Nightingale International Foundation:

Åberg, Elsa: "The 'Old Internationals,'" *Am. J. Nursing*, **39**:480, 1939.

Broe, Ellen; "The Educational Division of the International Council of Nurses (Florence Nightingale International Foundation)," *Internat. Nursing Bull.*, **8**:10, 1952.

Constitution and Bylaws. Florence Nightingale International Foundation, London, England, 1934.

Dunbar, Virginia: "Internationalists in the Making," *Am. J. Nursing,* **36**:433, 1936.

The Florence Nightingale International Foundation (pamphlet). Florence Nightingale International Foundation, London, England, 1935.

"The Florence Nightingale International Foundation," *Am. J. Nursing*, **36**:1001, 1936.

"The Florence Nightingale International Foundation Inaugurated," *Am. J. Nursing*, **34**:786, 1934.

"The FNIF Council Meets," *Am. J. Nursing*, **50**:381, 1950.

"FNIF Affiliates with the ICN," *Am. J. Nursing*, **49**:490, 1949.

Hamley, H. R., and Uprichard, Muriel: *A Study of the Florence Nightingale International Foundation*. Welbecson Press, Ltd., London, 1948.

"Report of the ANA Committee on the Florence Nightingale Foundation" (statement of quota contributions from state nurses' associations), *American Nurses' Association Proceedings*, House of Delegates, 1950, p. 123.

"Report of ANA Committee on the Florence Nightingale International Foundation," *American Nurses' Association Proceedings, Advisory Council Reports*, 1944, pp. 54–58.

"The Stockholm Conference," *Am. J. Nursing*, **49**:487, 1949.

The International Council of Nurses:

The Basic Education of the Professional Nurse. The International Council of Nurses, London, England, 1949.

Breay, Margaret, and Fenwick, Ethel Gordon: *The History of the ICN, 1899–1925*. The International Council of Nurses, Geneva, Switzerland, 1931.

Bridges, Daisy C.: "Events in the History of the International Council of Nurses," *Am. J. Nursing*, **49**:594, 1949.

"Forty Nations and One World," *Am. J. Nursing*, **47**:437, 1947.

"The ICN and Nursing Education," *Am. J. Nursing*, **50**:385, 1950.

Johns, Ethel: "The ICN's Responsibility for International Education of Nurses," *Internat. Nursing Bull.*, **7**:20, 1951.

"Report of the Committee on Public Health Nursing, ICN" (Mary S. Gardner, chairman), *Pub. Health Nursing*, **21**:540, 1929.

"Report of Executive Secretary to the Board of Directors, Brussels, August, 1951" (including the FNIF), *Internat. Nursing Bull.*, **7**:3, 1951.

Scher, Alice C.: "Report on the Work of the International Nurses' Screening Board," *Internat. Nursing Bull.*, **7**:6, 1951.

Schwarzenberg, Anna: "Activities and Programs of the ICN," *Am. J. Nursing*, **45**:718, 1945.

Seymer, Lucy Ridgely: "Nurses' Organizations," *A General History of Nursing*, 2nd ed. The Macmillan Company, New York, 1949, Chap. XVI.

"The Stockholm Conference," *Am. J. Nursing*, **49**:487, 1949.

"Structure of National Organizations and the International Council of Nurses," *Am. J. Nursing,* **49**:635, 1949.

Taylor, Effie J.: "The International Council of Nurses," *Am. J. Nursing,* **50**:615, 1950.

————: "The International Council of Nurses," *American Nurses' Association Proceedings, Special Sessions,* 1947–1948, p. 34.

"What the International Council of Nurses Does," *Am. J. Nursing,* **49**:131, 1949.

The League of Red Cross Societies:

Carter, Maynard L.: "International Courses at Bedford College, University of London," *The ICN,* **3**:25, 1928.

Dulles, Foster Rhea: *The American Red Cross, A History.* Harper & Brothers, New York, 1950.

Fox, Elizabeth G.: "The Nursing Service of the League of Red Cross Societies," *Thirtieth Annual Report of the National League of Nursing Education,* 1924, p. 208.

Hentsch, Yvonne: "Influence of the Red Cross on Professional Nursing," *Information Bulletin for Red Cross Nurses,* Geneva, May–August, 1947. Also in *Proceedings, 9th Congress, International Council of Nurses,* Atlantic City, 1947.

Kernodle, Portia B.: *The Red Cross in Action, 1882–1948.* Harper & Brothers, New York, 1949.

"Recommendations Made by LORCS Regarding Schools in Other Countries," *Am. J. Nursing,* **46**:428, 1946.

Seymer, Lucy Ridgely: *A General History of Nursing,* 2nd ed. The Macmillan Company, New York, 1949. Chapter VIII, "The Red Cross in Action," p. 101; also, Appendix B, "Delegates to the Nursing Section, Cannes Conference, 1919," p. 287.

United Nations Relief and Rehabilitation Administration:

Arnstein, Margaret: "Nursing in UNRRA Middle East Refugee Camps," *Am. J. Nursing,* **45**:378, 1945.

Crabtree, James A.: "Health Problems in Occupied Countries," *Tr. Am. Hosp. A.,* **45**:377, 1943.

Frazier, Mary Frances: "International Guests on Welfare Island," *Am. J. Nursing,* **47**:27, 1947.

Johnston, Lillian L.: "UNRRA Nurses in Europe," *Pub. Health Nursing,* **38**:333, 1946.

The Story of UNRRA. United Nations Relief and Rehabilitation Administration, Washington, D.C., 1948.

"What Is UNRRA?" *Am. J. Nursing,* **45**:713, 1945.

Chapter 51

THE WORLD HEALTH ORGANIZATION—AND
INTERNATIONAL HEALTH PROGRAMS

During the last three years, the world has seen greater improvement in health conditions than in any similar period in history. In spite of the troubled political outlook and precarious economic conditions, there is now far greater security of life in most free countries than ever before.[1]

IN OCTOBER, 1945, 51 nations, including the USA, bound themselves together as members of the United Nations. Within a few years the number has risen to 60, and an additional 29 countries were represented in the UN's specialized agencies of which the World Health Organization is one of the most important. Airplanes, radio, and other twentieth-century inventions had made the world so small, in terms of interrelationships, that no nation could remain uninfluenced by political, health, and economic conditions in the others. By mid-century, therefore, two thousand millions of people had become partners in the purposes set forth in the United Nations charter—one of the greatest documents of our times. Consideration of the corrosive influence of political and military rivalries on the idealistic purposes of the charter have no place in this volume. We are here concerned with world health and the rapidly growing significance of nursing in relation to it.

In the complex organization of the United Nations which is designed, among other things, "to work for social progress, higher living standards, better standards of life in larger freedom"[2] two agencies are primarily concerned with raising the standard of

[1] Annual Report of the Federal Security Agency, US Public Health Service, 1951, p. 67.
[2] Charter of the United Nations, 1945.

health throughout the world. They are the World Health Organization (WHO), which is one of the 13 separately organized but coordinated "Specialized Agencies" of the UN, and the United Nations International Children's Emergency Fund. As a participating member of the WHO, the US contributes to its support. As of 1952, it is also continuing its contributions to UNICEF. The US has also developed unilateral international health services which will be discussed later in this chapter. It must be noted, also, that many voluntary agencies established health programs in underdeveloped countries both before and after the WHO came into existence. The cumulative work of missionary groups, for example, is impressive. Protestant mission groups, by 1950, had established over 1100 mission hospitals and more than 2000 dispensaries, about one half of which were American. Catholic agencies under Mission-Humanity—a division of the Society for the Propagation of the Faith—had established over 1100 hospitals, over 3000 dispensaries, and 219 leprosaria.[3]

The WHO, having absorbed the functions of the earlier international health organizations, is now the directing and coordinating authority in international health work. All countries benefit from its technical services: epidemiology, statistics, standardization of drugs, and the like. It provides advisory service to national governments requesting it and gives emergency aid to governments in epidemics or disasters. The WHO program is facilitated by decentralization to six regional offices: at New Delhi, India, for Southeast Asia; Alexandria, Egypt, for Eastern Mediterranean area; and in Manila for the Western Pacific area. Europe is served from an office in Geneva and the regional office for Africa is at Brazzaville, French Equatorial Africa. The Pan American Sanitary Bureau in Washington serves as the regional office of WHO for the Americas. Olive Baggallay (Great Britain), well known for her work with the Florence Nightingale International Foundation and with UNRRA in Greece, is chief of the Nursing Section of WHO.

[3] *The Role of the Voluntary Agencies in Technical Assistance.* American Council of Voluntary Agencies for Foreign Service, Inc., Wilkie Memorial Bldg., New York 18, N.Y.

Associated with her at the offices in the Palais des Nations in Geneva is Lyle M. Creelman, a brilliant ex-president of the Canadian Nurses' Association. Each regional office has a nurse consultant on its staff; the only graduate of a school in the US is Elizabeth Hill (University of California) of the Western Pacific Area.

The immensity of the problem which confronted WHO has been succinctly stated by Dr. C.-E. A. Winslow as follows: "Two-thirds of the human race, living in Africa, Southeast Asia, the islands of the Pacific, and Latin America, have a mean annual income of $41 per person and an average length of life of 30 years. . . . Men and women in these lands are poor because they are sick, and sick because they are poor."[4] But "shortages of health personnel—whether doctor, nurse, sanitary engineer, laboratory technician or other workers—plague every single country in the world."[5] These two statements, coupled with one by Dr. Joseph W. Mountin, one of the greatest strategists of the USPHS, provide the key to all international nursing activities since nursing is part of a complex pattern in which the several categories of professional and nonprofessional health personnel work together in varying combinations. Dr. Mountin pointed out that in international planning, "the training of auxiliary workers should be given high priority in all organizations."[6]

Dr. Thomas Parran, then Surgeon General of the USPHS, headed the US delegation to the Public Health Conference of 1946, and became its chairman. At this conference the constitution of the World Health Organization was written and signed by representatives of 61 countries. By including a nurse in the group of technical experts who accompanied the delegation, Dr. Parran made a highly significant contribution to the prestige of nursing and therefore to its international advancement. Mrs. Elmira B. Wickenden, executive secretary of the National Nursing Council, who served as the technical expert on nursing at that conference, and Lucile Petry

[4] "The Global Problem: Inequality of Opportunity," *Pub. Health Rep.*, **67**: 318, 1952.

[5] *World Health Organization—Facts and Figures*, 2nd ed. Sept., 1952.

[6] Mountin, Joseph W.: "The Need for Sound Planning," *Pub. Health Rep.*, **67**:319, 1952.

(Leone),* who served in a similar capacity at the first assembly of the WHO in 1948 at Geneva, reported that members of the delegations of other countries sought many informal opportunities to discuss nursing with them. Since then distinguished nurses of Great Britain and Sweden have served as advisers to their respective delegations at the annual World Health Conferences. Other American nurses who have served successively in that capacity are Katharine Faville, Wayne University; Lillian B. Patterson, University of Washington; Anna M. Steffens, University of California at Los Angeles; and Ruth G. Taylor, US Children's Bureau (1952).

A function of the WHO is to bring into relationship all health activities, governmental and nongovernmental. At the first regular meeting of the Assembly of the WHO, a formal relationship between the nongovernmental ICN and the WHO was established. The privileges conferred are the "right to appoint a representative to participate without vote in the Assembly and the committees of WHO, particularly in respect to items with which the Council has an interest; access to nonconfidential documentation of the WHO, and the right to submit memoranda to the Director General."[7] Effie J. Taylor, ex-president of the ICN, was subsequently appointed by that organization to serve as its official representative at UN meetings in New York. Representatives of the ICN are invited to participate in WHO conferences and to attend meetings of the Expert Committee on Nursing which are usually held in Geneva.

The Expert Committee on Nursing is the mechanism employed by WHO to promote the development of nursing. Its function is: "To advise the World Health Assembly on measures to ensure the recruitment of nurses in proportion to the needs of each country" and (2) "to advise the World Health Assembly on measures to give nurses training in keeping with the numerous and complicated tasks which will devolve upon them."[8] Mary I. Lambie, formerly

---

* Miss Petry married Dr. Nicholas Leone, in 1952.
[7] Petry, Lucile: "World Health Organization and Nursing," *Am. J. Nursing*, **48**:611, 1948.
[8] *Expert Committee on Nursing. Report on the First Session.* World Health Organization Technical Report Series, #24, WHO, Geneva, 1951, p. 3.

director of the Division of Nursing of New Zealand's Department of Health, presided at the first session of this important committee in 1950. Tehmina K. Adranvala, chief nursing superintendent of the Directorate General of Health Services, New Delhi, India, was chairman of the second session. Lucile Petry was the American representative at both, serving as *rapporteur* at the first and as vice-chairman of the second session. Two reports of the work of the committee are available at this writing.

It is encouraging to note that some of the recommendations of the Expert Committee on Nursing have already been acted upon. Definitions were needed as a basis for action. The term *nurses* was defined as "the workers within any particular country who supply the most exacting, comprehensive, and responsible care of a nursing nature which is available in that country." The term "auxiliary nursing personnel" was accepted as indicating "those who give, in comparison, less exacting care which supplements that given by nurses, or whose duties are confined to some particular phase of nursing." The first report of the Expert Committee on Nursing pointed out that there is in the world today a need to review the functions variously accepted as those of nursing education and whether they succeed in meeting the real health needs of the people. In this connection it is of interest that a study is now being made in France and England under the joint auspices of the WHO and the Rockefeller Foundation "to ascertain the workers required for basic health and social welfare services within the family."

By 1950, with nurses moving more freely from country to country than ever before, labor laws and legislation restricting the practice of nursing were putting increasing pressure on the profession to reach some international standard of uniformity for nursing education. Of the 28 countries having legislation controlling the education of nurses, 20 were in the Western Hemisphere. Of a total of 3188 schools of nursing in 51 countries (1950) 91 per cent were hospital schools. (In the US the percentage had dropped to 86.3.) In 8 of the 48 countries reporting, all schools were independent institutions; in some of these nursing was in an early stage of development. As indicated in the preceding chapter, the WHO looks to the ICN for materials, research, and guidance in relation to the educational programs of nursing schools. The ICN referred the WHO's request for a comprehensive study of facilities for advanced nursing education to the FNIF. That study (1952) is well under way. A recommendation was made by the first Expert Committee of WHO that national governments be requested to make surveys of nursing as a preliminary step toward relieving the shortages. Margaret Arnstein (USPHS), who has directed many state surveys, worked with the staff in Geneva on the development of a survey guide.

A Working Conference on Nursing Education (1952) was developed on the basis of a committee recommendation.[9] The report of the conference was prepared by Kathleen Leahy, special consultant to WHO during a sabbatical leave from the University of Washington. "The basic need in most countries," the report states, "is for nurses capable of providing total nursing care in hospital and home and of undertaking public health nursing functions in an organized service." The report stresses the value of "the situation approach" in teaching. Materials on teaching methods, prepared by Hildegarde Peplau and others, for the use of the Expert Committee were circulated with the mimeographed news letter, *WHO Nursing News* (Oct., 1951). The materials and methods of visual education have an important place in such teaching. To encourage their use, WHO distributes copies of its reports to health officers in member countries and to many other readers. ICN distributes its reports on nursing to member associations.

The UN Commission on the Status of Women has been interested in nursing since the meeting in Beirut, Syria, in 1949 where Virginia Arnold of the USPHS, who had previously served with UNRRA and the ICN, was one of the three members of the delegation from the US. Lucile Petry represented the WHO at the commission's meeting in New York two years later, at which a report from the Expert Committee on Nursing was presented. She spoke to a resolution, which was voted unanimously, which requested

[9] *Working Conference on Nursing Education.* World Health Organization Technical Report Series, #60, Geneva, Feb., 1953.

the Secretary General of the WHO to draw the attention of member states to the need for ensuring wider recognition of the professional status of nursing and legal protection of the status.[10-11] "The transcendental importance of the training of midwifery personnel, especially for underdeveloped countries"[12] was considered by the Expert Committee on Maternity Care (1951). This committee recommended to the WHO that a joint expert committee, composed of members of the advisory panels on nursing and maternal and child health be convened and that further consideration be given to the training of midwifery personnel at all levels.

The voluminous report of WHO for 1951, the third full year of the program, indicates that an increasing number of governments were adding nursing divisions to their national health administrations and that nurses were being placed in charge of them. Most of the requests from member states were for assistance in increasing their facilities for the preparation of nurses and for improving the clinical teaching in hospitals and health services. Plans had been completed for assistance to 27 nursing schools. Special attention was given to the training of public health nurses and subprofessional workers in the programs sponsored jointly by WHO and UNICEF. The number of nurses employed by WHO is never large and varies in accordance with the number of projects in operation. In the spring of 1952, 93 nurses were working directly under WHO in many parts of the world; but only 13 of them were from the USA. This relatively low percentage has been attributed in part to lack of proficiency in languages.

Early WHO programs in underdeveloped countries were focused primarily on the problems of environmental sanitation and preventive medicine with increasing emphasis on the preparation of personnel for more personalized health programs. In its war on disease WHO gave priority to malaria, tuberculosis, and venereal

[10] *The Work of WHO, 1951.* Official Records of the World Health Organization, #38, 1952, p. 143.

[11] "UN Commission on the Status of Women Adopts Resolution on Nursing," *Am. J. Nursing,* 51:486, 1951.

[12] The Work of the World Health Organization Expert Committees, Maternity Care," *Pub. Health Rep.,* 67:364, 1952.

infections and treponemal diseases (such as yaws in which penicillin produces spectacular results). Its principal armaments, in these campaigns, are DDT and other insecticides, BCG vaccination, and penicillin. Maternal and child welfare programs developed in cooperation with UNICEF have an important place in WHO planning. UNICEF inherited enormous supplies from UNNRA, the wartime emergency agency. It is supported by gifts from national governments, individuals, and organizations. UNICEF has provided clothing and supplementary meals of protective foods for millions of children. It helps to fight yaws, malaria, and other diseases which are responsible for much childhood sickness and death. It has assisted the International Children's Center in Paris where people go from all over the world to learn up-to-date methods of maternal and child care.

As WHO programs developed, it was found that nurses should be included in practically all the teams sent out to make surveys and initiate programs. Even in malaria control, which is primarily a task for sanitarians, the value of the nurse came to be recognized because she can most readily, although not always easily, gain access to homes and persuade families to have their dwellings sprayed with DDT. When the usefulness of the spraying, in terms of comfort, has been demonstrated, the nurses logically and progressively have turned their attention to the development of the maternal and child welfare aspects of the health programs. WHO programs are coordinated with technical programs of other UN Specialized Agencies, such as UNESCO and the Food and Agriculture Organization (FAO) of the United Nations. With better health for example as a result of malaria control, workers can participate more vigorously in improved agricultural programs. When the combination results in greater production of food (as of rice in the Terai area in India), the vicious cycle cited by Dr. Winslow is broken and the standard of living can be perceptibly improved.

When the health needs of an area have been assessed and methods for the control of the most prevalent diseases have been instituted, it becomes necessary to develop long-range programs including the preparation of native workers to carry forward the programs which have been set in motion. By the end of 1951 most of the requests from member nations to WHO, in relation to nursing, were for assistance in increasing the facilities for the education of nurses and for improving the teaching in hospitals and health services. Special attention was given to the training of public health nurses and community midwives in the joint programs sponsored by WHO and UNICEF. Nurses of many nationalities are participating in these and other programs which sometimes involve changing 1000-year-old customs. In such situations, nurses are needed who have "the confidence, courage and vision to be original,"[13] coupled with the patience to proceed slowly until they have acquired a real and sympathetic understanding of the mores of the people with whom they are working.

Space permits the inclusion of only one or two examples of WHO methods which, it must be remembered, are constantly being augmented by the programs of other agencies. In Burma, after consultations in which the government, WHO, and UNICEF took part, a project was launched in 1951. A WHO team consisting of a pediatrician, five nurse-educators, and four public health nurses started work in Rangoon and Mandalay. UNICEF bore the cost of two members of the team and provided equipment and supplies for maternal and child health centers and maternity wards. Eight fellowships were awarded to nurses outside Rangoon to enable them to take a three-month course for nurse instructors in Rangoon which was conducted with the assistance of the WHO nurses. The instruction of auxiliary workers would be one of the important functions for which such nurses would be prepared.

Work now going forward in Costa Rica provides a quite different example of WHO activity. Since Costa Rica is in the area served by the Pan American Sanitary Bureau, a request for assistance from the health ministry was referred to that office. A nurse consultant was sent to Costa Rica to make a study with a view to the incorporation of public health nursing in the curriculum of an existing school. This was the School of Nursing and Midwifery of the Association of Physicians and Surgeons of Costa Rica. It had been estab-

[13] Hill, Elizabeth: *WHO Newsletter*, July, 1951.

lished in the century-old Hospital San Juan de Dios at San José where the apprentice method of teaching hospital nursing had been adopted. The report of the study was followed by a signed agreement providing for technical assistance from WHO in the reorganization of the school. The National School of Nursing of Costa Rica had its beginning in the fall of 1950 when a three-member WHO nursing team was assigned to it. The team leader came from Portugal, her two associates from Panama. A Spanish-speaking American nurse was added to the group to teach mental hygiene and psychiatric nursing. One-year fellowships for study in a North American university school were provided for small groups of graduates of the school for each of three successive years. They are being prepared to assist and ultimately to replace the members of the international team.

Among the many mid-century international health programs which were outside the direct administrative jurisdiction of the WHO were several programs developed by governmental agencies of the US. The Point Four and the later Mutual Security Agency programs are of particular significance. The Point Four program was so named because it is based on the fourth recommendation in President Truman's inaugural address (1949) of which he said:

This program will provide means needed to translate our words of friendship into deeds. . . . By patient diligent effort, levels of education can be raised and standards of health improved to enable the people of such areas to make better use of their resources. Their lands can be made to yield better crops. . . .[14]

By 1952 the program was in action in 35 countries of Asia, Africa, and Latin America. Technical assistance in public health was an important element in the programs developed in Europe (Greece and Turkey), the Middle East, Africa (Monrovia), South East Asia, the Caribbean area, and in South America.[15] The USPHS supplied technical support and much of the personnel in both programs.

[14] *Aspects of Point Four Program.* Reprint, Department of State Bulletin, Sept. 22, 1952.
[15] "International Technical Assistance in Public Health," *Pub. Health Rep.,* **67**:333, 1952.

The programs stemmed from a variety of motivations such as the development of strategic resources during World War II; relief, rehabilitation, and reconstruction of devastated areas; the containment of Communism and joint planning for long-range social advancement. The social lethargy of people in underdeveloped countries was shattered by the war. It quickly became apparent that the unhappy peoples of countries in which standards of living were extremely low might be responsive to propaganda which would be inimical to the free world. Programs designed to help people in such areas to improve their health in order that they might improve their standards of living may therefore be attributed to enlightened self-interest as well as to the humanitarianism we believe to be an American characteristic.

The Division of International Health of the USPHS participates in the multilateral programs of WHO and the Pan American Sanitary Bureau. It assists in developing the position to be taken by the United States in international health organizations in which the Surgeon General is the official representative. The division furnishes additional representatives. It participates in bilateral programs operating under the Technical Cooperation Administration (TCA) and the Mutual Security Agency (MSA), recruiting and assigning personnel for the health activities of missions sent to other countries by these agencies. The division collaborates in the development and evaluation of the health programs of the missions and provides technical consultation. It plans programs for international fellowship students and visitors in the health field who come to this country under TCA and MSA sponsorship, and for some who are referred by WHO, the United Nations, other foreign governments, and foundations. The division has developed a large amount of information on health conditions and programs in most countries of the world which is useful to other government agencies as well as to the USPHS. Virginia Arnold is chief nurse of this division. She assists with the operation of health programs in 21 countries in the Eastern Hemisphere.

The US has a relatively long history of cooperative relationships with the other American republics. The Children's Bureau had established informal relationships before World War I. This was accomplished through the Pan-American Child Congresses, initiated by Argentinian women in 1916, and by exchange of publications and correspondence. Specialists from the Latin American countries who visited the Children's Bureau were given consultative service. In 1928 the US gave formal adherance to the official Pan-American International Institute for the Protection of Childhood which had been established in Montevideo, Uruguay, the previous year as the result of recommendations of the various Pan-American Child Congresses.

Based on congressional action (which need not be detailed here), since 1941 there has been in the Children's Bureau a unit now known as the Division of International Cooperation. It recruits and assigns specialists in maternal and child welfare to other countries at their request and plans for training and observation by personnel in these fields who come to the US for further training.

In the period 1941 to 1951 the Children's Bureau sent nine professional persons, including nurses and nurse-midwives, physicians, and nutritionists, on 43 missions to South America in the field of maternal and child health. During the same period it sent 16 child welfare workers, group workers, and a medical social worker on 55 missions. Nineteen Latin-American countries received such services. A large number of personnel from those countries, including physicians, nurses, social workers, and other specialists in the fields of child health and welfare, were provided training in the US through the facilities of the Children's Bureau.

When in 1950, enabling legislation[16] was passed to set up the Point Four program, the types of Children's Bureau programs previously restricted to Latin America got under way in other parts of the world, notably in Egypt, Iraq, India, and Pakistan.

A bilateral technical assistance program was launched shortly after Pearl Harbor when 18 Latin-American countries and the United States cooperated in a program developed by the Institute for Inter-American Affairs. Just prior to this development, the 40-

[16] Public Law 535, Act for International Development, approved June 5, 1950.

year-old Pan American Sanitary Bureau added nurses to its staff, some of whom were later taken over by the Institute of Inter-American Affairs. Since 1947, Agnes Chagas has been the chief nurse consultant for PASB, which serves as the regional office for the Americas of the WHO. Its program is stimulating the development of nursing in the Western Hemisphere. Kathleen Logan, one of the nurses formerly with the PASB, became the chief nurse of the institute. The original purposes of the institute were (1) to promote friendly relations between the US and the Latin-American countries and (2) to improve and protect the health of workers in Latin America to ensure a flow of essential materials to North American industries.

The Inter-American program provided a pattern for the Point Four program and, under the Institute of Inter-American Affairs, was continued as a part of it. By 1952, 110 Latin-American nurses had received fellowship grants through the institute. Among them were 15 Catholic Sisters from a half-dozen countries for whom the institute, working in cooperation with the Catholic Hospital Association, made arrangements for a year of observation and study. Among the evidences of ten years of cooperative effort, in which the Latin-American countries bore a steadily increasing proportion of the costs, there were established approximately 150 hospitals and health centers, 12 schools of nursing, 4 graduate programs of sanitary engineering, and 3 graduate schools of public health. As noted in the preceding chapter, the Rockefeller and Kellogg foundations were providing scholarships and fellowships and otherwise promoting the development of nursing education in cooperation with national health and educational authorities in Latin America throughout this period.

The second step in the development of bilateral programs between the US and other nations occurred in 1944, also to meet a war-created problem. The government of Liberia, in which the US had established an enormous military base, requested assistance in the development of a health program to protect the military. The organization of the Tubman School of Nursing in Monrovia is one of the important outcomes of that program. It is of interest that in addition to a basic course in nursing, it also offers a two-and-a-half-year program in midwifery.

In 1947 the US responded to a request for aid from the Greek government and developed a program which included projects for the training of Greek nurses and for the construction and improvement of hospitals, sanitoriums, and nursing schools. By mid-1951 the status of nursing in Greece had been greatly improved, and the number of students enrolled in nursing schools had been increased two and a half times.

In Southeast Asia, following the overthrow of the Chinese government by Communists, the US began intensive efforts "to relieve the suffering of the people in this area and to assist the governments to develop sound economies which can include support for adequate health service."[17] Space permits consideration of a program in only one of the countries in this complex area with its many health problems. In Thailand, American experts (including nurses) are assisting the Ministry of Health in venereal disease, malaria, trachoma, and plague control programs, in rural sanitation, and professional education. Nurses are assisting in strengthening the nursing schools where they emphasize the preparation of teachers and supervisors, and help to establish demonstration health centers where midwives and nurses can receive field training. Under contract with the USA, the medical school at Washington University, St. Louis, provided key medical and nursing personnel to two medical and nursing schools in Bangkok. WHO and UNICEF have initiated a three-year yaws control program and are assisting in malaria and tuberculosis control. Early and spectacular results in the trachoma program helped to pave the way for less dramatic programs. A sound beginning in nursing education had been laid years earlier when the Rockefeller Foundation assisted with the development of a school of nursing at King Chulalongkorn Memorial Hospital in Bangkok.

The Rockefeller Foundation has frequently stated that the provision of fellowships is the most important part of its program because "a fellowship is an investment in leadership." For this reason fellowships, scholarships, and travel grants are an extremely impor-

[17] *Pub. Health Rep.*, **67**:349, 1952.

tant part of WHO and all other international programs. There are many sources of educational aid in addition to the foundations, the ARC, the FNIF committees, and the international agencies we have been discussing. Chief among them is the visitor-exchange program of the US. The Institute of International Education has the responsibility of making the preliminary selection of Fulbright scholars in "the graduate student and special categories" (which includes nursing). The universities of the US reported to the institute that 372 nurses from other countries had been enrolled for the academic year 1951–1952.[18] This obviously is far short of the total number who came to the US under various auspices for varying periods of study or observation. Furthermore, the international planning agencies were not sending all the nurses in need of additional preparation to the US. The resources of educational centers in Great Britain, Scandinavia, Canada, New Zealand, and other countries were also being utilized. Regional conferences and workshops, developed under the auspices of the regional offices of WHO, were also demonstrably valuable methods for promoting the development of nursing in underdeveloped countries. The scope and usefulness of international nursing activities cannot be described with precision. Their further development is a stimulating challenge to nurses who agree with Raymond B. Fosdick that "anything that contributes to the exchange of creative ideas across boundry lines contributes to the welfare of mankind."[19]

BIBLIOGRAPHY

Arnold, Virginia: "Your Stake in International Health," *New York State Nurse*, 24:3, 1952.

Aspects of Point Four Progress. Economic Cooperation Series #34. US Government Printing Office, Washington, D.C., 1952.

Barck, Oscar Theodore, Jr., and Blake, Nelson Manfred: *Since 1900. A*

[18] *Education for One World.* Institute of International Education, New York, March, 1952.

[19] *The Story of the Rockefeller Foundation—A Review for 1947.* The Rockefeller Foundation, New York, 1947.

History of the United States in Our Times, rev. ed. The Macmillan Company, New York, 1952.

Bowlby, John: *Maternal Care and Mental Health.* World Health Organization Monograph Series #2, World Health Organization, Geneva, 1952.

Calder, Ritchie: *The Lamp Is Lit—The Story of the World Health Organization* (pamphlet). World Health Organization, Geneva, 1951.

Chagas, Agnes W.: "A Workshop Experience in Latin America," *Am. J. Nursing,* **51:**374, 1951.

Cooperative Health Programs of the USA and Latin America. US Government Printing Office, Washington, D.C.

Cumming, Hugh S.: "The Work of the Pan American Sanitary Bureau in Relation to Child Welfare," *The Child,* **4:**261–63, 1940.

Dreisbach, Albert: "Inter-American Health Program Goes Forward," *Pub. Health Nursing,* **35:**445, 1943.

Education and Training of Medical and Public Health Personnel. World Health Organization, Geneva, May 3, 1951.

Enochs, Elisabeth Shirley: "To Promote Child Welfare in Other American Republics, Children's Bureau Gives Advisory Service to Children's Agencies on Their Request," *The Child,* **10:**122–23, 1946.

———: "One World in Social Welfare," *The Child,* **14:**170–74, 1950.

Faville, Katharine F.: "The Second World Health Assembly," *Am. J. Nursing,* **49:**766, 1949.

Feller, A. H.: *United Nations and World Community.* Little, Brown & Co., Boston, 1952.

Final Acts of the International Health Conference (includes constitution of the World Health Organization). United Nations, Lake Success, New York, 1946.

Forbes, Mary D., and Arnold, Virginia: "Federal Nursing Assignments outside the United States," *Am. J. Nursing,* **50:**465, 1950.

Fosdick, Raymond B.: *The Story of the Rockefeller Foundation.* Harper & Brothers, New York, 1952.

Goodman, Nelville M.: "Nursing and the WHO," *Am. J. Nursing,* **49:**134, 1949.

How Peoples Work Together: the United Nations and the Specialized Agencies. United Nations, New York, 1951.

International Health Organizations and Their Work. Blakiston Co., New York, 1952.

"International Technical Assistance in Public Health," *Pub. Health Rep.,* **67:**333, 1952.

Iverson, Kenneth R.: *The Servicio in Theory and Practice.* Institute of

Inter-American Affairs, Washington, D.C. Reprinted from *Pub. Administration Rev.*, Vol. 11, No. 4, Autumn 1951.

———: *Ten Years of Point 4 in Action in Latin America.* Institute of Inter-American Affairs, Washington, D.C. Reprinted from *Export Trade and Shipper*, Jan. 7 and 28, 1952.

Mackie, Janet W.: "Nursing in the Other American Republics," *Am. J. Nursing*, 45:355, 1945.

"Meeting Problems of World Health: A Symposium" (participants: C.-E. A. Winslow, Joseph W. Mountin, Gaylord W. Anderson, A. W. Dent, Frank G. Boudreau), *Pub. Health Rep.*, 67:317, 1952.

Morison, Samuel Eliot, and Commager, Henry Steele: *The Growth of the American Republic*, 4th ed. Oxford University Press, New York, 1950.

"My 50,000 Children," *WHO Newsletter*, Nov.-Dec., 1951.

Nevins, Allan: *America in World Affairs.* Oxford University Press, New York, 1942.

"The Objectives of the United States," *Pub. Health Rep.*, 67:334, 1952.

O'Brien, Bryan R.: "An Irish Brogue in Thailand," *Am. J. Nursing*, 51:590, 1951.

O'Hara, Hazel: "Public Health Nursing in Latin America," *Pub. Health Nursing*, 42:73, 1950.

Parran, Thomas: "National and International Horizons," *Pub. Health Nursing*, 38:583, 1946.

Patterson, Lillian B.: "The Third World Health Assembly," *Am. J. Nursing*, 50:760, 1950.

Petry, Lucile: "World Health Organization and Nursing," *Am. J. Nursing*, 48:611, 1948.

———: "Nursing on the World Health Front," *Am. J. Nursing*, 50:611, 1950.

"The Pride of San Juan De Dios," *WHO Newsletter*, Vol. 5, May, 1952.

Public Health Service, 1951 (annual report of the Federal Security Agency). US Government Printing Office, Washington, D.C., 1951.

The Public Health Service Today. Federal Security Agency, Washington, D.C., 1952.

Report. Expert Committee on Nursing, First Session. Technical Report Series #24, World Health Organization, Geneva, 1950.

Sleeper, Ruth: "What Kind of Nurse?" *Am. J. Nursing*, 52:828, 1952.

Steffen, Anna M.: "Fourth World Health Assembly," *Am. J. Nursing*, 51:747, 1951.

Stoegerer, Beatrice J.: "A Good Neighbor Fellowship Program," *Am. J. Nursing*, 48:440, 1948.

Taylor, Ruth G.: "Fifth World Health Assembly," *Am. J. Nursing*, 52:1463, 1952.

Two-Way Street. Report of the US Advisory Commission on Educational Exchange. US Government Printing Office, Washington, D.C., 1950.

The United Nations and the Specialized Agencies. United Nations, New York, 1951.

Wickenden, Elmira B.: "Magna Carta for Health," *Am. J. Nursing,* **46:** 613, 1946.

Williams, Ralph Chester: *The United States Public Health Service, 1798–1950.* US Public Health Service, Washington, D.C., 1950.

Winslow, C.-E. A.: *The Cost of Sickness and the Price of Health.* World Health Organization Monograph Series #7, World Health Organization, Geneva, 1951.

The Work of WHO, 1951. Official records of the World Health Organization, #38, World Health Organization, Geneva, March, 1952.

"The Work of the World Health Organization Expert Committees," *Pub. Health Rep.,* **67:**358, 1952.

Appendix I

IN HONOR OF . . .

THE VERY considerable number of nurses whose services have won them military and other awards is a matter of which the profession may well be proud. So, too, is the number whose valuable educational or community services have been recognized by the award of honorary degrees. No attempt has been made to prepare a classification of such awards for this volume. Neither has it been possible to make a comprehensive study of "memorials." The following discussion must, therefore, be recognized as suggestive rather than definitive. Most of the existing memorials may be said to be ecclesiastic, military, or educational. The fundamentally religious motivation of nursing has been memorialized in some of the nation's greatest churches, three of them in New York. The bas-relief of Mother Seton on the handsome bronze doors of St. Patrick's Cathedral is a reminder of the fundamental relationship of nursing to the Christian Church, also that Mother Seton is believed to be the founder of the first indigenous American Sisterhood.

Over the altar of Riverside Church, in a group which symbolizes Christ the Humanitarian, there is a statuette of Florence Nightingale. In this group are the figures of Walter Reed and Edward Jenner placed there, instead of in a group of physicians, because their "attitude and accomplishments were such as to classify them as friends of man first and physicians afterward." A place of honor with them was accorded Miss Nightingale because: "She has vicariously ministered in skillful and tender fashion to millions of men and women who have suffered the wounds of either war or peace."[1]

The figure of a nurse caring for a patient occupies a medallion in the "Glorification of Healing" window in the Cathedral of St. John the Divine. It was designed by the artists in stained glass who created the beautiful Florence Nightingale window in Washington Cathedral. Both remind the beholder of the glories of Chartres and other famous Gothic churches. In the Washington window the medallions which depict six phases of Miss Nightingale's life are wrought in richly glowing colors. That window was the gift of Mrs. William T. Hildrup, Jr. (of Boston) in memory of her husband.

[1] "Florence Nightingale Is Placed Among Mankind's Benefactors," *Am. J. Nursing,* **50**:265, 1950.

One of the most widely known of the many memorials to Miss Nightingale is the Florence Nightingale medal awarded by the International Red Cross. The medal was first proposed at a meeting of the International Red Cross in Washington in 1912. Awards are made on nomination from the National Red Cross Societies. Since 1921 when six American nurses received the medal, a total of 22 have been accorded that honor. In 1947, the regulation that awards should go only to professional nurses was changed. Helen Byrne Lippmann was honored for her superb service as director of the ARC's Volunteer Aide Program throughout World War II. The American nurses most recently honored (1951) are Col. Florence A. Blanchfield and Sophie C. Nelson.

A number of monuments bear mute testimony to the relationship between war and nursing. The earliest one known to the writer was dedicated in 1904 at Galesburg, Illinois, in honor of the redoubtable "Mother Bickerdyke" (Chap. 2) of whom General Sherman, commander of the Union forces in the War between the States, said, "She outranks me!" The memorial was so admired that, when the nurse practice act of Illinois was amended to require annual re-registration, the state nurses' association requested that the renewal certificates bear a reproduction of the monument. Just a year after its dedication, the Spanish-American nurses, who had organized under the energetic leadership of Dr. Anita Newcomb McGee, unveiled a monument, a Maltese Cross mounted on a granite pedestal, in Arlington National Cemetery in honor of their fallen comrades.

An impressive symbolic figure, the work of Frances Luther Rich, which stands guard over the beautifully located nurses' plot in Arlington, was placed there in 1938. At the dedication ceremonies Julia C. Stimson, superintendent of the Army Nurse Corps (retired) and then president of the ANA, called it a symbol of the spirit of nursing: "Their tenderness and compassion, their competence, courage and human qualities . . . the spirit of nursing of the past, of today, and of the years to come."[2]

In Miami, Florida, the figure of a nurse, in a uniform of the period of World War I, is one of four figures surrounding the shaft of a memorial honoring the armed forces which was erected by an American Legion post. Across the country a few years later women's units of Legion posts in California planned a beautiful memorial to Army and Navy nurses, a fountain surrounded by stone benches, for the Veterans Administration Cemetery in Los Angeles.

Immediately after the death in France of Miss Delano (April 15, 1919) nurses still in service "over there" began sending contributions for a memorial although no plan was formulated until after the biennial

[2] "Nurses' Monument Unveiled in Arlington," *Am. J. Nursing,* 39:90, 1939.

convention of 1920. A large committee representing the nursing organizations and the ARC was appointed. A decision about the type of memorial which would be pleasing to a majority of friends and contributors was delayed by technicalities related to the placement of works of art in Washington. No more suitable site could have been found than that finally chosen. The impressive bronze memorial stands in a handsome garden surrounded on three sides by buildings of the American Red Cross. The open side faces the beautiful building of the Daughters of the American Revolution. Two of the Red Cross buildings are themselves memorials (1) to the women of the North and the South who served in the War Between the States and (2) to the women of World War I. A column on the latter is dedicated to the nurses of World War I. Dr. R. Tait McKenzie's transcendent "Spirit of Nursing" was unveiled during the biennial convention of 1934. It honors "Jane A. Delano and 296 nurses who died in the War, 1914–1918." In spirit and in deeply graven words the memorial reminds all who visit it that "Blessed Are the Merciful." Miss Delano and the spirit of her times are memorialized in other ways, especially by the several nurses' posts of the American Legion which bear her name.

The emotional climate of World War I was charged with a crusading spirit. The nursing profession emerged from it with a deep sense of pride in its accomplishments and with an optimistic outlook. And so it came to pass that nurses who lost their lives during that war are honored by two memorials—the monument in Washington and the American Nurses' Memorial which houses "the Bordeaux School" in France. This is L'École Florence Nightingale which is affiliated with the Hopital la Maison de Santé Protestante. While a medical student, Dr. Anna Hamilton, the Scotch-French directrice of the hospital, had made an intensive study of the work of Miss Nightingale. The school she established was the only one in France which attempted to follow Miss Nightingale's teachings (French nursing, in general, is heavily weighted with social service). It was therefore a logical choice for a memorial to American followers of the Nightingale tradition. The school had been named after personal permission had been granted by Miss Nightingale. During World War I the badly overcrowded little hospital became heir to a beautiful estate on the outskirts of Bordeaux. But, in shattered France, there were no resources available for the erection of a hospital on the new site. Visiting the US in 1919 in search of funds for the hospital, Dr. Hamilton failed to arouse interest in the hospital, but did arouse interest in the school among nursing leaders. Under the leadership of a joint committee of the three national nursing organizations, a goal of $50,000 was quickly oversubscribed. The cornerstone of the substantial nursing school building which bears the name—American Nurses' Memorial—above its portal was laid in 1921, and two units of the building were dedicated the following year. Building costs had gone up (!) since the initial estimates were made. An additional $25,000 was raised to add the wing which completed the structure in 1931. Because the committee served in an advisory as well as a fund-raising capacity, the school was chartered, a training school committee was organized, and an alumnae association founded. Surplus funds were used to provide faculty members with opportunities for travel and study.

The school was not, however, the first building to be erected on the new site. That honor goes to a dispensary, built by the Rockefeller Foundation, which was an outgrowth of the work of the wartime Commission on Tuberculosis with which Elisabeth Crowell had begun her international career. A visiting nurse service operated in connection with the dispensary provides experience in public health nursing for student nurses. Impressed by the American contribution to the school, the French government supplied funds for the construction of the much needed new hospital. Graduates of the school had been eagerly sought by Mary Breckinridge when she was establishing a visiting nurse service under the auspices of the American Committee for Devastated France. American nurses who visited the school in the thirties were impressed by the excellent planning of both hospital and school, the quality of the care given patients, and by the fine type of young women who were enrolled in the school. A map showing the location of graduates of the school in France and throughout Europe was proudly shown to American visitors. There was a gratifying demand for them as administrators and teachers. It was self-evident that Dr. Hamilton and her associates had dedicated themselves to maintaining the school in accordance with the needs of the times and in consonance with the traditions they and the American donors had inherited from Miss Nightingale. An informal liaison with the school was maintained by the Advisory Committee until World War II cut off all communication.

A tragically heroic story was revealed when relationships were renewed after the war. True to her trust, Dr. Hamilton had kept the school going throughout the war although the enemy had occupied the memorial building and students lived wherever they could find shelter. She had courageously faced the enemy and insisted on retaining control of a small section of the hospital in order that teaching might be carried on. There could be no greater tribute to the school than the quick response of young women to the opportunity to enroll, as soon as Dr. Hamilton regained full control of the institution which is now a living memorial to her vision and devotion. The buildings had been badly used and were left in a shocking condition. Equipment which could not be carried off or completely destroyed was made unfit for use. The Advisory Committee secured estimates of the cost of rehabilitation and promptly began working through the state nurses' associations to secure funds for this purpose. Nurses responded magnificently, and the state associations have turned over more than $60,000 for the committee's use. Over $40,000 went to the rehabilitation of the building. The nurses, students and graduates, like those in many other parts of Europe, needed uniforms and accessories. (Through a special committee the ANA was also able to ship case after case of uniforms to other parts of Europe.) The "Bordeaux School Committee," as it was generally known, sent linens and other supplies, food and clothing to the school. Supplementary food and all types of clothing were tragically needed by the seriously undernourished and scantily clothed nurses. When the school requested assistance in augmenting its faculty, the committee persuaded Jeanne LaMotte (later director of the ANA's International Unit) to accept that assignment and financed the position for two years. It also provided a scholarship for a member of the faculty who, after study in this country, is doing excellent work. The committee, which had been operating as an independent committee, has now been reorganized as a "special committee of the ANA" and is charged with responsibility for maintaining effective liaison with the school. The American Nurses' Memorial in Bordeaux is far more than a durable structure of brick and stone. It is dedicated today, as when it was built: ". . . . To the Higher Education of Nurses—for Humanity and for France."[3]

Many memorials to individual nurses reveal the practical idealism that is one of the outstanding characteristics of nurses. The earliest and best known are the Robb Scholarship and the McIsaac Loan Funds. As many fellowships, scholarships, and loan funds now bear the names of individual nurses, the example set by these funds has had a far wider influence than the relatively limited amount of assistance they have been able to provide for ambitious nurses. The sudden accidental death of Isabel Hampton Robb in 1910 was a stunning blow to the profession which owed so much to her brilliant leadership. "It seems," said Isabel McIsaac, "that Providence had given Isabel Hampton so many gifts to work out our salvation. To a lesser woman the obstacles and the dreary work of overcoming them would have been overwhelming, but like Pilgrim, Miss Hampton saw only the delectable mountains; her far-seeing brain and her warm heart leaped over the heart-breaking drudgery and weariness of the way, and always she saw what was to be gained for

[3] "Dedication of the American Nurses' Memorial, Florence Nightingale School, Bordeaux, France," *Am. J. Nursing*, **22**:799, 1922.

the good of the sick and the betterment of the nurse. The two were never separated in her mind; the higher education of the nurse was never to her simply a means of bettering the nurse for her own sake, but always that the nurse might be better fitted for the work she had to do."[4] Mrs. Robb was a distinguished founder of the National League of Nursing Education and had been the first president of the American Nurses' Association. At the Illinois Training School and the Johns Hopkins Hospital Training School she had developed standards for schools of nursing which, although accepted in principle, were often reluctantly followed in practice by other schools. Then, too, Miss Nutting always gave Mrs. Robb credit for getting the foot of nursing, as it were, inside the door of Teachers College!

The two organizations agreed that a scholarship fund would be the most suitable memorial for a person so intensely interested in adequate preparation of nurses. The Isabel Hampton Robb Memorial Fund, which was proposed at the first joint meeting of the two national nursing organizations in 1910, was established by the self-perpetuating Isabel Hampton Robb Memorial Committee in 1915. A $50,000 goal was set for the fund. The president of the Bellevue Board of Managers, a generous and understanding friend of nursing education, contributed $5,000 the following year. In general, however, the fund has been built up by the contributions of individual nurses and the state nursing organizations.[5]

Isabel McIsaac, who had spoken so eloquently of Mrs. Robb, was the first chairman of the Robb Committee. She died (1915) a very short time after ill health forced her to leave her desk in the War Department where she was superintendent of the Army Nurse Corps. Miss McIsaac had been president of the Associated Alumnae and a hard-working member of practically every important committee of the two organizations. After her retirement as principal of the Illinois Training School, she had been persuaded to take on the arduous work of field secretary for the ANA. This was a composite position in which she served the two organizations, the ARC Nursing Service and the *American Journal of Nursing* for two years before going to the Army Nurse Corps. The McIsaac Loan Fund which was established in her honor in 1917 is administered by the Robb Committee.[6]

The Robb Fund has never achieved the original goal set for it. At the beginning of 1950, its assets totaled a little less than $38,000. Those of the McIsaac Fund added up to slightly less than $24,000. Twenty-nine nurses were then being assisted by modest loans. Some of the 81 nurses

[4] *Proceedings of the American Society of Superintendents of Training Schools for Nurses*, 1910, p. 20; also pp. 26 and 89.
[5] "Report of the Robb Memorial Committee," *Am. J. Nursing*, 15:932, 1915.
[6] *Am. J. Nursing*, 17:1004, 1917.

who have been awarded Robb scholarships have reimbursed the fund. In retrospect, it would seem that an "independent" committee, even when created by vote of the national organizations, lacks the drive which is characteristic of committees which have the continuous stimulation, service, and support of one or more of the professional organizations.

The urgent need for more scholarship and loan funds has been discussed elsewhere. The cost of nursing education has risen enormously since these funds were established. In 1952 the Robb Committee decided that out of its limited resources one good-sized scholarship ($1000–$1200) might be more useful than several small ones such as it had been granting. Both funds have truly been "living" memorials as many of the nurses aided by them have achieved distinction.

All of the funds we have been discussing are used for the advancement of nursing in the US. But mid-century interest in giving needed assistance to nurses of other countries caused the alumnae of the Presbyterian Hospital School of Nursing (New York) to establish the Anna C. Maxwell Fellowship Fund, in honor of the founder of the school, through which each year a nurse from another country is invited to spend a year of study at Columbia University. The West Virginia State Nurses' Association offered somewhat similar assistance to nurses of other countries for several years in honor of the editor emeritus of the *American Journal of Nursing*.

A considerable number of residences for nurses bear the names of distinguished nurses, some of whom were honored during their lifetime. Among them are Delano Hall at the Army's Walter Reed Hospital, Maxwell Hall at the Presbyterian Hospital in New York, Hampton Home at Johns Hopkins, Powell Hall at the University of Minnesota, Greenwood Hall at Cincinnati's Jewish Hospital, and McLaughlin Hall at Harper Hospital in Detroit. The Education Unit at the Johns Hopkins School proudly bears the name of Mary Adelaide Nutting.

Probably the first nursing school library to be named for a beloved teacher was Bellevue's excellent Carrie J. Brink Library. That at the Massachusetts General bears the names of two members of the class of '77 who gave the *American Journal of Nursing* its start in life—Mary E. P. Davis and Sophia F. Palmer. The library at national nursing headquarters, for which the *Journal* library is providing a nucleus, is now the Sophia F. Palmer Memorial Library. A few nursing school libraries, such as those at the Rhode Island Hospital and the University of Cincinnati, are endowed but not in honor of nurses.

Relatively little attention had been given to the libraries of schools of nursing when the second collegiate school of nursing in the United States was organized by Laura R. Logan in 1916. This was the school now known as the College of Nursing and Health of the University of Cin-

cinnati. The Solomon W. Levi Memorial Library, named for a generous
donor and subsequently endowed by his widow, was a conspicuous attribute of the new school. An interesting feature of the library of some
4000 volumes is the Phoebe Miller Kandel Historical Section. Miss
Kandel, a former member of the faculty, contributed funds and her
professional library to the school in 1950. At the time alumnae and friends
presented the portrait of Miss Kandel. A display case was presented in
honor of Marguerite E. Fagan, director of the school prior to its reorganization.

Eleven years after the heroic death of Clara Louise Maass from the
experimental bite of a mosquito carrier of yellow fever, her alumnae
association endowed and named in her honor a room for sick nurses in
the German Hospital, Newark, N.J., which has been renamed the Clara
Maass Memorial Hospital. Was it the first endowed room to be named
for a nurse? We do not know.

The prestige value of awards by national or other organizations necessarily depends on the character and objectivity of the criteria used in
making them. The national nursing organizations have proceeded cau-
tiously and constructively in this matter. The two awards now in existence
are highly valued. They are the Mary Adelaide Nutting Award of the
NLNE (now NLN) and the Mary Mahoney Award of the National
Association of Colored Graduate Nurses now awarded by the ANA. For
a brief period during the celebration of the Golden Jubilee of Nursing
(1949) the ANA offered Linda Richards Achievement Awards.

The influence on the evolution of nursing education of Miss Nutting—
scholar, humanitarian, and educational strategist—had gained world-wide
recognition long before ill health forced her retirement from Teachers
College. It was not, however, until the NLNE was preparing to celebrate
its own fiftieth anniversary that a plan for the Mary Adelaide Nutting
Award was formulated. It was announced at the convention of 1943. The
purposes of the award are:

(1) To honor Miss Nutting as a distinguished leader in nursing
education;

(2) To recognize and encourage outstanding leadership in nursing
education;

(3) To stimulate scholarly investigation and research in the field of
nursing education.[7-8]

[7] "Adelaide Nutting Awards," *Am. J. Nursing,* 47:259, 1947.
[8] Taylor, Effie J., and Stewart, Isabel M.: "Presentation of the Mary Adelaide Nutting Plaque to the National League of Nursing Education," *Forty-
ninth Annual Report, NLNE,* 1943, p. 220.

The award, a silver medal for individuals, a bronze plaque for organizations, was designed by the renowned sculptor Malvina Hoffman. The medal bears a profile likeness of Miss Nutting on one side and the lamp of knowledge on the other. Miss Nutting was herself the first recipient. No other awards were made until after World War II when Isabel M. Stewart was the first to be honored. In 1952 the plaque was awarded to the Maternity Center Association and the medal to the Honorable Frances Payne Bolton. A number of other methods for honoring Miss Nutting have also been established. On the occasion of the twentieth anniversary of the Department of Nursing Education of Teachers College students and alumnae presented Miss Nutting, an ardent bibliophile and collector of historical materials, with a small fund which was designated the Adelaide Nutting Historical Fund. Transferred to Teachers College, the fund was used to augment the collection of historical materials on nursing which Miss Nutting had built up through the years—named the Adelaide Nutting Historical Nursing Collection. In celebration of the thirtieth anniversary of the department, a catalogue[9] of the collection was published to stimulate further growth of the collection and to encourage a spirit of emulation in other educational institutions. The FNIF has received the nucleus of a fund, named for Miss Nutting, which is to be used for historical research. The NLN also has a small fund for similar purposes which it inherited from the NLNE. The League's interest in historical research has been demonstrated chiefly through the republication of historic materials in order that they may become more widely known.[10]

The NACGN instituted the Mary Mahoney Award in 1936 to honor the memory of the first Negro nurse to complete a formal course in nursing (Training School of the New England Hospital for Women and Children, 1879) and to give recognition to outstanding work by Negro nurses. The ANA fell heir to the privilege of granting the award when the NACGN was integrated with it at mid-century.

[9] *The Adelaide Nutting Historical Nursing Collection of Teachers College.* Columbia University, New York, 1929.

[10] The volumes now available are:

1. Hampton, Isabel A., and others: *Nursing of the Sick 1893.* McGraw-Hill Book Co., New York, 1949. This volume contains the papers on nursing presented at the International Congress of Charities, Correction, and Philanthropy, Chicago, 1893.

2. *A Century of Nursing.* G. P. Putnam's Sons, New York, 1950. This volume is named for a remarkable report by Abby Howland Woolsey to a committee of the State Charities Aid Association, 1876.

3. *Source Materials in Nursing Education.* NLNE, New York, 1952. The articles were selected from the AJN, 1900–1910, and reports of the American Society of Superintendents of Training Schools for Nurses (later the NLNE) for approximately the same period.

The Linda Richards Achievement Award was a medallion bearing a likeness of Miss Richards on one side and the letters ANA on the other. It was presented by the ANA, in connection with the Diamond Jubilee Celebration, to the young nurse designated by each state association as meriting that distinction, and who was graduated, or registered, between August 1, 1948, and July 31, 1949.[11]

Between 1930 and 1942 the Walter Burns Saunders Medal "for distinguished service in the cause of nursing" (writing excepted) was awarded ten times. The handsome medals were the gift of the publisher, W. L. Saunders II, in honor of his father. Instead of setting up an independent committee to formulate plans and develop the intricate mechanisms essential to the formulation of impartial judgments, that responsibility was delegated to the ANA. The presidents of the three national nursing organizations, with Mr. Saunders, served as the Committee on Awards.

The first award was made posthumously to S. Lillian Clayton— "Educator, Administrator, Humanitarian"—director of the nursing school and nursing service of the Philadelphia General Hospital. At the time of her death Miss Clayton was president of the ANA. Six other distinguished nurses received the medal: the Misses Adda Eldredge, Mary S. Gardner, Annie W. Goodrich, Annabelle McCrea, M. Helena McMillan, and Clara D. Noyes. The Committee on Awards then decided that recognition was due the many who have devoted their professional lives to sympathetic and intelligent bedside nursing. In a colorful ceremony at the biennial convention of 1938, in which bedside nurses were represented by private duty nurses and by public health and institutional staff nurses, each state nurses' association received an attractively framed bronze replica of the gold medal. In 1942 when Army and Navy nurses had been assigned to installations encircling the globe and the horrors and heroisms of Bataan and Corregidor were vivid in memory, the tenth award medals were presented to the Nurse Corps of the Army and the Navy.

Endowed lectureships have long been effectively used to honor eminent members of other professions. A distinguished precedent has been established in nursing. The Annie W. Goodrich Lectureship Foundation was made possible by students and alumnae of the Division of Nursing, Teachers College, in tribute to that much loved teacher when she was about to embark on her crowning life work as dean of the Yale School of Nursing. In the midst of mid-century interest in international affairs it is noteworthy that the first series of lectures made possible by the foun-

[11] "Linda Richards—1949 Version," *Am. J. Nursing*, 49:457–687, 1949. "Linda Richards Achievement Awards," *Am. J. Nursing*, **50**:30, 1950.

dation, delivered in 1931, was on International Aspects of Nursing Education. A similar fund was established at Teachers College in honor of Elizabeth C. Burgess on the occasion of her retirement (1948) which coincided with that of Isabel M. Stewart who was honored by the nucleus of a scholarship fund.

Doubtless a considerable number of memorial tablets, such as the one to S. Lillian Clayton at the Philadelphia General Hospital, to which she gave extraordinarily devoted and constructive service, are in existence.[12] But the flame of devotion to the afflicted which inspired that great life has been kept alive in other ways by her followers.

The restless, seeking mid-century spirit needs to be reminded of the vision, spirit, and fortitude with which the foundations of modern nursing have been laid. Living memorials such as fellowships, scholarships, and funds for special lectures or for research are usefully linking the achievements of the past with the potentialities of the future. They are tangible evidences of the profession's continuous effort to make its tomorrows greater than its yesterdays while striving to meet the needs of each demanding day.

BIBLIOGRAPHY

"American Nurses' Memorial, Florence Nightingale School of Nursing, Bordeaux, France," *Proceedings of the American Nurses' Association, Special Sessions,* 1947–1948, pp. 30–33.

"American Nurses' Memorial, Florence Nightingale School of Nursing, Bordeaux, France," *Proceedings of the Thirty-seventh Convention of the American Nurses' Association,* Vol. 1, House of Delegates, 1950, p. 126.

"The Bordeaux School," *Internat. Nursing Rev.,* **10**:6, 1936.

Breckinridge, Mary: *Wide Neighborhoods.* Harper & Brothers, New York, 1952, Chap. 11.

"Dedication of the American Nurses' Memorial, Florence Nightingale School, Bordeaux, France," *Am. J. Nursing,* **22**:799, 1922.

"Dedication of the Bordeaux School Building," *Am. J. Nursing,* **22**:635, 1922.

"The Delano Memorial Unveiled," *Am. J. Nursing,* **34**:523, 1934.

Erlandson, E. V.: "The Story of Mother Bickerdyke," *Am. J. Nursing,* **20**:628, 1920.

"Florence Nightingale Is Placed Among Mankind's Benefactors," *Am. J. Nursing,* **50**:265, 1950.

[12] Goodrich, Annie W.: *The Social and Ethical Significance of Nursing.* The Macmillan Company, New York, 1932, pp. 384–392.

"The Glorification of Nursing," *Internat. Nursing Rev.*, **13**:211, 1939.

Guinther, Leopoldine: "A Nurse Among the Heroes of the Yellow Fever Conquest [Clara Maass]," *Am. J. Nursing*, **32**:173, 1932.

Hamilton, Anna: "An Open Letter to American Nurses," *Am. J. Nursing*, **21**:378, 1921.

International Aspects of Nursing Education. Teachers College, Columbia University, New York, 1931.

"Isabel Hampton Robb Memorial Fund," *Fifty-sixth Annual Report of the National League of Nursing Education*, 1950, p. 288.

"Isabel Hampton Robb Memorial Fund," *The Oregon Nurse*, **17**:11, 1952.

"Isabel Hampton Robb Memorial Fund, Inc.," *Proceedings of the Thirty-seventh Convention, American Nurses' Association*, Vol. 1, House of Delegates, 1950, p. 177.

"The McIsaac Fund," *Am. J. Nursing*, **17**:1004, 1917.

"Mary Adelaide Nutting Medal," *Am. J. Nursing*, **44**:587, 1944.

"Mary Mahoney Award," *Proceedings of the Thirty-eighth Convention of the American Nurses' Association*, Vol. 1, House of Delegates, 1952, p. 12.

"Memorial Plaque—Mary Eugènie Hibbard in the Canal Zone," *Am. J. Nursing*, **52**:406, 1952.

"Miami's Memorial," *Am. J. Nursing*, **30**:7, 1930; see also frontispiece in same issue.

Noyes, Clara D.: "To the Bordeaux School," *Am. J. Nursing*, **31**:1059, 1931.

"Our Memorial Requires Rehabilitation," *Am. J. Nursing*, **46**:327, 1946.

Rath, Elizabeth H.: "A Scholarship Committee in Action," *Am. J. Nursing*, **51**:174, 1951.

Reynolds, Joseph G., Jr.: "The Florence Nightingale Window," *The Cathedral Age*, **13**:15, 1938.

Stimson, Julia C.: "The History of the Delano Memorial," *Am. J. Nursing*, **33**:671, 1933.

"Unveiling of the Monument to Spanish War Nurses," *Am. J. Nursing*, **5**:555, 1905.

Walker, Evelyn T.: "A Visit to the American Nurses' Memorial," *Am. J. Nursing*, **32**:1168, 1932.

Walter Burns Saunders Medal:

Announced, *Am. J. Nursing*, **30**:477, 1930.

Requirements for candidates, *Am. J. Nursing*, **31**:389, 741, 1446, 1931.

"Whose House Is This?" (American Nurses' Memorial), *Am. J. Nursing*, **31**:947, 1931.

Appendix II

CONCLUSIONS

OF THE COMMITTEE FOR THE STUDY OF NURSING EDUCATION,
BASED ON THE REPORT OF A SURVEY
BY JOSEPHINE A. GOLDMARK.[1-2]

CONCLUSION 1. That, since constructive health work and health teaching in families is best done by persons:

(a) capable of giving general health instruction, as distinguished from instruction in any one specialty; and

(b) capable of rendering bedside care at need; the agent responsible for such constructive health work and health teaching in families should have completed the nurses' training. There will, of course, be need for the employment, in addition to the public health nurse, of other types of experts such as nutrition workers, social workers, occupational therapists, and the like.

That as soon as may be practicable all agencies, public or private, employing public health nurses, should require as a prerequisite for employment the basic hospital training, followed by a postgraduate course, including both class work and field work, in public health nursing.

[1] *Nursing and Nursing Education in the United States.* Report of the Committee for the Study of Nursing Education and a Report of the Survey by Josephine A. Goldmark. The Committee for a Study of Nursing Education. The Macmillan Company, New York, 1923, pp. 11–30.

[2] The committee:

C.-E. A. Winslow, Dr. P. H., Chairman

Mary Beard, R.N.
H. M. Biggs, M.D.
S. Lillian Clayton, R.N.
Lewis A. Conner, M.D.
David L. Edsall, M.D.
Livington Farrand, M.D.
Annie W. Goodrich, R.N.
L. Emmett Holt, M.D.
Julia C. Lathrop

Mrs. John Lowman
M. Adelaide Nutting, R.N.
C. G. Parnall, M.D.
Thomas W. Salmon, M.D.
Winford H. Smith, M.D.
E. G. Stillman, M.D.
Lillian D. Wald, R.N.
W. H. Welch, M.D.
Helen Wood, R.N.

Josephine Goldmark, Secretary

CONCLUSION 2. That the career open to young women of high capacity, in public health nursing or in hospital supervision and nursing education, is one of the most attractive fields now open, in its promise of professional success and of rewarding public service; and that every effort should be made to attract such women into this field.

CONCLUSION 3. That for the care of persons suffering from serious and acute disease the safety of the patient, and the responsibility of the medical and nursing professions, demand the maintenance of the standards of educational attainment now generally accepted by the best sentiment of both professions and embodied in the legislation of the more progressive states; and that any attempt to lower these standards would be fraught with real danger to the public.

CONCLUSION 4. That steps should be taken through state legislation for the definition and licensure of a subsidiary grade of nursing service, the subsidiary type of worker to serve under practicing physicians in the care of mild and chronic illness, and convalescence, and possibly to assist under the direction of the trained nurse in certain phases of hospital and visiting nursing.

CONCLUSION 5. That, while training schools for nurses have made remarkable progress, and while the best schools of today in many respects reach a high level of educational attainment, the average hospital training school is not organized on such a basis as to conform to the standards accepted in other educational fields; that the instruction in such schools is frequently casual and uncorrelated; that the educational needs and the health and strength of students are frequently sacrificed to practical hospital exigencies; that such shortcomings are primarily due to the lack of independent endowments for nursing education; that existing educational facilities are on the whole, in a majority of schools, inadequate for the preparation of the high grade of nurses required for the care of serious illness, and for service in the fields of public health nursing and nursing education; and that one of the chief reasons for the lack of sufficient recruits, of a high type, to meet such needs lies precisely in the fact that the average hospital training school does not offer a sufficiently attractive avenue of entrance to the field.

CONCLUSION 6. That, with the necessary financial support and under a separate board or training school committee, organized primarily for educational purposes, it is possible, with completion of a high school course or its equivalent as a prerequisite, to reduce the fundamental period of hospital training to 28 months, and at the same time, by eliminating unessential, noneducational routine, and adopting the principles laid down in Miss Goldmark's report, to organize the course along intensive and coordinated lines with such modifications as may be necessary for practical application; and that courses of this standard would be reasonably certain to attract students of high quality in increasing numbers.

CONCLUSION 7. Superintendents, supervisors, instructors, and public health nurses should in all cases receive special additional training beyond the basic nursing course.

CONCLUSION 8. That the development and strengthening of university schools of nursing of a high grade for the training of leaders is of fundamental importance in the furtherance of nursing education.

CONCLUSION 9. That when the licensure of a subsidiary grade of nursing service is provided for, the establishment of training courses in preparation for such service is highly desirable; that such courses should be conducted in special hospitals, in small unaffiliated general hospitals, or in separate sections of hospitals where nurses are also trained; and that the course should be of eight or nine months' duration; provided the standards of such schools be approved by the same educational board which governs nursing training schools.

CONCLUSION 10. That the development of nursing service adequate for the care of the sick and for the conduct of the modern public health campaign demands as an absolute prerequisite the securing of funds for the endowment of nursing education of all types; and that it is of primary importance, in this connection, to provide reasonably generous endowment for university schools of nursing.

Appendix III

PRESIDENTS AND EXECUTIVE OFFICERS
OF THE THREE NATIONAL
NURSING ORGANIZATIONS

PRESIDENTS OF THE AMERICAN NURSES'
ASSOCIATION

Mrs. Hunter Robb (Isabel Hampton)	1897–1901
Annie Damer	1901–1902
Mary M. Riddle	1902–1905
Annie Damer	1905–1909
Jane A. Delano	1909–1911
Sarah E. Sly	1911–1913
Genevieve Cooke	1913–1915
Annie W. Goodrich	1915–1918
Clara D. Noyes	1918–1922
Adda Eldredge	1922–1926
S. Lillian Clayton	1926–1930
Elnora E. Thomson	1930–1934
Susan C. Francis	1934–1938
Julia C. Stimson	1938–1944
Katharine J. Densford	1944–1948
Pearl McIver	1948–1950
Mrs. Elizabeth K. Porter	1950–

DIRECTORS AT HEADQUARTERS OF THE ANA

Agnes G. Deans	1922–1925
Janet M. Geister	1926–1933
Alma H. Scott	1933–1946
(Acting Director, 1933–1935)	
Ella M. Best	1946–

PRESIDENTS OF THE NATIONAL LEAGUE
OF NURSING EDUCATION

Linda Richards	1894
M. E. P. Davis	1895
M. Adelaide Nutting	1896
Mary Agnes Snively	1897
Isabel McIsaac	1898
Isabel Merritt	1899
Emma J. Keating	1900
Mrs. Lystra E. Gretter	1901
Ida F. Giles	1902
Georgia M. Nevins	1903–1904
Annie W. Goodrich	1905
Maud Banfield	1906
Mary Hamer Greenwood	1907
Mrs. Isabel Hampton Robb	1908
M. Adelaide Nutting	1909
Mary M. Riddle	1910
Mary C. Wheeler	1911–1912
Clara D. Noyes	1913–1915
Sara E. Parsons	1916
S. Lillian Clayton	1917–1919
Anna C. Jammé	1920–1921
Laura R. Logan	1922–1924
Carrie M. Hall	1925–1927
Elizabeth C. Burgess	1928–1931
Effie J. Taylor	1932–1935
Nellie X. Hawkinson	1936–1939
Stella Goostray	1940–1943
Ruth Sleeper	1944–1947
Agnes Gelinas	1948–1950

EXECUTIVE SECRETARIES OF THE NATIONAL
LEAGUE OF NURSING EDUCATION

Effie J. Taylor	1923
Blanche Pfefferkorn	1924–1928
Nina D. Gage	1929–1931
Claribel A. Wheeler	1932–1942
Adelaide A. Mayo	1942–1950
Julia M. Miller	1951–1952

PRESIDENTS OF THE NATIONAL ORGANIZATION
OF PUBLIC HEALTH NURSING

Lillian D. Wald	1912–1913
Mary S. Gardner	1913–1916
Mary Beard	1916–1919
Katharine Tucker	1919–1920
Edna L. Foley	1920–1921
Elizabeth G. Fox	1921–1926
Mrs. Anne L. Hansen	1926–1930
Sophie C. Nelson	1930–1934
Amelia Grant	1934–1938
Grace Ross	1938–1942
Marion G. Howell	1942–1944
Marion Sheahan	1944–1946
Ruth W. Hubbard	1946–1950
Emilie Sargent	1950–1952

GENERAL DIRECTORS NATIONAL ORGANIZATION
OF PUBLIC HEALTH NURSING

Ella Phillips Crandall	1912–1921
Florence Patterson	1921–1922
Anne A. Stevens	1922–1926
Jane C. Allen	1926–1928
Katharine Tucker	1929–1935
Dorothy Deming	1935–1942
Ruth Houlton	1942–1948
Anna M. Fillmore	1948–1952

Appendix IV

CHRONOLOGY

1633—St. Vincent de Paul founded Sisters of Charity.

1798—An organized course of instruction in nursing given at New York Hospital.

1809—Sisters of Charity, established by Mother Seton and believed to be the first indigenous North American Order. Incorporated by Act of the Maryland legislature January 1817.

1836—Pastor Fliedner initiated modern order of Deaconesses at Kaiserswerth.

1847—American Medical Association organized.

1849—Rev. William A. Passavant brought four Lutheran Deaconesses to Pittsburgh.

1854—Miss Nightingale went to the Crimea.

1859—First District Nursing Association established in Liverpool, England.

1860—Nightingale Training School established at St. Thomas's Hospital, London.

First American edition of Miss Nightingale's *Notes on Nursing*.

1861–65—The War Between The States.

1864—Treaty of Geneva—International Red Cross.

1872—The American Public Health Association founded.

Training schools for nurses established by New England Hospital for Women and Children, and Woman's Hospital of Philadelphia.

1873—Three "Nightingale" schools established in the US at Bellevue Hospital, New York City; Massachusetts General Hospital, Boston; and the New Haven Hospital, New Haven, Conn.

1877—For first time in the United States, nurses sent into homes of sick poor by the New York City Mission.

1881—American Red Cross established.

1884—Elizabeth McKechnie, first American missionary nurse, to China.

1885—Buffalo District Nursing Association established—first in the US. Clara S. Weeks (Shaw) published first textbook by a nurse for nurses.

1889—Johns Hopkins Hospital and Training School for Nurses established.

Donor of institutions had stipulated that a "training school for female nurses" be established.

1893—Henry Street Settlement established by Lillian D. Wald.

Nursing subsection of International Congress of Charities, Correction, and Philanthropy met in Chicago during World Columbian Exposition.

American Society of Superintendents of Training Schools for Nurses. (Renamed National League of Nursing Education, 1912.)

1895—First industrial nurse employed by Vermont Marble Works.

X-rays discovered by German scientist, Roentgen.

1897—Nurses Associated Alumnae of the United States and Canada (renamed American Nurses' Association, 1911).

1898—Beginning of municipal nursing service in Los Angeles.

Spanish-American War. Dr. Anita Newcomb McGee organized Army nursing service.

1899—International Council of Nurses organized.

Teachers College, Columbia University, offered course in hospital economics.

Association of Hospital Superintendents organized (renamed American Hospital Association, 1907).

1900—*American Journal of Nursing*, first issue appeared in October.

American Federation of Nurses organized.

1901—Army Nurse Corps authorized by Army Reorganization Bill.

American Medical Association organized Council on Medical Education and Hospitals.

State nurses' associations organized in New York, Virginia, and Illinois.

1902—Pan American Sanitary Bureau founded.

First school nurses employed (by New York City).

1903—Nurse Practice Acts secured by state nurses' associations of New York, New Jersey, North Carolina, and Virginia.

Wright Brothers' first flight at Kittyhawk.

An automobile crossed the US for the first time.

Discovery of radium announced by the Curies.

1904—National Organization for the Study and Prevention of Tuberculosis (now the National Tuberculosis Association) founded.

New York School of Philanthropy offered one-year program in social work.

1905—Medical social work inaugurated at the Massachusetts General Hospital.

1907—Volumes I and II of the Nutting and Dock *History of Nursing* published.

1908—Navy Nurse Corps authorized by Navy Appropriations Act of 1908.

National Association of Colored Graduate Nurses organized.

1909—Nurses Associated Alumnae affiliated with ARC; national committee on Red Cross nursing service appointed.

American Association for the Study and Prevention of Infant Mortality organized.

Metropolitan Life Insurance Company inaugurated visiting nurse service.

University of Minnesota School of Nursing established.

Department of Nursing and Health of Teachers College endowed by Mrs. Helen Hartley Jenkins.

1910—Public health nursing added to offerings of Department of Nursing and Health, Teachers College.

Robb Scholarship Fund established.

State leagues of nursing education organized in Massachusetts and New York.

"The Flexner Report" (*Medical Education in the United States and Canada*) published.

1911—First contributions to ANA Relief Fund.

1912—The American Federation of Nurses ceased to exist.

ANA became sole owner of *American Journal of Nursing* stock.

Children's Bureau established.

Rural nursing service (later Town and Country Nursing Service) established by the ARC.

National Organization for Public Health Nursing founded.

Report: *Educational Status of Nurses*, by M. Adelaide Nutting, published by US Bureau of Education.

1913—*Visiting Nurse Quarterly* presented to NOPHN and published as the *Public Health Nurse Quarterly*, later became monthly *Public Health Nurse*.

ARC nurses called for flood relief in Ohio.

New York first state to establish a Division of Public Health Nursing in a state department of health.

1914—A shot at Sarajevo led to World War I.

1915—125 ARC nurses sailed for Europe on "The Mercy Ship" (S.S. *Red Cross*).

The first Health Center (under that name) established in New York.

Catholic Hospital Association founded.

National Council for Mental Hygiene financed study of nursing care of the insane.

1916—"Is Social Work a Profession?" by Abraham Flexner. First edition of *Public Health Nursing* by Mary S. Gardner published.

ANA began the restructuring (completed in 1922) which made it a federation of state nurses' associations. Private Duty and Mental Hygiene Sections first to be organized.

University of Cincinnati School of Nursing and Health offered (first to do so) a five-year program leading to a degree.

1917—US declared war on Germany, April 6.

Committee on Nursing of the General Medical Board of the Council of National Defense organized.

NLNE published *Standard Curriculum.*

1918—Army School of Nursing organized.

First national census of nurses.

ARC established Bureau of Public Health Nursing.

Preliminary nursing course for college graduates at Vassar College.

American Council on Education established.

Public health nursing organized in 22 extra-cantonment zones under direction of US Public Health Service.

Pandemic influenza.

Maternity Center (New York) founded.

Armistice, November 11.

1919—American College of Surgeons released first list of "approved" hospitals.

League of Red Cross Societies founded.

Nursing Service, Hospital Division, US Public Health Service, established.

ARC set up bureau of information for ex-service nurses in New York.

1920—LORCS inaugurated international nursing education program, London.

NOPHN initiated program for approving university programs in public health nursing.

National Hospital Day inaugurated on one-hundredth anniversary of Miss Nightingale's birth.

Hospital Progress launched by the Catholic Hospital Association.

NOPHN organized Industrial and School Nursing Sections.

Army nurses granted relative rank.

1921—National Health Council organized.

National nursing headquarters established.

Sheppard-Towner Maternity and Infancy Act.

Nursing Service, Veterans Bureau, established.

1922—First time-study of hospital nursing by New York Academy of Medicine.
1923—Winslow-Goldmark Report, *Nursing and Nursing Education in the United States.*

Public Health Nursing Section of the APHA organized.

Collegiate schools of nursing established at Yale and Western Reserve Universities.

Nurses classified as subprofessional by US Civil Service Commission.
1924—Protestant Hospital Association organized.

Nursing Service, Indian Bureau, established.

NOPHN made first census of public health nurses.
1925—John Hancock Mutual Life Insurance Co., established visiting nurse service.
1926—The three national nursing organizations consider, and reject, proposal to amalgamate.

NOPHN published *Manual of Public Health Nursing.*

Committee on the Grading of Nursing Schools began studies of nursing.

NOPHN published minimum qualifications for those appointed to public health nursing positions.
1927—International Hospital Association organized.

Journal of the American Medical Association published data on nursing.

ARC nurses called out for Mississippi Valley floods.

A Curriculum for Schools of Nursing (rev. ed.).
1928—Grading Committee published *Nurses, Patients, and Pocketbooks.*
1929—ANA study of registries.

The three national nursing organizations endorsed the Harmon Plan for annuities for nurses.

N.Y. stock market crash (October). Beginning of "the Great Depression."
1930—NOPHN published *Board Members' Manual.*

White House Conference on Child Health and Protection.

Council on Nursing of Catholic Hospital Association organized.

NLNE published manual, *Nursing School Faculty.*
1931—Standards of employment for private duty and institutional nurses formulated by Sub-committee of Joint Committee on Distribution.

American Nurses' Memorial dedicated, Bordeaux, France.

Army School of Nursing suspended.

American Association of Nurse Anesthetists organized.

ANA institute for state executive secretaries.

ANA, *Use of Graduate Nurse on a Staff Basis.*

Nursing Education. Bulletin #6, Catholic Hospital Association.

1932—NLNE established Department of Studies.

NOPHN published *Principles and Practice of Public Health Nursing.*

ANA decentralized Relief Fund to state nurses' associations.

Association of Collegiate Schools of Nursing organized.

Final report of Commission on Medical Education published.

Committee on Costs of Medical Care published final report (Vol. 28), *Medical Care for the American People.*

Survey of public health nursing by NOPHN in cooperation with Commonwealth Fund.

Midwest Nurse Placement Service established in Chicago.

1933—*Public Health Nursing in Industry* published by NOPHN.

Federal Emergency Relief Administration (FERA) provided employment and salaries for unemployed nurses.

National Recovery Act.

Rosenwald Fund sponsored study of hourly nursing in Chicago.

The "Dust Bowl" created by storms and drought in the Southwest.

American College of Hospital Administrators organized.

AHA endorsed principle of voluntary hospital insurance.

1934—ICN published first edition of *Educational Programme for the School of Nursing.*

Grading Committee published (1) *An Activity Analysis of Nursing* and (2) *Nursing Schools—Today and Tomorrow* (final report).

Delano Memorial unveiled (Washington).

Maternity Center Association (New York) assumed responsibility for the midwifery school established by the Lobenstine Midwifery Clinic.

NACGN established headquarters in New York.

First public health nurse appointed by USPHS.

Nursing Information Bureau of the ANA established by *American Journal of Nursing.*

National campaign by ANA to establish eight-hour day as regular working day for nurses.

First collegiate program in hospital administration at University of Chicago.

Florence Nightingale International Foundation established in London; took over educational program of LORCS.

1935—ICN office transferred from Geneva to London.

Social Security Act.

FERA succeeded by Works Progress Administration.

National Labor Relations Act.

NIB published first edition of *Facts about Nursing.*

1936—AHA began publication of official organ, *Hospitals.*

AHA and NLNE published *Manual of the Essentials of Good Hospital Nursing Service.*

NLNE published *Essentials of a Good School of Nursing.*

ANA made study of services and placement of practical nurses.

NOPHN set up Orthopedic Council.

Regional nurse supervisors appointed by USPHS and Children's Bureau.

American Psychiatric Association and NLNE sponsored study of nursing in mental hospitals.

Personnel Policies in Public Health Nursing published by NOPHN.

1937—*Curriculum Guide* published by NLNE.

Red Cross nurses called out for Mississippi Valley flood.

1938—ANA study of *Incomes, Salaries and Employment Conditions of Nurses* (exclusive of those in public health nursing).

NTA and nursing organizations sponsored study of nursing in institutions for tuberculosis.

NLNE set up accreditation program.

National Health Conference.

1939—School of Nurse Midwives, Frontier Nursing Service, Hyden, Kentucky.

ANA adopted policy favoring "licensure of all who nurse for hire."

ICN office transferred from London to New Haven, Conn.

Invasion of Poland by Germany, September, began World War II.

1940—Practical Nurses of New York, Inc., organized.

Nursing Council on National Defense organized.

Nurse Practice Acts and Board Rules—A Digest, (ANA).

NLNE published *Fundamentals of Administration for Schools of Nursing.*

Men Nurses' Section ANA organized.

Brief Historical Review and . . . Information about ANA.

AHA and NLNE published *Cost Analysis of Nursing Service and Nursing Education.*

Joint Orthopedic Nursing Advisory Service subsidized by the National Foundation for Infantile Paralysis, now (1952) Nursing Advisory Service for Orthopedics and Poliomyelitis of the NLN.

First peacetime draft in American history.

1941—National census of nursing resources by USPHS in cooperation with state nurses' associations.

Sub-Committee on Nursing of the Health and Medical Committee of the Office of Defense, Health and Welfare appointed.

Federal aid for nursing education provided by act—Training for Nursing—National Defense.

The General Staff Nurse, Report of study by ANA and NLNE in cooperation with the hospital associations.

National Association for Practical Nurse Education organized.

Dec. 7, Japan bombed Pearl Harbor.

1942—*Public Health Nursing Curriculum Guide;* prepared by NOPHN in cooperation with USPHS.

American Association of Industrial Nurses organized.

Bulletin, *Nursing Education in Wartime*, published by NLNE.

APHA set up Merit System Study as an administrative unit.

Relative rank granted Army and Navy nurses.

ANA—*Study of Organization, Control and Financing of Nurses' Professional Registries.*

Institute of Inter-American Affairs established.

1943—*Public Health Nursing Care of the Sick* (report of NOPHN's survey of needs and resources for home care in 16 communities).

Nursing Division of Procurement and Assignment Service of War Man Power Commission.

US Cadet Nurse Corps created by Nurse Training Act ("Bolton Act") of 1943.

Emergency Maternity and Infant Care Program of Children's Bureau (EMIC).

ANA—Bureau of State Boards of Nurse Examiners.

1944—NOPHN—Midwifery Section.

Nursing Practices in Industry, prepared by USPHS.

Army and Navy nurses granted temporary commissioned rank.

Public Health Service Act included provision (1) for Division of Nursing in USPHS and (2) commissioned rank for nurses.

School for Nurse-Midwives established by Medical Mission Sisters, Santa Fe, New Mexico.

June 6, D-Day (the invasion of Normandy).

ICN office transferred to New York.

1945—President Roosevelt asked Congress for legislation to draft nurses.

ANA Professional Counseling & Placement Service, Inc., established.

"Comprehensive Program for Nation Wide Action in the Field of Nursing," released by National Nursing Council.

ANA undertook rehabilitation of American Nurses' Memorial in Bordeaux, France.

Hiroshima and Nagasaki bombed.

V-J Day, Sept. 2.

Admission of Cadet Nurses discontinued in October.

Charter of United Nations in effect, Oct. 24, 1945.

1946—Joint Tuberculosis Nursing Advisory Service established. (By NTA, NLNE, NOPHN.)

Industrial Nurse Section, ANA, established.

Hospital Survey and Construction (Hill-Burton) Act.

ANA launched Economic Security Program.

Nurses classified as professional by US Civil Service Commission.

Report on Structure of Organized Nursing by Raymond Rich Associates.

Mental Health Act.

1947—ICN re-established in London.

Cost Analysis for Schools of Nursing (USPHS).

National Security Act.

ANA cooperating with exchange-nurse program of ICN.

Army and Navy nurses permanently commissioned.

The Economic Status of Registered Professional Nurses 1946–1947 (US Government Printing Office).

ANA established Public Relations Unit.

Montefioré Hospital (New York) instituted home care program.

ICN congress, Atlantic City.

Practical Nursing—An Analysis, US Office of Education.

Special meeting, ANA, House of Delegates (re structure).

Report of Commission on Hospital Care, *Hospital Care in the United States*.

1948—National Nursing Council dissolved.

Universal Declaration of Human Rights (UN).

ANA celebrated Diamond Jubilee of Nursing.

Joint Commission for Improvement of Care of the Patient.

A Program for the Nursing Profession (Ginzberg report).

World Health Organization permanently established in Geneva (Sept. 1).

First World Health Assembly.

ARC announced new basis for nurse enrollment.

National Committee for Improvement of Nursing Services.

Southern regional conference of state leagues.

National Committee on Careers in Nursing organized.

Nursing for the Future (Brown report).

ICN in official relationship with WHO.

A Guide for Supervision of State Approved Schools of Nursing (ANA).

Permanent commission for Nurse Corps, Army and Navy.

1949—Interim classification of schools offering basic nursing programs.
US Air Force Nurse Corps (commissioned) established.
Department of State *Regulations for US Exchange-Visitor Program.*
FNIF affiliated with ICN.
National Nursing Accrediting Service superceded all other nursing accreditation programs.
President Truman's Point Four Program.
National Federation of Licensed Practical Nurses.
ANA's First Inventory of Nurses.

1950—Professional Registration of Displaced Nurses transferred from International Refugee Organization to ICN.
Cost Analysis for Public Health Nursing Services (NOPHN).
Manual, *Hospital Nursing Services* (AHA and NLNE).
Nursing Schools at the Mid-Century (NCINS).
First meeting Expert Committee on Nursing, WHO.
Civil Defense Act.
Communist invasion of South Korea.
American Red Cross, Metropolitan Life Insurance Co., and John Hancock Mutual Life Insurance Co. announced dissolution of visiting nurse services to be completed by 1953.
ANA launched five-year program of studies of nursing function.
Practical Nurse Curriculum, US Office of Education.
All state boards nurse examiners members of NLNE State Board Test Pool.
NACGN integrated with ANA and legally dissolved the following year.
An American Challenge (ANA).

1951—Seminar, "Nursing Service Administration," at University of Chicago.

1952—ANA adopted Code of Ethics.
Nursing Research, first issue, June.
Program of Joint Commission on Hospital Accreditation superseded hospital approval program of American College of Surgeons.
National League for Nursing organized; NLNE, NOPHN, and ACSN dissolved.
Public Health Nursing magazine discontinued.
Nursing Outlook, first issue planned for January, 1953.

Glossary

AAIN	American Association of Industrial Nurses
AANA	American Association of Nurse Anesthetists
ACS	American College of Surgeons
ACSN	Association of Collegiate Schools of Nursing
AEF	American Expeditionary Forces
AHA	American Hospital Association
AJN	American Journal of Nursing
AMA	American Medical Association
ANA	American Nurses' Association
ANC	Army Nurse Corps
APA	American Psychiatric Association (formerly Medico-Psycho-logical Association)
APHA	American Public Health Association
ARC	American Red Cross
AWH	American Women's Hospitals
BEF	British Expeditionary Forces
CMB	Central Midwives' Board (certificate of)
DAR	Daughters of the American Revolution
EMIC	Emergency Maternity and Infant Care Program
ETO	European Theater of Operations
FAO	Food and Agriculture Organization (of the UN)
FERA	Federal Emergency Relief Act
FNIF	Florence Nightingale International Foundation
ICN	International Council of Nurses
ITS	Illinois Training School
JONAS	Joint Orthopedic Nursing Advisory Service
JTNAS	Joint Tuberculosis Nursing Advisory Service

LORCS   League of Red Cross Societies

MCWR   Marine Corps Women's Reserve
MLI   Metropolitan Life Insurance Company
MSA   Mutual Security Agency

NACGN   National Association of Colored Graduate Nurses
NAPNE   National Association for Practical Nurse Education
NASOP   Nursing Advisory Service for Orthopedics and Poliomyelitis
(of the NLN)
NCINS   National Committee for the Improvement of Nursing Services
NFIP   National Foundation for Infantile Paralysis
NFLPN   National Federation of Licensed Practical Nurses
NIB   Nursing Information Bureau
NLN   National League for Nursing
NLNE   National League of Nursing Education
NNAS   National Nursing Accrediting Service
NNC   Navy Nurse Corps
NOPHN   National Organization for Public Health Nursing
NRA   National Recovery Act
NTA   National Tuberculosis Association
NYA   National Youth Administration

OCD   Office of Civil Defense

PASB   Pan American Sanitary Bureau
P&AS   Procurement and Assignment Service
PC&PS   Professional Counseling & Placement Service (ANA)

SPAR   Women's Reserve of the US Coast Guard Reserve

TC   Teachers College
TCA   Technical Cooperation Administration
TERA   Temporary Emergency Relief Administration (state of New
York)

UN   United Nations
UNESCO   United Nations Educational, Scientific, and Cultural Organ-
ization
UNICEF   United Nations International Children's Emergency Fund
UNRRA   United Nations Relief and Rehabilitation Administration
USPHS   United States Public Health Service

VA	Veterans Administration
V-E Day	Victory in Europe Day
V-J Day	Victory in Japan Day
VNA	Visiting Nurse Association
VNS	Visiting Nurse Service
WAAC	Women's Army Auxiliary Corps
WAC	Women's Army Corps
WASP	Women's Air Force Service Pilots
WAVES	Women's Reserve of the US Naval Reserve
WLB	War Labor Board
WHO	World Health Organization
WPA	Works Progress Administration (later, Work Projects Administration)
YWCA	Young Women's Christian Association

INDEX

Hay, Helen Scott, 156
Health insurance, 94, 272, 469
Heintzelman, Ruth A., 271
Henry, Muriel C., 544
Henry Street Settlement, 3
  Visiting Nurse Service, founded, 14
Hentsch, Yvonne, 614
Hersey, Mabel F., 602
Hibbard, Mary Eugènie, 35, 36
Hickey, Mary A., 173
Higbee, Lenah S., 146
Hilbert, Hortense, 581
Höjer, Gerda, 478
  president, ICN, 607
Holtzhausen, Erma A., 493
Home nursing, 337, 339, 499, 500
Hospital Library and Service Bureau, 444
Hospitals, Commission on Hospital Care, 475, 539
  educational programs, 167, 261, 539, 540
  hospital care programs, 260, 300
  number *1873*, 15; *1909*, 15; *1928*, 164
  nursing service, 258, 262, 263
  social service, 51, 167
  studies, Harper, 491, 492; "pilot," 523, 524
Hospitals, psychiatric, 95, 263, 264
  nursing school, first, 50
Hourly nursing, 225, 226
Household Nursing Association (Boston), 460
Howell, Marion C., 357
Hubbard, Ruth, 582
  quotation, 484
Hughes, Dorothea, 159
Hume, Edward H., 33
Hurd, Henry M., 21

ICN. See International Council of Nurses
Illinois Training School for Nurses (ITS), 14, 21, 68; discontinued, 182, 183
India, nursing in, 32, 34
Industrial nursing. See Occupational nursing
Institute of Inter-American Affairs, 599, 634

Institute of International Education, 636
Institutional nursing. See General duty nursing
Inter-Association Committee on Health, 505
Interim Classification of Schools. See National Committee for the Improvement of Nursing Services
International Congress of Charities, Correction, and Philanthropy meeting, 21
  report, *Hospitals, Dispensaries, and Nursing,* 24, 25
International Council of Nurses (ICN), 468, 590, 591
  international health, 598–621
  organized, 78–81
International Council of Women, 79
International health, 597–639. See also World Health Organization
International Office of Public Health, 598
International Red Cross Committee, 608
International relations. See American Nurses' Association, International Unit; International Council of Nurses; International health; League of Red Cross Societies; United Nations
Inventory of Professional Registered Nurses. See American Nurses' Association
ITS. See Illinois Training School

Japan, nursing in, 33
Jenkins, Helen Hartley, 67
John Hancock Mutual Life Insurance Company, 265, 474, 498, 499
Johns Hopkins Hospital School of Nursing, 63
Johnson, Sally, 477
Joint Commission for the Improvement of the Care of the Patient, 471, 504
Joint Committee on Careers in Nursing, 473, 543, 544, 545
  placed in NLN, 588, 589
Joint Committee on Distribution, 155, 159

NNAS. *See* National Nursing Accrediting Service

NNC. *See* Navy Nurse Corps

NOPHN. *See* National Organization for Public Health Nursing

North American Conference of State and Territorial Health Officers, 497

Noyes, Arthur P., 264

Noyes, Clara D., 146, 156, 203, 219
  awarded Walter Burns Saunders Medal, 650
  death, 301

NRA. *See* National Recovery Act

NTA. *See* National Tuberculosis Association

Nurse practice acts. *See* Legislation

Nurse's aides. *See* Auxiliary workers

Nurses, definition, legal, of "nurse," 75
  number, registered *1918*, 134
  "shortage," 468, 469, 470, 485, 486, 525

Nurses' Associated Alumnae of the United States and Canada, membership, 41
  organized, 26
  purpose, 72
  renamed American Nurses' Association, 72
  See also American Nurses' Association

"Nurses' House, Inc.," 203

Nursing, definition, legal, 75

Nursing, status of, relation to other professions, 48–52

Nursing Council for National Defense, 301–10. *See also* National Nursing Council for War Service

Nursing education, Committee for the Study of Nursing Education (Winslow-Goldmark report), 178
  development, 20–30, 48–52, 54–69, 512–53
  faculty, 535, 536; instructor, rise of, 62, 63, 67, 78; university professor, first, 66
  financing, 15, 16, 57, 112; federal aid, 537, 538; legislation, 538, 539

Ginzberg report. *See* Ginzberg, Eli

Interim Classification of Schools of Nursing Offering Basic Programs, 517–19

Nursing Schools at the Mid-Century, 513, 517, 535, 538

"School Data Analysis," 517

studies, progress, 176–89

Winslow-Goldmark report. *See* Goldmark, Josephine

Nursing Information Bureau (NIB), 293–98, 366
  organized, 293; discontinued, 297, 476

Nursing Outlook, 479

Nursing practice, Atomic Age, 554–74

Nursing Research, 479

Nursing service, development, 7–17, 20–30, 48–52, 177, 258, 262, 263, 468–71, 477, 484–511; seminar, 513, 540, 541; study *1952*, 471
  See also National Committee for the Improvement of Nursing Services

Nutting, M. Adelaide, 5, 26, 27, 42, 63, 64, 66, 67, 77, 81, 96, 130, 131, 145, 170, 179, 202, 212, 218, 219, 282
  Adelaide Nutting Historical Nursing Collection, memorial, 649
  international health, 599, 600, 602, 604
  Mary Adelaide Nutting Award, 477, 648
  president, American Federation of Nurses, 78
  quotation, 54, 61, 83, 312
  university professor, first nurse, 66

NYA. *See* National Youth Administration

Occupational nursing, development, 85, 86, 278, 300, 331, 431, 488, 584
  study, 430
  See also American Association of Industrial Nurses

OCD. *See* US Office of Civilian Defense

O'Donnell, Mary, 35